Physical Activity & Well-being

Vern Seefeldt, Editor

Sponsored by the
National Association for
Sport and Physical Education

An Association of the
American Alliance for Health,
Physical Education, Recreation,
and Dance

Copyright © 1986

American Alliance for Health,
Physical Education, Recreation,
and Dance
1900 Association Drive
Reston, Virginia 22091

ISBN 0-88314-335-6

About the Alliance

The American Alliance is an educational organization, structured for the purposes of supporting, encouraging, and providing assistance to member groups and their personnel throughout the nation as they seek to initiate, develop, and conduct programs in health, leisure, and movement-related activities for the enrichment of human life.

Alliance objectives include:

1. Professional growth and development—to support, encourage, and provide guidance in the development and conduct of programs in health, leisure, and movement-related activities which are based on the needs, interests, and inherent capacities of the individual in today's society.
2. Communication—to facilitate public and professional understanding and appreciation of the importance and value of health, leisure, and movement-related activities as they contribute toward human well-being.
3. Research—to encourage and facilitate research which will enrich the depth and scope of health, leisure, and movement-related activities; and to disseminate the findings to the profession and other interested and concerned publics.
4. Standards and guidelines—to further the continuous development and evaluation of standards within the profession for personnel and programs in health, leisure, and movement-related activities.
5. Public affairs—to coordinate and administer a planned program of professional, public, and governmental relations that will improve education in areas of health, leisure, and movement-related activities.
6. To conduct such other activities as shall be approved by the Board of Governors and the Alliance Assembly, provided that the Alliance shall not engage in any activity which would be inconsistent with the status of an educational and charitable organization as defined in Section 501(c) (3) of the Internal Revenue Code of 1954 or any successor provision thereto, and none of the said purposes shall at any time be deemed or construed to be purposes other than the public benefit purposes and objectives consistent with such educational and charitable status.

Bylaws, Article III

Preface

This book reviews evidence in the biological and behavioral sciences relating physical activity to human well-being. It is intended for beginning level graduate students, but upper division undergraduate students also may find that some of the chapters are appropriate for their purposes. In addition, scholars and practitioners in disciplines and professions that focus on developing and aging organisms will benefit from this information.

The book contains 18 chapters, divided into five sections by the compatibility of their content. All of the manageable inconsistencies have been resolved, but some of the redundancies have been retained, deliberately, because of the various perspectives used by the authors in the presentation of their material. Several other topics were considered, but eventually omitted because of space limitations. The book, nonetheless, exceeds our initial allocation of pages; I appreciate the commitment of Jack Razor and Ross Merrick to publish what was written, despite the writers' zeal.

The need for this book grew out of the frustrations of many individuals, including physical education teachers who had watched their programs erode for lack of local and state support, curriculum specialists who may have believed, intuitively, in the value of physical activity, but could not find sufficient reasons to retain the programs under their supervision, administrators who were under siege by parents wanting more of the school day for "academic subjects," and students who had been promised much and received little in their physical education classes. Each of these groups has requested an answer to the basic question, "What are the beneficial and detrimental effects of physical activity on the human organism?" In the 1980's, when more evidence of physical activity's positive contribution to human health is available than ever before, it seems imperative to answer the question.

The impetus for this book was provided by the Executive Cabinet of the National Association For Sport and Physical Education (NASPE) and its executive director, Ross Merrick. Prompted by persistent requests to assist in the nationwide defense by beleaguered physical education programs, the NASPE cabinet responded by launching what has become known as the "Justification Project." Initially, the goal of the Justification Project was to marshall sufficient evidence to defend school-based physical education programs from further erosion or elimination. This initiative was subsequently expanded to a more comprehensive plan involving three phases.

The first phase of the Justification Project was concluded with the publication of this book. Phase II will be the contents of this book as part of the bases for developing a description of a physically educated person at various developmental levels. This description will serve to develop demonstrable and reproducible outcomes associated with elementary and secondary physical education programs. A final phase will be to use these outcomes as a means to encourage excellence in K-12 physical education by encouraging their adoption and by recognizing those schools who meet these standards.

The initial selection of the authors and their topics was the responsibility of the editor. Subsequently, 16 authors met for several days in the fall of 1984 to exchange outlines and identify additional topics and writers. The title of the book, its contents, sequence of chapters, and writing style were determined at that meeting. Credit for whatever success was achieved in amalgamating the evidence concerning physical activity's contribution to human well-being, as reflected in the behavioral and biological sciences, should go to this committee of writers.

The authors were selected because of their knowledge in a specific area. Most of their names will be immediately recognized by the readers because of their long history as contributors to the topics for which they provided reviews in this book. Several authors are emerging young scientists who have established themselves as frontrunners, despite the relatively short time they have spent in their academic discipline. All of them gave of their time, without remuneration, so that this book could be printed. Their willingness to answer the call of a struggling profession is greatly appreciated.

Vern Seefeldt
Editor

Contents

Section I. Growth and Motor Function

Chapter		Page Number
1	Physical Growth and Maturation *Robert M. Malina,* University of Texas, Austin	3

2	Acquisition of Motor Skills During Childhood
	    John L. Haubenstricker and *Vern D. Seefeldt,*
	    Michigan State University, East Lansing
		41

3	Development of Sensory-Motor Function in Young Children *Harriet G. Williams,* University of South Carolina, Columbia	105

4	Memory Development and Motor Skill Acquisition
	    Jerry R. Thomas, Louisiana State University, Baton Rouge
	    Jere Dee Gallagher, University of Pittsburgh
		125

5	Physical Activity and the Prevention of Premature Aging *Waneen W. Spirduso,* University of Texas, Austin	141

Section II. Biological Perspective

6	Physical Activity and Body Composition *Pat Eisenman,* University of Utah, Salt Lake City	163
7	Neuromuscular Adaptations to High-Resistance Exercise *Gary Kamen,* Indiana University, Bloomington	185
8	Menstruation, Pregnancy, and Menopause *Christine L. Wells,* Arizona State University, Tempe	211
9	Nutrition and Ergogenic Aids *Emily M. Haymes,* Florida State University, Tallahassee	237
10	Cardiorespiratory Adaptations to Chronic Endurance Exercise *Russell R. Pate* and *J. Larry Durstine,* University of South Carolina, Columbia	275

Section III. Social and Psychological Perspectives

11	Mental Health *Rod K. Dishman,* University of Georgia, Athens	303

12	Social Development	343
	George H. Sage, University of Northern Colorado, Greeley	
13	Moral Development	373
	Maureen R. Weiss, University of Oregon, Eugene	
	Brenda Jo Bredemeier, University of California, Berkeley	

Section IV. Special Applications

14	Disabling and Handicapping Conditions	393
	Alfred F. Morris, Armed Forces Staff College, Norfolk, Virginia	
15	Cardiorespiratory Diseases	415
	Patty S. Freedson, University of Massachusetts, Amherst	
16	Metabolic Disease: Diabetes Mellitus	425
	Kris Berg, University of Nebraska, Omaha	

Section V. Organized Delivery Systems for Physical Activity

17	The Relation of Movement and Cognitive Function	443
	Jerry R. Thomas, Louisiana State University, Baton Rouge	
	Katherine T. Thomas, Southeastern Louisiana University, Hammond	
18	Effects of Physical Education Programs on Children	455
	Paul Vogel, Michigan State University, East Lansing	

List of Contributors

Kris Berg, School of Health, Physical Education and Recreation, University of Nebraska at Omaha, Omaha, Nebraska.

Brenda Bredemeier, Department of Physical Education, University of California, Berkeley, California.

Rod K. Dishman, Department of Physical Education, University of Georgia, Athens, Georgia.

J. Larry Durstine, Department of Physical Education, University of South Carolina, Columbia, South Carolina.

Patricia A. Eisenman, College of Health, University of Utah, Salt Lake City, Utah.

Patty Freedson, Department of Exercise Science, University of Massachusetts at Amherst, Amherst, Massachusetts.

Jere Dee Gallagher, Department of Health, Physical and Recreation Education, University of Pittsburgh, Pittsburgh, Pennsylvania.

John L. Haubenstricker, School of Health Education, Counseling Psychology and Human Performance, Michigan State University, East Lansing, Michigan.

Emily Haymes, Department of Movement Science and Physical Education, Florida State University, Tallahassee, Florida.

Gary Kamen, School of Health, Physical Education and Recreation, Indiana University, Bloomington, Indiana.

Robert M. Malina, Department of Anthropology, University of Texas at Austin, Austin, Texas.

Alfred F. Morris, Director, Health and Fitness Programs, Armed Forces Staff College, Norfolk, Virginia.

Russell R. Pate, Department of Physical Education, University of South Carolina, Columbia, South Carolina.

George H. Sage, School of Health, Physical Education and Recreation, University of Northern Colorado, Greeley, Colorado.

Waneen W. Spirduso, Department of Physical and Health Education, University of Texas at Austin, Austin, Texas.

Vern D. Seefeldt, Institute for the Study of Youth Sports, School of Health Education, Counseling Psychology and Human Performance, Michigan State University, East Lansing, Michigan.

Jerry R. Thomas, School of Health, Physical Education, Recreation and Dance, Louisiana State University, Baton Rouge, Louisiana.

Katherine T. Thomas, Division of Health, Physical Education, Recreation and Dance, Southeastern Louisiana University, Hammond, Louisiana.

Paul G. Vogel, Institute for the Study of Youth Sports, School of Health Education, Counseling Psychology and Human Performance, Michigan State University, East Lansing, Michigan.

Maureen Weiss, College of Human Development and Performance, University of Oregon, Eugene, Oregon.

Christine L. Wells, Department of Health and Physical Education, Arizona State University, Tempe, Arizona.

Harriet G. Williams, The Motor Development/Motor Control Laboratory, Department of Physical Education, University of South Carolina, Columbia, South Carolina.

Section I

GROWTH AND MOTOR FUNCTION

- Physical Growth and Maturation
- Acquisition of Motor Skills During Childhood
- Development of Sensory-Motor Function in Young Children
- Memory Development and Motor Skill Acquisition
- Physical Activity and the Prevention of Premature Aging

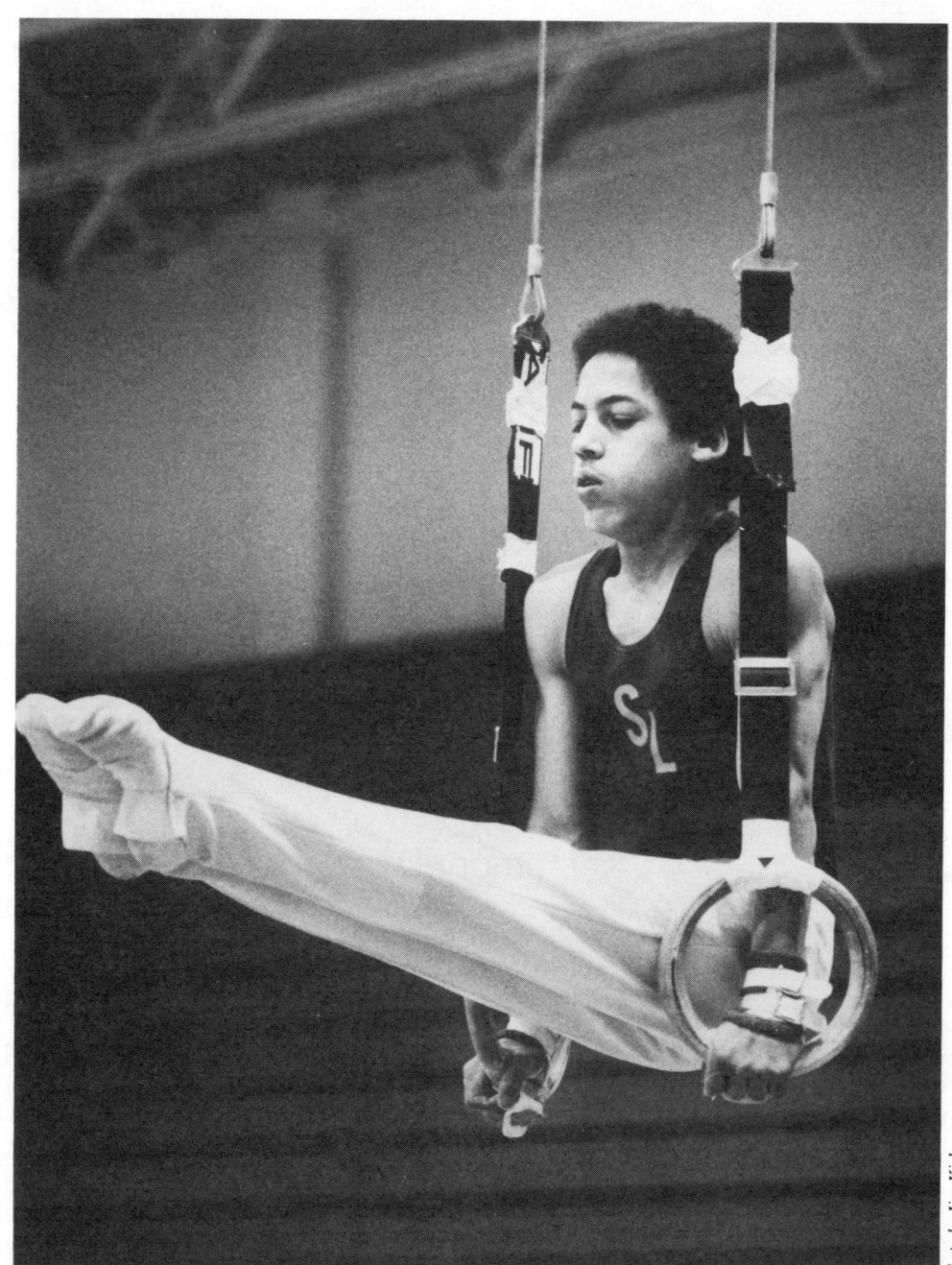

photo by Jim Kirby

CHAPTER ONE

Physical Growth and Maturation

Robert M. Malina
Department of Anthropology
University of Texas
Austin, Texas

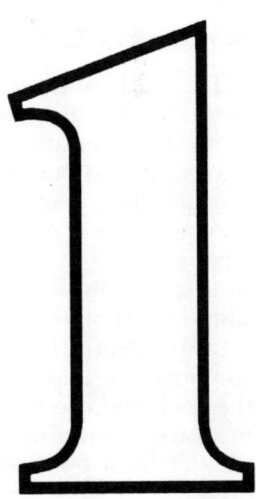

Regular physical activity during childhood and youth is often viewed as necessary for normal growth and maturation, and as having favorable influences on the body during growth and into adulthood. Some effects of regularly repeated physical activity on the growing person are considered here. However, two limitations must be recognized at the outset. First, physical activity is only one of many factors that may affect the growing individual; and second, it is quite difficult to differentiate activity-related changes from those associated with normal growth and maturation.

Growth and Maturation

Growth and maturation are dominant biological activities during the first two decades of life. These activities, however, are fundamentally different from each other in concept. Growth implies changes in size. The changes are the result of the underlying processes of increase in cell number (hyperplasia), increase in cell size (hypertrophy), and increase in intercellular materials (accretion). Maturation implies progress towards the mature state, which varies with the biological system involved. Skeletal maturity, for example, is a fully ossified skeleton; sexual maturity is reproductive capability. The concept of maturity relates to the child's inborn chronometer, or biological clock, which regulates his/her progress towards the mature state. Thus, all individuals end up as adults, skeletally and sexually mature, but all end up as adults with different heights. This is the fundamental distinction between growth and maturity, that is, progress towards maturity versus ultimate size. Both processes are probably under separate genetic control; yet, they are related.

The biological processes of physical growth and maturation are the focus of this chapter. However, the processes are not ordinarily studied; rather, the *results* of the underlying processes are observed and/or measured. For example, size attained is measured, rather than the activities at the growth plate of specific long bones. A stage of skeletal maturation, rather than the process of ossification occurring in a particular bone, is assessed.

Indicators of Growth and Maturation

The study of growth and maturation implies measurement and observation of the outcomes of these processes. The following summarizes several more commonly used indicators of growth and maturation.

Weight and stature (height) are the two most often used measurements of growth. *Body weight* is a measure of body mass, a composite of independently varying tissues. Although weight should be measured with the child nude, it is frequently taken with the individual attired in ordinary, indoor clothing (e.g., gym shorts) without shoes. *Stature* or standing height is a linear measurement of the distance from the floor or standing surface to the vertex of the skull. It is measured with the subject in standard erect posture, without shoes. Stature is a composite of linear dimensions contributed by the lower extremities, the trunk, the neck and the head. From birth to age two or three, an individual's stature is measured as *recumbent length*, i.e., the length of the child's body while lying in a standardized position. As a rule, we are longer lying down than while standing erect.

Sitting height, as the name implies, is the height of the child while sitting. It is measured as the distance from the sitting surface to the top of the head with the child seated in a standard position. This measurement is of particular value when used with stature. Stature minus sitting height provides an estimate of the length of the lower extremities *(subischial length)*. Or, expressing sitting height as a percentage of stature, the sitting height/stature ratio provides an estimate of relative leg length. Two individuals, for example, can have the same stature; yet, one has a sitting height/standing height ratio of 54%, while the other has a ratio of 51%. In the former, sitting height accounts for 54% of stature and by subtraction the lower extremities account for 46%. This individual is said to be relatively short-legged. In contrast, in the other child sitting height accounts for 51% of the standing height and by subtraction the legs account for 49%. This child is relatively long-legged compared to the other child.

Breadth or width measurements are usually taken across specific bone landmarks and therefore provide an index of skeletal robusticity. *Biacromial breadth* measures the distance across the right and left acromial processes of the scapulae and thus provides an indication of shoulder breadth. *Bicristal breadth* measures the distance across the most lateral parts of the iliac crests and thus provides an indication of hip breadth. These two breadth measurements provide information on the width of the upper and lower trunk, and are commonly used in the form of a ratio (biacromial breadth/bicristal breadth × 100) to illustrate proportional changes in shoulder-hip relationship during growth. Breadth across the bony condyles of the femur *(bicondylar breadth)* and the humerus *(biepirondylar breadth)* provide general information on the robusticity of the extremity skeleton. The former is a measure of bone breadth across the knee, while the latter is a measure of bone breadth across the elbow.

Limb circumferences are indicators of relative muscularity. Note, however, that a circumference includes bone, surrounded by a mass of muscle which is ringed by a layer of subcutaneous fat. The two more commonly used limb measurements are the *arm* and *calf circumferences*. The former is measured with the arm hanging loosely at the side at the point midway between the acromial (see above) and olecranon (tip of the elbow) processes. The latter is measured as the maximum circumference of the calf most often with the subject in a standing position and the weight distributed evenly on both legs.

Skinfold thicknesses are used as indicators of subcutaneous fat, i.e., that portion of body fat which is located immediately beneath the skin. This thickness, in the form of a double fold of skin and underlying subcutaneous tissue, can be determined with special calipers. The resultant measurement is a skinfold thickness, which can be taken at any number of sites on the body. Most often, skinfolds are measured on the extremities and on the trunk, as body fat shows a differential pattern of distribution. Two of the more commonly used sites in growth studies are the *triceps skinfold*, on the back of the arm over the triceps muscle, and the *subscapular skinfold*, on the back just beneath the inferior angle of the scapula.

The selection of measurements described above provides information on the size of the child as a whole and of specific parts and tissues. More specific study of bodily tissues falls within the area labeled *body composition*, which attempts to partition the body mass (i.e., weight) into its basic tissue components. To this end, a two-compartment model is most often used: Body Weight = Lean Body Mass + Fat. A variety of techniques are available to estimate total body fatness and/or lean body mass. Many of them require specialized equipment and procedures. In additon, many of the procedures are not amenable to use over the entire growth period, i.e., infancy through adolescence, and the models and assumptions underlying most methods are derived from adults. For example, recent evidence indicates that fatness is overestimated by at least four percent when adult equations for estimating fat from density are used for children (Boileau et al., 1984). Further, most methods for estimating body composition yield information only for the body as a whole, i.e., total body fat or lean body mass, and do not provide information on changes in specific tissues (e.g., muscle or bone) or changes in specific regions of the body which accompany growth. Nevertheless, they do provide important growth data, but the limitations must be recognized.

The specific tissue which has received most attention is subcutaneous fat as measured by skinfold thicknesses at any number of body sites. Fat, muscle, and bone on the upper and lower extremities have most often been approached in growth studies by means of radiographs.

The concept of physique or body build is important in studies of growth. Physique refers to the general configuration of the body as a whole. There have been numerous attempts at physique classification. Most are derived from studies of adults, and all describe physique in two or three components. The approach to physique assessment that has influenced the direction of studies in the United States is that of Sheldon (Sheldon et al., 1954), which is built upon the premise that there is continuous variation in physique based on the contribution of varying components to the conformation of the entire body. These components are *endomorphy*, referring to a relative preponderance of the digestive organs and of softness and roundness of contour throughout the body, as in an individual who tends toward fatness and obesity; *mesomorphy*, referring to a predominance of muscle, bone, and connective tissue so that muscles are prominent with sharp contours, as in a muscular individual; and *ectomorphy*, referring to a general linearity and fragility, poor muscle development, and a preponderance of surface area over body mass, as in an extremely thin individual. A clear-cut dominance of one of these three components defines the individual's physique, which is called a *somatotype*. In Sheldon's approach, the method used in assessing physique is basically photographic, visual (anthroposcopic), and subjective, although stature and weight measurements are used in the form of a weight/stature ratio.

Each of the three components of an individual's physique is assessed individually from three standardized photographs. Rating is based on a 7-point scale, with 1 representing the least expression and 7 the fullest expression of the specific component. Emphasis is placed on the contribution of each component to total physique, which can be extreme or balanced. The ratings of each component represent the individual's somatotype.

The basic principles underlying Sheldon's approach to the assessment of physique have been modified. Heath and Carter (Carter, 1980), for example, use both the anthroposcopic procedures (if photos are available) and anthropometric procedures to estimate an individual's somatotype, which is expressed as three digits as noted above. In practice, however, the anthropometric procedures of the Heath-Carter method are most often used. The anthropometric estimate of somatotype is derived from the sum of three skinfolds (triceps, subscapular, and suprailiac) to estimate endomorphy; stature adjusted for biepicondylar and bicondylar breadths and for arm and calf circumferences corrected for the triceps and medial calf skinfolds, respectively, to estimate mesomorphy; and a height-weight ratio (height divided by the cube root of weight) to estimate ectomorpy.

Two types of maturity assessments are most commonly used in growth studies. *Sexual maturation* refers to the state of development of the primary and secondary sex characteristics (e.g., breast development and menarche in females, penis and testes growth in males, and pubic hair development in both sexes). Scales are available for the assessment of sexual maturation using these criteria (Tanner, 1962). Each trait is rated on a 5-stage scale. Note, however, that breast, genital, and pubic hair development are continuous processes upon which arbitrary discontinuities are imposed. Further, outside the clinical setting, such assessments are extremely difficult to use for primarily social/cultural reasons. Age at menarche is the most commonly reported maturational event and is often used to classify girls into maturational categories for comparison. There can be, however, considerable error in reported ages at menarche and extreme care must be used in obtaining such information. In addition to practical difficulties in obtaining sexual maturity information, these maturity indicators are basically time-limited, that is, they are useful only during the adolescent years.

Skeletal maturation is perhaps the best method for the assessment of biological age or maturity status of the child. The skeleton is an ideal indicator of maturity in that its development spans the entire period of active growth and maturation. All children start with a skeleton of cartilage and have a fully developed bony skeleton in early adulthood. In other words, both the beginning and end points of the maturation process are known, since the skeletal structure of all indivduals progresses from cartilage to bone.

The primary limitation of skeletal maturation as an indiactor of a child's maturity status at present is that it requires the use of an x-ray of the hand and wrist. This area contains many separate centers of bone growth and maturation. Although some variation is apparent, the hand-wrist area is fairly typical of the remainder of the skeleton. Two procedures are commonly used to assess skeletal maturity, the Greulich-Pyle method (Greulich and Pyle, 1959) and the Tanner-Whitehouse method (Tanner et al., 1975). Both methods involve comparison of the x-ray of a child, with skeletal maturity reference criteria for American (in the case of the Greulich-Pyle system) or for British (in the case of the Tanner-Whitehouse method) children. Both methods provide a bone age or skeletal age, which is expressed relative to the child's chronological age. Thus, a child can be 10.5 years chronologically, but may be 12.3 years skeletally.

In addition to sexual and skeletal maturity, age at peak height velocity, percentage of adult height attained at a given chronological age, or age at which a specific percentage of adult height is attained are useful maturity indicators. Estimates of these indicators require longitudinal data, which present specific logistical problems in data collection and analysis. Dental maturation is another occasionally used indicator, but it tends to proceed independently of the other more commonly used maturity indicators.

Age and Age Periods

Growth and maturation operate over a time framework, that is, the outcomes are measured at a single point in time or over time. The point of reference for time is the child's chronological age, which is measured relative to the birthday. Although chronological age is the point of reference, it should be emphasized that biological processes have their own clocks. Biological time does not necessarily proceed in concert with the calendar; hence, we can have children of the same chronological age who may differ by several years in skeletal age, age at menarche, and so on.

Postnatal growth is ordinarily divided into three age periods. *Infancy* comprises the first year of life and is a period of rapid growth in most bodily systems. *Childhood* covers the span from one year of age until adolescence. It is often divided into *early childhood*, which includes the preschool years (approximately 1 through 5 years), and *middle childhood*, which includes approximately the elementary school years (6 through the beginning of adolescence) in our culture. Childhood is a period of relatively steady progress in growth and maturation. *Adolescence* is defined in a number of ways due to variation in the time of its onset and termination. The age ranges 8 to 19 years in girls and 10 to 22 years in boys are often given as limits for normal variation in the onset and termination of adolescence in the human species. It is the period during which most bodily systems become adult or mature both structurally and functionally. Structurally, it begins with an acceleration in the rate of growth in stature which represents the adolescent growth spurt. The rate of statural growth then merges into a slowing or decelerative phase, and finally terminates with the attainment of adult stature. Functionally, adolescence usually is viewed in terms of sexual maturation, which begins with the initial development of the secondary sex characteristics (i.e., breasts and pubic hair in girls; genitalia and pubic hair in boys), and terminates with the attainment of mature reproductive function. Although menarche or the first menstrual flow is perhaps the most commonly used indicator of sexual

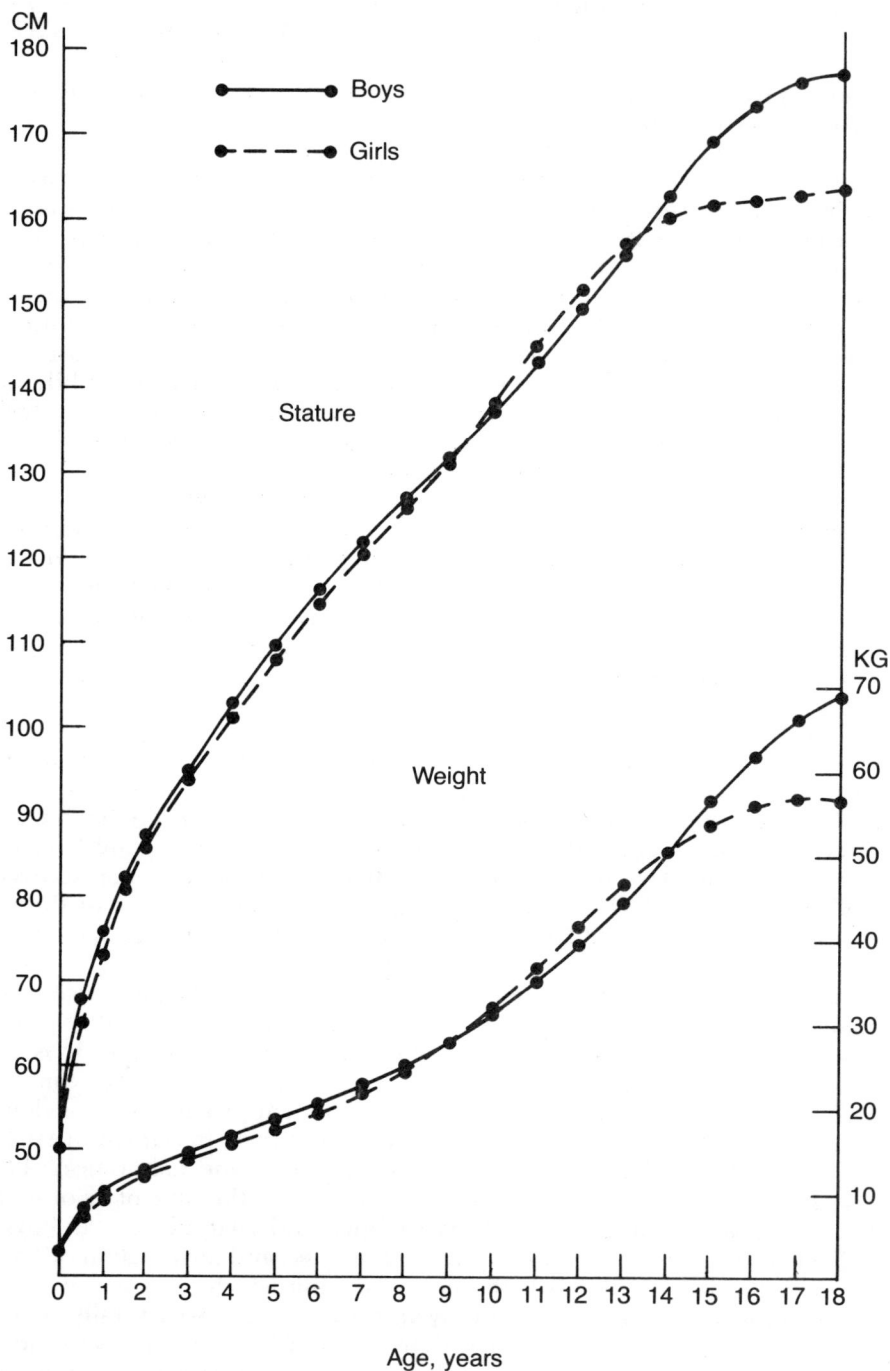

Fig. 1. Median recumbent length/stature and body weight for American boys and girls from birth to 18 years of age. Recumbent length from birth to 2 years, and then stature. Drawn from the data of the National Center for Health Statistics (1977).

maturity in girls, it does not necessarily mean reproductive maturity (fertility). The latter may not be achieved until the late teens or early twenties.

Age Changes and Sex Differences in Size, Proportions, and Body Composition

The general course of growth in stature and weight from birth to 18 years is shown in Figure 1. From birth to early adulthood, both stature and weight generally follow a four-phased growth pattern: rapid gain in infancy and early childhood, rather steady gain during middle childhood, rapid gain during adolescence, and slow increase and eventual cessation of growth at the attainment of adult stature. Note, however, that body weight usually continues to increase into adult life. Both sexes follow the same course of growth. Sex differences before the adolescent growth spurt are consistent, though minor. Boys, on the average, tend to be slightly longer/taller and heavier than girls. During the early part of adolescence, girls are temporarily taller and heavier than boys, which indicates their earlier adolescent spurt. Girls soon lose the size advantage as the male adolescent spurt occurs and they catch up and eventually surpass females in body size. The type of growth curve illustrated in Figure 1 is a distance curve. It indicates the size attained by the child at a given age or the distance the child has traversed on his or her path of growth. Such curves are indicators of growth status at a given age. This is the most commonly used growth curve for assessing the growth status of children in pediatric clinics and in schools.

Rate or velocity of growth, in centimeters or kilograms per year, differs for stature and weight during the pre-adolescent years. Stature growth occurs at a constantly decelerating rate. The child gets taller, but at a constantly slower rate. Weight growth, on the other hand, occurs at a slightly but constantly accelerating rate, except for a deceleration in early infancy.

During the adolescent growth spurt, growth in both stature and weight accelerate sharply. The adolescent spurt occurs earlier and is slightly less dramatic in girls than in boys. Sex differences in adult stature, therefore, are due primarily to the fact that boys, on the average, grow over a longer period of time than do girls. Girls, on the average, stop growing in stature by about 16 years of age, while boys continue to grow for another two years or so.

In order to derive a velocity curve, it is necessary to observe the same child over a considerable period of time, especially if observations on the adolescent phase of growth are desired. Estimating the adolescent spurt is further complicated by the fact that children vary in the timing of this event, and the event occurs, on the average, about two years earlier in girls. In longitudinal studies of American children, mathematically estimated average ages of peak velocity (i.e., the age of maximum growth during adolescence) varies between 11.0 and 11.6 years in girls and between 12.9 and 13.7 years in boys (Malina, 1967). Estimated ages vary with the procedures used. Menarche almost invariably occurs after peak height velocity in girls. The average age at menarche for American girls is about 12.8 years (National Center for Health Statistics, 1973).

Most body dimensions follow the same general pattern of growth in terms of size attained and rate of growth as do stature and weight. In general, sex differences are minor prior to adolescence. In the early part of adolescence, girls may have a temporary size advantage due to their earlier adolescent growth spurt, but eventually boys surpass girls in size attained in most body dimensions. As an example, size attained curves of arm and calf circumferences are shown in Figure 2, while similar curves for biacromial and bicristal breadths are shown in Figure 3. Note, however, that in bicristal breadth, boys catch up to girls in absolute size late in adolescence and the sex difference in size is not nearly as large as it is for biacromial breadth.

There are several exceptions to the general pattern of growth of the body as a

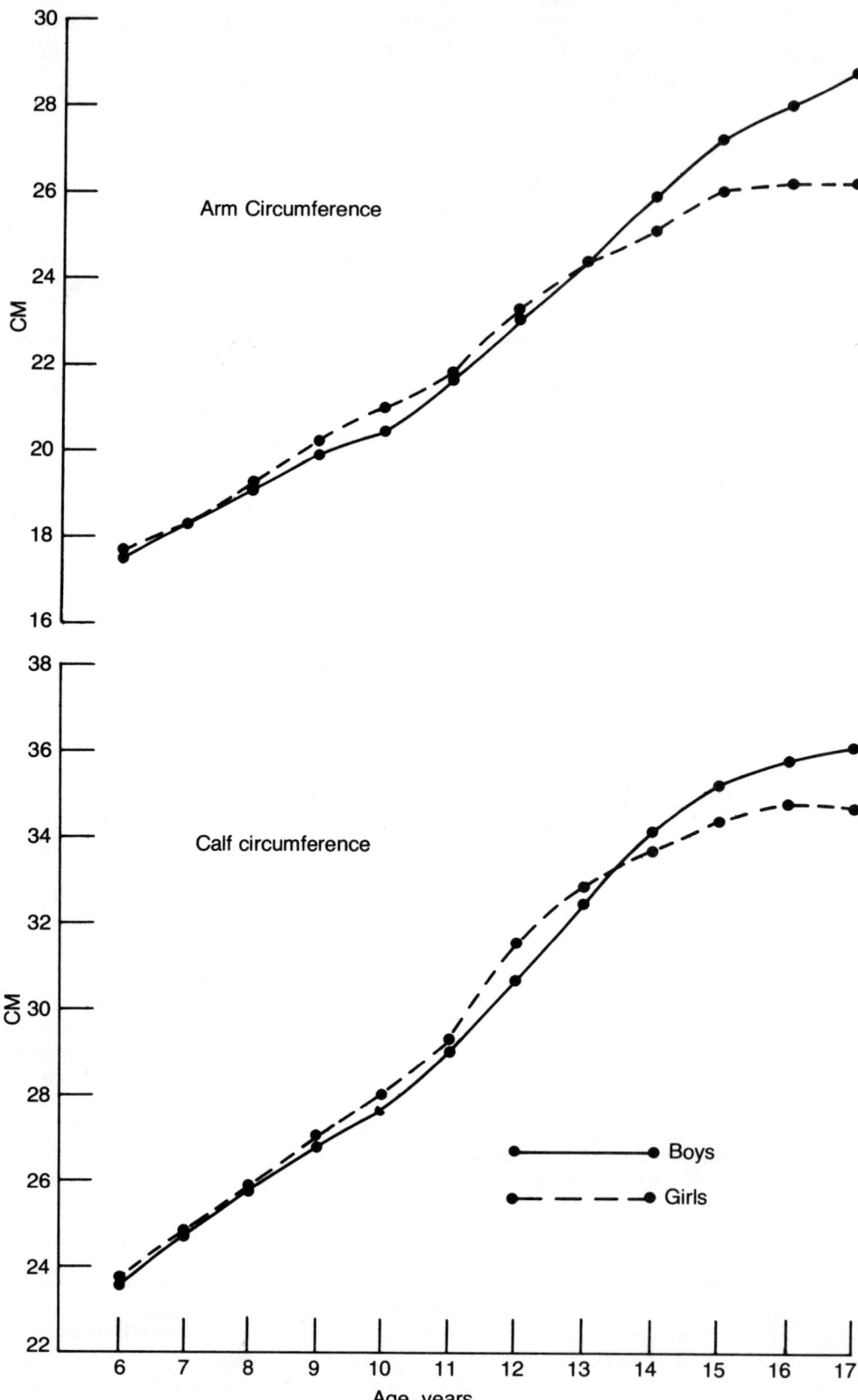

Fig. 2. Mean arm and calf circumferences for American children from 6 through 17 years of age. Drawn from the data of the National Center for Health Statistics published in Roche and Malina (1983).

whole and most of its external dimensions. These deal with specific body tissues and have been described by Scammon (1930) many years ago. The brain and its parts, the head, and upper face experience extremely rapid growth early in life so that by the age of 7 years the brain and its related structures have attained approximately 95% of their adult size. In contrast, the reproductive system and related structures, the testes, penis, ovary, uterus, prostate, and so on, show a slight increase early in postnatal life, followed by a latent period through childhood, and then an extremely rapid growth spurt during adolescence. The lymph tissues of the body, the thymus, lymph nodes, and intestinal lymphoid masses, which are associated in part with the body's immunity to disease, experience a rapid rise during infancy and childhood. By about 12 years of age there is almost twice as much lymphoid tissue as at 20 years of age. The relative decrease in the second decade of life reflects the gradual involution (degeneration) of the thymus gland, whose secretory function is considerably reduced. The amount of lymphoid tissue further decreases during adulthood. Fat tissue also follows a different postnatal growth pattern (see Figure 6). The preceding, however, serves to illustrate the differential but orderly nature of postnatal growth.

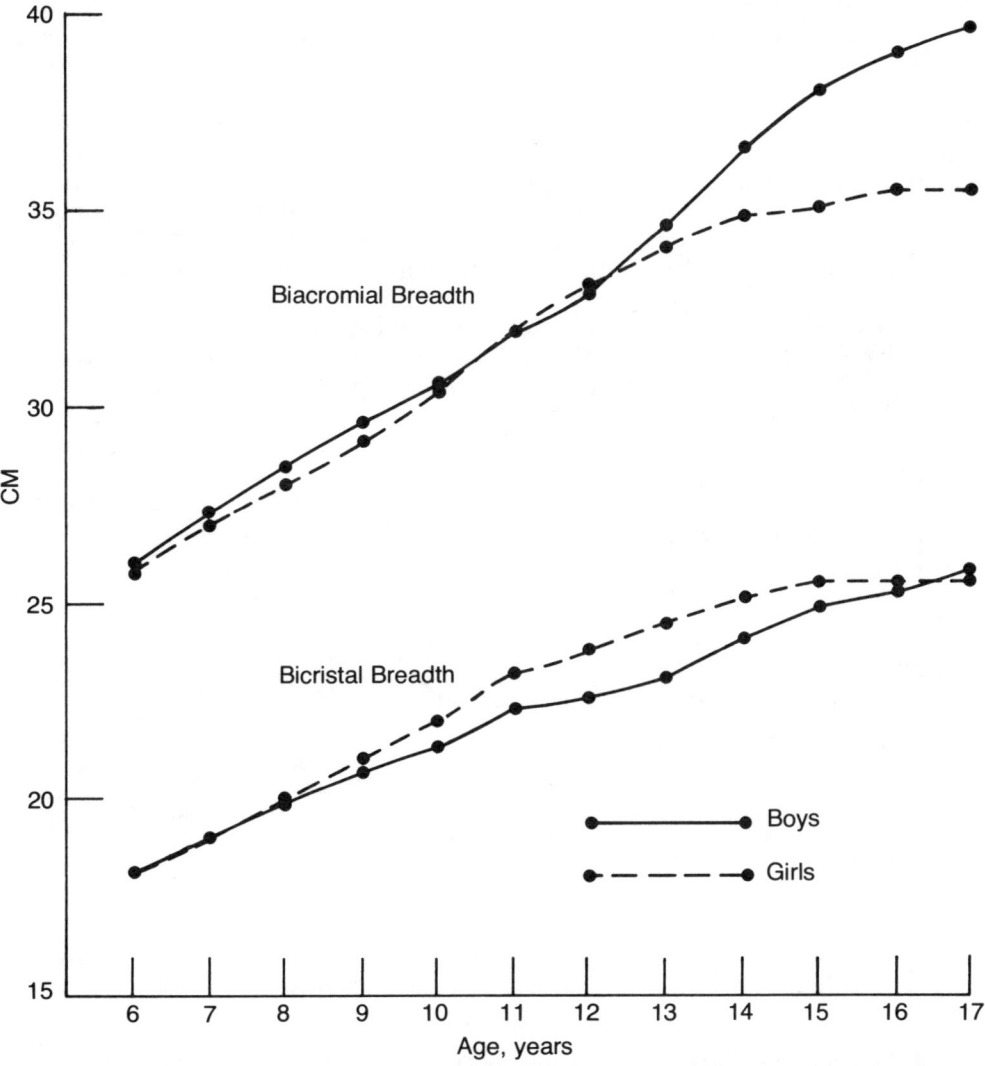

Fig. 3. Mean biacromial and bicristal breadths for American children from 6 through 17 years of age. Drawn from the data of the National Center for Health Statistics published in Roche and Malina (1983).

A consideration of the relationship between specific measurements permits an examination of body proportions, that is, the size of one part of the body relative to another. Proportions are ordinarily viewed in terms of ratios, and two in particular contribute to the understanding of sex differences in body build and the impact of the adolescent growth spurt on body proportions.

The obvious broadening of the shoulders relative to the hips is characteristic of male adolescence, while the broadening of the hips relative to the shoulders and waist is characteristic of female adolescence. The development of these proportional differences is shown in the ratio of biacromial to bicristal breadths in Figure 4. From 6 to 11 years, the ratio is almost constant in boys and then shows a marked increase from 11 to 16 years of age. The rise in the ratio is due to the fact that biacromial breadth is getting larger at a faster rate than bicristal breadth during male adolescence, that is, the numerator in the ratio increases at a faster rate than the denominator. In girls, on the other hand, the ratio declines slightly but consistently from 7 through 17 years. Note that these ratios are derived from cross-sectional data so that the curve is not necessarily smooth because different children are represented at each age. Because girls are developing broader hips relative to their shoulders, the ratio declines as the denominator (bicristal breadth) increases at a faster rate than the numerator (biacromial breadth).

The sex difference in the biacromial/bicristal ratio is especially apparent in longitudinal data obtained during adolescence. In growth studies, this is ordinarily done annually before adolescence, and at three-monthly or six-monthly intervals during the adolescent phase of growth. In a longitudinal study of British children, the estimated adolescent gain in biacromial breadth was 8.5 cm in boys and 6.2 cm in girls. The estimated adolescent gain in bicristal breadth was only 4.8 cm in boys and 6.0 cm in girls (Tanner et al., 1976). Thus, boys on the average gain more in shoulder breadth, while girls gain more in hip breadth during adolescence, and this differential magnitude of gains during adolescence contributes to the sex differences in proportions observed at this time.

Similar proprotional differences are apparent in relative length of the extremities. This is illustrated in growth studies using the ratio of sitting height to

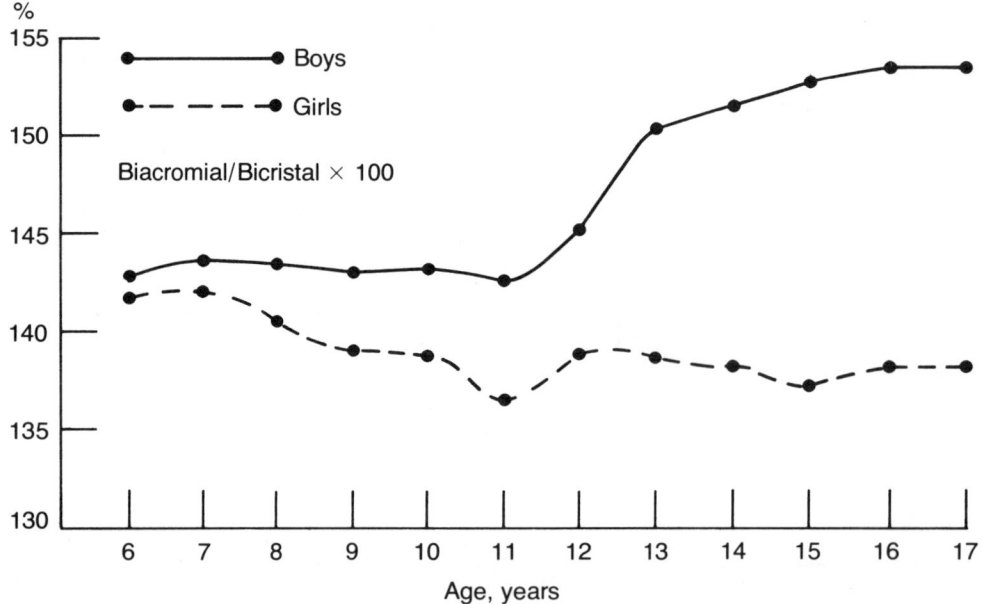

Fig. 4. The biacromial breadth/bicristal breadth ratio for American children from 6 through 17 years of age. Drawn from the mean values plotted in Figure 3.

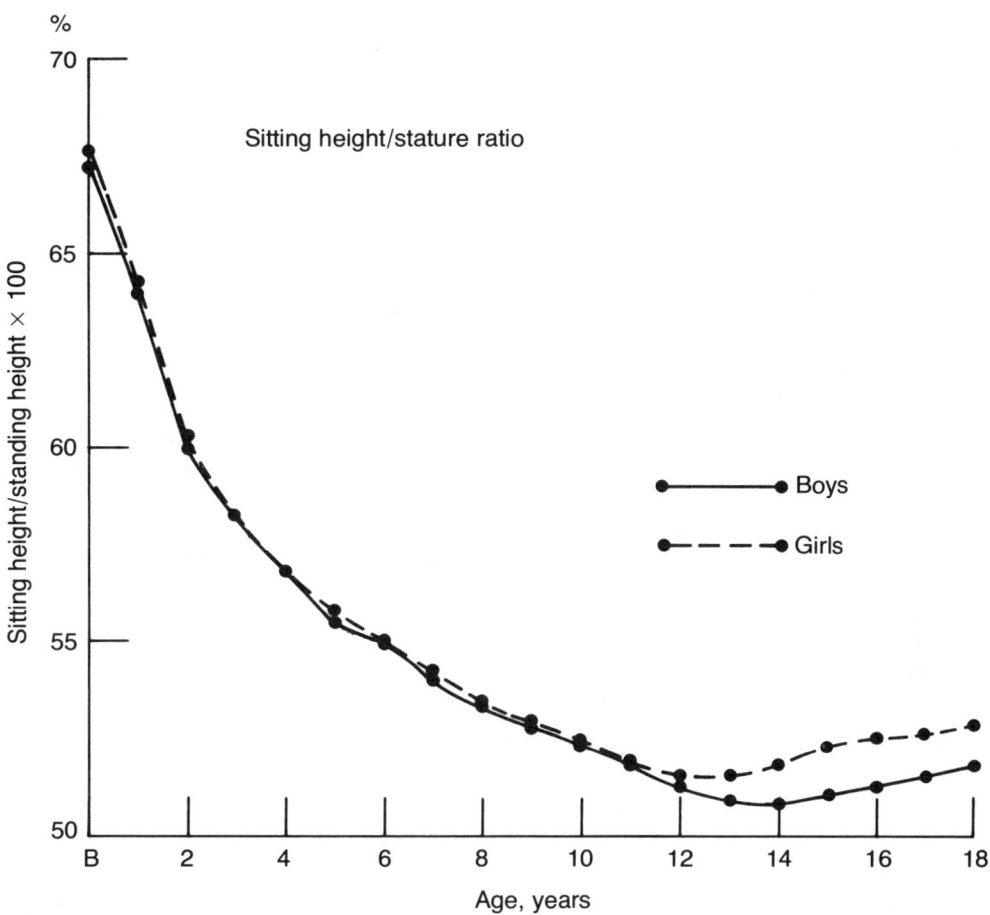

Fig. 5. The sitting height/standing height ratio for Denver children from birth to 18 years of age. Drawn from the data of Hansman (1970).

stature, an index of the contribution of the trunk and legs to stature. The growth curve for this proportion is shown in Figure 5. The ratio is highest in infancy and declines throughout childhood into adolescence. The ratio is lowest during the midst of adolescence, that is, 12 to 13 years of age in girls and 13 to 15 years of age in boys, and is then followed by an increase. During infancy and childhood, the legs are growing faster than the trunk; as result, sitting height contributes progressively less to stature with age and the ratio declines. The ratio reaches its lowest point during adolescence, earlier in girls than in boys. During the adolescent growth spurt, the legs experience their spurt earlier than the trunk. In British girls, for example, the age of peak velocity (maximum growth) for leg length is 11.6 years, while that for sitting height is 12.2 years. Corrresponding ages for boys are 13.6 years and 14.3 years respectively (Tanner et al., 1976). The slight increase in the ratio in later adolescence indicates late adolescent growth in trunk length at a time when growth in the lower extremities has already ceased.

The sitting height/stature ratio is identical for boys and girls until about 10 or 11 years of age, when it becomes slightly higher in girls and remains so through adolescence and into adulthood. Thus, prior to adolescence, both boys and girls are proportionately similar in terms of relative leg length or relative trunk length. However, during adolescence and in adulthood, females have, for an equal stature, relatively shorter legs than males.

Changing body proportions during growth and maturation contribute to age-

Table 1
Size and relative fatness (means) for samples of children in the U.S.[a]

Sample	n	Age (yrs)	Weight (kg)	Stature (cm)	Fatness (%)	Method[b]
MALES:						
Illinois, White	49	8-11	34.9	141.6	20.0	D
					19.2	K 40
					21.5	Skf
Arizona & Illinois,						
White-prepubescent	31	10.1	33.9	139.6	21.5	D, TBW[c]
-pubescent	11	12.3	45.1	157.0	19.1	
-postpubescent	34	15.5	63.1	170.9	17.3	
Black-pubescent	10	12.8	45.3	154.0	13.7	
-postpubescent	18	15.5	63.2	172.2	12.0	
New York, White	20	10	32.0	140.6	17.8	K 40
	57	12	40.0	150.3	17.8	
	41	14	56.6	165.8	14.8	
	20	16	63.0	172.3	11.7	
	18	18	70.3	180.9	10.8	
Louisiana, White	79	12.1	41.5	148.8	23.5	D
Black	49	13.1	44.6	152.7	19.4	
Minnesota, White	21	12-14	50.6	160.2	14.7	D[c]
	19	14-16	66.8	171.8	11.2	
	17	16-18	69.0	177.2	11.2	
Minnesota, White	20	17.2	66.7	172.1	14.9	D
California, White	48	17.2	72.1	178.6	11.6	D
Texas, Mexican American	15	9.4	26.7	128.3	11.8	D
	19	10.5	29.6	132.4	13.6	
	16	11.5	34.4	137.7	16.7	
	15	12.5	37.9	145.3	14.3	
	15	13.6	42.9	149.1	15.6	
	15	14.5	46.3	155.9	12.7	
FEMALES:						
Arizona & Illinois,						
White-prepubescent	12	10.1	34.3	140.2	24.5	D, TBW[c]
-pubescent	17	12.1	45.1	152.2	27.5	
-postpubescent	29	15.3	55.2	161.8	25.5	
Black-pubescent	12	10.8	42.0	148.3	24.5	
-postpubescent	26	14.9	57.7	162.5	24.4	
New York, White	19	9-10	33.0	139.2	24.2	D[c]
	21	12	45.2	155.4	25.6	
	14	14	50.0	162.0	27.0	
	12	16	55.9	166.0	27.8	
New York White	24	10	33.7	139.2	23.4	K 40
	36	12	43.0	151.0	21.7	
	15	14	50.0	158.2	22.2	
	31	16	54.8	161.7	23.6	
	19	18	56.0	163.2	22.7	
Louisiana, White	64	12.5	48.9	155.1	29.1	D
Black	50	12.5	48.1	153.8	25.7	
Minnesota, White	21	12-14	45.7	157.0	15.2	D[c]
	19	14-16	52.0	162.1	18.7	
	13	16-18	56.5	164.8	24.8	

[a] Adapted from Malina et al. (1978) which contains the primary references except for the data from Arizona and Illinois (Boileau et al., 1984).

[b] Method refers to the method of estimating body fatness: D = densitometry; K 40 = potassium 40; TBW = total body water; Skf = predicted from skinfolds. With densitometry, the equations of Siri and Brožek and colleagues are the two used.

[c] Fatness estimated from mean or median values in the original reports.

and sex-associated variation in physique. When viewed in the traditional three-component somatotype, the following summarizes changes in physique during growth and maturation. Diri childhood, girls have, on the average, higher endomorphy and boys have higher mesomorphy. The sexes differ little in ectomorphy. The distributions of somatotypes within a sample of boys and girls show the sex difference in physique somewhat more clearly. For example, in a study of preschool children, Walker (1962) noted that only 25% of the boys' somatotype ratings reached or exceeded a value of 4 for endomorpy, while more than one-half of the girls' ratings reached or exceeded this value for endomorphy. In mesomorphy, on the other hand, over one-half of the boys reached or exceeded a rating of 4, while only 16% of the girls' ratings reached or exceeded this value.

Although the preceding suggests reasonably clear-cut sex differences in physique during childhood, it should be emphasized that the physiques of male and female endomorphs, or of male and female mesomorphs are much alike. The important point is that there are more endomophic girls and more mesomorphic boys.

During adolescence, sex differences in physique are somewhat magnified. Male adolescence is characterized by major development in the mesomorphic component, a reduction in the endomorphic component, and an increase in the ectomorphic component. Female adolescence, on the other hand, involves primary development in endomorphy, slight increase in mesomorphy, and a reduction in ectomorphy. The effects of adolescence on somatotype are such that in young adulthood as in childhood, there are more endomorphic females than males, and more mesomorphic males than females.

Age trends and sex differences in lean body mass and fatness as derived from measurements of potassium-40 (a natually occurring radio-isotope in the body) are shown in Figure 6. At all ages from 6 through 17 years, boys have, on the average, a greater lean body mass than girls. Note that the difference between the sexes is reduced during early adolescence. However, in contrast to the growth curve for body weight (see Figure 1), which show a temporary female size advantage, the growth curve for lean body mass does not. By inference, the temporary body weight advantage of females during early adolescence is most likely due to greater fatness in females. This is shown in the middle and lower parts of Figure 6. On the average girls exceed boys in absolute and relative amounts of fat during growth. The differences are not great during childhood, but as adolescence approaches, the differences are magnified and persist through adolescence and into adulthood. It should be recalled at this point that the values shown in Figure 6 probably overestimate relative fatness by at least four percent.

Estimates of relative fatness in samples of school age American children and youth are shown in Table 1. Variation among samples, as well as among estimates based on different techniques to assess body compositon, should be noted. Further, the statistical constants used to estimate body compositon are based on adults and do not take into consideration child-adult differences in body composition. Hence, the averages probably overestimate relative fatness by about four percent (Boileau et al., 1984).

Estimates of total lean body mass and fatness treat the body as a whole and do not illustrate changes in different areas of the body. Growth in arm and calf musculature is shown in Figure 7. Sex differences, though apparent, are small during childhood, boys having slightly wider muscles. By about 11 years of age, girls begin their adolescent spurt and have a temporary size advantage in muscle width measures of the calf (as is the case for body weight). There is, however, no temporary size advantage for girls in arm musculature. Boys then have their adolescent spurt in muscle mass, and have considerably wider extremity muscles than girls. Sex differences in muscle widths, established during adolescence, persist into adulthood and are more apparent for musculature of the upper extremities.

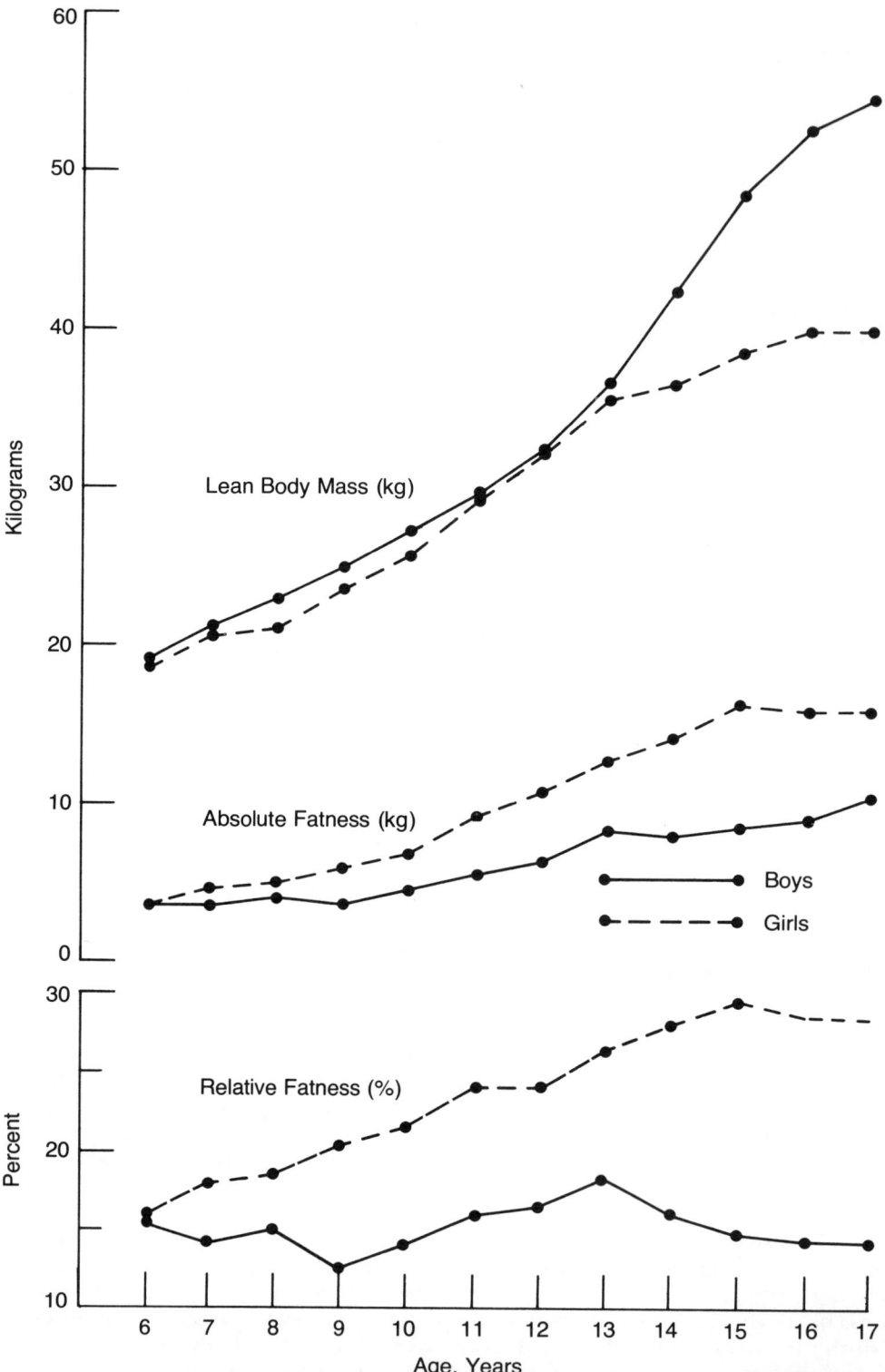

Fig. 6. Median lean body mass (determined from potassium-40), absolute amount of fat, and percentage of body weight as fat in German children from 6 through 17 years of age. Drawn from the data of Burmeister (1965).

When longitudinal data for radiographic muscle widths are aligned on peak height velocity (Tanner et al., 1981), sex differences in the magnitude and perhaps timing of the adolescent muscle tissue spurt are apparent. Boys have a spurt in arm muscle width that is approximately twice the magnitude of that in females. In contrast, the peak in calf muscle width is only slightly greater in males. Peak velocities of arm and calf musculature occur after peak height velocity. For the arm, it occurs about three to four months after peak height velocity in boys and about six months after peak height velocity in girls. When muscle widths are plotted relative to peak muscle velocities, it is apparent that the adolescent spurt in arm and calf muscle occurs over a two year period, which is about the same duration as the adolescent height spurt (Tanner et al., 1981).

To illustrate regional changes in subcutaneous fatness during growth, age- and sex-associated variation in the triceps (an extremity fat site) and subscapular (a trunk fat site) skinfolds are shown in Figure 8. Both skinfolds are thicker and increase with age in girls. In contrast, the subscapular skinfold increases with age in boys, while the triceps skinfold shows a decrease in thickness during male adolescence. Thus, adolescent sex differences are more apparent for the extremities than for the trunk, which in turn indicates differential fat patterning of subcutaneous fat on the extremities and on the trunk. Thus, summing the two skinfolds to indicate fatness as in the National Children and Youth Fitness Study (Ross and Gilbert, 1985) may have merit, but it does not address the issue of fat

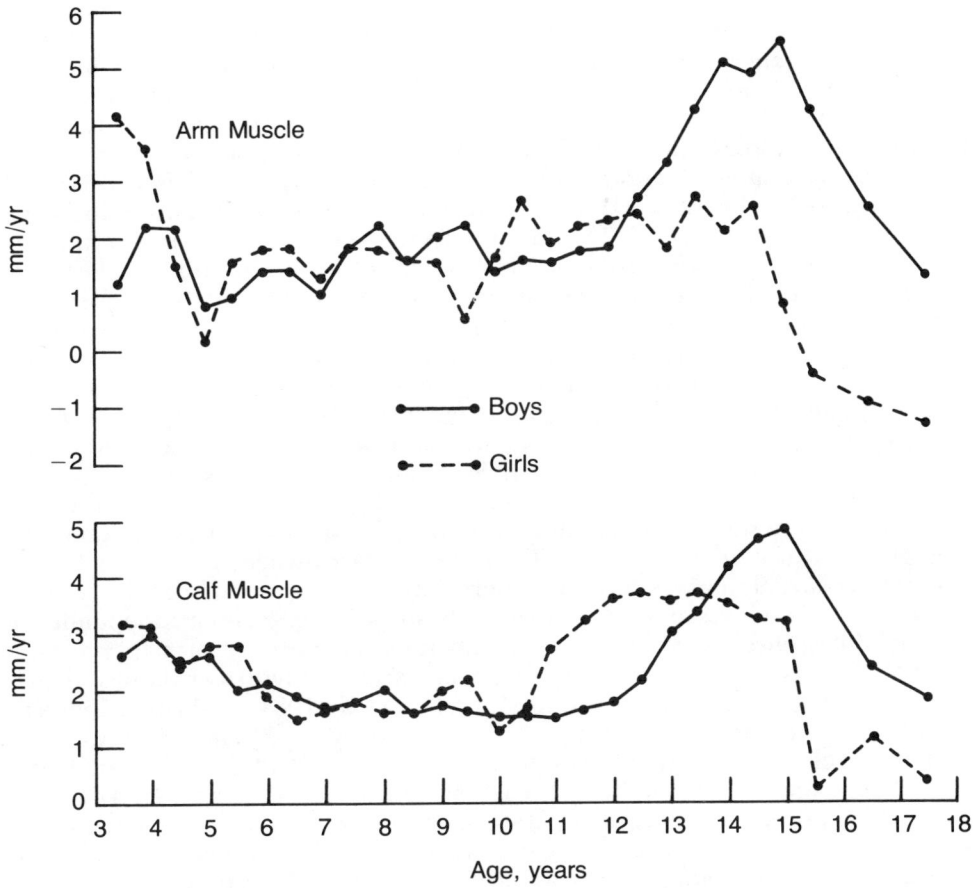

Fig. 7. Mean widths of muscle tissue in the arm and calf for British children 3 through 17 years of age. Drawn from the data of Tanner et al. (1981).

patterning, that is, where the fat is distributed. A large subscapular skinfold (20mm) summed with a small triceps skinfold (8mm) gives a identical indication of fatness (28mm) as subscapular and triceps skinfolds of the same thickness (14mm each). The estimated fatness is the same, but the distributions differ.

Maturity-Associated Variation

In the preceding discussion, the child's chronological age is used as the point of reference. Children also have an inborn biological clock, which sets the pace of their growth rate and maturation. Hence, the child may not necessarily proceed in tempo with his or her biological clock. The net result is a considerable degree of biological maturity-associated variation in size, physique, and body composition during growth. This is especially apparent in samples of 12-year-old girls and 14-year-old boys. Such groups may include youngsters who are physically and sexually close to adulthood, some who are physically and sexually children, and some who are at various stages of transition from childhood to adulthood.

The sequence of events occurring during adolescence is shown in Figure 9 for British children. Several features should be noted. Girls, on the average, mature in advance of boys. The sex difference, however, varies with the criterion used. It is about two years for age at peak height velocity but only a fraction of a year between mean ages at attaining other maturity stages. Ages at the onset of different pubertal stages or attaining peak height velocity and menarche are quite variable and may span several years. This is apparent in the range of variation about the means in Figure 9. Finally, the sequence of somatic and sexual maturation during adolescence is generally quite uniform. The rate of maturation or the timing, that is, ages at onset, is quite variable as is the rate of passage from one stage to another.

Maturity-associated variation in size, physique, and composition, though apparent prior to adolescence, is most pronounced during this period of accelerated growth and sexual maturation. Two questions are of importance in considering maturity-associated variation. First, do the maturity indicators measure the same kind of biological maturity? That is, if a youngster is rated as maturationally advanced by one indicator, is he or she rated as advanced by another? With the exception of dental maturity, which tends to proceed independently, other indicators of maturity are positively related. This is shown in Table 2 for certain indices of maturity during adolescence. Stage 2 of breast or genital development is generally accepted as the first overt sign of sexual maturation. All correlations are moderate to high, although data are more extensive for girls than for boys. Thus, youngsters advanced or delayed in sexual maturation are also advanced or delayed in the adolescent growth spurt. Skeletal maturity is also related to the development of secondary sex characteristics and growth during adolescence.

The second question relates to the consistency of maturity ratings over time. Is a youngster maturationally delayed at 6 years of age also delayed at 11 years of age? The answer is generally yes, although there may be variation during adolescence.

The interrelatedness among maturity indicators as well as their independence during adolescence are reasonably well illustrated in results of principal components analyses of indices of somatic, sexual, and skeletal maturity in boys and girls 8 through 18 years of age (Bielicki, 1975; Bielicki et al., 1984). Indices included in the analyses were ages at attaining peak height velocity, peak weight velocity, peak leg length velocity, peak trunk length velocity, 80% of adult height, genital and pubic hair stages 2 and 4 in boys, breast and pubic hair stages 2 and 4 in girls, menarche, and skeletal maturity at 10 through 15 years of age. The sex-specific analyses resulted in two principal components. The first, which accounted for 77% and 68% of the total sample variance in boys and girls respectively, had high loadings on almost all indices. It appears to be a general maturity factor, which discriminates among individuals who are early-, average-, or late-maturing. The

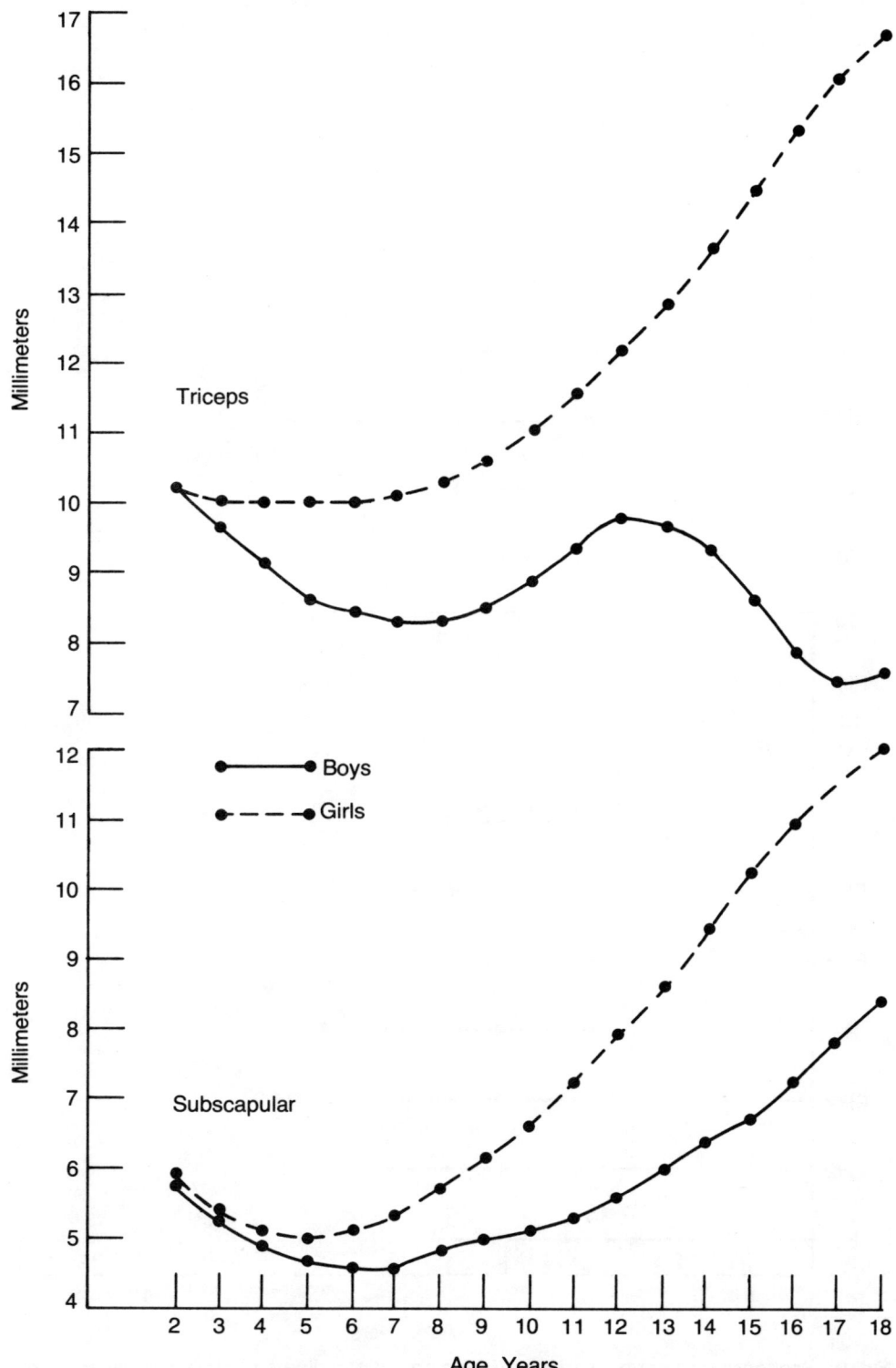

Fig. 8. Median triceps and subscapular skinfold thickness for American children from 2 through 18 years of age. Drawn from the data of the National Center for Health Statistics (1981).

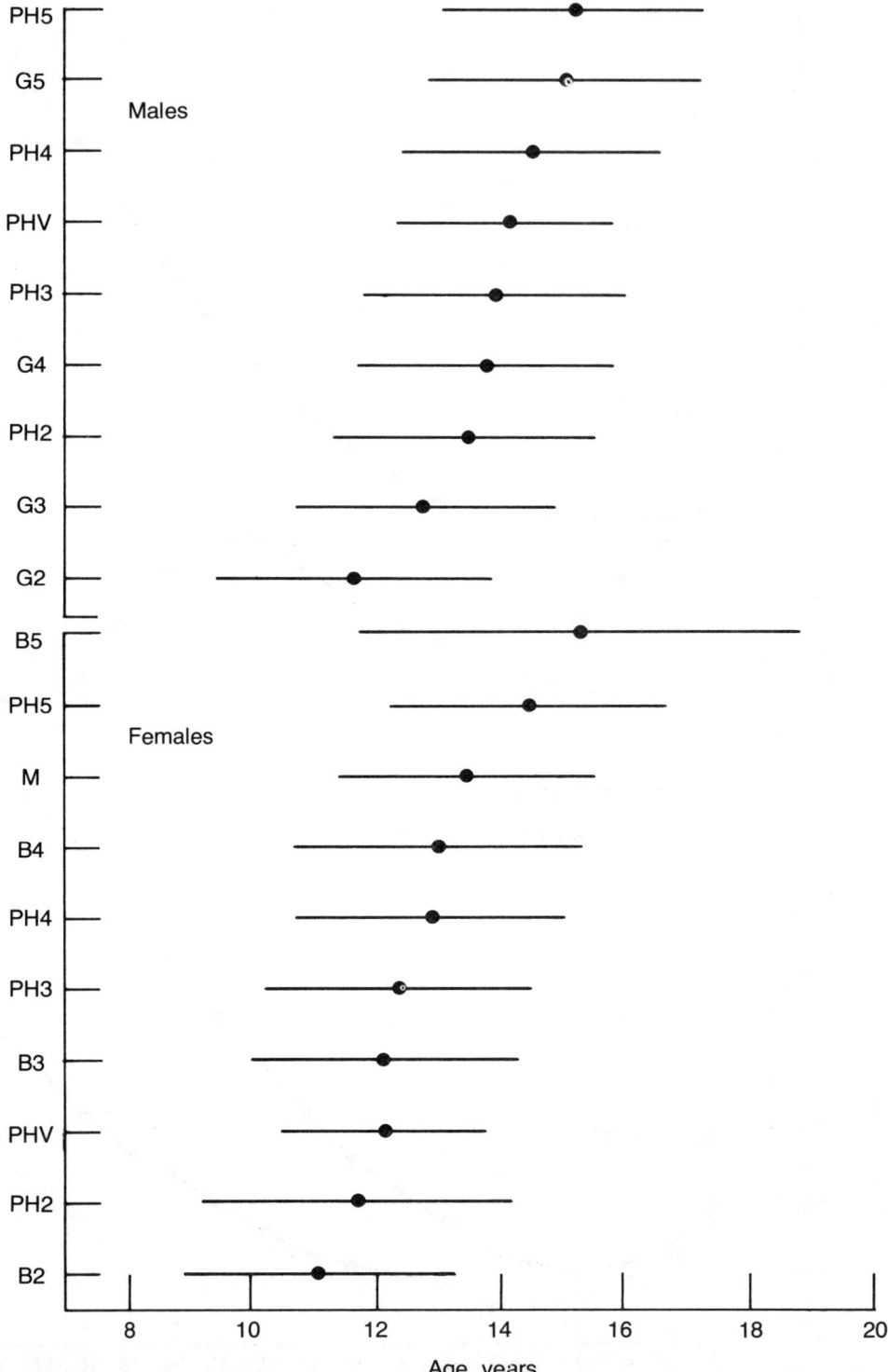

Fig. 9. Sequence and normal variation (mean age at attaining a particular stage or event, plus and minus two standard deviations) of pubertal development in British boys and girls. Drawn from the data of Marshall and Tanner (1969, 1970). B2-B5 = stages of breast development, G2-G5 = stages of genital development; PH2-PH5 = stages of pubic hair development; M = menarche; PHV = peak height velocity.

second principal component accounted for 12% and 7.5% of the total sample variance in boys and girls, respectively. Among boys, this component, which had high positive loadings on skeletal maturity at 11 and 12 years, and lower loadings at 13, 14, and 15 years of age, appears to be a rather specific factor which refers to the rate of skeletal maturation during pre-adolescence. The second component in girls was somewhat similar, in that it had moderate loadings for skeletal maturity scores which systematically decreased from 10 through 14 years of age. The second component also differed between the sexes, particularly in the magnitude and sign of loadings for indices of linear growth and secondary sex characteristic development.

Although there are some differences in the two separate analyses, the results show similar patterns. Indices of linear growth, sexual maturation and skeletal maturation are sufficiently interrelated to indicate a general maturity factor during adolescence. However, in contrast to the notion of a general maturity factor, the evidence also suggests variation within and between the somatic, sexual, and skeletal indicators of growth and maturity. Hence, although there is a general maturity factor underlying the tempo of growth and maturation during adolescence in both sexes, there is variation so that no single system provides a complete description of the tempo of growth and maturation of an individual boy or girl during adolescence.

The apparent "disharmony" among indicators probably reflects real biological variation, for example, the nature of hormonal control in prepubertal and pubertal phases of development. It may also reflect methodological issues, for example, secondary sex characteristics are rated on 5-stage scales, although the development of there characteristics is a continuous process upon which discontinuities, or stages, are imposed. The variation also relates to individual variability in the timing and duration of the events used to document pubertal growth, sexual maturation and skeletal maturation. Some boys may pass from genital stages 2 through 5 in about two years, while others may take about five years (Marshall, 1978). Further, there is no consistent relationship between the age at which secondary sex character development begins and the rate of progress through the stages. Another example is the observation that skeletal age varies as much as chronological age at the first overt signs of puberty in boys (genital stage 2) and girls (breast stage 2).

Table 2
Correlations between ages at reaching certain maturity indicators during adolescence[a]

	Girls						Boys	
	PHV			B2		PH2	PHV	
Sample	B2	PH2	M	PH2	M	M	G2	PH2
United States				.66	.86	.70		
United States	.80	.75	.71	.75	.74	.74	.67	
United States	.78		.93					.56
England	.82		.91			.64		
England	.78	.77	.84				.47	.84
Denmark	.80	.73	.84	.70	.74	.58	.78	.49
Poland	.76	.77	.76	.77	.72	.73	.87	.84

[a] Adapted from Malina (1978), which contains the primary references except for the data for Polish boys (Bielicki et al., 1984). PHV = peak height velocity; B2 = stage 2 of breast development; PH2 = stage 2 of pubic hair development; M = menarche; G2 = stage 2 of genital development.

Maturity-associated variation is clearly observed when grouping children by their skeletal age or according to the stage of development of secondary sex characteristics. Youngsters are generally grouped into maturity categories as "early," "average", and "late" maturers. Early-maturing children are those in whom the maturity indicators are in advance of their chronological age. For example, a child with a chronological age of 9 and a skeletal age of 11 would be early maturing, as would a girl experiencing menarche at a chronological age of 11. In contrast, late-maturing children are those in whom the maturity indicators lag relative to chronological age. A child having a chronological age of 9 years and a skeletal age of 7 years would be late maturing, as would a girl experiencing menarche at 15 years of age. It should be emphasized that maturity associated variations are best noted at the extremes of early and lateness. Average-maturing children comprise the broad middle range of normal variation, with normal variation in growth studies often defined as plus or minus one to two years of an individual's chronological age.

Early-maturing children are generally taller and heavier for their age from early childhood through adolescence than their late-maturing peers (Figure 10). Late maturers, however, catch up to early maturers in height in late adolescence or early adulthood, but they do not catch up in body weight. Early maturers thus have more weight for their statures than late maturers. This can be translated into physique differences; early maturers have stockier, more mesomorphic physiques in the case of boys, and stockier, more endomorphic physiques in the case of girls. On the other hand, late maturers of both sexes tend to have less weight for height and tend to be extremely ectomorphic or linear in build. Such maturity-associated physique differences can be extended to body composition. Early maturing children of both sexes, as compared to late-maturing children, generally have larger amounts of fat and lean tissue, reflecting to a great extent their overall larger body sizes. On a relative basis (i.e., when expressed as a percentage of body weight), early maturing children are fatter and not as lean as late maturers. It should be noted that differences between late-maturing children and those in the average category of the maturity continuum are generally not as apparent as differences between average-maturing and early-maturing children, and between early-maturing and late-maturing children. This would seem to suggest that the marked maturity-associated variation in physique and body composition is more associated with early maturation.

Regulation of Growth and Maturation

The integrated nature of growth and maturation is maintained by the interaction of genes, hormones, nutrients, and the environments in which the individual lives. This complex interaction regulates a person's growth and their sexual maturation, and physical metamorphosis in general.

A comprehensive review of the regulatory mechanisms and influence is beyond the scope of this chapter. Only a brief overview of genetic, endocrine and nutritional factors is given.

An individual's genotype can be viewed as representing potential. Whether a child attains this growth potential depends on the environments in which he or she is reared. In a growth study or in the classroom, the child is observed in phenotypic form, that is, a product of his gentotype and environments. The partitioning of genotypic and environmental components as well as their interaction in growth and maturation is important to understanding these processes.

Linear body measurements (e.g., stature, leg length) tend to have a higher genetic influence than breadths or circumferences. Circumferences, skinfolds and body weight have a lower genetic influence than bone dimensions because the former are subject to short term changes with the environment (e.g., training or

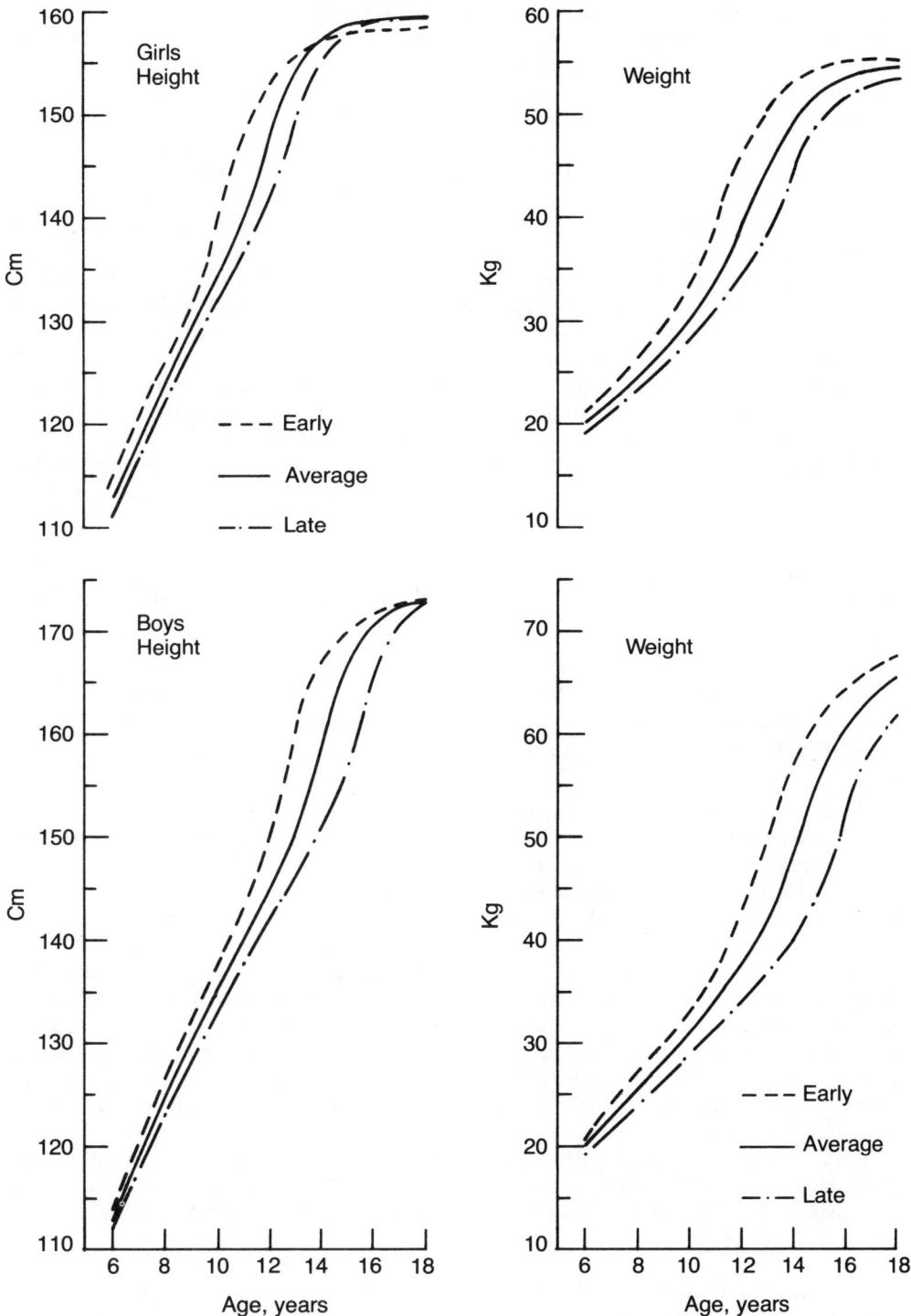

Fig. 10. Mean statures and weights of boys and girls classified as early, average and late maturing on the basis of age at maximum growth. Drawn from the data of Shuttleworth (1939).

nutritional stress). However, the pattern of fat distribution on the body is highly influenced by heredity, as are indices of biological maturity, that is, menarche, skeletal age, secondary sex characteristics, and age at peak height velocity. Hence, the genetic contribution to individual differences in growth and maturation is significant.

Endocrine secretions are basically regulatory and have an important function in growth and maturation processes. Some growth, however, will occur in the absence of growth promoting hormones, emphasizing the organism's inherent tendency to grow. Endocrine secretions are themselves strongly influenced by genetic mechanisms. These hormones are essential for the full expression of the genetically determined patterns of growth and maturation of tissues and systems, and thus the individual. The nervous system, in turn, is intimately involved in regulating endocrine secretions, and since the nervous system mediates our interactions with the external environments which the individual encounters, the sources for potential variation may be many.

The neuroendocrine hypothesis for the regulation of sexual maturation involves changes in the hypothalamus, anterior pituitary, and gonads. Gonatropin releasing hormone (GnRH) is secreted by the hypothalamus and results in the secretion of gonadotropins by the anterior pituitary. The latter in turn initiate the maturation of the gonads and the process of sexual maturation (Wierman and Crowley, 1986). The process is gradual and probably begins in the late prepubertal period, long before any overt signs of sexual maturation are evident.

The initiation of the changes in the hypothalamic-pituitary-gonadal axis resides in the central nervous system. Wierman and Crowley (1986, p. 238), however, find that:

> At this time, however, no definite statement can be made as to the precise trigger (or triggers) of sexual maturation. Although the final common pathway of this effect is clearly mediated by modulation of hypothalamic secretion of GnRH, little else is clear.

The anterior pituitary, for example, can apparently modify the "CNS initiative", while as sexual maturation progresses, the gonad can "amplify the pituitary gonadotropin message" (Wierman and Crowley, 1986, p. 235).

The adolescent growth spurt and changes in skeletal maturation are influenced by adrenal sex steroids in addition to the gonadal steroids which underlie sexual maturation. Hence, there is considerable potential for variation among indicators of somatic, sexual and skeletal maturity during adolescence. For example, the earlier phases of skeletal maturation are principally dependent upon the stimulation of growth hormone, while the later phases, which include epiphyseal capping and fusion, are chiefly under the influence of steroid hormones among others (Tanner et al., 1975). The later phases of skeletal maturation are thus under the control of the same factors which underlie the adolescent growth spurt and sexual maturation.

The control of sexual maturation and the adolescent growth spurt is genetically determined. Grumbach shows that "when socioeconomic and environmental factors are optimal for growth and development, the age of onset of puberty is normal children is determined principally be genetic factors" (1980, p. 250). However, the timing of the growth spurt and puberty can be influenced by environmental factors. This is especially evident in populations living under conditions of chronic undernutrition. Clinical observation of ". . . unusually 'fractured' curves of growth and pubertal development in girls translated to unfamiliar boarding schools at various times in puberty" (Tanner, 1978, p. 102), would seem to implicate stressful life events as a factor contributing to variation in pubertal development. A logical question, which will be addressed later in this chapter, is whether regular physical training is sufficiently stressful to influence growth and maturation.

Interacting with the individual's genotype and endocrine secretions is his/her nutritional status. Nutrient requirements are many, and from the developmental perspective are often viewed in terms of energy and proteins for growth, maintenance, and repair. Nutrient requirements vary considerably with age, sex, and body size, and in the growing organism they vary with stage of growth. Energy needs to support growth processes are greatest during infancy and progressively decline with age. The energy needs for maintenance, on the other hand, increase during growth. In other words, as the individual gets bigger, more energy is necessary to support this size. However, with age, the rate of growth declines so that the amount of energy necessary to support the growth processes, per se, is progressively reduced. The effects of chronic undernutrition on growth and maturation are well documented and need no further discussion here.

The preceding has provided a brief overview of the major factors influencing growth and maturation. There are, in addition, other growth influencing factors whose direct effects are more difficult to identify or are of less overall importance. Of these, physical activity is often viewed as a favorable influence on growth and maturation. It should be noted, however, that physical activity is only one of many factors that may affect growth and maturation so that the precise role of properly graded activity programs in influencing these processes is not completely understood.

Activity, Growth and Maturation

The Need to Quantify Activity and Training

Physical activity is not necessarily the same as regular physical training. Physical activities are obviously a part of training programs, but not all physical activities qualify as training. Physical training refers to the regular, systematic practice of specific physical activities such as calisthenics, lifting weights, isometric exercises, running, games/sports activities, and so on, performed at specific intensities and for different durations. Training programs vary in kind or type, and may emphasize endurance, strength, speed, or skill. The effects of such programs are generally specific to the type of training stimulus, although training effects induced by one kind of program may be more general. Running, for example, apparently has more general effects than cycling. Thus, training is not a single entity, but varies in kind, intensity, and duration. It can be viewed as a continuum, ranging from relatively mild work to severely stressing activity.

In studies of training during growth, programs vary in type, intensity, and duration, and are often described as mild, moderate, or severe, without more specific definiton. At times, children are simply defined as "active" or "inactive." These labels are often based upon teacher and/or coach assessment of frequency and duration of sports participation, and self-reported activity levels. There is a need to qualify and quantify training programs (e.g., how many sessions per week, duration of workouts, how many meters swam during a workout and at what intensity, how many miles run per workout and at what time or pace, and so on). Age-group swimmers 9 through 12 years of age in some programs may swim about 4500 meters per session at varying time intervals six days per week, while in other programs they may swim only 2500 meters per session.

Designs Used in Activity Studies

Data from a variety of studies have been used to make inferences about the effects of regular physical activity on human growth and maturation. Thus, results may be of unequal value and may have limitations in making inferences on the role of activity in growth and maturation.

Experimental studies compare trained (treatment) and untrained (control) groups. The training stimulus usually varies in type, intensity and duration, so that problems are generally encountered in defining and quantifying the training stimulus within and across studies. Selection of subjects, motivation to train and control of outside activity are also critical factors. In addition, variable and composite age groups of children and youth are used as are small samples. Attrition rates tend to be high, and most studies are short term. There is a lack of experimental studies in which the training factor has been regularly applied and changes monitored over a sufficiently long period during growth. Difficulties inherent in conducting longitudinal programs with children and youth are obvious. Hence, a significant amount of experimental data are derived by extrapolation from studies of animals. Although reasonable generalizations can be made for human growth, the concept of species specificity must be recongnized.

A limitation of studies monitoring changes associated with regular training during youth is that the focus is not ordinarily the growth and maturation of children. Many studies have as their focus physiological changes associated with training such as maximal oxygen consumption and metabolic substrates. Growth observations are usually made in passing or indirectly, while maturity status is generally not included.

Comparisons of athletes and non-athletes during childhood and adolescence are commonly used to make inferences about the effects of physical training on growth and maturation. It is assumed that the athletes had been training regularly, and differences in growth and maturation relative to non-athletes are attributed to the training programs required for the specific sports. Problems with such an approach are the definition of an athlete at young ages and subject selection. Youngsters proficient in sports are undoubtedly selected for their motor skills and in some sports, for their size. Size, physique, strength and motor skill proficiency are related, and an individual's strength and motor ability may in turn influence his/her level of habitual activity. Maturity differences also characterize youngsters who excel in sports, and these differences are especially apparent during and around puberty. Males who are successful in sports competition are often advanced in biological maturity status. This probably reflects the size, strength, and performance advantages associated with earlier maturation. In contrast, females who excel in sports tend to be average or late in biological maturity status. Swimmers tend towards the average, while female athletes in other sports tend to be late maturing. Late maturing girls tend to be more linear in physique and leaner, both factors which may be more suitable for sports performance. Another factor which must be considered in comparing young athletes and non-athletes is the role of social circumstances, that is, socialization into or away from sports. Social factors may interact or vary with a youngster's growth and maturity progress, and in turn influence his/her sporting or activity pursuits. Hence, young athletes, especially the elite, are most likely not a random sample, and may not be representative of the general population of children and youth.

The limitations of studies of young athletes should be considered. The study of Astrand and colleagues (1963) on the growth and functional capacity of elite female swimmers is often cited as suggesting that training stimulates growth in stature. A close examination of the data for the 30 swimmers, however, indicates that the girls were in fact taller than the average since seven years of age, and apparently entered adolescence slightly earlier than average. Mean stature was +0.4 standard deviation units at seven years of age and +0.6 standard deviation units at the time of the study when the girls ranged in age from 11.9 to 16.4 years. The apparent acceleration in statural growth was not related to the intensity of training. Rather, it was probably related to the swimmers' somewhat earlier maturation: eight girls attained menarche between 11.0 and 11.9 years, seven between 12.0 and 12.9 years, 10 between 13.0 and 13.9, and four at 14.0 years. The average age at menarche for the group was 12.9 years, and menarche generally follows peak height velocity so that one might expect the young swimmers to be somewhat taller. Their tallness most likely represents earlier maturation and not the effects of intensive swimming training.

In the study of young boys (11-13 years of age) selected for swimming training, Milicer and Denisiuk (1964) noted slightly greater average increments in stature over two years of training compared to a control sample. The apparent rate differences in statural growth most likely reflect maturity variation. The young swimmers included a greater percentage of early maturers (25%) compared to the control sample (17%), and did not include any late maturers.

Similar trends are evident in small samples of boys 10 to 15 years of age engaged in endurance running training. Measures of maturity status are not included, so that short term changes in height which occur during the training program cannot be attributed to the training. The youngsters could have experienced all or part of their adolescent spurts, given the normal variation in the timing and intensity of the male growth spurt.

Young female gymnasts tend to be shorter than the average and delayed in biological maturation. Concern has been expressed over the possible growth and maturation stunting effects of intensive training. However, analysis of their heights at three years of age indicates that young gymnasts are already shorter than the average. Hence, it is difficult to implicate intensive training as the cause of their short stature.

Comparisons of adult athletes with non-athletes or the general population are also used to make inferences on the effects of regular physical activity during growth. It is assumed that the adult athletes began training during their youth, and the differences relative to non-athletes reflect training effects on growth and maturation processes. Most recently, such an approach was used to make inferences on the effects of early training on the sexual maturation of young girls (Frisch et al., 1981). Problems associated with subject selection, age of onset of training, motivation to persist in training programs, and so on are similar to those already mentioned.

Some activities such as tennis and baseball pitching require *extreme levels of unilateral effort*. This specialized activity is occasionally used to illustrate training effects. The individual is his/her own control, as the dominant limb (trained) is compared to the non-dominant (untrained). Observations from such studies are ordinarily limited to skeletal and muscular observations of the upper extermity.

The co-twin control method involves comparisons of monozygotic (identical) twins discordant for regular physical activity. One member of the twin pair is regularly trained while the other is not and/or follows his/her usual pattern of activity. Data from such studies consider primarily physiological variables. Twin studies, however, have several limitations (see Bouchard and Malina, 1983).

Clinical and experimental observations of prolonged bed rest, immobilization with casts, and muscular inactivation as in nerve injuries also provide insights into the role of physical activity in developing and maintaining the integrity of skeletal and muscular tissues. These are perhaps most apparent in the muscular atrophy and loss of skeletal mineral associated with prolonged inactivity or disuse.

Effects of Activity on Growth

Stature. Regular physical activity has no apparent effect on stature in growing individuals. Although some early data suggest an increase in stature with regular training, the observed changes are usually quiet small and are derived from studies that did not control for subject selection and for maturity status at the time of training or at the time of making the comparison. As noted above in the discussion of young athletes, the literature is based almost entirely on the growth of generally small samples of youngsters participating in sport activities. Comparisons of larger samples of youth, including both athletes and non-athletes, grouped by degree of physical activity give similar results.

Although the preceding indicates that regular training does not stimulate growth in stature, it is likewise apparent that the experience of training and competition in sports does not have a negative effect on statural growth. This is relevant to the frequently misquoted early study of Rowe (1933), who compared the growth in stature and weight of male athletes and non-athletes, 13.7 to 15.7 years, over a two year period. Rowe noted that the athletes were taller, but grew at a slower rate over the two year period. This observation is occasionally taken at face value without heeding Rowe's (p. 115) qualifying comment that the observed differences could reflect differential timing of the adolescent spurt: ". . . since the athletic group is composed of boys who have matured earlier, age considered, than the group of non-athletic boys, the athletic boy is not going to grow as much as the non-athletic boys, over the period studied."

Body Weight and Composition. Regular physical activity is an important factor in the regulation and maintenance of body weight. Body weight is a heterogeneous mass, quite often partitioned into lean body mass and fat. Regular training generally results in an increase in lean body mass and a corresponding decrease in body fat in children and youth. Training produces similar effects in adults, quite often without any appreciable change in body weight. Results, however, are not consistent across studies. The magnitude of change in body composition with regular activity varies with the intensity and duration of the program, and the changes are dependent on continued activty.

Body composition changes considerably during normal growth and maturation so that it is difficult to separate effects of training from those associated with normal growth. Further, the continuity of fatness levels from childhood through adolescence is rather weak, which emphasizes the variation in fatness associated with growth and maturation.

In one of the more comprehensive studies of training and body composition, Pařizkova (1977) followed boys engaged in different levels of sports participation and training over a seven year period from 11 to 18 years. Three levels of training were compared: regularly trained (intensive, 6 hr/week); trained but not on a regular basis (in sport schools, about 4 hr/week), and untrained (about 2.5 hr/week, including school physical education). Sample sizes for the three groups at the conclusion of the study, however, were small: 8, 18 and 13 respectively. The groups did not differ in anthropometric characteristics at the beginning of the study nor in body composition. During the course of the study and at its end, the most active boys had significantly more lean body mass and less fat than the least and moderately active boys, who differed between themselves only slightly.

In a similar study, V. Dobëln and Eriksson (1972) reported significant body composition changes in nine boys (11-13 years) after an endurance training program. Using potassium measurements, they observed average gains of 0.5 kg in weight and 12 grams in potassium at the end of the training program. A 12 gram increase in potassium corresponds to a gain of about 4 kg of muscle mass, which would indicate that the 0.5 kg gain in body weight was accompanied by a loss of about 3 kg of fat during the training program. Relative to statural growth, the increase in potassium was about six percent greater than expected, while the gain in body weight was about five percent less than expected. These changes are perhaps the result of training and growth. The boys gained, on the average, 3.5 cm in stature over the 16 week program, which may indicate that the adolescent spurt occurred during the progam. And, male adolescence is accompanied by a significant increase in muscle mass.

The results of these two studies summarize quite well the information on training and body composition. Children regularly engaged in physical activity programs, be they formal training for sport or recreational activities, are generally leaner (have more lean body mass and less fat) than those who are not regularly active. Two questions, however, remain. First, are the changes in body composition associated with regular activity greater than those associated with normal growth and maturation? And second, how persistent are the training-associated changes? The increase in lean body mass observed in youth regularly trained over a several year period would seem to suggest an increase greater than expected with normal growth. It should be noted, however, that muscle mass and thus lean body mass continues to increase into the mid-twenties. On the other hand, most of the variation in body composition with activity or inactivity is associated with fatness, which fluctuates inversely with the training stimulus. Changes in response to short-term training programs are most likely related to fluctuating levels of fatness, with only minimal changes in lean body mass.

Physique. In an analysis of the stability of anthropometric estimates of somatotypes in a sample of 39 boys engaged in different levels of regular physical activity from 11 to 18 years of age, Pařizkova and Carter (1976) did not observe any changes in the distribution of somatotypes in the three activity groups. This would suggest no effect of the training programs on somatotype. Individual boys changed considerably in somatotype over the seven year period. The changes occurred in a random manner and were not attributable to physcial activty. All boys changed in somatotype ratings at least once, and 67% changed in component dominance. Thus, individual variation in somatotype stability during adolescence confounds the evaluation of possible training-related changes. In a follow-up of a subsample (n = 14) of the original series at 24 years of age, mesomorphy increased from 18 to 24 years of age, even though the boys had ceased regular training (Carter and Pařizkova, 1978).

Several studies of teenagers indicate beneficial effects of short-term training on muscular development, especially in those body parts specifically trained, for example, thoracic and arm measurements of gymnasts, muscular development in the shoulder region of swimmers, muscular development in response to weight training, and so on.

Specific Tissues. There is a reasonably extensive literature in the exercise and sport sciences that considers the effects of activity programs on specific tissues and functions. Many of these efforts are approaching the level at which growth processes occur, and may thus contribute to our understanding of regular activity on the processes of growth. The subsequent discussion considers some of the available informaton dealing with the effects of regular training on bone, muscle and fat tissues, as these three tissues account for a significant degree of variation in body composition.

Experimental studies of developing animals indicate greater skeletal mineralization and density, and wider, more robust bones with prolonged physical training. Observations on adult humans engaged in prolonged unilateral activity, as in tennis or baseball pitching, indicate similar results: wider, more robust bones, and increased bone mineral in the preferred arm compared to the non-preferred arm. Since the majority of adults began formal training during childhood, the evidence would suggest a training-mediated response. Activity-related bone mineralization data for children are limited. In a study of bone mineralization of the dominant and non-dominant arms of amateur baseball players 8 to 19 years of age, Watson (1973) reported significant mineralization and width differences between the dominant and non-dominant humeri, but not for the radii and ulnae. The differences in mineral content between the dominant and non-dominant humeri increased with age, which would suggest a training effect, assuming that the older boys participated in the specialized throwing activity longer than the younger boys in the sample. It should be noted that these studies of unilateral activities indicate rather localized increases in bone mineralization.

Experimental literature on training and specific bone lengths indicates reduced bone lengths in rats and mice exposed to voluntary or forced swimming, and moderate or intensive running. Corresponding data for humans are not available. The observations of Kato and Ishiko (1966) suggest that excessive compressive forces on the epiphyses of the knee may obstruct growth and thus reduce stature. The sample upon which this suggestion is based, however, came from an economically poor and nutritionally substandard background. The experimental and clinical data of Viteri and Torun (1981), on the other hand, suggest that regular activity during rehabilitation from protein-energy malnutrition facilitates recovery, including linear growth. Buskirk et al. (1956) reported longer bones of the dominant compared to the non-dominant arm of elite tennis players, and suggested that the difference is attributable to the effects of vigorous activity on bone growth during the adolescent years.

Given the evidence on activity and growth of a bone in length, it seems that the conclusion of Steinhaus (1933) presented over 50 years ago may still be plausible: the pressure effects of physical activity may stimulate epiphyseal growth to an optimal length, but excessive pressure can retard linear growth. There is an obvious need to evaluate the effects of activity on the epiphyseal growth plate. When dealing with children, it is difficult, of course, to define excessive pressure. As noted earlier, elite young athletes grow as well in stature as non-athletes even after controlling for maturity differences and recognizing the possible role of selection for body size in some sports.

Growth of muscle tissue postnatally is characterized by constancy in number of muscle fibers, an increase in fiber size, and a considerable increase in number of muscle nuclei which are apparently derived from satellite cells. Regular physical training commonly results in hypertrophy of skeletal muscle. The degree of hypertrophy varies with the intensity of the training stimulus. Hypertrophy is accompanied by an increase in contractile substances, myofibrils, enzyme activity, and strength. The concept of the specificity of training must be emphasized. Muscular hypertrophy is associated primarily with high-resistance training activities such as weight training, and may not occur with endurance training. Hypertrophy occurs in the existing muscle fibers and not as a result of an increase in fibers. However, experimental evidence with adult animals indicates that muscle fibers will divide by longitudinal fission (fiber splitting) under the stress of excessive, prolonged training.

Data on muscle tissue responses to training in developing organisms are not as extensive as that for adults. Nevertheless, results of several studies indicate similar findings as those for adults. There is a need to more carefully consider the effects of different kinds of training on muscle tissue in developing organisms so that training-associated changes can perhaps be partitioned from those which accompany normal growth.

Studies of high-resistance weight training in children and youth indicate muscular hypertrophy of the exercised muscle groups. Persistence of the changes with the cessation of training is not ordinarily considered. Studies of DNA content and thus number of muscle nuclei in growing animals undergoing regular training indicate a significant rise in DNA above that expected from normal growth. The normal pattern of change in DNA content of skeletal muscle tissue with growth is one of steady increase until puberty with a rather constant level thereafter. The increased DNA in trained animals would seem to suggest that training is a significant factor influencing nuclear number during growth.

Among five boys, 11 years of age, who were endurance trained for six weeks, Eriksson (1972) observed no change in the muscle fiber population of the muscle tissue sampled, but did note a marked increase in the oxidative potential of both slow- and fast-twitch fibers. Succinate dehydrogenase (SDH) activity increased by 30%, while phosphofructokinase (PFK) increased by 83%, a marked increase with the short term training program. It should be noted that PFK activity in the boys was low compared to adult values, which would suggest differences in magnitude of response between children and adults. More recently, Fournier et al. (1982) compared the responses of 12 adolescent boys, 16-17 years of age, to three months of sprint and endurance training and six months of detraining. There were no changes in fiber distribution in both groups, but the endurance trained group showed an increase in the surface area. The endurance trained group showed a 42% increase in SDH activity and no change in PFK activity. In contrast, the sprint trained group showed a 21% increase in PFK activity and no change in SDH activity. After six months of detraining, SDH activity in the endurance trained group and PFK activity in the sprint trained group fell to lower values than at the start of training; however, the mean values did not differ significantly. The results of both studies thus illustrate the specificity of training in youth and demonstrate responses which are similar in direction to those observed in adults. The magnitude of the responses, however, differs.

Given the current interest in adipose tissue cellularity during growth and the generally favorable influence of training on body fatness, one can inquire into the possible effects of regular training during growth on adipose tissue cellularity. Björntorp et al. (1972) reported a training-associated reduction in fat cell size in young adult soccer athletes and middle-aged endurance athletes. Krotkiewski et al. (1979), on the other hand, observed a reduction in subcutaneous fat thickness with strength training in adult women, but no significant changes in estimated fat cell size. Rather, the evidence suggested that the decreased thickness of subcutaneous tissue was a function of altered muscle thickness, meaning that the same amount of fat surrounded an increased muscle volume.

Some experimental evidence suggests that training initiated early in the life of rats (at preweaning ages) effectively reduced the rate of fat cell accumulation and thus resulted in a significant reduction in the number of fat cells and body fatness later in life. On the other hand, endurance running began after 7 weeks of age in rats did not affect adipose cell number, but significantly reduced adipose cell size. These results thus indicate an important role for regular activity in regulating fat cell size; however, for training to influence fat cell number, the program must be initiated very early in life of rats. By about 7 weeks of age in rats, the pattern of fat cell proliferation is apparently established so that adipose cells continue to increase in number even though a training stimulus may be present.

It is difficult to apply the preceding experimental observations to developing children. If so, it may require that training programs be initiated early in life, perhaps in early childhood, to have an influence on adipose tissue cellularity. However, the present information on developmental age trends and sex differences is variable across studies. Further, methodological limitations and regional variability in estimated adipose cell number and size render the currently available information difficult to interpret (see Kirtland and Gurr, 1979; Roche, 1981).

Effects of Activity on Maturation

Skeletal maturation. Although regular activity functions to enhance skeletal mineralization and density, it does not accelerate or delay skeletal maturity as assessed in growth studies, that is, initial ossification, shape changes in epiphyseal centers and eventual union of epiphyses and diaphyses in the hand-wrist. Three studies from Czechoslovakia provide data which address this issue. Černy (1969) monitored the skeletal maturity of the boys engaged in the training project of Pařizkova (1977) discussed earlier. There were no significant skeletal maturity differences among the three groups at the start, during and at the completion of the study. Rather, variation in skeletal maturity within the different activty groups was greater than between. Novotny (1981) compared the progress of skeletal maturation in elite young female athletes in several sports over periods of three to four years between 12 and 17 years of age. Athletes were grouped as having accelerated, average or delayed skeletal ages at the start and at the end of the study. There was little variation in category changes among sports after the period of regular training. Only 19 (21%) of the 89 girls changed categories, while 70 (90%) remained in the same skeletal maturity category. And, given the error in assessing skeletal age and normal variation in the timing of the adolescent spurt and sexual maturation, the changes are quite small. Of the small number who changed categories, 11 shifted from advanced to normal or from normal to delayed, while 8 shifted from delayed to normal or from normal to advanced. In addition, at the beginning and end of the study, mean chronological and skeletal ages of the young athletes did not differ significantly. Hence, gains in chronological and skeletal age were also very similar over the period of training and competition. Similar results were reported by Kotulán et al. (1980) on young males training regularly for cycling, rowing and ice hockey from 12 to 15 years of age. Over the three year period, the gains in skeletal maturity varied, on the average, between 2.6 and 3.3 years in the athletes, and did not differ from the control subjects and from youngsters who trained irregularly during the project.

The preceding would suggest, therefore, that the process of skeletal maturation as reflected in the hand and wrist is not affected by regular training for sport in adolescent boys and girls. It may also be inferred from these observations that skeletal maturity is stable over a time; those advanced at one age are most likely advanced at later ages, and vice versa.

Sexual maturation. Much of the discussion on training and sexual maturation focuses on the observation of delayed menarche in athletes (i.e., intensive training is suggested as a factor which may delay menarche). The data dealing with the inferred relationship between training and delayed menarche are, however, associational, generally based on small samples, and limited to observations of post-menarcheal samples. The training load is not ordinarily specified, other factors which are known to influence menarche are not considered, and other maturity indicators receive no mention.

The suggested mechanism for the association between training and delayed menarche in athletes is hormonal. It is suggested that intensive training and perhaps associated energy drain influence circulating levels of gonadotrophic and ovarian hormones, and in turn menarche. And, exercise is a highly effective means of stressing the hypothalamic-pituitary-gonadal axis. Most of the data, however, are derived from studies of post-menarcheal women (both athletes and non-athletes). The evidence indicates short term exercise-related increases in serum levels of almost all gonadotrophic and sex steroid hormones. The many factors, in addition to exercise, capable of influencing hormonal levels must also be considered, for example, diurnal variation, state of feeding or fasting, emotional states, and so on. In addition, virtually all hormones are episodically secreted. Hence, studies of hormonal responses should not be based on single serum samples. They most likely do not reflect the overall pattern. What is needed are studies in which 24-hour levels of hormones are monitored, or in which actual pulses are sampled every 20 mintues or so in response to exercise. Otherwise, the evidence from the available studies on the hormonal response to exercise stress is inconclusive.

Hormonal data for active prepubertal or pubertal youth are limited. Warren (1980) noted extremely low gonadotrophin secretion in association with only "mild" growth stunting in premenarcheal ballet dancers. In 11-year-old prepubertal athletes, Peltenburg et al. (1984) reported lower plasma levels of estrone, testosterone and androstenedione in gymnasts than in swimmers who had been training since 4.8 and 7.2 years respectively, but no differences in gonadotrophins and dehydroepiandrosterone-sulphate. On the other hand, plasma levels of the seven hormones assayed did not differ in early pubertal (stage 2 of breast development) gymnasts and swimmers, who had been training since 5.0 and 8.0 years respectively. The similar levels of dehydroepiandrosterone-sulphate in the prepubertal gymnasts and swimmers suggest a similar stage of adrenarche, although the gymnasts have been training for a significantly longer period. This observation thus does not support the suggestion of Brisson et al. (1982) that training delays adrenarche and prolongs the prepubertal state. Moreover, recent evidence does not support the view that secretion of adrenal androgens triggers sexual maturation (Wieman and Crowley, 1986).

The acute hormonal responses to exercise are apparently essential to meet the stress which intense exercise imposes upon the organism. More information is needed on changes, if any, in basal levels of hormones with training in young athletes. In small samples of pre- and post-menarcheal competitive female swimmers 13 to 18 years of age, Carli et al. (1983a) noted similar basal levels of ACTH, cortisol, prolactin and testosterone during a 24-week training season. In the combined sample, ACTH levels gradually increased, prolactin levels tended to increase, testosterone levels decreased, while cortisol levels showed a variable pattern during the season. As expected, basal estradiol levels differed between the pre- and post-menarcheal swimmers, and both groups experienced a decrease in basal levels during the first 12 weeks of training, which was followed by a rise at 24 weeks. In the pre-menarcheal swimmers, the basal level at 24 weeks was lower than that at the start of training. Thus, levels of all hormones studies were influenced by training, and there were similar patterns of response to training in pre- and post-menarcheal girls.

In a subsequent study of competitive male swimmers 12 to 16 years of age (presumably pubertal), Carli et al. (1983b) noted variable results during two competitive seasons. For example, basal plasma levels of ACTH and testosterone were not altered by training during one season, but were significantly altered in the next season. ACTH decreased from 4 to 43 weeks of training after an initial rise during the first four weeks. Testosterone, on the other hand, showed no change after 4 weeks of training, increased significantly to 12 weeks, changed negligibly from 12 to 24 weeks, and then decreased below initial values at the end of the season (43 weeks). In contrast, plasma levels of growth hormone and gonadotrophic hormones were not affected by training. Thus, changes in basal hormonal levels were observed during training in young male swimmers. The changes, however, were variable and within the physiological range.

The results of these studies of young athletes are variable and not conclusive. They are based upon observations of plasma levels. However, the simple presence of a hormone does not necessarily imply that it is physiologically or biochemically active. There also is variation in tissue responsiveness, and in developing children, the tissue probably must be sufficiently mature in order to respond. In other words, for a hormone to have its effect, the tissue, or more specifically the cells, must be capable of responding.

The preceding is largely concerned with female athletes. Training and maturity associations in males, on the other hand, are not considered. It is somewhat puzzling why one would expect training to delay the maturation of girls and not boys, even though the underlying processes are quite similar. Further, there is a reasonable body of literature which suggests that males may be more susceptible to environmental stresses while females are better buffered against environmental stresses (Stinson, 1985).

With the exception of studies of growth hormone responses to exercise, data on other hormonal responses of boys to exercise are generally limited. Variable results in a small sample of young swimmers were mentioned earlier. In a sample of boys who were not athletes, Fahey et al. (1979) did not observe any differences in post-maximal exercise concentrations of serum testosterone and growth hormone among boys grouped into different stages of puberty. This would suggest that a critical pubertal state with enhanced hormonal responsiveness to exercise does not exist.

In summary, menarche is a rather late maturational event, and menstruation cannot occur unless the hypothalamus, anterior pituitary and the ovaries are functioning and the genital ducts are patent. Given the available data on hormonal responses to training in children and youth, it is difficult to implicate regular training as a critical factor. What is specifically relevant for pre-menarcheal girls is the possible cumulative effects of hormonal responses to regular training. Such data are presently lacking.

A corollary of the suggestion that training delays menarche is that the weight or body composition changes associated with training may function to delay menarche, that is, delay maturity of young girls by keeping them lean. This is, in turn, related to the critical weight or fatness hypothesis that a certain level of fatness must be attained for menarche to occur. This hypothesis has been discussed at length by many, with the conclusion that the data do not support the specificity of weight or fatness as the critical variable for menarche.

In contrast, there appears to be little concern for the effects of regular training on the sexual maturation of boys. The data for both sexes are derived largely from young athletes, who as indicated earlier, are a select group and most likely are not representative of the general population of youth. Nevertheless, the available evidence, with its limitations, suggests that regular training has no apparent effect on biological maturation as commonly assessed in growth studies.

Principles

1. Sex differences in body size and most anthropometric indicators of physique and body composition are, on the average, minor prior to the adolescent growth spurt. Boys, on the average, tend to be larger in most dimensions, more mesomorphic and larger in muscle and lean body mass. Girls, on the average, tend to be more endomorphic and to have greater amounts of subcutaneous fat. Note, however, that there is considerable overlap in the distributions of most measurements during childhood.

2. Sex differences apparent in childhood become magnified during the adolescent growth spurt. Males become, on the average, especially leaner and more muscular.

3. Females, on the average, mature in advance of males at all ages, and the sex difference reaches its maximum during adolescence when girls are almost two years in advance of boys in the timing of primary adolescent events.

4. Given the nature of the data and study designs, the following generalizations on physical activity and growth seem warranted:
   a) Physical activity has no apparent effect on stature in growing individuals and on maturation as commonly assessed by skeletal and sexual maturation.
   b) Physical activity is an important factor in the regulation and maintenance of body weight. Regular activity generally results in an increase in lean tissue and a corresponding decrease in body fat, quite frequently without any appreciable change in body weight. Most of the changes with training are, however, associated with fat tissue.
   c) Regular physical activity is a significant factor influencing the growth and integrity of bone and muscle tissue. Activity functions to enhance skeletal mineralization and density, and to stimulate bone growth in width. Activity

can result in muscular hypertrophy, an increase in contractile proteins and enhanced oxidative enzyme activity in muscle tissue. However, such changes are specific to the type of training program, for example, endurance versus strength training.

d) The preceding generalizations on changes in body composition and specific tissues in association with regular physical activity are a function of the intensity and duration of training and of continued activity. More active individuals generally show greater changes in association with training programs than less active individuals. Nevertheless, responses to regular activity tend to be highly individualized.

e) In growing individuals, it is essential to partition out the effects of maturity-associated variation from those attributed to an activity program, especially during adolescence.

f) Changes in response to short term training programs are generally not permanent, and vary with the quantity and type of training. This is especially clear in fluctuating levels of fatness commonly observed with regular activity. During the active training period, fat levels generally decrease; however activity levels begin to decline, fat levels may slowly increase.

g) The effects of regular activity on biological maturation are less well known, but limited evidence suggests little if any effect.

5. Since studies of young athletes are often considered in the context of the effects of activity on growth and maturation, the available data indicate that young athletes of both sexes grow as well as non-athletes. The experience of athletic training and competition does not apparently harm the physical growth and maturation of the youngster.

Author's Note

The materials presented in this chapter are derived from a number of reviews the author has prepared over the past few years. Hence, the chapter is not heavily documented. The primary references upon which the report is based can be found in the following reviews by the author:

Malina, R.M. (1969). The quantification of fat, muscle and bone in man. *Clinical Orthopaedics, 65*, 9-38.

Malina, R.M. (1978). Adolescent growth and maturation: Selected aspects of current research. *Yearbook of Physical Anthropology, 21*, 63-94.

Malina, R.M. (1979). The effects of exercise on specific tissues, dimensions and functions during growth. *Studies in Physical Anthropology, 5*, 21-52.

Malina, R.M. (1980). The measurement of body composition. In F.E. Johnston, A.F. Roche & C. Susanne (Eds.), *Human Physical Growth and Maturation: Methodologies and Factors* (pp. 35-59). New York: Plenum.

Malina, R.M. (1980). Physical activity, growth and functional capacity. In F.E. Johnston, A.F. Roche & C. Susanne (Eds.), *Human Physical Growth and Maturation: Methodologies and Factors* (pp. 303-327). New York: Plenum.

Malina, R.M. (1982). Physical growth and maturity characteristics of young athletes. In R.A. Magill, M.A. Ash & F.L. Smoll (Eds.), *Children and Sport*, 2nd edition (pp. 73-96). Champaign, IL: Human Kinetics.

Malina, R.M. (1983) Menarche in athletes: A synthesis and hypothesis. *Annals of Human Biology, 10*, 1-24.

Malina, R.M. (1983). Human growth, maturation and regular physical activity. *Acta Medica Auxologica, 15*, 5-23.

Malina, R.M. (1984). Physical growth and maturation. In J.R. Thomas (Ed.), *Motor Development during Childhood and Adolescence* (pp. 2-26). Minneapolis: Burgess.

Malina, R.M. (1985). Growth of muscle tissue and muscle mass. In F. Falkner & J.M. Tanner (Eds), *Human Growth. Volume 2. Postnatal Growth,* revised edition (pp. 77-99). New York: Plenum.

Malina, R.M. Meleski, B.W., & Shoup, R.F. (1982). Anthropometric, body composition, and maturity characteristics of selected school-age athletes. *Pediatric Clinics of North America, 29*, 1305-1323.

References

Åstrand, P.O., Engstrom, L., Eriksson, B.O., Karlberg, P., Nylander, I., Saltin, B., & Thoren, C. (1963). Girl swimmers. *Acta Paediatrica,* Supplement 147.

Bielicki, T. (1975). Interrelationships between various measures of maturation rate in girls during adolescence. *Studies in Physical Anthropology, 1*, 51-64.

Bielicki, T., Koniarek, J., & Malina, R.M. (1984). Interrelationships among certain measures of growth and maturation rate in boys during adolescence. *Annals of Human Biology, 11*, 201-210.

Björntorp P., Grimby G., Sanne H., Sjöström L., Tibblin G., & Wilhelmsen L., (1972). Adipose tissue fat cell size in relation to metabolism in weight-stable, physically active men. *Hormone and Metabolic Research, 4*, 178-182.

Boileau, R.A., Lohman, T.G., Slaughter, M.H., Ball, T.E., Going, S.B., & Hendrix, M.K. (1984). Hydration of the fat-free body in children during maturation. *Human Biology, 56*, 651-666.

Bouchard, C., & Malina, R.M. (1983). Genetics for the sport scientist: Selected methodological considerations. *Exercise and Sport Sciences Reviews, 11*, 275-305.

Brisson, G.R., Dulac, S., Perronet, F., & Ledoux, M. (1982). The onset of menarche: A late event in pubertal progression to be affected by physical training. *Canadian Journal of Applied Sport Sciences, 7*, 61-67.

Burmeister, W. (1966). Body cell mass as the basis of allometric growth function. *Annales Paediatrici, 204*, 65-72.

Buskirk, E.R., Andersen, K.L., & Brožek, J., (1956). Unilateral activity and bone and muscle development in the forearm. *Research Quarterly, 27*, 127-131.

Carli, G., Martelli, G., Viti, A., Baldi, L., Bonifazi, M., & Lupo di Prisco, C. (1983a). The effect of swimming training on hormon levels in girls. *Journal of Sports Medicine and Physical Fitness. 23*, 45-51.

Carli, G., Martelli, G., Viti, A., Baldi, L., Bonifazi, M., & Lupo di Prisco, C. (1983b). Modulation of hormone levels in male swimmers during training. In A.P. Hollander, P.A. Huijing & G. de Groot (Eds.), *Biomechanics and Medicine in Swimming* (pp. 33-40). Champaign, IL: Human Kinetics Publishers.

Carter, J.E.L. (1980). *The Heath-Carter Somatotype Method* (revised edition). San Diego: San Diego State University.

Carter, J.E.L., & Pařizkova, J. (1978). Changes in somatotypes of European males between 17 and 24 years. *American Journal of Physical Anthropology, 48*, 251-254.

Černy, L. (1969). The results of an evaluation of skeletal age of boys 11-15 years old with different regimes of physical activity. In *Physical Fitness Assessment* (pp. 56-59). Prague: Charles University Press.

Eriksson, B.O. (1972). Physical training, oxygen supply and muscle metabolism in 11-13 year old boys. *Acta Physiologica Scandinavica,* Supplement 384.

Fahey, T.D., del Valle-Zuris, A., Oehlsen, G., Trieb, M., & Seymour, J. (1979). Pubertal stage differences in hormonal and hematological responses to maximal exercise in males. *Journal of Applied Physiology, 46*, 823-827.

Fournier, M., Ricci, J., Taylor, A.W., Ferguson, R.J., Montpetit, R.R., & Chairman, B.R. (1982). Skeletal muscle adaptation in adolescent boys: Sprint and endurance training and detraining. *Medicine and Science in Sports and Exercise, 14*, 453-456.

Frisch, R.E., Gotz-Welbergen, A.V., McArthur, J.W., Albright, T., Witschi, J., Bullen, B., Birnholz, J., Reed, R.B., & Hermann, H. (1981). Delayed menarche and amenorrhea of college athletes in relation to age of onset of training. *Journal of the American Medical Association, 246*, 1559-1563.

Gruelich, W.W., & Pyle, S.I. (1959). *Radiographic Atlas of Skeletal Development of the Hand and Wrist* (2nd edition). Stanford: Stanford University Press.

Grumbach, M.M. (1980). The neuroendocrinology of puberty. In D.T. Krieger & J.C. Hughes (Eds.), *Neuroendocrinology* (pp. 249-258). Sunderland, MA: Sinauer Associates.

Hansman, C. (1982). Anthropometry and related data. In R.W. McCammon (Ed.), *Human Growth and Development* (pp. 101-154). Springfield, IL: C.C. Thomas.

Kato, S., & Ishiko, T. (1966). Obstructed growth of children's bones due to excessive labor in remote corners. In K. Kato (Ed.), *Proceedings of International Congress of Sport Sciences* (p. 479). Tokyo: Japanese Union of Sports Sciences.

Kirtland, J., & Gurr, M.I., (1979). Adipose tissue cellularity: A review. 2. The relationship between cellulartiy and obesity. *International Journal of Obesity, 3*, 15-55.

Kotulan, J., Řezničkova, M., & Placheta, Z. (1980). Exercise and growth. In Z. Placheta (Ed.), *Youth and Physical Activity* (pp. 61-117). Brno: J.E. Purkyne University Medical Faculty.

Krotkiewski, M., Aniansson, A., Grimby, G., Björntorp, P., & Sjöström, L. (1979). The effect of unilateral isokinetic strength training on local adipose and muscle tissue morphology thickness and enzymes. *European Journal of Applied Physiology, 42*, 271-281.

Malina, R. M. (in press). Competitive youth sports and biological maturation. In V. Seefeldt (Ed.), *CIC Symposium on the Effects of Competitive Sports on Children and Youth*. Champaign, IL: Human Kinetics Publishers.

Marshall, W.A. (1978). Puberty. In F. Falkner & J.M. Tanner (Eds), *Human Growth. Volume 2. Postnatal Growth* (pp. 141-181). New York: Plenum.

Marshall, W.A., & Tanner, J.M. (1969). Variations in pattern of pubertal changes in girls. *Archives of Disease in Childhood, 44*, 291-303.

Marshall, W.A., & Tanner, J.M. (1970). Variations in the pattern of pubertal changes in boys. *Archives of Disease in Childhood, 45*, 13-23.

Milicer, H., & Denisiuk, L. (1964). The physical development of youth. In E. Jokl & E. Simon (Eds.), *International Research in Sport and Physical Education* (pp. 262-285). Springfield, IL: C.C. Thomas.

National Center for Health Statistics (1973). Age at menarche, United States. *Vital and Health Statistics,* Series 11, No. 133.

National Center for Health Statistics (1977). NCHS growth curves for children birth - 18 years, United States. *Vital and Health Statistics,* Series 11, No. 165.

National Center for Health Statistics (1981). Basic data on anthropometric measurements and angular measurements of the hip and knee joints for selected age groups, 1-74 years of age, United States, 1971-1975. *Vital and Health Statistics,* Series 11, No. 219.

Novotny, V. (1981). Veränderungen des Knochenalters im Verlauf einer mehrjahrigen sportlichen Belastung. *Medizin und Sport, 21*, 44-47.

Pařizkova, J. (1977). *Body Fat and Physical Fitness.* The Hague: Martinus Nijhoff.

Pařizkova, J., & Carter J.E.L. (1976). Influence of physical activity on stability of somatotypes in boys. *American Journal of Physical Anthropology, 44*, 327-339.

Peltenburg, A.L., Erich, W.B.M., Thijssen, J.J.H., Veeman, W., Jansen, M., Bernink, M.J.E., Zonderland, M.L., van den Brande, J.L., & Huisveld, I.A., (1984). Sex hormone profiles of premenarcheal athletes. *European Journal of Applied Physiology,* 52, 385-392.

Roche, A.F. (1981). The adipocyte-number hypothesis. *Child Development, 52*, 31-43.

Roche, A.F., & Malina, R.M. (1983). *Manual of Physical Status and Performance in Childhood. Volume 1*. New York:Plenum.

Ross, J.G., & Gilbert, G.G. (1985). The National Children and Youth Fitness Study: A summary of findings. *Journal of Physical Education, Recreation, and Dance, 56*(1), 45-50.

Rowe, F.A. (1933). Growth comparisons of athletes and non-athletes. *Research Quarterly, 4*, 108-116.

Scammon, R.E. (1930). The measurement of the body in childhood. In J.A. Harris, C.M. Jackson, D.G. Paterson & R.E. Scammon (Eds.), *The Measurement of Man* (pp. 173-215). Minneapolis: University of Minnesota Press.

Sheldon, W.H., Dupertuis, C.W., & McDermott, E. (1954). *Atlas of Men: A Guide for Somatotyping the Adult Male of All Ages*. New York: Harper.

Shuttleworth, F.K. (1939). The physical and mental growth of girls and boys age six to nineteen in relation to age at maximum growth. *Monographs of the Society for Research in Child Development*, Serial No. 22.

Steinhaus, A.H. (1933). Chronic effects of exercise. *Physiological Reviews, 13*, 103-147.

Stinson, S. (1985). Sex differences in environmental sensitivity during growth and development. *Yearbook of Physical Anthropology, 28*, (in press).

Tanner, J.M. (1962). *Growth at Adolescence* (2nd edition). Oxford: Blackwell Scientific Publications.

Tanner, J.M. (1978). *Fetus into Man. Physical Growth from Conception to Maturity*. Cambridge, Massachusetss: Harvard University Press.

Tanner, J.M., Hughes, P.C.R., & Whitehouse, R.H. (1981). Radiographically determined widths of bone, muscle and fat in the upper arm and calf from age 3-18 years. *Annals of Human Biology, 8*, 495-517.

Tanner, J.M., Whitehouse, R.H., Marshall, W.A., Healy, M.J.R., & Goldstein H. (1975). *Assessment of Skeletal Maturity and Prediction of Adult Height*. New York: Academic Press.

Tanner, J.M., Whitehouse, R.H., Marubini, E., & Resele, L.F. (1976). The adolescent growth spurt of boys and girls of the Harpenden growth study. *Annals of Human Biology, 3*, 109-126.

V. Döbeln W., & Eriksson, B.O. (1972). Physical training, maximal oxygen uptake and dimensions of the oxygen transporting and metabolizing organs in boys 11-13 years of age. *Acta Paediatrica Scandinavica, 61*, 653-660.

Viteri, F.E., & Torun, B. (1981). Nutrition, physical activty, and growth. In M. Ritzen, A. Aperia, K. Hall, A. Larsson, A. Zetterberg, & R. Zetterström (Eds.), *The Biology of Normal Human Growth* (pp. 265-273). New York: Raven Press.

Walker, R.M. (1962). Body build and behavior in young children. I. Body build and nursery school teachers' ratings. *Monographs of the Society for Research in Child Development*, Serial No. 84.

Warren, M.P. (1980). The effects of exercise on pubertal progression and reproductive funtion in girls. *Journal of Clinical Endocrinology and Metabolism, 51*, 1150-1157.

Watson, R.C. (1973). *Bone growth and physical activity in young males*. Unpublished doctoral dissertation, University of Wisconsin, Madison.

Wierman, M.E., & Crowley, W.F. Jr. (1986). Neuroendocrine control of the onset of puberty. In F. Falkner & J.M. Tanner (Eds.), *Human Growth, Volume 2: Postnatal Growth,* revised edition, (pp. 225-241). New York: Plenum.

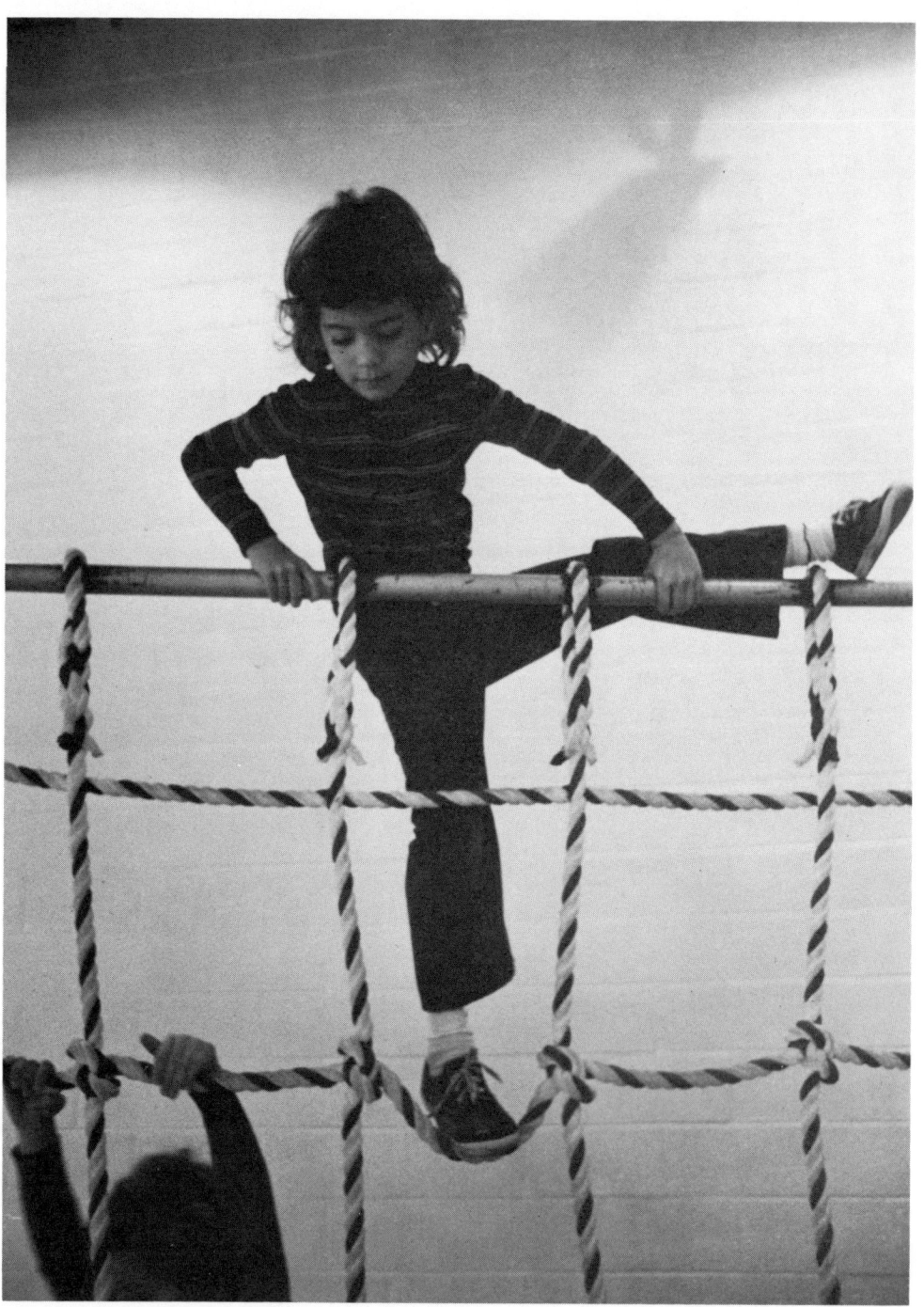

CHAPTER TWO

Acquisition of Motor Skills During Childhood

John Haubenstricker and Vern Seefeldt
School of Health Education, Counseling
Psychology and Human Performance
Michigan State University
East Lansing, Michigan

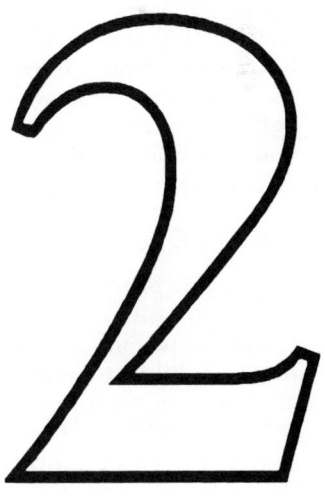

Although considerable progress has been made in describing the motor behavior of children and youth, little is understood about the mechanisms that bring about skill acquisition. The development of motor behavior in the human being begins within a few months after conception. It changes radically over time, yet follows predictable patterns in stable environments. The extent to which the development of these inherent patterns can be enhanced or modified through education or training during the early years of life has received extensive study in the past two decades. Available evidence suggests that the quality of motor development in early life may have a significant impact on the quality of life experienced in later years.

The purpose of this chapter is to summarize what is known about the development of motor skills and their relationship to the total welfare of the growing child. The first section will provide an overview of motor development. The next section will focus on the development of motor behavior from the early moments of life through the late childhood years. In subsequent sections, the influence of biological age, and the variability and stability of motor behavior will be examined. The chapter will conclude with a series of summary statements.

Overview of Motor Skills Development

The systematic study of motor behavior in infants and children began in the 1920s and intensified in the 1930s. Most of these early investigations were conducted by physicians and specialists in child development such as Cunningham (1927), Gesell (1928), Shirley (1931), Bayley (1935) and McGraw (1940). Concurrently, the motor achievements of older children were being examined by physical education specialists, including Atkinson (1924, 1925) and Bliss (1927). Although the study of motor skill acquisition in children continued to receive some attention during the 1940s and 1950s, it was not until the late 1960s that a resurgence of interest in motor development, particularly its qualitative aspects, took place.

Today, a number of textbooks dealing with the motor development of children and youth are available. They include the work of Espenschade and Eckert (1967, 1980), Wickstrom (1970, 1977, 1983), Ridenour (1978), Corbin (1980), Gallahue (1982), Williams (1983), Roberton and Halverson (1984), Thomas (1984), and Keogh and Sugden (1985). In addition, the first volume of current research in motor development was recently published (Clark and Humphrey, 1985). Space in this chapter permits only a limited overview of motor behavior during infancy and childhood. The reader is referred to the above publications for more detailed information.

The Study of Motor Development

Several approaches have been used to document the course of motor development in infants and children. Among the earliest of these was the establishment of chronological milestones which focused on the systematic observation and assessment of children's motor achievements, placed in the order of their appearance, along an age continuum. The identification of chronological milestones yielded several significant contributions to our knowledge about motor development: (a) significant motor behaviors common to all normal individuals were identified; (b) the orderliness of motor development during the early years of life was determined; (c) numerous interskill or intertask sequences were developed; and (d) a basis for comparing the rate at which individual children achieved significant motor behaviors was established. Research using this approach resulted in the publication of developmental scales, which were subsequently used to assess motor progress during the first two to three years after birth (Bayley, 1936; Gesell and Armatruda, 1941).

The approach of equating behavior with chronological milestones was limited by the focus of investigators on the presence or absence of particular behaviors and not on the age range across which they emerged. Furthermore, little attention was given to the quality of a skill exhibited by a child. Improvement generally was noted quantitatively in terms of frequency, distance, accuracy or time. Motor scales based on chronological milestones are still in common use, but they are supplemented by various criterion-referenced scales which emphasize current progress in relation to previous achievements, in lieu of comparing current status with established norms. An improvement in the current norm-referenced instruments is the inclusion of age ranges within which the specific motor behaviors occur.

A second approach focused on the qualitative changes that took place as a specific skill developed. Changes in body configurations and/or the movement patterns of body parts, or the timing of those movements, were observed as children progressed from rudimentary performance to efficient, mature execution of a skill. Developmental levels or stages were identified within the skill. These were either movement patterns of the whole body or components of the body that could be readily identified by a trained observer. Each stage in this process represents progress along a continuum toward mature performance. A series of stages within a skill is called an intraskill or intratask sequence. Reserach using this approach is best exemplified by the work of Halverson (1931), Wild (1938), Seefeldt, Reuschlein and Vogel (1972), Roberton (1977), and McClegnaghan and Gallahue (1978).

Advantages of the intratask sequence approach are that it: (a) permits the assessment of progress toward mature form of a skill; (b) provides clues for instructors concerning changes in form that must be made before individuals can progress to the next level; and (c) allows the comparison of individual progress with that of peers through the use of age-stage norms. Current disadvantages include: (a) a lack of agreement regarding the nature and number of developmental levels in specific skills; (b) the issue of whether to use the whole body or body components to identify levels of development; (c) the lack of identified sequences for many basic motor skills; and (d) the lack of competence by teachers and parents in the skills of observation and task analysis in order to accurately assess the quality of performance.

A third approach to the study of motor behavior in children is to examine the impact of environmental variables and/or instruction on the acquisition of skills. Early investigators examined the effects of restricted activity on infants (Dennis, 1935, 1938, 1940) or the effects of additional practice (Gesell & Thompson, 1929; Hilgard, 1932; Mirenva, 1935; McGraw, 1935) on skill acquisition. More recent studies have focused on the effects of systematic training programs and the manipulation of environmental variables on skill learning (Dusenberry, 1952; Halverson, Roberton, Safrit & Roberts, 1977; Werner, 1974; Miller, 1978; DuRandt, 1985). Major benefits of this approach are (a) the ability to determine to what extent specific skills can be modified; and (b) at what age and under what conditions intervention is most effective. Obvious disadvantages include the difficulty of controlling the numerous variables that could influence skill acquisition, the number of skills to be studied and the myriad of intervention strategies that could be introduced.

Models of Motor Development

At present, there is no commonly accepted, comprehensive theory of motor development, influenced by the fact that most of the research has been largely descriptive in nature. Description has led to an accumulation of facts and the generation of principles, but has not stimulated a formulation of theories that explain the behavior observed. However, several models have been proposed which attempt to provide some organization and direction to what is currently known about the course of motor development in children and youth.

A model proposed by Seefeldt (1979) contains four levels in a progression for achieving motor efficiency (see Fig. 1). The first level represents the reflexes and reactions with which an individual is endowed at birth. Many of these reflexes and reactions must be inhibited, replaced or integrated into higher levels of motor functioning, while others must emerge during infancy, if progress toward motor proficiency is to be made. The second level contains the fundamental movements and skills associated with locomotion, object manipulation and postural control. Mastery of these skills by infants and children is necessary if optimum development of higher level skills is to occur. A proficiency barrier is placed between the

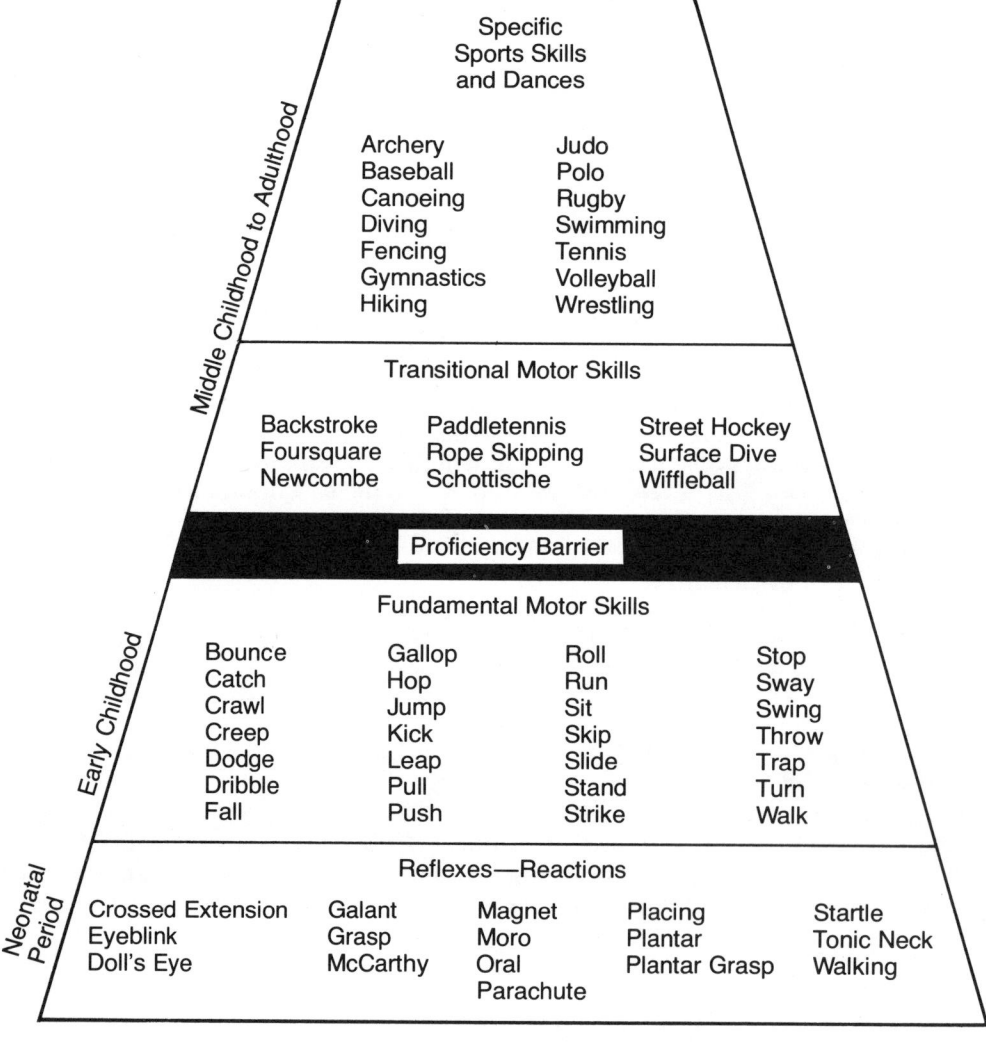

Fig. 1. Sequential progression of skill levels in the achievement of motor proficiency. (Adapted from "Developmental motor patterns: Implications for elementary school physical education" by Vern Seefeldt. In C. Nadeau. W. Holliwell, K. Newell & G. Roberts (Eds.), *Psychology of motor behavior and sport* (p. 317), 1979, Champaign, IL: Human Kinetics Publishers. Adapted by permission.)

second and third levels to indicate the importance of these skills to later skill development. The third level contains transitional skills and activities which may be ends in themselves or which may lead to activities at the fourth level. The skills at level two may be combined or modified in various ways, with or without the use of equipment, to generate specific sport or dance skills that can be practiced alone or incorporated into simplified activities at the third level. The fourth level includes the more complex sports and dance skills and their application in highly organized games, contests and activities. According to this model, the success achieved at any level (except the first) is dependent, at least in part, on the degree of proficiency attained at each of the levels beneath it.

A similar, but slightly more comprehensive model has been proposed by Gallahue (1982). This model also contains four levels called phases of motor development, each containing two or three stages (see Fig. 2). The reflexive movement phase contains an information gathering stage and an information

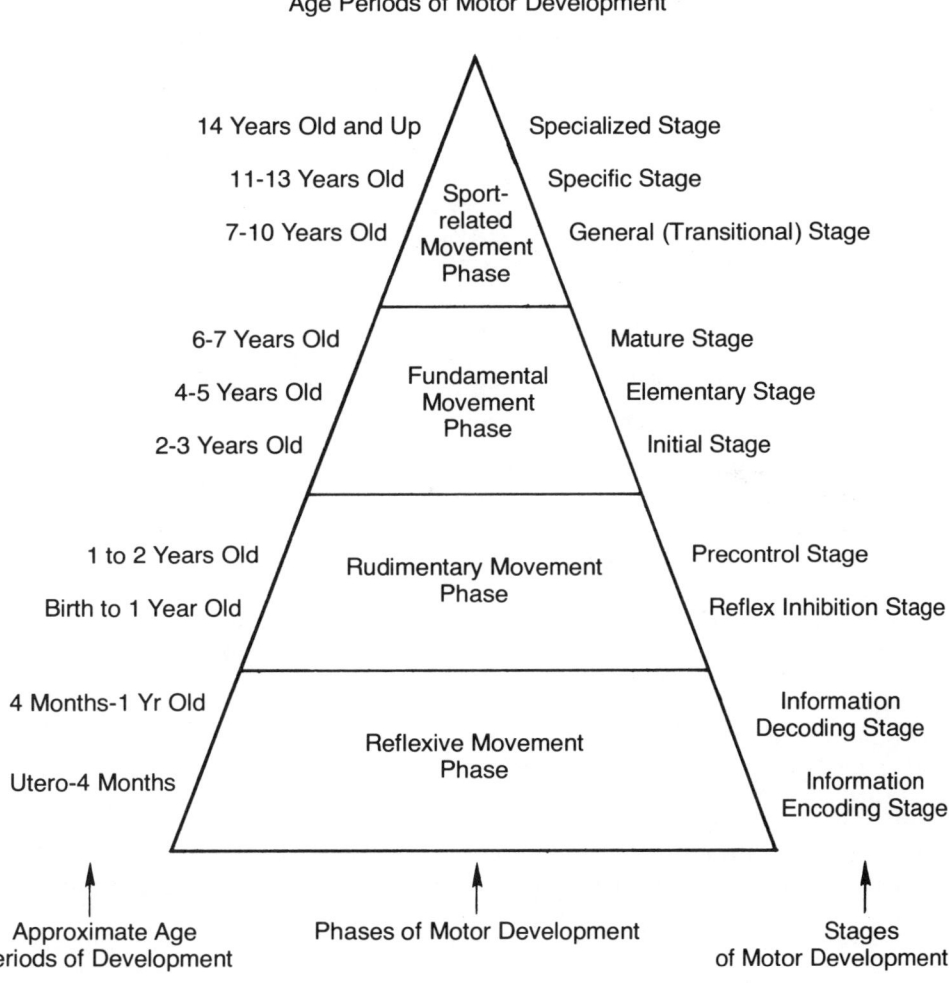

Fig. 2. The phases of motor development. (Reprinted with permission of Macmillan Publishing Company, from *Understanding Motor Development in Children* by David L. Gallahue, originally published by John Wiley & Sons, Inc. New York: Macmillan, 1982.)

processing stage. The next level, the rudimentary movement phase, includes stages of reflex inhibition and precontrol, both of which are largely under the control of maturational processes. The third level, or fundamental movement phase, involves the acquisition of locomotion, stability and manipulation. Each category of skills is divided developmentally into initial, elementary and mature stages. The fourth level is called the sport-related movement phase. This phase contains a transitional stage which involves the conversion or application of fundamental movements to sport-related skills; a specific movement skills stage where individuals select the specific activities in which they wish to become proficient; and, a specialized movement skill stage which represents the final choice of activities that a person intends to pursue into the adult years. General age ranges for each stage within each phase also are provided in the model.

Development of Motor Behavior

Motor Behavior of the Fetus and Neonate

The quality of motor development that occurs in the womb and shortly after birth has both immediate and long range effects on the welfare of the developing human being. The absence of appropriate reflexes and reactions at birth is a sign that the central nervous system (CNS) and/or other systems of the body are inadequately developed. In extreme cases, inappropriate development may place the life of the neonate in immediate jeopardy or may even result in a stillbirth. In other instances, inadequate development of the CNS may result in a variety of handicapping conditions that manifest themselves in the physical, mental, perceptual, sensory and/or psychosocial development of the individual (Fiorentino, 1973).

Most of the severe handicapping conditions (mental and neurological) found in preschool children are attributable to prenatal factors, many of which can be controlled or eliminated through proper prenatal care (Hagberg, 1975). Thus, the quality of life of many young children is dependent, to a large extent, on the nature of the prenatal environment in which their initial development occurs, rather than on genetic factors over which there is no control. Prenatal factors that adversely influence subsequent growth and development must be eliminated if the opportunity for optimum progress is to be assured. (For further information on the effects of various prenatal factors on the development of the fetus, see the reference to Gallahue, 1982).

The structural and functional development of the unborn child has been summarized by Espenschade and Eckert (1980), as presented in Table 1. Reactive behavior involving striated muscle begins at about eight weeks after conception, and spontaneous movements are observed two weeks later. Although these initial movements tend to be somewhat generalized in nature (the response includes body parts other than the specific site stimulated), specific reflex behavior such as the grasp and plantar reflexes have been observed by the eleventh week (Hooker, 1944). The nature of the response, whether generalized or specific, may also be a function of the strength of the stimulus, with a weak stimulus evoking a more specific response than a strong stimulus. As the fetus continues to develop, more complex reflexes and motor patterns emerge, including contralateral reflexes (13 weeks), reciprocal innervation in movements (16 weeks), head turning (22 weeks), tendon reflexes (24 weeks), sucking and sneezing (24 weeks), and synergistic muscle action (28 weeks). By the end of 40 weeks, the normal fetus has acquired a plethora of reflexes and reactions including all the processes required by the new born infant to sustain independent existence (Espendschade & Eckert, 1980).

Assessment of reflexes and reactions in the neonate by pediatricians provides valuable information concerning the integrity and previous development of the

Table 1
Summary of prenatal development

Age in Weeks	Structural Development	Functional Development*
2.5 weeks	Neural groove indicated	
3.5 weeks	Primitive blood vessels and heart; neural crest formed	Heart beat begins
4 weeks	All somites present; limb buds form; neural tube closes; optic cup and lens pit forming	
5 weeks	Premuscle masses in head, trunk, and limbs	
6 weeks	Limbs recognizable; semicircular ducts become outlined	
7 weeks	Muscles differentiate rapidly—assume final shapes and relations; cerebral hemispheres becoming large; eyelids forming	Contralateral neck flexion (7.5)
8 weeks	Digits well formed; first ossification in middle of long bones; cerebral cortex begins to get typical cells; well-represented, definitive muscles in trunk, limbs and head; olfactory nucleus appears	Contralateral neck and trunk flexion (8.5) Spontaneous movement (9.5) Mouth opening (9.5) Stretch reflex (9.5)
10 weeks	Limbs nicely modeled; ossification spreading; spinal cord attains definitive internal structure; eyelids fused	Eyelid squint (10) Ventral head flexion (10) Incomplete finger closure (10.5) Plantar flexion of all toes (11) Ipsilateral head rotation (11)
12 weeks	Sex determined by external inspection; brain attains general structural features; spinal cord shows cervical and lumbar enlargements; internal ear formed; some bones well outlined; taste buds appear	Lip closure and swallowing (12) Dorsiflexion of big toe and toe fanning: Flexion at foot, knee, hip (12) Elevate angle of mouth (13) Complete finger closure (13) Contralateral responses established (13) Vestibular and proprioceptive influence on responses (13)
16 weeks	Face looks "human"; hair on head; most bones distinctly indicated; joint cavities appear; cerebellum assumes some prominence; general sense organs differentiating (cutaneous)	Muscular movements can be detected in utero; reciprocal innervation in movements (16) Diagonal responses (16) "Scowl" combined with head extension (16) Temporary diaphram contraction (17) Effective but weak true grasp (18.5)
20 weeks	Myelination of cord begins; nail plate begins	Side-to-side head turning (22) Weak vocal sounds (22)

*Based mainly on data presented by T. Humphrey. Some correlations between the appearance of human fetal reflexes and the development of the nervous system. In Purpura, D.P. and J.P. Schade (Eds.), *The Growth and Maturation of the Brain.* New York: Elsevier Publishing Co., 1964.

Note: From *Motor Development* (2nd ed.), (pp. 64-65) by A.S. Espenschade and H.M. Eckert (as revised by H.M. Eckert), 1980, Columbus, OH. Charles E. Merrill Books, Inc. Copyright 1980 by Charles E. Merrill Books, Inc. Reprinted by permission.

Table 1 (continued)
Summary of prenatal development

Age in Weeks	Structural Development	Functional Development*
24 weeks	Cerebral cortex layered typically	Sucking (24)
		Sneezing (24)
		Tendon reflexes (24)
		Palpebral reflex (25)
		Permanent respiration if delivered (27)
28 weeks	Cerebral fissures and convolutions appearing rapidly; eyelids reopen	Synergic muscle action (28)
		Corneal reflexes (28)
		Audible sucking (29)
32 weeks		Taste sense present; olfactory present
36 weeks	Most general sense organs completed	
40 weeks	Myelination of brain begins	Iris reflexes

*Based mainly on data presented by T. Humphrey. Some correlations between the appearance of human fetal reflexes and the development of the nervous system. In Purpura, D.P. and J.P. Shade (Eds.), *The Growth and Maturation of the Brain.* New York: Elsevier Publishing Co., 1964.

CNS. Early diagnosis of persistent abnormal reflexes is important in the treatment of infants and children with neurological dysfunction (Bobath, 1980). The persistence of special reflexes and lower brainstem reflexes may interfere with the development of important righting reflexes and equilibrium reactions which are necessary for the development of locomotion (Fiorentino, 1973). Moreover, even children with only mild neurological dysfunction often are delayed in their acquisition of gross motor skills and display a lack of confidence in their ability to acquire motor skills (Haubenstricker & Seefeldt, 1974; Haubenstricker, Seefeldt, Fountain & Sapp, 1981, April).

Reflexes present in the neonate generally are classified as primitive or postural. Primitive reflexes usually are related to infant survival (i.e. protection or nourishment), while postural reflexes are regarded as precursors to the development of subsequent voluntary movements (Gallahue, 1982). Table 2 contains a listing of diagnostic human reflexes and reactions that are present at birth or emerge shortly thereafter. These reflexes are under subcortical control and must disappear, diminish, or be modified in some way in order for higher patterns of behavior to develop (Fiorentino, 1973).

Primitive reflexes. The sucking and the searching or rooting reflexes are necessary for obtaining nourishment. The former can be evoked by the insertion of an object (finger or nipple) in the newborn's mouth; the latter by contacting the cheeks or skin surrounding the lips. The sucking reflex usually disappears within two or three months and is replaced by voluntary sucking. The rooting reflex may persist throughout the first year of life.

Most of the reflexes of the eye, such as the blink reflexes and pupil response to light are protective in function and probably persist throughout life. However, some of them (e.g. naso-palpebral, ciliary and corneal) can be controlled or inhibited voluntarily by older children and adults. The importance of these protective reflexes to the visual system is readily apparent, as is the importance of vision in the acquisition of motor skills. (The role of vision in motor skill learning is discussed in chapter 3 by Williams.)

The foot and leg reflexes, according to Fiorentino (1973), "coordinate muscles of the extremities in patterns of either total flexion or extension" (p. 8). Uncontrolled extension or flexion of the limb upon stimulation of the foot or leg is

Table 2
Reflexes and reactions of the neonate and infant

Protection/Nourishment	Posture/Manipulation
Oral 1. Sucking 2. Searching (rooting)	*Eye* 1. Doll's eye 2. Response to rotation

Eye
 1. Blink
    a. cochleo-palpebral
    b. visuo-palpebral
    c. cutaneo-palpebral
    d. naso-palpebral
    e. optic (opisthotonos)
    f. ciliary
    g. corneal
    h. McCarthy's
 2. Pupil response to light
 3. Photic sneeze
 4. Resistance to passive opening
	Foot
	 1. Plantar grasp
	 2. Babinski's
	 3. Heel
	
	 Other Body
	 1. Palmar grasp
	 2. Placing
	 3. Walking
	 4. Crawling
	 5. Swimming
	 6. Hip (amphibian)
	 7. Landau

Foot/Leg 1. Withdrawal (flexor) 2. Crossed extension 3. Extensor thrust	*Tonic* 1. Tonic neck-asymmetrical 2. Tonic neck-symmetrical 3. Tonic labyrinthine-supine 4. Tonic labyrinthine-prone
Other Body 1. Moro 2. Startle 3. Protective extensor thrust (arms)	*Tendon* 1. Knee 2. Biceps 3. Heel (achilles) *Righting* 1. Neck 2. Labyrinth (acting on head) 3. Body (acting on body) 4. Optic 5. Positive supporting (leg straightening) *Equilibrium* 1. Supine 2. Prone 3. Kneeling (upright) 4. Standing (forward, backward, right, left) 5. Squatting

Note: Compiled primarily from material presented in *The Development of the infant and young child: Normal and abnormal* (4th ed.), (pp. 116-132) by R.S. Illingworth, 1970, Baltimore: Williams and Wilkins. Copyright 1970 by E. & S. Livingstone LTD; and, in *Reflex testing methods for evaluating C.N.S. development* (2nd ed.), (pp. 3-37) by M.R. Fiorentino, 1973, Springfield, IL: Charles C. Thomas. Copyright 1973 by Charles C. Thomas.

normal in the newborn, but such behavior beyond the age of two months is considered a sign of delayed reflexive maturation.

    The Moro and startle reflexes often are confused with each other. The Moro reflex is best elicited by a sudden movement of the cervical region, whereas the startle reflex is usually evoked by a sudden, loud noise. Furthermore, the elbows are extended and the hands opened in the Moro reflex, but the elbows are flexed and the hands remain closed in the startle reflex (Illingworth, 1970). The Moro reflex normally disappears by about three months of age, while the startle reflex remains throughout life.

A protective (also postural) reflex that does not emerge until about six months of age is the protective extensor thrust or parachute reaction. This reflex or reaction is elicited throughout life as a protective measure when balance is lost while engaging in various forms of upright locomotion. It is tested by holding the child in an inverted position and then suddenly lowering the child toward the floor. The typical response is extension of the arms and the fingers to keep the head from contacting the floor (Fiorentino, 1973).

Postural reflexes. Postural responses involving the eyes include doll's eye and rotational nystagmus. Doll's eye (delayed movement of the eyes in response to movement of the head) is normally present the first ten days after birth. Asymmetrical eye responses indicate paralysis of ocular muscles served by the abducens nerve. The ntagmus reaction (alternating lateral movement of the eyes) to body rotation has oeen used to determine the presence of occular palsies in newborn children (Illingworth, 1970).

The Babinski, plantar grasp, and heel reflexes are primitive reflexes of the foot that are used to assess neurological integrity. However, the first two also are premanipulative, whereas the heel reflex may be regarded as prepostural. The Babinski reflex (fanning of the toes upon stimulation of the sole) normally disappears within three months after birth, but the plantar reflex (flexion of the toes upon stimulation of the ball of the foot) often persists for the first year. The heel reflex, caused by percussion on the heel or pressure on the sole, results in extension of the leg (Illingworth, 1970). This reflex may be modified later by higher neural centers and incorporated into voluntary behaviors such as standing and walking.

Other reflexes that appear to be precursors to later voluntary movements are the palmar grasp, placing, walking, crawling and swimming reflexes. All of these reflexes are normally present at birth and must disappear or be suppressed before the corresponding voluntary behaviors can be learned. A direct connection between these early reflexes and subsequent voluntary behavior has not been established. However, McGraw (1954) believed that neuromuscular mechanisms underlying reflexive swimming are the same as those used in reflexive crawling and stepping. Furthermore, Zelazo (1972) found that infants who practiced the stepping and placing reflexes daily (four 3 minute sessions) for a period of seven weeks learned to walk sooner then subjects who did not have this experience.

Two types of reflexes under the control of the brain stem are the tonic neck reflexes (TNR) and the tonic labyrinthine reflexes (TLR). The asymmetrical TNR is assessed by placing the child in a supine position and then turning the head to one side. Characteristically, the near arm and leg extend while the opposite arm and leg flex. The response of the upper limbs is stronger than that of the lower limbs. This reflex response also is referred to as the "fencer's position." The symmetrical TNR often is tested by placing the subject in a prone position across the thighs of the examiner. Extension (dorsiflexion) of the head in midline position produces extension of the arms and flexion of the knees. Ventriflexion of the head causes the opposite effects (Fiorentino, 1973). TLR responses are examined with the child in a supine or in a prone position. When in a supine position with the head in mid-position and the arms and legs extended, the child will exhibit dominant extensor tone in response to attempts at passively flexing the limbs. When placed in a prone position, the child is unable to raise the head and retract the shoulders and also cannot extend the trunk, arms and legs (Fiorentino, 1973).

Normally, both the TNRs and the TLRs should be inhibited by higher neural centers after four months of age. When these reflexes remain dominant, the individual is confined to prone- and supine-lying positions and unable to crawl, creep or walk (Fiorentino, 1973). Inhibition of these reflexes appears to be necessary for complex skills to be learned. Swartz and Allen (1975) reported that improper inhibition of the asymmetrical TNR led to difficulties in learning the breaststroke because the movements of the head and arms were yoked together, inappropriately.

A group of responses known as righting reflexes are controlled at the midbrain level. They are integrated with each other to establish normal head-body relationships, as well as the relationship of the body to the force of gravity. They enable a child to roll over, sit, crawl and creep (Fiorentino, 1973). The neck righting reaction normally is present during the first six months after birth. When the infant is placed in supine position, active or passive rotation of the head to one side will result in a "block" rotation of the body toward that side. The neck righting reaction should be supplanted by the body righting reaction, which is characterized by a segmental (sequential) rotation of the shoulders and pelvis in response to the turning of the head. The body righting reaction normally continues until 18 months of age.

Labyrinthine righting reactions orient the head to gravity. The child is blindfolded and then held in prone, supine or upright position by the examiner. When the child is placed in a prone or supine position, the head should automatically raise to a normal position, with the face vertical and the mouth horizontal. This response should be present by two months of age for the prone position and by six months of age for the supine position. When the body is tilted to the right or left from an upright position, the head should right itself in a child who is eight months of age. Optical righting reactions are tested in the same manner as the labyrinthine righting reactions, except that the child is not blindfolded. These reactions usually are not tested unless the labyrinthine righting reactions are not functional (Fiorentino, 1973). The Landau reaction permits the infant to extend its trunk, arms and legs by dorsiflexing its head. This righting reaction is present from about 6 to 30 months of age (Fiorentino, 1973).

Equilibrium reactions constitute the highest level of involuntary responses. They are mediated by the cerebral cortex, basal ganglia and cerebellum. Their function is to adapt the position of the body when its center of gravity is displaced. Well developed equilibrium reactions enable the child to engage in upright locomotion (Fiorentino, 1973). Tasks to assess these reactions include tilting, pulling or moving a child who is: a) lying on a tiltboard either in a prone or supine position; b) on hands and knees; c) sitting in a chair; d) kneeling upright; e) standing; and f) squatting in a Simian position. On each task, the child is expected to respond by righting the head and thorax and by adjusting the arms and legs to maintain balance and provide protection. When standing, positive responses may include hopping to maintain balance when the child is pulled or tilted. Equilibrium reactions for the prone and supine positions emerge as early as six months of age. However, those for the upright positions do not appear until 15 or 18 months of age.

The postural reflexes appear to be the most directly related to voluntary movement. The righting and equilibrium reactions undoubtedly play a major role in voluntary skill acquisition by enabling the child to maintain static and dynamic balance while learning new skills. In some instances, however, it may be necessary to "override" these normal reactions when learning skills where the requirements for body position and movement are contrary to the normal upright orientation to gravity, such as in gymnastics and diving. A thorough knowledge of primitive reflexes and postural reactions should be of great value to teachers of movement skills, not only for the purpose of remediating gross motor dysfunction, but also because their presence or absence can either help or hinder the process of learning gross motor skills.

Motor Behavior In Infancy and Early Childhood

Infancy. The first 12 to 24 months after birth are characterized by radical changes in motor behavior. Primitive reflexes disappear or become subordinated to higher neural centers. Righting and equilibrium reactions emerge and become stabilized, and voluntary movements become the dominant form of motor behavior. Infancy is the age period for mastering skills such as sitting, grasping, creeping and walking (Touwen, 1971).

The development of voluntary motor patterns in infancy is frequently associated with a substrate of reflexes and patterned reactions (Milani-Comparetti & Gidoni, 1967). Progressive refinements of selective behaviors are dependent on the breakdown of massive functional units of primitive reflex patterns into smaller units so that they may be used for the construction of new patterns. For example, Twitchell (1965) showed that increasingly complex forms of voluntary grasping are associated with the evolution of three kinds of automatic grasping response— the traction response, grasp reflex, and instinctive grasp reaction. Bruner (1973) suggested that patterned behaviors of an instinctive or reflex nature are converted by the infant into intentional actions as soon as the infant observes the results of these behaviors; and that, although the building blocks of volitional behavior are provided through development and maturation, their application to environmental situations must be learned.

Bruner also stressed the importance of mastery play and adequate social environments in order for appropriate skill development to occur in infants. Mastery play involves the extension of a newly acquired skill, such as grasping and holding an object, in which the child develops variations of the act (i.e. mouthing, banging, shaking and dropping the object). These variations are then applied to other objects as they are secured. Such play has the effect of developing routines which later can be incorporated into more complex programs of action. The importance of adequate environmental stimulation in a social context for normal motor development has been demonstrated by Dennis (1935) and Dennis and Najarian (1957). Moreover, even though many of the early voluntary behaviors of infancy are heavily dependent upon the maturation of the nervous system, the acquisition of rudimentary forms of fundamental motor skills by most infants and young children does not guarantee that the mature forms of these skills will be attained (Halverson, 1966).

The motor development of infants has been well documented. Gesell (1928), Shirley (1931), Halverson (1931), Bayley (1935) and McGraw (1940), among others, have identified the sequential order in which infants gain postural control, upright locomotion and manipulative skills. Because space does not permit a discussion of these behaviors, the reader is referred to the most recent edition of *Manual of the Bayley Scales of Infant Development* (Bayley, 1969) for a representative sample of the motor achievements of infants and the age ranges during which they are normally achieved.

Studies, such as those cited in the previous paragraph, have established several facts about motor achievements in infants. First, the order in which specific motor behaviors appear is common to nearly all infants, although slight variations in the order do occur. Second, early voluntary behaviors are closely related to the maturation of the neuromuscular system in the infant. Third, there is greater variability in both the appearance and performance of voluntary behavior in infants as age advances. This is likely due to a variety of reasons, including differential maturation rates among the infants, a greater capacity for varied responses with maturation, and to the greater impact of environmental variables on the type and quality of responses as the infant grows older. There is greater similarity among infants in the performance of some skills (e.g. locomotor skills) than in the performance of others (e.g. manipulative skills).

Of interest to researchers has been the capacity of infants and young children to learn motor skills and the extent to which early motor behavior is predictive of subsequent skill learning. Although the studies are not numerous, the capacity of infants to adapt or learn as a result of intervention has been demonstrated. Lipsitt and Kaye (1964) found that the sucking response of three and four day old infants could be conditioned. Zelazo (1972) advanced the timetable for walking without assistance by applying a daily exercise program involving the walking and placing reflexes of one week old newborns for a period of seven weeks. Stimulation of vestibular apparatus of infants by spinning them also has resulted in accelerated motor development (Clark, Kreutzberg & Chee, 1977).

On the other hand, studies of twins such as those by Gesell and Thompson (1929) and McGraw (1939) cast doubt on the value of early training sessions because of the control twin in each study was able to "catch up" to the trained twin at a later age with much less practice time. Three points should be noted, however. First, practice opportunities were necessary for "catch up" to occur. Second, the trained twin in McGraw's study was able to learn ontogenetic skills (skills not generic to life) such as roller skating and swimming at a very early age. Third, both twins who received the early training were judged to be more coordinated and more daring than the untrained twins.

Some positive links between early motor behavior and subsequent motor behavior have been identified. In one study, fetal activity accounted for 30 to 70% of the variance in infant performance on the Gesell Schedules at six months of age (Richards & Newberry, 1938). Total fetal activity during the last trimester also correlated significantly with motor items in the Gesell Schedules at 12, 24 and 36 weeks after birth (Walters, 1965). Apgar scores obtained shortly after birth were significantly related to the gross and fine motor coordination of 147 children at four years of age (Edwards, 1968). Unfortunately, reports that relate the impact of early motor behavior on skill learning in late childhood, adolescence and adulthood are not available.

Early childhood. The time period of two to seven years of age is of particular importance for the development of motor skills in the growing child. During this time the rudimentary, postural, locomotor, and object control skills attained in infancy become refined and many new skills emerge. Table 3 contains the gross motor skills generally associated with early childhood, as identified by investigators who have examined the motor achievements of young children. Space does not permit a discussion of each skill separately; therefore, only general comments will be made regarding the assessment of these skills, their general course of development, gender differences, and the effects of intervention on skill acquisition. For more detailed information, the reader is referred to the original reports cited in the references or to the texts cited at the beginning of this chapter.

Several approaches have been used to study the motor achievements of young children. One method has been to define a series of age-related tasks, each of increasing difficulty, for a given set of skills. Test batteries are usually comprised of the common motor tasks of early childhood. Children are assessed to determine how many of the specified tasks they can perform. Scoring is done on a pass/fail basis. Level of motor development is determined by the extent to which the children "pass" tasks that are commensurate with, above, or below expectations for their chronological age. This approach was used in the studies of Cunningham (1927), Bayley (1935, 1969), McCaskill and Wellman (1938), Gesell (1940), and Frankenberg and Dodds (1967) cited in Table 3. The results of these studies often were used to establish developmental scales or screening tests. Examples of two task series, with their accompanying age equivalents for each item, are presented in Table 4.

A second, less frequently used approach is to establish criteria for rating the performance of children on individual motor skills. For example, Gutteridge

Table 3
Gross motor skills of early childhood

	Cunningham (1927) 1.0–3.5 years	Jenkins (1930) 5.0–7.0 years	Bayley (1935) Birth–3.0 years	McCaskill & Wellman (1938) 2.0–6.0 years	Gutteridge (1939) 2.0–7.0 years	Gesell (1940) 1.25–7.0 years	Hartman (1943) 4.0–6.5 years	Keogh (1965) 5.0–11.0 years	Frankenberg & Dodds (1967) Birth–6.0 years	Bayley (1969) Birth–2.5 years	Sinclair (1971) 2.0–6.0 years	Vilchkovsky (1972) 3.0–17.0 years	Morris et al. (1982) 2.0–6.0 years
CLIMBING													
Equipment (Chairs, boxes, stools)	X			X	X								
Stairs—ascending	X		X	X	X	X				X	X		
Stairs—descending	X		X	X	X	X					X	X	
Ladders—ascending				X	X	X					X		
Ladders—descending				X	X	X							
WALKING													
Form/Patterns	X				X				X		X		
Variations/Directions			X		X				X	X			
Accuracy/Control (Lines, circles, etc.)	X			X	X		X		X	X			
Balance/Control (Beams, blocks, boards)	X				X		X		X	X			
RUNNING													
Start/Stop/Control	X				X								
Form/Speed		X			X	X	X			X	X	X	X
Agility/Coordination						X				X		X	X
JUMPING													
From heights	X		X	X	X	X				X			
Two-foot continuous			X	X	X	X			X	X			
Standing long jump		X	X	X	X	X	X	X	X	X	X	X	X
Running long jump		X				X						X	
Jump and reach	X				X	X	X						
Over obstacles (Hurdles, cables, etc.)	X		X		X		X	X		X			
Running high jump											X	X	
GALLOPING					X						X		
HOPPING	X	X	X	X	X	X		X	X	X	X		
SKIPPING				X	X	X				X			
SLIDING													
Inclines					X								
Sideways											X		
TRICYCLING				X	X				X				
THROWING													
Rolling a ball	X												
Form/Distance		X		X	X	X	X	X	X	X	X	X	X
Accuracy	X	X						X					
CATCHING				X	X	X			X		X		X
KICKING		X		X	X				X		X		
STRIKING											X		

Table 3 (continued)
Gross motor skills of early childhood

	Cunningham (1927) 1.0-3.5 years	Jenkins (1930) 5.0-7.0 years	Bayley (1935) Birth-3.0 years	McCaskill & Wellman (1938) 2.0-6.0 years	Gutteridge (1939) 2.0-7.0 years	Gesell (1940) 1.25-7.0 years	Hartman (1943) 4.0-6.5 years	Keogh (1965) 5.0-11.0 years	Frankenberg & Dodds (1967) Birth-6.0 years	Bayley (1969) Birth-2.5 years	Sinclair (1971) 2.0-6.0 years	Vilchkovsky (1972) 3.0-17.0 years	Morris et al. (1982) 2.0-6.0 years
BOUNCING (Ball)				X	X						X		
BALANCING (Static)			X			X		X	X	X			X
HANGING (Hands)											X		
FORWARD ROLL											X		
PUSHING/PULLING											X		
LIFTING & CARRYING											X		
BOUNCING (Board)											X		

Table 4
Levels of achievement for walking on stairs and walking on a line

Tasks	Mean Age
WALKING ON STAIRS	
Walks up stairs with help	20.3 months
Walks down stairs with help	20.5 months
Walks up stairs alone; marks time	24.3 months
Walks down stairs alone; marks time	24.5 months
Walks up stairs; alttino forward foot	35.5 months
Walks down stairs; alternating forward foot	50.0 months
WALKING ON LINE	
Walks on tiptoes	30.1 months
Walks on line, general direction	31.3 months
Walks backward, three meters	33.2 months
Walks tiptoe, three meters	36.2 months
Keeps feet on line, three meters	38.5 months

Note: Adapted from "The development of motor abilities during the first three years" by N. Bayley, 1935, Monographs of the Society for Research in Child Development, 1-26. Copyright 1935 by the Society for Research in Child Development.

(1939) established a series of ten hierarchical behaviors for rating performance on skills such as climbing, jumping, galloping, and throwing. The ten behaviors were assessed by four criteria, used to determine: (a) when children made no attempt to perform the skill; (b) when they were in the process of developing the skill; (c) when the skill was essentially achieved and, (d) when the skill was used with variations. Thus, a certain percent of children at a given age were rated as "skillful," "basic achievers," "developing," or "non-performers." Sinclair (1971) established performance criteria for "success" and "mature pattern" for each of 25 motor tasks, based on the elements of each skill. The movement performance of each child was then filmed and analyzed, followed by the assignment of a score, on a five point scale, that was based on the degree of success achieved and the number of critical elements exhibited. Sinclair's method allowed for comparisons, by age and gender, on the basis of the scores.

A third, and the most common, method for determining the motor achievement of young children is to measure skill performance, quantitatively. This method measures the product of performance, such as the distance jumped, the time required to complete a run over a known distance, or the number of volleys made in a specified amount of time. Using quantitative data, individual performances can be compared to those of children who represent a similar age and gender. In addition, the same skills may be examined at various ages and changes in performance over time can be recorded. The studies by Jenkins (1930), Hartman (1943), Keogh (1965), Vilchkovsky (1972), and Morris et al. (1982) listed in Table 3 are representative of this method.

Change in motor achievements over time, without the benefit of direct instruction, is considered to be the product of maturation and general interaction with one's environment. Each of the three approaches discussed above have demonstrated age-related changes in the motor development of young children. For example, 4-year-old children run faster than 2-year-old children (Fortney, 1983); 5-year-old children jump higher (Cowan & Pratt, 1934) and farther (Haubenstricker, Branta, Ulrich, Brakora & E-Lotfalian, 1984) than children who are three years of age. Children who are six years old are more adept at galloping than children who are four years old (Gutteridge, 1939).

Most year-to-year changes in the motor skills of young children tend to be linear in nature, but not without exception. Young children tend to exhibit more trial-to-trial variation than older children. In addition, there is substantial variability in the performance of specific skills within age groups, reflecting differential rates of maturation, skill learning ability and environmental experiences. The data reported in Figure 3 are representative of the change and variability that occur when young children perform gross motor skills.

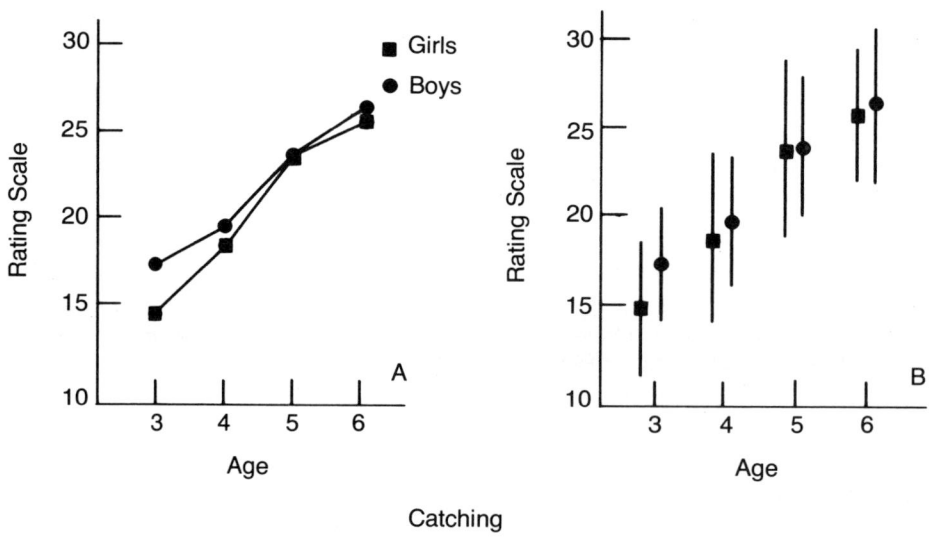

Catching

Fig. 3. Means (A Graphs) and standard deviations (B Graphs) for the performance of young children on selected motor skills. (From "Age and sex differences in motor performance of 3 through 6 year old children" by A.M. Morris, J.M. Williams, A.E. Atwater & J.H. Wilmore, 1982 by American Alliance for Health, Physical Education, Recreation and Dance. Reprinted by permission.)

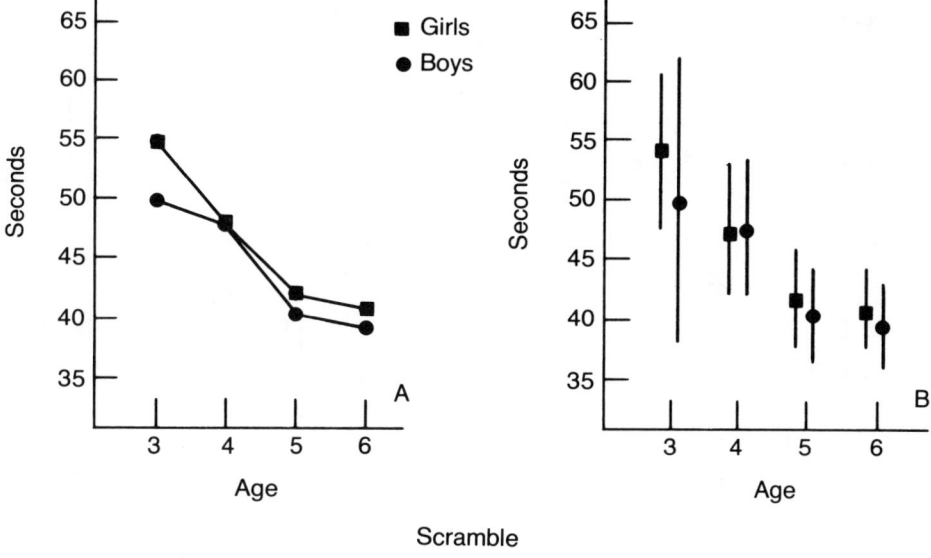

Scramble

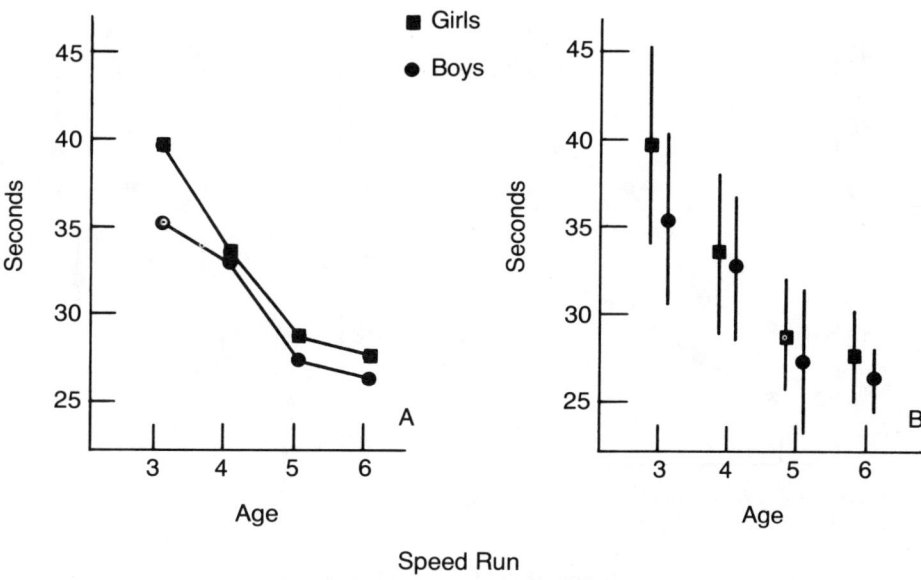

Speed Run

Fig. 3 (continued). Means (A Graphs) and standard deviations (B Graphs) for the performance of young children on selected motor skills. (From "Age and sex differences in motor performance of 3 through 6 year old children" by A.M. Morris, J.M. Williams, A.E. Atwater & J.H. Wilmore, 1982 by American Alliance for Health, Physical Education, Recreation and Dance. Reprinted by permission.)

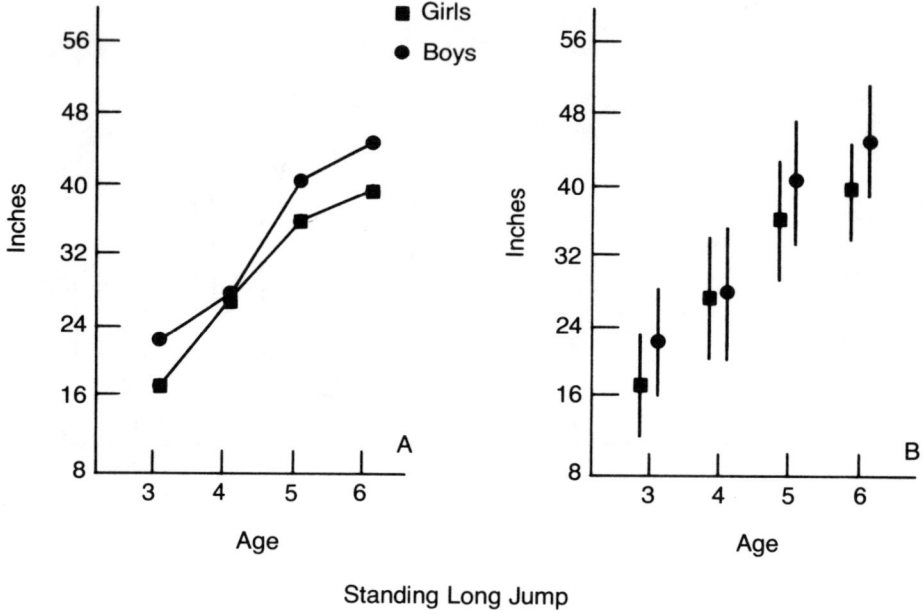

Standing Long Jump

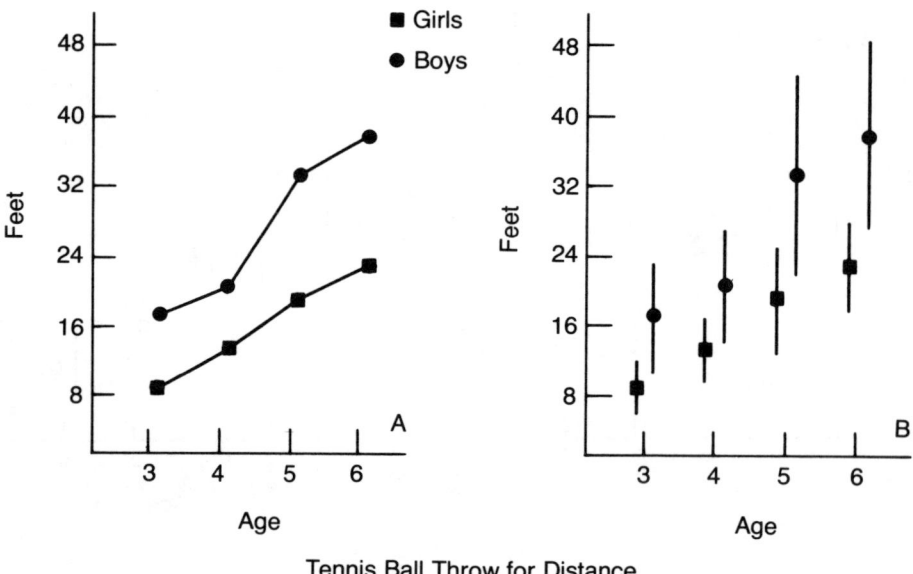

Tennis Ball Throw for Distance

Fig. 3 (continued). Means (A Graphs) and standard deviations (B Graphs) for the performance of young children on selected motor skills. (From "Age and sex differences in motor performance of 3 through 6 year old children" by A.M. Morris, J.M. Williams, A.E. Atwater & J.H. Wilmore, 1982 by American Alliance for Health, Physical Education, Recreation and Dance. Reprinted by permission.)

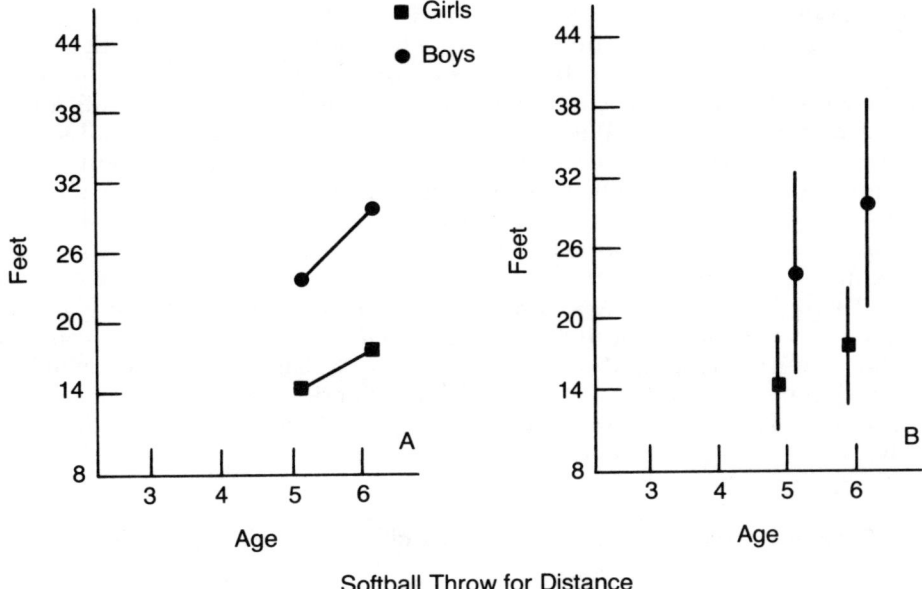

Softball Throw for Distance

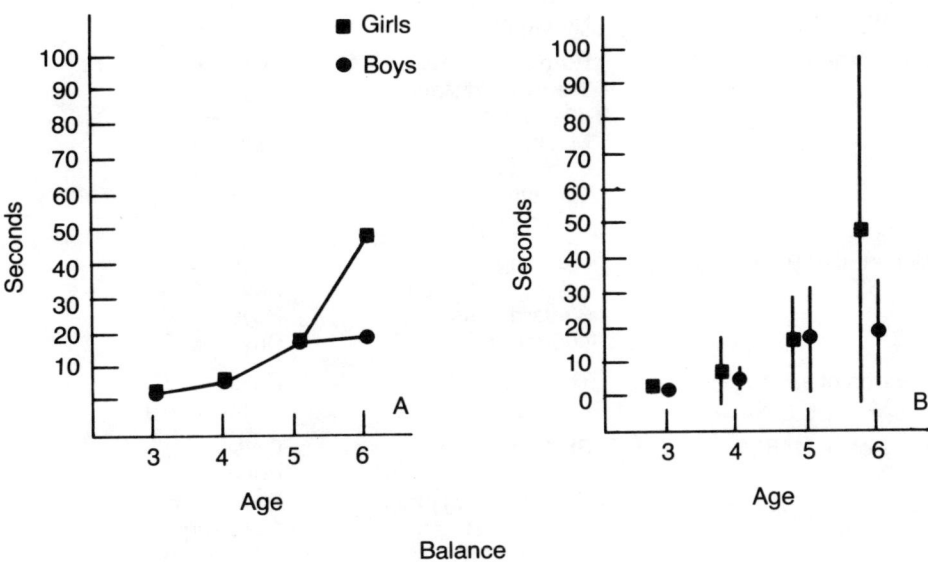

Balance

Fig. 3 (continued). Means (A Graphs) and standard deviations (B Graphs) for the performance of young children on selected motor skills. (From "Age and sex differences in motor performance of 3 through 6 year old children" by A.M. Morris, J.M. Williams, A.E. Atwater & J.H. Wilmore, 1982 by American Alliance for Health, Physical Education, Recreation and Dance. Reprinted by permission.)

Considerable controversy surrounds the issue of gender differences in the motor skill performance of young children. The practice of some investigators to claim gender differences on the basis of raw score means, without the support of appropriate statistical analysis to determine if the differences are significant or due to chance, has contributed to the problem. Reports that include small sample sizes and data that are difficult to analyze, statistically, are also prevalent.

A summary of published reports leads to the conclusion that gender differences in motor skill performance do exist at very young ages. Table 5 is a compilation of those studies which have reported significant gender differences in gross motor skills. Note that except for conflicting results on the hurdle jump (Hartman, 1943; Keogh, 1965) there is agreement among the various studies concerning gender superiority in performing specific gross motor skills. Girls are superior to boys on tasks that require balance and coordination (i.e. static balance, hopping, mat hop and cable jump), whereas boys excel on power dependent events such a throwing, long jumping, kicking, running and changing the direction of the entire body quickly.

Table 5
Studies that reported significant gender differences in early childhood

Study	Tasks	Gender/Age
Jenkins (1930) N = 231	50 - foot hop Throw for distance Toss for accuracy Running long jump Kick for distance	Girls—7 Boys—5, 6, 7 Boys—5, 6, 7 Boys—5, 6, 7 Boys—5, 6, 7
Hartman (1943) N = 36	Throw for distance Hurdle jump	Boys—6 Boys—6
Keogh (1965) N = 1171	Hurdle jump Throw for distance 50 - foot hop Mat hop Cable jump Grip strength (R) Grip strength (L)	Girls—7 Boys—6, 7 Girls—7 Girls—6, 7 Girls—6, 7 Boys—6, 7 Boys—5, 6, 7
Milne et al. (1976) N = 553	Standing long jump Agility shuttle run 30-yard dash 400-foot run	Boys—5, 6, 7 Boys—5, 6, 7 Boys—5, 6, 7 Boys—5, 7
Roberton et al. (1979) N = 54	Throw for velocity	Boys—6, 7 (longitudinal)
Morris et al. (1982) N = 269	Static balance 40-foot run Standing long jump Ball throw (tennis) Ball throw (softball)	Girls—6 Boys—6 Boys—3-6 (combined) Boys—3, 4, 5, 6 Boys—5, 6
Haubenstricker et al. (1984) N = 1352	Standing long jump	Boys—2½-5 (combined)

It should be noted, however, that the majority of studies reviewed did not include tests for determining significant differences between boys and girls. Yet, in most instances, the direction of raw score outcomes were in agreement with the significant results reported. The presence of gender differences does not explain the relative impact of cultural conditioning and biological processes. However, it seems logical to presume that the younger the detection of gender differences in motor performance, the greater is the relative impact of genetic and constitutional influences.

Although information on age-related tasks, general skill ratings, and quantitative performance data has been useful to determine the status of a child in relation to that of other children of a similar age on a specific motor skill, it has provided little information on how to change or improve motor behavior. However, research which focused on the qualitative aspects of motor skill development has made a major contribution in solving this dilemma.

Developmental sequences. Information concerning the qualitative development of a motor skill was first reported in the early 1930s by Halverson (1931). He examined the development of prehension in infants, describing 10 distinct stages, with their related model ages. The first published report of changing motor patterns in a motor skill involving the total body is the classic study of the overhand throw by Monica Wild (1938). These early investigators established that fundamental motor skills developed in an orderly manner and that the changes which occur could be recorded in the form of identifiable motor patterns. These developmental motor patterns occur in sequence and are called stages (Seefeldt et al., 1972) or steps (Roberton, 1978). Individual skill sequences are referred to as intraskill sequences. Each successive motor pattern is more complex than the previous one. The intraskill sequences are age-related, but not necessarily age-dependent, because individual children acquire gross motor skills at different rates. Thus, at a given age, some children may exhibit an initial stage, whereas others may already have advanced to the mature stage.

During the last two decades, developmental sequences have been proposed for many of the fundamental gross motor skills. Table 6 contains a listing of gross motor skills for which two or more developmental sequences have been suggested. Major attention has been focused on locomotor and object control skills. However, developmental sequences also have been proposed for the forward roll (Roberton & Halverson, 1977, 1984; Williams, 1980; Gallahue, 1982), horizontal ladder travel (Gabbard & Patterson, 1981), and rope jumping (Wickstrom, 1974). In addition, Gallahue (1982) has hypothesized three-stage sequences for jumping from heights, leaping, climbing, ball rolling, ball trapping, ball volleying, axial movements, inverted supports, dodging, the one-foot balance, and beam walking.

Table 6
Developmental sequences of fundamental motor skills

Skill	Sequence Proponents
WALKING	Wickstrom* (1977, 1983); Gallahue (1982); Williams (1983).
RUNNING	Wickstrom (1970, 1977, 1983); Seefeldt, Reuschlein & Vogel (1972); Roberton & Halverson (1977, 1984); McClenaghan & Gallahue (1978); Gallahue (1982); Williams (1983); Roberton (1984).
STANDING LONG JUMP	Hellebrandt, et al. (1961); Wickstrom (1970, 1977, 1983); Seefeldt et al. (1972); Roberton & Halverson (1977, 1984); McClenaghan & Gallahue (1978); Gallahue (1982); Williams (1983); Haubenstricker et al. (1983); Roberton (1984); Clark & Phillips (1985).

*Wickstrom's three editions of Fundamental Motor Patterns (1970, 1977, 1983) contain comprehensive literature reviews for most of the skills listed. However, Wickstrom does not propose his own developmental sequences.

Table 6 (continued)
Developmental sequences of fundamental motor skills

Skill	Sequence Proponents
VERTICAL JUMP	Wickstrom (1970, 1977, 1983); Poe (1976); Gallahue (1982); Williams (1983).
HOPPING	Seefeldt & Haubenstricker (1976a); Roberton & Halverson (1977, 1984); Gallahue (1982); Wickstrom (1983); Williams (1983); Roberton (1984); Halverson & Williams (1985).
GALLOPING	Sapp (1980); Gallahue (1982); Williams (1983).
SKIPPING	Haubenstricker & Seefeldt (1976); Gallahue (1982); Williams (1983).
THROWING	Wild (1938); Deach (1950); Wickstrom (1970, 1977, 1983); Seefeldt et al. (1972); Seefeldt & Haubenstricker (1976d); Roberton & Halverson (1977, 1984); McClenaghan & Gallahue (1978); Gallahue (1982); Haubenstricker et al. (1983, May); Williams (1983); Roberton (1984).
CATCHING	Deach (1950); Wickstrom (1970, 1977, 1983); Seefeldt (1972, March); Seefeldt et al. (1972); Roberton & Halverson (1977, 1984); McClenaghan & Gallahue (1978); Gallahue (1982); Haubenstricker et al. (1983, May); Williams (1983); Roberton (1984).
KICKING	Deach (1950); Wickstrom (1970, 1977, 1983); Seefeldt & Haubenstricker (1974); McClenaghan & Gallahue (1978); Haubenstricker et al. (1981, March); Gallahue (1982); Williams (1983).
PUNTING	Wickstrom (1970, 1977, 1983); Seefeldt & Haubenstricker (1976b); Roberton & Halverson (1977, 1984); Roberton (1984).
STRIKING	Deach (1950); Wickstrom (1970, 1977, 1983); Seefeldt & Haubenstricker (1976c); Roberton & Halverson (1977, 1984); Gallahue (1982); Williams (1983).
DRIBBLING	Deach (1950); Gallahue (1982); Wickstrom (1983); Williams (1983).

Intraskill sequences generally are expressed according to one of two models. In one model, called the whole body model, each developmental stage is described as a configuration involving the whole body. The movement patterns of selected body segments and other factors (i.e. weight transfer) are identified within each stage. In this model, the movement pattern of a particular body segment may or may not change from one stage to the next, but it will change at one or more stages in the sequence. The model does not require simultaneous change in the movement patterns of all body segments from one stage to the next (as interpreted by some). However, the total body movement configuration does change and is clearly distinguishable from those of the adjacent stages. Configurations that are not in full compliance with one of the decribed stages are considered to be in transition between stages.

There is general agreement that motor skill development occurs on a continuum and not in a staircase or stepwise manner (which is why some investigators prefer to use the term stage rather than step in describing the developmental levels). Table 7 contains a developmental sequence for the standing long jump, using this model

Table 7
Developmental sequence of the standing long jump

Stage 1	The vertical component of force may be greater than horizontal. The resulting jump is then upward rather than forward. Arms move backward, acting as brakes to stop the momentum of the trunk as the legs extend in front of the center of mass.
Stage 2	The arms move in an anterior-posterior direction during the preparatory phase, but move sideward (winging action) during the "in-flight" phase. The knees and hips flex and extend more fully than in stage one. The angle of take-off is still markedly above 45°. The landing is made with the center of mass above the base of support, with the thighs perpendicular to the surface rather than parallel as in the "reaching" position of stage four.
Stage 3	The arms swing backward and then forward during the preparatory phase. The knees and hips flex fully prior to take-off. Upon take-off the arms extend and move forward, but do not exceed the height of the head. The knee extension may be complete but the take-off angle is still greater than 45°. Upon landing, the thigh is still less than parallel to the surface and the center of mass is near the base of support when viewed from the frontal plane.
Stage 4	The arms extend vigorously forward and upward upon take-off, reaching full extension above the head at "lift-off." The hips and knees are extended fully with the take-off angle at 45° or less. In preparation for landing the arms are brought downward and the legs are thrust forward until the thigh is parallel to the surface. The center of mass is far behind the base of support upon foot contact, but at the moment of contact the knees are flexed and the arms are thrust forward in order to maintain the momentum to carry the center of gravity beyond the feet.

Note: From "Sequencing motor skills within the physical education curriculum" by V. Seefeldt, P. Reuschlein and P. Vogel, 1972, March. Paper presented at the national convention of the American Association for Health, Physical Education and Recreation, Houston, Texas. Reprinted by permission.

The second model is called the component model. In this model, developmental changes are identified for individual body parts (i.e. arms, legs, trunk in jumping). Thus, when assessing the performance of a child on a particular motor skill, the observer assigns a developmental level for each body component under consideration. The rationale for the component approach is based on the assumption that the movement patterns of individual body segments do not develop at the same rate, therefore each segment should be assessed independently. In addition, since body segments may exhibit different movement patterns during critical phases in the execution of a skill (i.e., windup, force production, follow through), several assessments for each body segment may be necessary. For example, the sequences proposed by Roberton (1984) for the standing long jump, presented in Table 8, require that six assessments be made for each child in order to determine the level of development.

Proponents of each model have attested to the practical utility of the developmental sequences. First, they can be readily learned by observers. Second, they can be observed and assessed quite accurately in children by individuals who have learned the sequences. Third, they provide a basis for initiating change through teaching because the next "step" of a component sequence or the next "stage" of a whole body sequence becomes an instructional goal. Fourth, instructional strategies can be applied to achieve these goals. Fifth, the achievement of the goals and/or the effectiveness of the instructional strategies can be verified through observation.

Effects of intervention. A fundamental question is, "Can the motor patterns of young children be changed through intervention or are they almost entirely

Table 8
Developmental Sequences for the Standing Long Jump

	Takeoff: Leg Action Component
Level 1	One foot leads in asymmetrical takeoff.
Level 2	Both feet leave ground symmetrically, but hips or knees or both do not reach full extension by takeoff.
Level 3	Takeoff is symmetrical, with hips and knees fully extended.

	Takeoff: Trunk Action Component
Level 1	Trunk is inclined forward less than 30 degrees from vertical. Neck is hyperextended.
Level 2	Trunk leans forward less than 30 degrees, with neck flexed or aligned with trunk at takeoff.
Level 3.	Trunk is inclinded forward 30 degrees or more at takeoff, with neck flexed.
Level 4	Trunk is inclined forward 30 degrees or more. Neck is aligned with trunk, or slightly extended.

	Takeoff: Arm Action Component
Level 1	Arms move in opposition to legs or are held at side, with elbows flexed.
Level 2	Shoulders retract, arms extend backward in winging posture at takeoff.
Level 3	Arms are abducted about 90 degrees, with elbows frequently flexed, in high or middle guard position.
Level 4	Arms flex forward and upward with minimal abduction, reaching incomplete extension overhead by takeoff.
Level 5	Arms flex forward, reaching full extension overhead by takeoff.

	Flight and Landing: Leg Action Component
Level 1	Legs assume asymmetrical run pattern in flight, with one-footed landing.
Level 2	Legs assume asymmetrical run pattern, but swing to two-footed landing.
Level 3	During flight, hips and knees flex in a synchronous fashion. Knees then extend for two-footed landing.
Level 4	During flight, flexion of both knees precedes hip flexion. As hips flex, knees extend, reaching forward to two-footed landing.

	Flight and Landing: Trunk Action Component
Level 1	Trunk maintains forward inclination of less than 30 degrees in flight, then flexes for landing.
Level 2	Trunk corrects forward lean of 30 degrees or more by hyperextending. It then flexes forward for landing.
Level 3	Trunk maintains forward lean of 30 degrees or more from takeoff to midflight, then flexes forward for landing.

	Flight and Landing: Arm Action Component
Level 1	Arms move in opposition to legs as if child were running in flight and on landing.
Level 2	Shoulders retract and arms extend backward (winging) during flight and move forward (parachuting, page 51) during landing.
Level 3	During flight, arms assume high or middle guard positions and may move backward in windmill fashion. They parachute for landing.
Level 4	Arms lower or extend from flexed position overhead, reaching forward at landing.

Note. From "Changing motor patterns during childhood" by M.A. Roberton. In *Motor development during childhood and adolescence* (p. 69) by J.R. Thomas (Ed.), 1984, Minneapolis: Burgess Publishing Company. Copyright 1984 by Burgess Publishing Company. Reprinted by permission.

controlled by maturational forces?" The evidence is reasonably clear that, when given appropriate tasks and sufficiently guided practice, gross motor skill learning in young children can be effectively enhanced through planned instruction. However, the number of studies dealing with the effects of training on the gross motor skill acquisition of young children is limited. Furthermore, not all studies reported positive results. For example, Hicks (1930) studied the effects of an eight-week training program on the ability of young children to hit a moving target with a thrown ball. The training consisted of 10 practice throws per week. Post-test results were similar for both the practice and the control groups, although both groups improved in their performance over the eight-week period. Hicks concluded that maturation and general practice accounted for the improvement. It should be noted, however, that no instruction in throwing was provided the children during the practice sessions. Thus, learning was essentially trial-and-error in nature. Furthermore, a stationary target, in lieu of a moving one, would seem to be more appropriate for young children. Moreover, attribution of observed changes to maturation and general practice does not seem to be a warranted conclusion in an experiment of eight weeks duration.

Similar results were reported by Hicks and Ralph (1931) after studying the effects of training on the ability of young children to trace mazes. Although significant gains were made by both the experimental and control groups after a seven-week training period, the difference in gains between the two groups was negligible. Again, no meaningful instruction was provided to the students during the practice sessions.

Positive training effects on the acquisition of gross motor skills have been reported by several investigators. Hilgard (1932) found that after 12 weeks of instruction, ten 2-year-old children were significantly more proficient than a matched control group in buttoning, cutting with scissors and climbing. The fact that one week of intensive practice permitted the control group to develop the same level of proficiency as the trained group does not negate the value of guided practice for the trained group. Rather, it points out that there may be periods during the early childhood years when certain skills are learned more efficiently than at other times. In other words, there may be critical or sensitive periods for learning motor skills. Mirenva (1935), after 4½ months of daily training, was able to effect large performance gains in 4-year-old twins on tasks of jumping and throwing. These gains were significantly greater than those obtained by their identical twin controls.

Significant practice effects were obtained with young subjects on the throw for distance (Dusenberry, 1952) and on throwing form (Halverson & Roberton, 1979), but not on throwing velocity (Halverson, Roberton, Safrit & Roberts, 1977). In addition, Werner (1974) reported that an eight-week program of guided instruction in locomotor, stability and manipulative movement patterns involving 18 nursery school children resulted in a superior performance by these children when compared to 18 control subjects. Motor skills assessed were the standing long jump, soccer volley kick, ball bounce, and static balance on a balance board. Finally, a study by Miller (1978) demonstrated that guided instruction in gross motor skills provided by a motor development specialist or trained parents produced significantly greater performance changes in nursery school age children when compared to children who used the same time period for free play sessions in the same physical environment as the children receiving the instruction. Children who attended local nursery schools did not differ in motor skill acquisition from those in free play sessions, but both groups were significantly inferior to the children who had received the instruction. Thus, the evidence suggests that in appropriate learning environments, motor skill acquisition can be enhanced during the early childhood years.

Summary. The attainment of reasonable proficiency in a wide variety of gross motor skills during the early childhood years is important for several reasons. First, early childhood seems to be the most efficient time to learn the fundamental motor skills, because the capacity to learn and the motivation to practice motor tasks are present at this time. There is sufficient evidence to conclude that gross motor skills can be taught effectively to young children if guided instruction, appropriate task sequences and sufficient practice time are provided. Second, skills and activity habits acquired in early life often persist into the adult years (Beach & Jaynes, 1954; Rarick, 1964). The importance of remaining physically active throughout life is a well recognized fact. Enjoyment of movement resulting from successful skill acquisition can contribute toward this goal. Third, careful analysis of the motor skills required in the games, sports and dances of our culture reveals that most of these skills are combinations and/or modifications of two or more basic locomotor, postural or object control skills. Therefore, children who have a large repertoire of movement skills have an advantage over children without those skills, when confronted with the task of learning complex motor skills. The former individuals need only to recognize learned units of behavior, whereas the latter must learn the basic movements before they can reorganize them into complex entities (Rarick, 1964). Motorically skilled children are more relaxed and willing than unskilled children to attempt new motor challenges (McGraw, 1939; Rarick, 1964). The rationale for teaching motor skills to young children is compelling when one considers the alternate consequences of delaying or withholding instruction. The quality of life that can be attained through efficiency of movement and the healthful benefits of vigorous activity have their foundation in the fundamental motor skills of infancy and childhood.

Motor Behavior in Middle and Late Childhood

The line of demarcation between the end of early childhood and the beginning of middle childhood is not clearly established. Children 6 or 7 years of age are often arbitrarily classified into either category depending on the definitions established by the specific investigator or writer (see Chapter 1 for definitions by Malina). For the purpose of this chapter, middle and late childhood will include the age range from 8 to 14 years or grades 3 to 8. However, when cited studies of motor behavior include data that extend beyond this age range, they will be included in this section.

Motor behavior in middle and late childhood is marked by the refinement of the fundamental motor skills acquired during early childhood and by the development of basic dance and sports skills, including the application of these skills to low organized games, lead-up activities to sports and to highly structured sport and dance activities. Due to limitations of space, the acquisition of specific sports skills will not be discussed in this section. However, the exclusion of these skills from this section does not in any way diminish the need for sound physical education programs in our nation's schools to ensure that all children receive ample opportunity to learn and practice the skills that are inherent in the games, dances and sports of their culture.

Continued attention to the development of fundamental motor skills during middle childhood is necessary for several reasons. First, children continue to increase in physical size and strength. As body coordination improves due to maturational processes, boys and girls are able to apply more force to their movements. Thus, their bodies or other objects can be projected farther and faster, requiring greater control for successful execution and safety of the performer. However, individual differences in the rate of physical growth and maturation often contribute to tremendous performance differences in these basic skills among boys and girls of the same chronological age. (The topics of stability and variability in performance will be discussed later in this chapter.) The nature of these changes and the magnitude of performance differences among children is essential information for movement educators if they are to provide optimum environments for the development and application of these skills.

A second and perhaps more important reason for continued attention to the fundamental motor skills is that by the end of third grade, many children still cannot demonstrate mature patterns when asked to do so (Reuschlein & Vogel, 1985, Reuschlein & Haubenstricker, 1985). The presence of both mature and immature skill patterns among similar aged children also contributes to the increased variability in skill performance for a specific age group. In addition, immature skill patterns are likely to interfere with the acquisition of more complex motor skills that are dependent upon the basic skills (Seefeldt, 1979, Gallahue, 1982). Repeated practice without corrective instruction can lead to the fixation of these immature skill patterns. During this age period, when successful participation in group games and team sport activities becomes increasingly important (McCraw and Tolbert, 1953), the need for effective physical education programs in the late elementary and middle schools becomes apparent.

Product or quantitative performance changes in gross motor skills, as a function of age and gender, have received considerable attention. A comprehensive review of such performance changes for running, jumping, throwing, and balancing skills prior to 1960 was reported by Espenschade (1960). A review of skill performance during the decade of the 1960s is presented by Keogh and Sugden (1985), and a review of post-1960 performance changes has been conducted by Branta et al. (1984). Other recent reviews appear in the publications of DeOreo and Keogh (1980), Espenschade and Eckert (1980) and Williams (1983). The most comprehensive treatment of changes in fundamental motor patterns was compiled by Wickstrom (1983).

The purpose of this section is to summarize and contrast what is known about performance changes in the more common skills of running, jumping, throwing, kicking, and striking. (The acquisition of balance will be discussed in Chapter 3 by Williams.) Particular attention will be directed at the pre-1960 and post-1960 performance comparisons within and between gender groups for running, jumping, and throwing. Composite means (unweighted) for these skills are presented in Table 9 and are depicted graphically in Figures 4 through 7. The composite means, representing pre-1960 performance, are based on 18 studies reported by Espenschade (1960). The values for post-1960 performances were calculated from the 14 sources listed in Table 10. Selection of these reports was based on the age range studied, availability, measurement protocol used and geographic representation. The studies also represent a blend of cross-sectional, mixed-longitudinal, and longitudinal data. Unweighted composite means were used because accurate information on the number of subjects within specific studies was not always available and the nature of the composite means (weighted or unweighted) reported by Espenschade was not known.

Running. The most common method used to assess running speed in children is the dash. The length of the dashes for children generally range from 30 to 60 yards and are administered by using either a running or a stationary start. By converting timed scores for the run to units of feet per second, reasonable comparisons can be made between data sets that reflect the same starting approach, although the distance of the dash will have some impact on the size of the units obtained. Therefore, to eliminate the influence of the type of start, only those studies that reported using a stationary start have been included in calculating the composite means for the post-1960 data presented in Table 9. Tests of running ability that also measure other primary components such as agility (shuttleruns, side stepping and figure eight runs) and cardiovascular endurance (distance runs) will not be reviewed here.

There is systematic improvement in the running speed of children during the

Table 9
Composite means for pre-1960 and post-1960 performance of males and females on selected motor skills

AGE	Run (Yds/Sec.)		Standing Long Jump (Inches)		Jump & Reach (Inches)		Distance Throw (Feet)	
	Pre-1960	Post-1960	Pre-1960	Post-1960	Pre-1960	Post-1960	Pre-1960	Post-1960
				MALES				
5	3.8	4.2	33.7	39.6	2.5	7.0	23.6	—
6	4.2	4.8	37.4	44.5	4.0	7.5	32.8	39.0
7	4.6	4.9	41.6	49.2	6.1	8.4	42.3	46.7
8	5.1	5.2	46.7	52.3	8.3	9.5	57.4	58.5
9	—	5.6	50.4	56.0	8.5	10.4	66.6	69.6
10	5.9	5.7	54.7	60.3	11.0	11.5	83.0	85.6
11	6.1	6.0	61.0	63.7	11.5	12.2	95.0	101.7
12	6.3	6.2	64.9	66.3	12.2	13.5	104.0	111.9
13	6.5	6.4	69.3	69.7	12.5	14.4	114.0	140.0
14	6.7	6.7	73.2	75.5	13.3	16.4	123.0	155.0
15	6.8	7.0	79.5	81.9	14.8	—	135.0	171.0
16	7.1	7.4	88.0	85.5	16.3	—	144.0	180.0
17	7.2	7.5	88.4	86.4	16.9	—	153.0	190.0
				FEMALES				
5	3.6	4.2	31.6	36.6	2.2	6.7	14.5	—
6	4.1	4.7	36.2	42.1	3.5	7.2	17.8	22.0
7	4.4	4.9	40.0	46.3	5.7	8.3	25.4	25.4
8	4.6	5.1	45.9	49.5	7.7	8.8	30.0	32.8
9	—	5.4	51.3	52.6	8.7	9.7	38.7	38.7
10	5.8	5.6	—	57.4	10.5	10.9	47.0	46.9
11	6.0	5.9	52.0	61.3	11.0	11.5	54.0	57.9
12	6.1	6.0	—	64.2	11.2	12.9	61.0	65.4
13	6.3	6.0	62.1	64.8	11.0	12.3	70.0	70.0
14	6.2	6.1	62.7	65.9	11.8	13.5	74.5	75.0
15	6.1	6.2	63.2	62.5	12.2	12.2	75.7	78.0
16	6.0	6.2	63.0	62.0	12.0	11.6	74.0	75.0
17	5.9	6.2	—	64.0	—	12.0	—	75.0

Table 10
Sources used to prepare post-1960 composite means for running, jumping and throwing skills

Source	Age Range (Years)	Run* (Dashes)	Standing Long Jump	Jump & Reach	Throw For Distance
Glasgow & Kruse (1960)	6-14[1]		X		
Johnson (1962)	6-11			X	
Cureton (1964)	7-13[2]	X	X	X	
Fleishman (1964)	13-17	X	X		
Hanson (1965)	7-12	X	X	X	X
Keogh (1965)	5-11	X	X		X
Vincent (1968)	12-17[1]			X	
Keogh (1969)	7-10, 9-12	X, X	X, X		X, X
Clarke (1971)	6-17[2]		X		
Curtis (1975)	5-12	X	X	X	X
Ellis et al. (1975)	10-16[2]		X		
AAHPERD (1976)	9-17	X	X		X
Hardin & Garcia (1982)	6-9	X	X		X
Branta et al. (1984)	5-9, 8-14		X, X	X, X	

* = Standing start   1 = Females only   2 = Males only

middle and late childhood years (Figure 4a-4d). This improvement in running speed continues during the teenage years for males (Figure 4c). The running speed of post-1960 females increases until age 15, after which time it appears to plateau (Figure 4d). This is in contrast to the pre-1960 running performance for females, where maximum speed was achieved at age 13, followed by a gradual decline thereafter. The post-1960 running speed of females more closely approximates that of the males for the age span of 5 to 11 years (Figure 4b) than did their pre-1960 running speed (Figure 4a). However, it never exceeded that of the males during either time period. The smaller discrepancy in the post-1960 male-female running performance may be the result of greater cultural stimulation for girls to be more physically active during the early and middle childhood years. In contrast, male-female running speed differences after age 11 have remained relatively unchanged.

Gender differences in the running form of school age children are small, particularly at the fourth grade level (Reuschlein & Haubenstricker, 1985). About 66% of the fourth grade boys and 64% of the fourth grade girls were rated as having good running form. However, among seventh graders only 51% of the boys and 43% of the girls met the six performance criteria for good running form. The results of this study suggest that running form does not necessarily impove as a function of maturation and experience, but that it may well deteriorate across time. Other plausible reasons for the apparent decline in form could be sampling error or observer bias, because not all subjects were assessed by the same individual.

Some interesting within-gender patterns are present in the pre-1960/post-1960 performance curves (Figure 4c-4d). For both boys and girls, post-1960 running speed was faster than pre-1960 running speed for ages 5 through 9 years and after age 14, but it was slightly lower from age 10 to 14 years. The improved performance during the early years might be explained, in part, by the earlier maturation of post-1960 children when compared to the pre-1960 children (Malina, 1975). The decline in performance from age 10 to 14 may reflect: (a) a loss of interest in events such as dashes; (b) the cumulative effects of a sedentary lifestyle; (c) the loss of middle school physical education programs; and (d) the earlier maturation of females, which often results in a loss of interest in vigorous physical activities.

The general improvement in the post-1960 running speed of males during the high school years may be a reflection of more personalized physical education offerings in high schools and greater interest in personal physical fitness. The same arguments can be advanced for high school females, although their performance stabilized at age 15. However, the lack of a decline in running performance during this time period may mean that a greater percentage of adolescent girls are remaining active today than in the decades prior to 1960.

Jumping. The jumping capacity of children and youth characteristically is assessed via the standing long jump or some form of a vertical jump. Although other methods for testing jumping ability are available (e.g. running long jump, hurdle jump, cable jump and high jump), only the first two will be presented here.

Performance on the standing long jump improves steadily until age 14 for both males and females (Figure 5a-5d). Thereafter, the performance of the males continues to improve (Figure 5c) while that of the females either declines or plateaus (Figure 5d). The male-female patterns for distance jumping are similar for both the pre-1960 (Figure 5a) and the post-1960 (Figure 5b) data. Interestingly, in contrast to running ability, male-female differences on the standing long jump during early and middle childhood (5 to 9 years) increased rather than decreased, after 1960. Comparisons between ages 9 and 13 are difficult to make due to the limited data on females available prior to 1960. Male-female differences in distance jumping at age 13 and thereafter are comparable for both data sets.

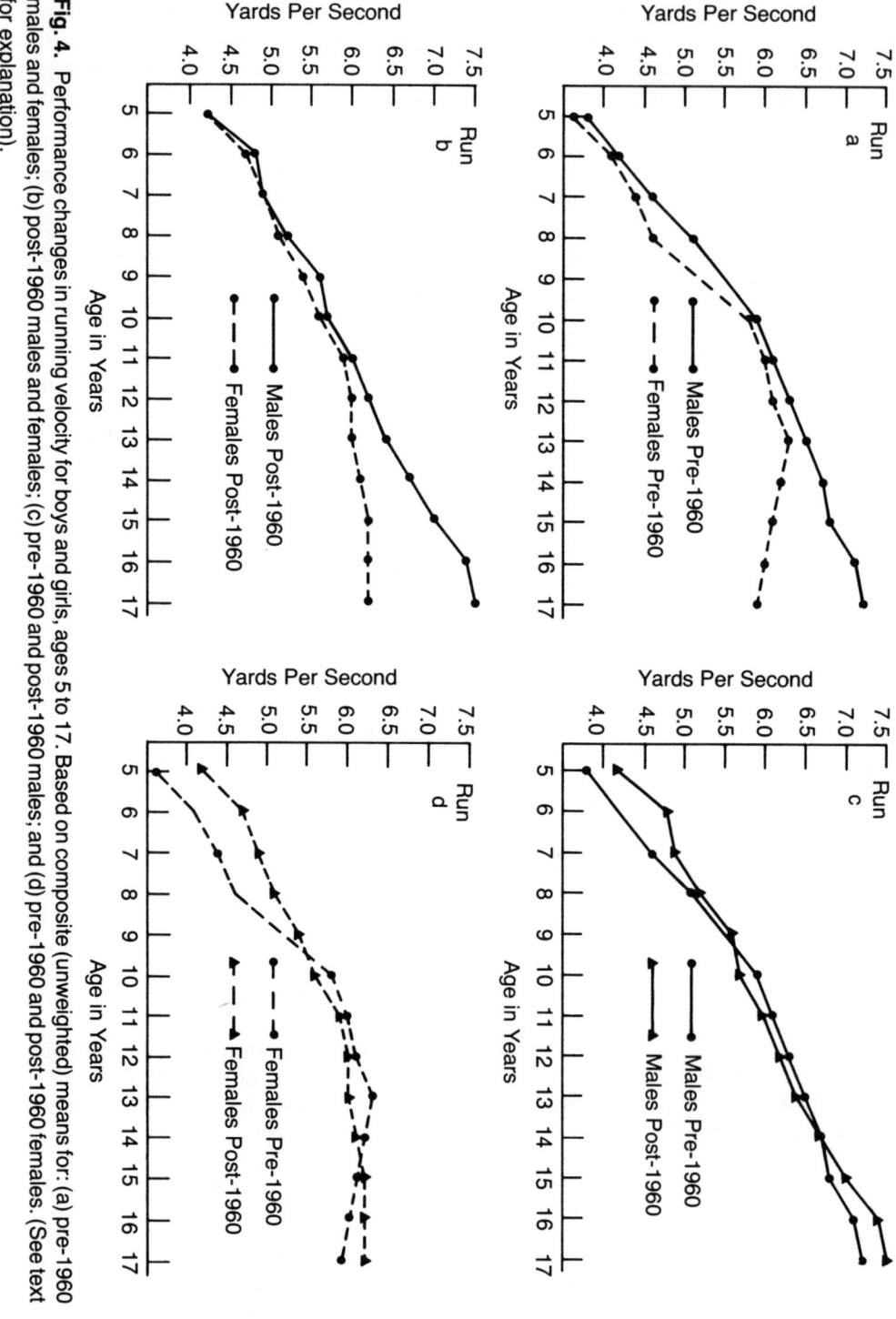

Fig. 4. Performance changes in running velocity for boys and girls, ages 5 to 17. Based on composite (unweighted) means for: (a) pre-1960 males and females; (b) post-1960 males and females; (c) pre-1960 and post-1960 males; and (d) pre-1960 and post-1960 females. (See text for explanation).

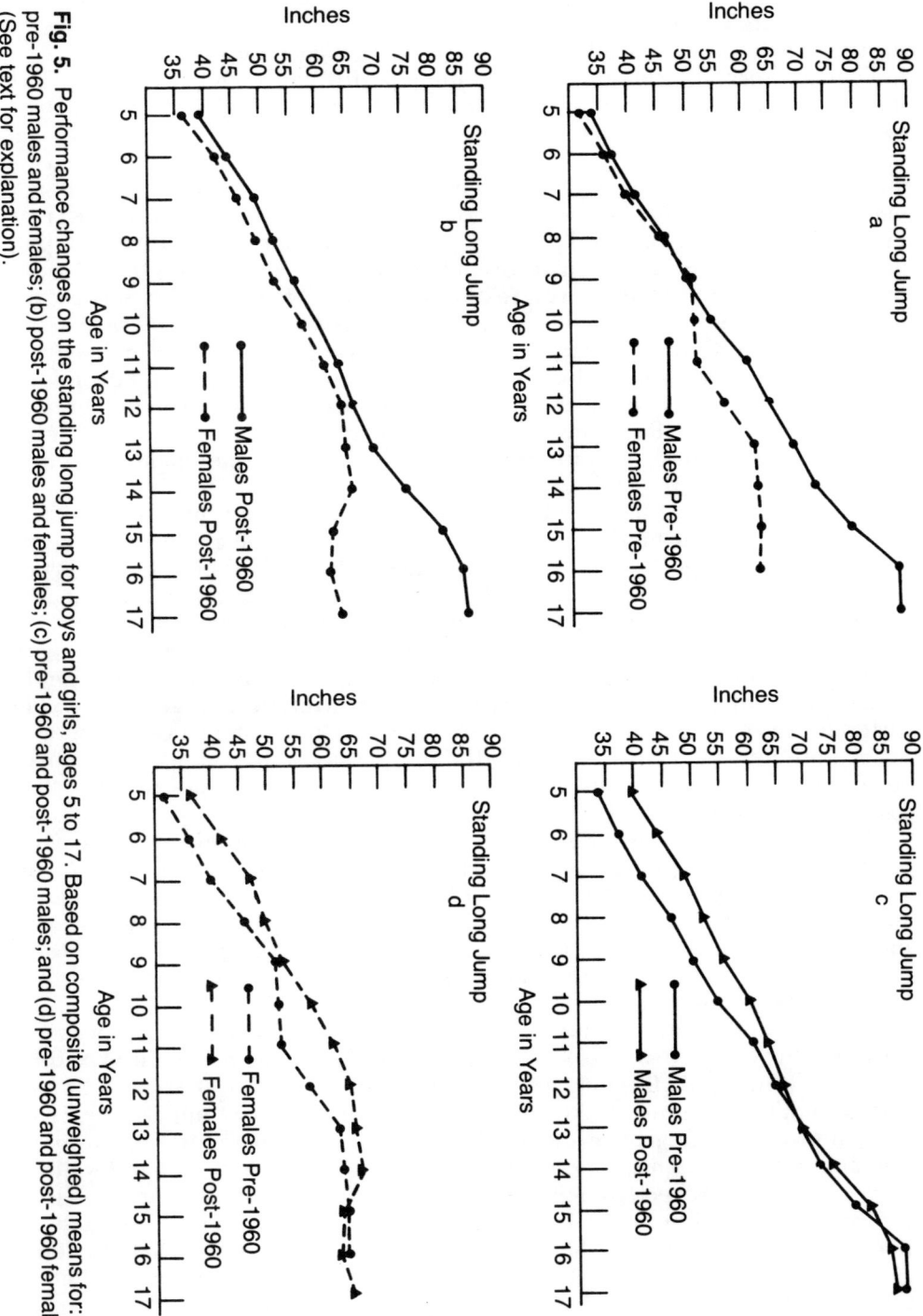

Fig. 5. Performance changes on the standing long jump for boys and girls, ages 5 to 17. Based on composite (unweighted) means for: (a) pre-1960 males and females; (b) post-1960 males and females; (c) pre-1960 and post-1960 males; and (d) pre-1960 and post-1960 females. (See text for explanation).

General improvement in jumping form occurs during the elementary and middle school years, but gender differences also are apparent (Reuschlein & Haubenstricker, 1985). Over 56% of the seventh grade boys jumped with good form, compared to only 34% of the fourth grade boys. Comparative figures for the seventh and fourth grade girls were 52 and 25%, respectively.

There is a secular trend toward better jump performance for both boys and girls during the childhood years (Figures 5c and 5d, respectively). The long jump performance of post-1960 boys exceeded that of pre-1960 boys across the age span of 5 to 15 years. The same relationship existed for pre-1960 and post-1960 girls until age 14. The secular differences were greatest during the early and middle childhood years, but diminished during late childhood. The earlier maturation of boys and girls noted previously may account for the improved jumping performance. However, since maturational differences between boys of today and those of earlier generations are greatest at age 15 (Malina, 1975), secular differences theoretically should be the greatest for boys at this age. Plausible explanations for the declining differences at the later ages are increased sedentary lifestyles for teenagers and a decline in physical education programs at the middle school level. The lack of a positive secular trend during the high school years may be due to the ceiling effect of more individuals maturing at earlier ages and/or to a greater emphasis on aerobic fitness in preference to the development of strength and power.

The patterns of performance for children on the jump and reach are similar to those for the standing long jump (Figure 6a-6d). Jumping height increased yearly for boys through age 17 and at least until age 14 for girls. The average vertical jump performance of males exceeded that of females at all ages, except age 9 on the pre-1960 data (Figure 6a and 6b). The vertical distance jumped by post-1960 males and females was greater than that jumped by their pre-1960 counterparts from age 5 through 14 years. The pattern of secular differences was similar for the males and females, which is characterized by large differences at ages 5 and 6. The differences diminished until age 10 and 11, and then systematically increased again until age 14 (Figure 6c and 6d). The previous reasons used to explain standing long jump performance also can be applied to the patterns of vertical jump performance.

The majority of fourth and seventh grade children used immature form when jumping for height (Reuschlein and Haubenstricker, 1985). Only 36% of the fourth grade girls and 39% of the seventh grade girls could demonstrate mature form when jumping vertically. The percentage of boys who jumped with good mechanics actually decreased from 48 at the fourth grade to 37 at the seventh grade. This regression in form can only be attributed to a lack of practice in this fundamental motor task.

Throwing. The throwing ability of children has been assessed in numerous ways, including throws for distance, velocity, accuracy, and frequency per unit of time. Tests of throwing for frequency and accuracy for children lack standardization across studies; therefore, it is difficult to make meaningful comparisons. However, improved performance is generally associated with increasing age. Johnson (1962) found that the mean performance of children on an underhand wall toss and catch task improved from grade 1 through grade 6. Boys also improved their performance on an accuracy throwing task from age 7 to age 9, although the performance of girls across the same age range was inconsistent (Keogh, 1965). An accuracy throwing test and a wall ball test administered by Vincent (1968) to girls 12 to 18 years of age yielded improved mean scores until age 15, but there was a slight decrease in performance at succeeding ages.

Based on the frequency of its occurrence in the scientific literature, the throw for distance is the test used most often to assess throwing ability in children. Data are available for the past half century. Because of differences in the size and

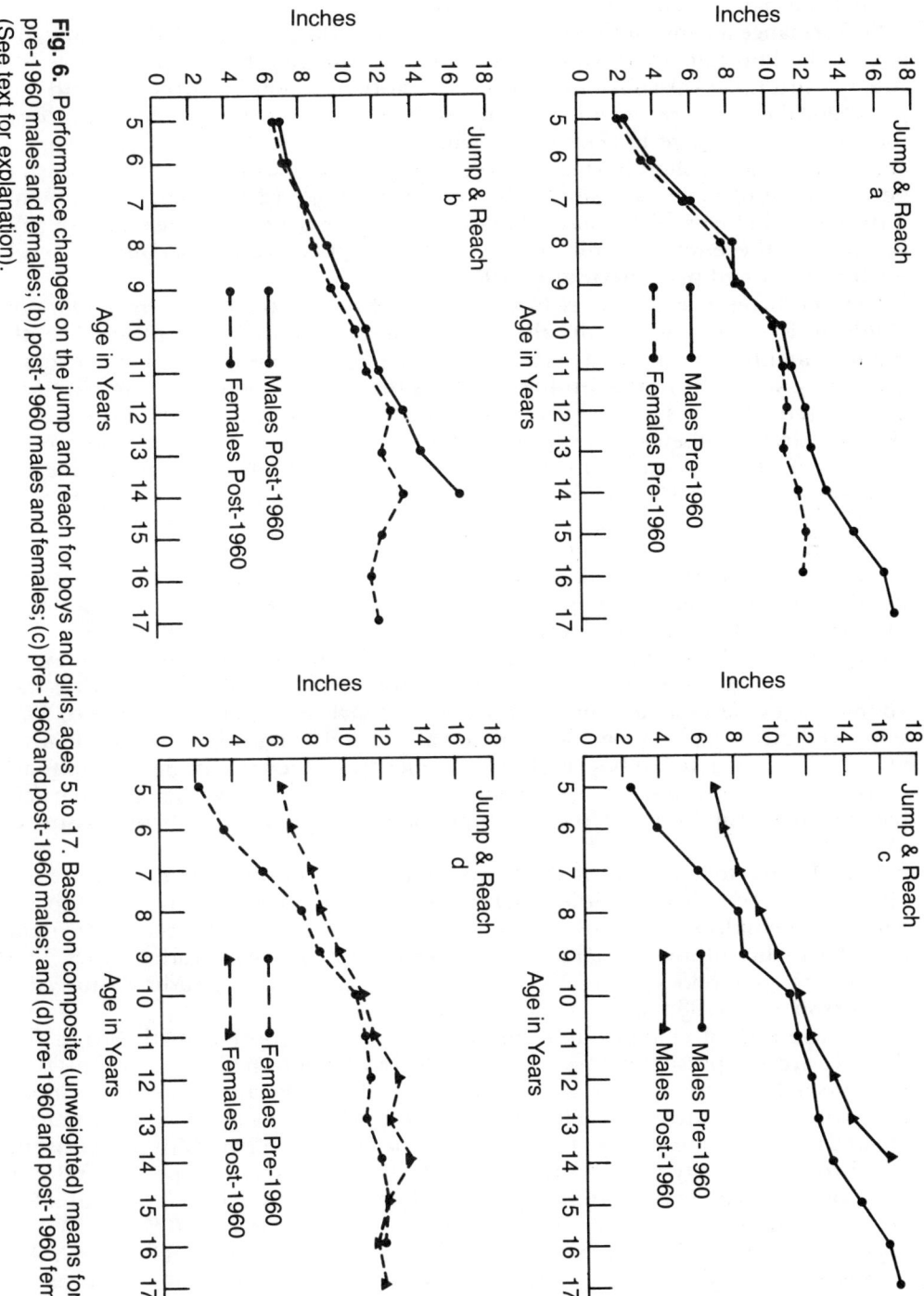

Fig. 6. Performance changes on the jump and reach for boys and girls, ages 5 to 17. Based on composite (unweighted) means for: (a) pre-1960 males and females; (b) post-1960 males and females; (c) pre-1960 and post-1960 males; and (d) pre-1960 and post-1960 females. (See text for explanation).

weight of the objects thrown, as well as in the administrative protocols used, studies included for comparative purposes were limited to those that used a 12-inch softball and similar testing procedures.

Performance means for the overhand throw for distance improved annually for both males and females during the middle and late childhood years (Table 9). Gender differences are obvious at all age categories for both the pre-1960 and the post-1960 data (Figure 7a and 7b). Throwing performance continued to improve for the males until age 17 (Figure 7c), while that of the females peaked at age 15 and then declined slightly (Figure 7d). The pre-1960 and post-1960 throwing performance of males was similar for ages 6 through 12 years, but substantial differences, in favor of the post-1960 males, were present thereafter (Figure 7c). In contrast, there was little difference in throwing performance at any age level for females tested prior to or after 1960.

Gender differences also were evident in the throwing form used by school age children. In a study where the throwing patterns of fourth, seventh and tenth grade students were assessed, 51% of the fourth grade boys, 61% of the seventh grade boys and 70% of the tenth grade boys threw with good form compared to 15, 19 and 23%, respectively, for the fourth, seventh and tenth grade girls (Reuschlein & Haubenstricker, 1985). Of interest is the fact that even though the percentage of children who threw well increased from grade to grade within each gender group, the difference between boys and girls within each grade increased as age advanced, indicating that the boys were making more progress toward mature throwing form than girls.

The lack of a positive secular trend in distance throwing during the early and middle childhood years is unexpected because of the greater relative physical size of post-1960 children. This increased size should result in higher performance scores than would be expected from the pre-1960 children. However, it may be that the existence of immature throwing patterns in more children during the younger ages places a limit on the distance a 12-inch softball can be thrown. The improved throwing performance of males after age 12 may reflect the cumulative effects of instruction that boys receive in agency sponsored programs, rather than school physical education programs. Proportionately more boys than girls participate in baseball and softball in non-school sponsored programs (Michigan Study, 1976).

Few investigators have studied the throwing velocity of children. Roberton et al. (1979) reported only five studies, including their own, that examined the velocity with which children can throw a ball. Table 11 presents a composite of the data available to the authors on ball throwing velocity or children in grades K to 8. The mean throwing velocities of 22 boys and 17 girls in a longitudinal study by Halverson et al. (1982) are depicted in Figure 8.

The age-related changes and gender differences reported in throwing for distance are also present in the throwing velocity of children (Table 11). This is to be expected because velocity, along with angle of release, are important components of distance throwing. The mean ball throwing velocity of boys increased about 212% from age 4 to age 12, or 6.59 feet per second per year. In comparison, the throwing velocity of girls increased only 172%, or 3.95 feet per second per year, over the same age span. Four-year-old boys threw a ball with 25% greater velocity than girls of a similar age. The gender gap increased to 40% during the early elementary years and expanded to 50% by grade 7. These data match the trends noted for distance throwing. Not only were significant gender differences present at an early age, but these differences became larger as the children became older.

Kicking. Although research on kicking behavior during the elementary and middle school years is limited, the evidence available reveals that rather consistent developmental trends are present during this time period. Reviews of product

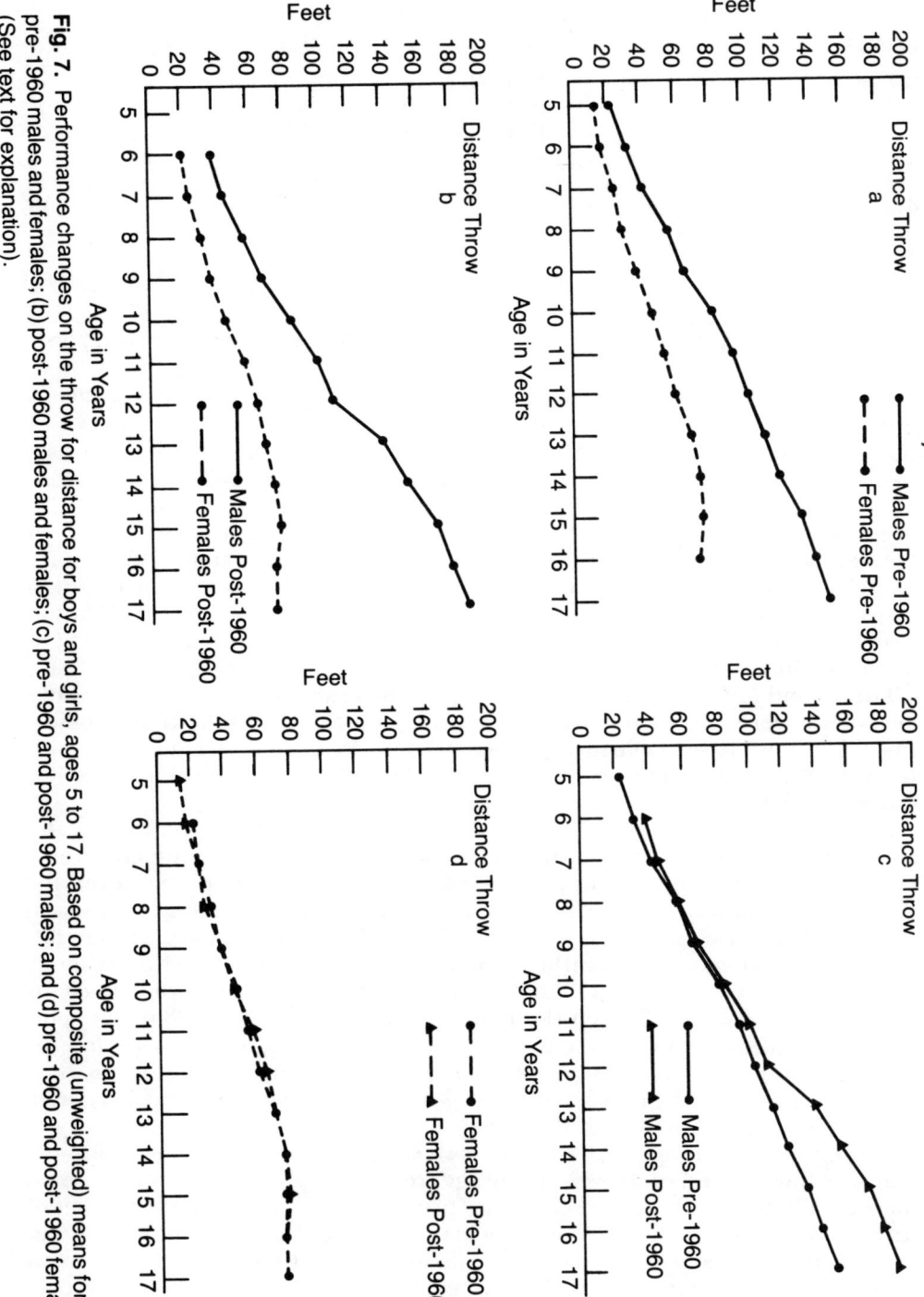

Fig. 7. Performance changes on the throw for distance for boys and girls, ages 5 to 17. Based on composite (unweighted) means for: (a) pre-1960 males and females; (b) post-1960 males and females; (c) pre-1960 and post-1960 males; and (d) pre-1960 and post-1960 females. (See text for explanation).

Table 11
Ball velocities (weighted means in ft./sec.) for the overhand throw performed by children in grades K-8

GRADE	Males		Females		Male/Female Velocity Ratio
	N	Mean	N	Mean	
K-4 yrs.	14	24.9	19	20.0	1.25
K-5 yrs.	66	35.2	59	25.3	1.40
1	95	40.4	105	29.0	1.39
2	95	46.4	130	33.0	1.41
3	—	—	72	34.5	—
4	—	—	69	38.7	—
5	—	—	61	41.9	—
6	—	—	50	47.2	—
7	22	77.6	64	51.6	1.50
8	—	—	31	54.3	—

Note: Based on data reported by Glassow & Kruse (1960), Roberton et al. (1979) and Halverson et al. (1982).

(quantitative) changes in kicking by DeOreo and Keogh (1980) and Williams (1983) show the existence of three such trends. First, despite the method of evaluation, the kicking performance of children improves with age. For example, the distance a ball can be kicked or punted by children increased annually (Jenkins, 1930; Hanson, 1965; Williams et al., 1971; Williams & Breihan, 1979). DeOreo and Keogh (1980) reported yearly gains in kicking distance of six to seven feet for boys and a range of two to seven feet for girls (Figure 9). Similar age-related gains also were obtained by Williams et al. (1971) when the criterion measure was ball kicking velocity (Figure 10), and by Latchaw (1954), Johnson (1962) and Hanson (1956) when timed or untimed ball kicking accuracy tests were administered.

The second and third trends in kicking behavior are related to gender. Boys consistently perform better than girls on product measures for kicking (Jenkins, 1930; Latchaw, 1954; Dohrman, 1964; Hanson, 1965). Gender differences in kicking skill also tended to become greater as the children became older (DeOreo & Keogh, 1980).

Gender differences in kicking proficiency often are attributed to cultural influences (Williams, 1983). These include advantages for males in practice time, experience, motivation and encouragement from support groups. However, the differences in kicking performance also may be due to the advantage of males in strength, body size and body tissues (Eckert 1973). Furthermore, gender differences in kicking form may influence quantitative outcomes. Males consistently showed better mechanics on a kicking task that was not practiced much by elementary school age children (Reuschlein & Haubenstricker, 1985). The percentage of children demonstrating good kicking mechanics, however, was low for both boys and girls, undoubtedly reflecting the lack of instruction in this skill. Only 37% of the fourth grade boys and 43% of the seventh grade boys kicked well, compared to only 25% of both the fourth and seventh grade girls.

Striking. Published reports of changes in striking behavior during the childhood years are few in number. However, the age trends and gender differences noted for the skills discussed previously also are present in striking behavior. Studies of striking with implements (bats or racquets) involving children indicate that improvement occurred with increasing age (Seils, 1951; Johnson, 1962; Williams et al., 1971; Williams & Breihan, 1979). For example, age-related increases in striking velocity for elementary age children are illustrated in Figure 11. Increased performance with age also was obtained on a timed wall volley test (Latchaw, 1954), a volleyball serve for distance (Hanson, 1965) and a volleyball serve for accuracy (Curtis, 1975).

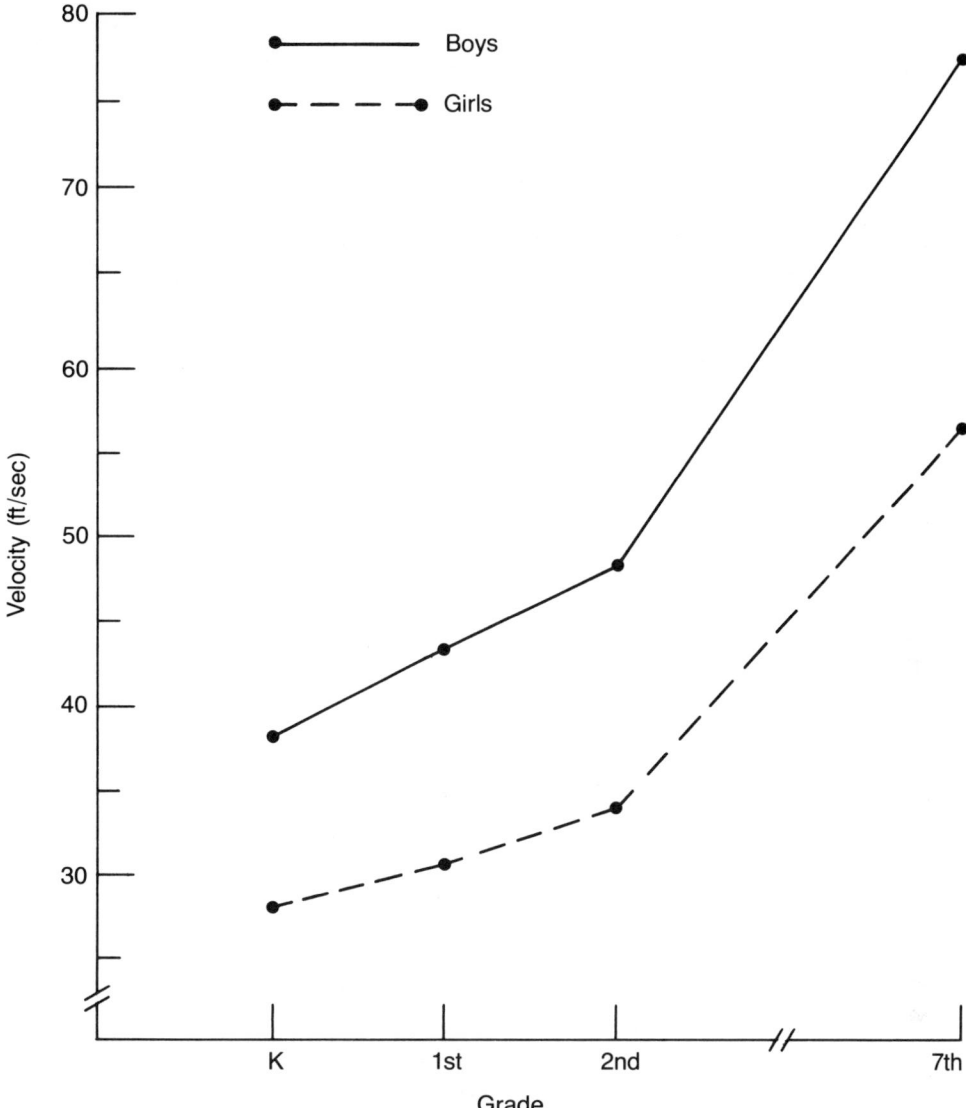

Fig. 8. Performance changes in throwing a ball for velocity—boys and girls, grades K to 7 (longitudinal data). (From "Changing motor patterns during childhood" by M. A. Roberton. In J. R. Thomas (Ed.), *Motor development during childhood and adolescence* (p. 73), 1984, Minneapolis: Burgess. Copyright 1984 by Burgess Publishing Company. Reprinted by permission.)

Improvement in striking form does not necessarily occur as a function of age. Only about 34% of both fourth and seventh grade boys demonstrated good form when striking a ball with a racquet, although 50% of the tenth grade boys showed good form. In contrast, 19% of the seventh grade girls had acceptable striking form, compared to only 9% of the fourth grade girls and 11% of the tenth grade girls (Reuschlein and Haubenstricker, 1985).

Gender differences in favor of the males were recorded in all of the studies cited above, whether the assessment focus was quantitative or qualitative in nature. Although some of the tasks may be culturally biased toward boys (e.g. the use of bats), others, such as serving a volleyball or striking one-handed with a racquet, do

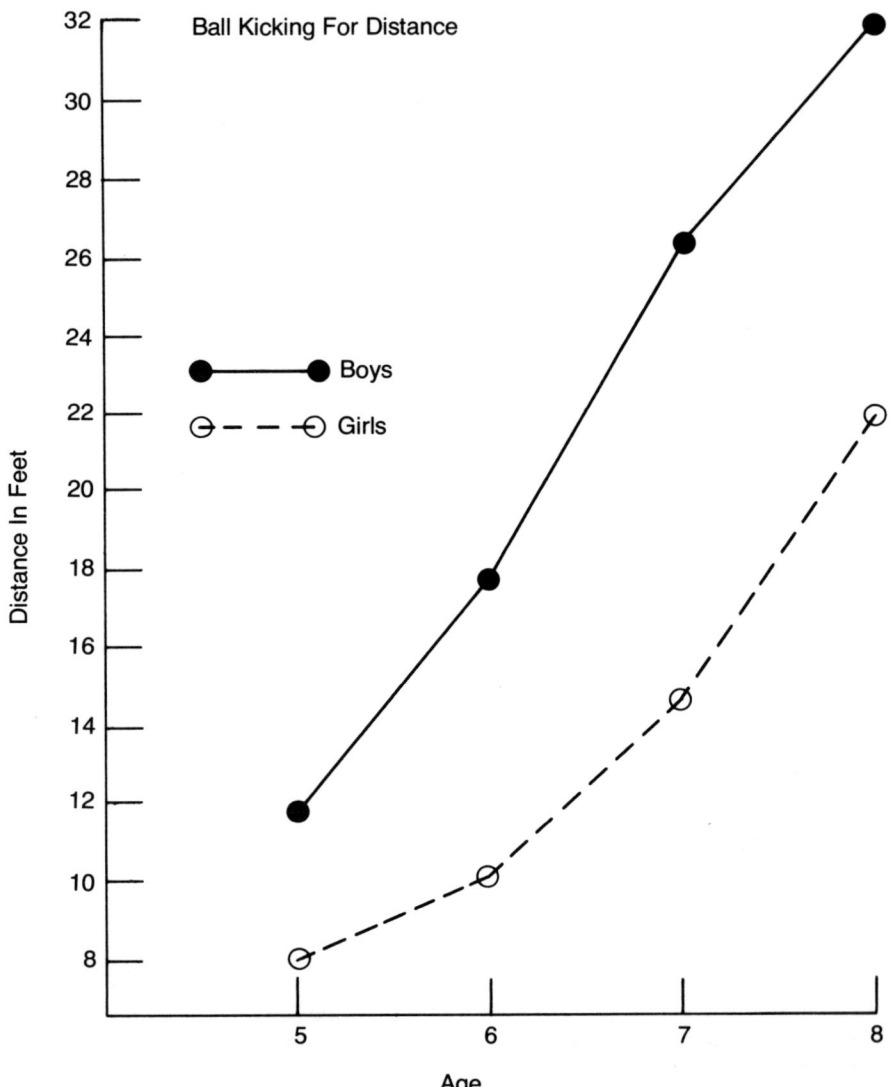

Fig. 9. Performance changes in kicking a ball for distance—boys and girls, ages 5 to 8. (From "Performance of fundamental motor tasks" by K. DeOreo & J. Keogh. In Corbin, Charles B., *A Textbook of Motor Development,* 2nd ed. © 1973, 1980 Wm. C. Brown Publishers, Dubuque, Iowa. All rights reserved. Reprinted by permission.

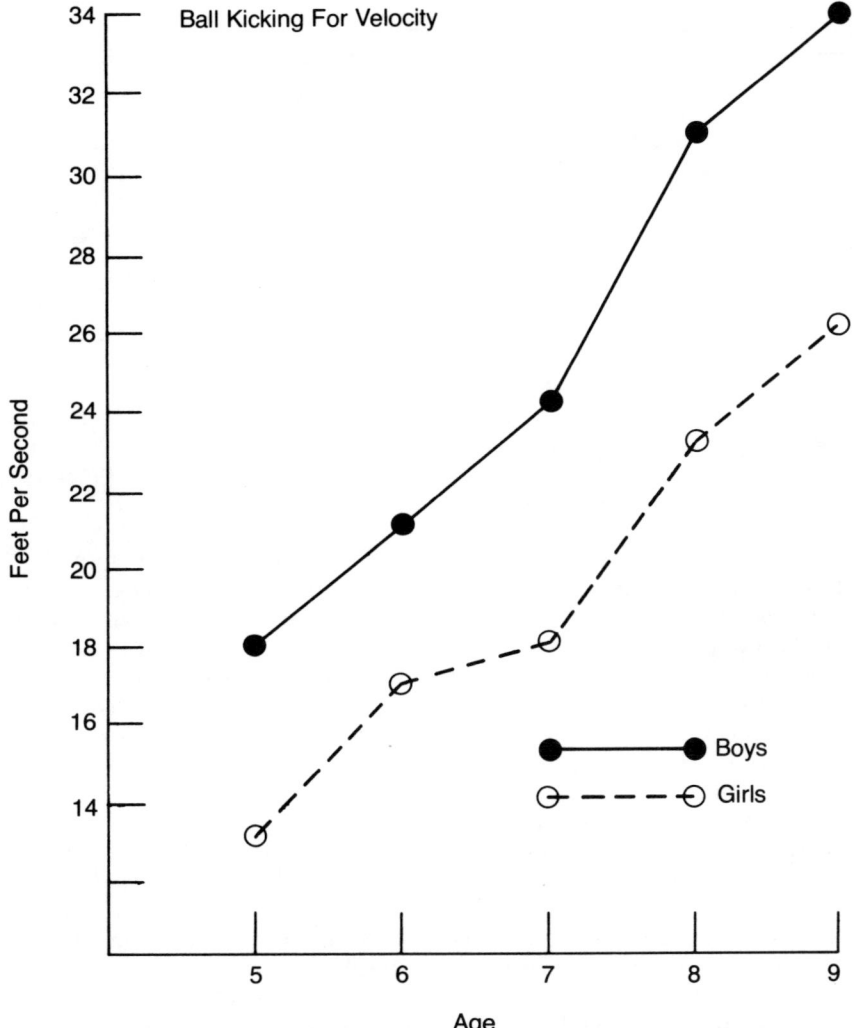

Fig. 10. Performance changes in kicking a ball for velocity—boys and girls, ages 5 to 9. (From "Performance of fundamental motor tasks" by K. DeOreo & J. Keogh. In Corbin, Charles B., *A Textbook of Motor Development,* 2nd ed. © 1973, 1980 Wm. C. Brown Publishers, Dubuque, Iowa. All rights reserved. Reprinted by permission.

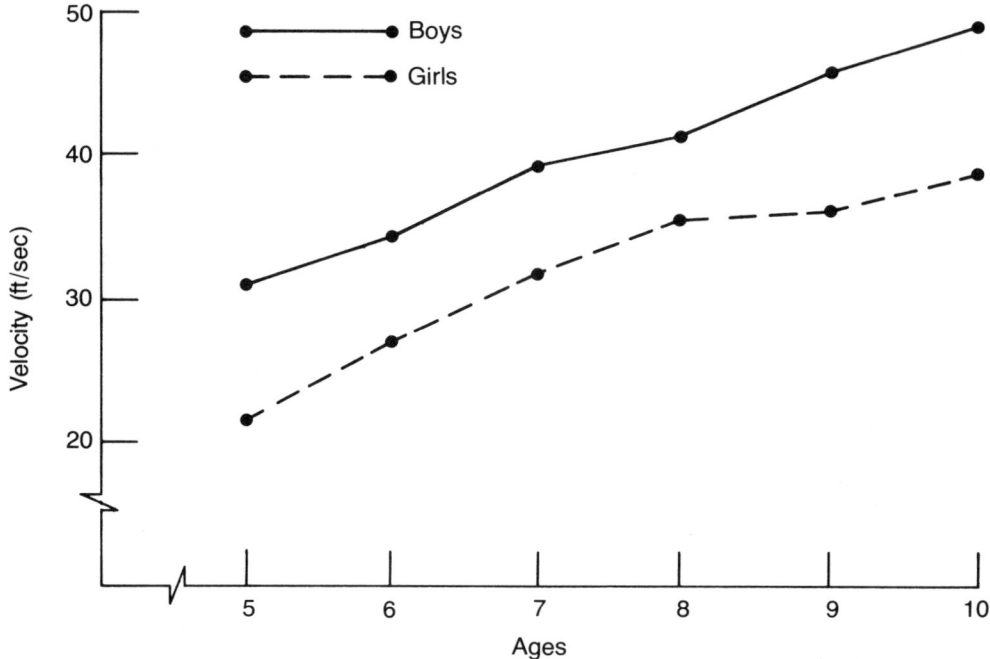

Fig. 11. Performance changes in striking a ball for velocity—boys and girls, ages 5 to 10. (From *Perceptual and motor development* (p. 254) by H. G. Williams, 1983, Englewood Cliffs, NJ: Prentice-Hall. Reprinted by permission.)

not appear to favor boys. Yet the gender differences existed. It is likely that influences other than culture were contributing to these differences.

Effects of intervention. There is general agreement that children attending elementary and middle schools can learn new motor skills and that their acquisition can be enhanced through appropriate instruction. Some improvement in the performance of skills (e.g. distance, speed, accuracy) can be expected as a function of maturation and general experience due to increased body size, strength and body coordination. However, the existence of physical education programs in schools does not guarantee adequate skill instruction or improved skill performance (Reuschlein & Haubenstricker, 1985).

Studies investigating the effects of instruction on motor skill development have produced mixed results. For example, Miller (1957) failed to obtain a differential advantage for a group of first grade children who received instruction in the overhand throw for accuracy over a comparison group that engaged in ball throwing games without instruction in throwing. However, because the nature of the instruction and the nature of the throwing games were not described, and because both groups improved significantly over twenty-six 20-minute lessons conducted within a two-month period, it is possible that the games required throwing accuracy, thereby benefitting the comparison group and offsetting the instruction for the treatment group. Certainly, the significant gains made by both groups cannot be attributed entirely to maturational factors because of the relatively short duration of the study. Extra daily training in throwing and kicking over a nine-week period did not significantly benefit a group of 8-year-old children over a control group (Dohrman, 1964). Because the time spent on throwing and kicking in the regular physical education program was not reported, it is difficult to evaluate the relative importance of the extra practice.

Other studies involving intervention have produced positive results. Whittle (1961) found that 12-year-old boys who attended schools with good physical education programs performed significantly better on various fitness and strength tasks than boys who attended schools where the physical education programs were rated as poor. Studies by Earls (1975, March), by Goldbergher, Gerney and Chamberlain (1982), and by Toole and Arink (1982), using different methods of instruction, all produced significant motor skill improvement in children beyond the levels that could be expected due to maturation and general experience. (A comprehensive review of school-based programs is provided by P. Vogel in Chapter 17.)

Summary. Performance of the fundamental motor skills that emerge during early childhood generally improves during the middle and late childhood years. This improvement occurs more consistently in product or quantitative performance than in assessments of form or qualitative performance. Boys are superior to girls in the performance of game-related skills such as running, jumping, throwing, kicking and striking. Gender differences are present during early and middle childhood and become accentuated during the late childhood and early teenage years. The secular trend toward enhanced product performance by post-1960 children is probably attributable to earlier maturation and greater opportunities for involvement in physical activities.

The capacity of children to learn gross motor skills provides strong support for the establishment of sound physical education in elementary and middle schools. The fact that not all physical education programs produce the desired changes in motor behavior underscores the need for carefully planned programs that provide specific objectives, appropriate instructional strategies, corrective feedback and objective-related evaluation. Inherent in the provision of desirable learning environments is the assumption that instruction will be provided by individuals who understand the needs and capabilities of children.

Influence of Biological Age on Motor Behavior

The distinction between chronological and developmental, or biological, age (see definitions of constructs such as skeletal and sexual maturation in Malina, Chapter 1) and the implications of using them to classify children and youth in educational programs and athletic competition has been known to physicians and educators for decades. Recognizing the difference in size and abilities of pre- and post-pubescent children of the same chronological age, C. Ward Crampton (1908) correlated their body sizes with assessments of scholarship and physical strength. In the same year Rotch wrote:

> When, however, the question of age is brought to bear on our school systems, whether in classifying and grading children as to their studies, or in pitting them against each other in athletic sports, it becomes a very serious question as to whether chronological age is a wise decision during the formative period of early life. (Rotch, 1909, p. 1197)

The relationship between developmental age and motor skill acquisition exists because of the correlation between body size, gross body coordination and cognitive ability in the performance of motor tasks and sport skills (Espenschade, 1940; Jones, 1949; Malina and Rarick, 1973). The association between developmental age and motor skill performance is greatest during the pubertal years, with some indication that the relationship becomes less direct when the combined events of skeletal maturity in earlier maturing individuals and a catch-up phenomenon in the later maturing subjects occurs in late adolescence (Malina, 1982). Thus, adolescent children within a chronological age group who excel in motor tasks or sports skills requiring combinations of strength, power, and total body coordination are also likely to be advanced in developmental age.

There appears to be a differential relationship between developmental age and proficiency in gross motor tasks and sports skills, depending on the gender and age of the subjects and the sport and level of competition being studied. Rarick and Oyster (1964) reported that skeletal maturity was not a factor when explaining individual differences in the strength and motor proficiency of second grade boys and girls. Howell and Seefeldt (1981) detected a significant relationship between skeletal ages and seven motor performance tests for 9-year-old boys, but not for the age groups at 10, 11, and 12 years. However, the more mature boys in each age group were taller and heavier than their later maturing peers. Clarke and Peterson (1962) reported that outstanding male athletes at both the elementary and junior high levels had higher mean skeletal ages than males who did not participate in athletics. Strength also was a consistent indicator of athletic ability.

Numerous reports document the close association between advanced biological age and successful sports experience in children and youth. Krogman (1959) noted that 71% of the boys who participated in the 1955 Little League world series had skeletal ages in advance of their chronological ages; nearly one-half had skeletal ages a year or more in advance of their chronological ages. Hale (1956) reported that nearly one-half of the boys who participated in the 1955 Little League World Series, all chronologically 12 years or younger, were postpubescent in terms of secondary sex characteristics. Similarly, Rochelle, Kelleher and Thornton (1961) noted that 71% of the boys on a junior high school football team had skeletal ages in advance of their chronological ages. Cummins, Garand and Borysyk (1972) reported that skeletal age was a better predictor of success in track and field events for boys and girls than was the combination of height and weight, without any indication of maturity in the prediction equations.

There are indications that the advantages of advanced biological age in acquiring gross motor skills may be temporary and specific to certain skills or sports. Attainment of a critical level of central nervous system organization, in combination with a ceiling effect of the association between skeletal age and motor prowess, may permit individuals who were relatively unskilled in childhood to exceed the proficiency level of their age peers during adolescence. Clark (1968) reported that coaches' ratings of boys changed markedly during a longitudinal study of athletic ability. Of the boys who were rated as outstanding athletes between 9 and 15 years, only 25% received this rating at both the elementary and junior high school level. Forty-five percent of the sample were rated as outstanding in elementary, but not in junior high school, and 30% were rated as outstanding in junior high, but not in elementary school. Thus, an over-emphasis on sports skills in childhood, to the detriment of other dimensions in cognitive and social development, and the converse situation, deprivation of opportunities to learn motor skills because of an initially low proficiency level, should be avoided for several reasons: (1) the accuracy of prediction motor proficiency or foretelling success in sports during childhood and adolescence is low; and, (2) the benefits of learning motor tasks and sports skills are related to the relative, and not the absolute, levels of achievement (see Chapters 3, 10, 12, 14 and 18).

Trends in biological maturity levels for male sports participants are available in football, ice hockey and soccer. Football players apparently require the muscular strength and power associated with the mesoendormorphic physique and are, therefore, early maturing (Rochelle et al., 1961; Clarke, 1971). Ice hockey players in the age range of 12 to 15 years appear to be average or slightly delayed, biologically (Cunningham, Telford & Sward, 1976; Kotulan, Riznickova & Placheta, 1980). Swimmers were generally slightly advanced in skeletal age (Bugyi and Kausz, 1970) and, within a group, those who were most proficient had the most advanced skeletal ages (Thompson, Blanksby & Doran, 1974; Kanetz & Bar-Or, 1974; Malina, 1982).

Most of the data relating biological maturity to the sports performance of girls involves swimming, gymnastics and track. Limited data on the maturity of team sport participants is likely due to the short history of girls in agency-sponsored and interscholastic sports. Girl swimmers matured at average or slightly advanced ages (Astrand, Engstrom, Eriksson, Karlberg, Nylander, Saltin & Thoren, 1963; Bugyi and Kausz, 1970; Thompson et al., 1974; Bar-Or, 1975; Malina, 1982; Bernink et al., 1983). There was an inverse relationship between skill level and maturity in gymnastics; gymnasts who were the most skillful had the greatest maturational delay. Track athletes tended to be of average maturity or slightly delayed, depending on the skill in which they participated (Cummins et al., 1972; Malina, 1983).

This review indicates that developmental age shares its influence on motor skill acquisition with such variables as gender, body build, body composition, specific requirements of the task or sport and age of the performer. All of these determinants must be considered whenever one attempts to predict the outcome of a learner's interaction with a motor task. Predictions of motor performance or success in sports based on biological maturity alone are apt to be incorrect and, therefore, detrimental to the athletes involved.

Variability and Stability of Motor Behavior

Two important issues confront those who are concerned with the development of motor behavior in children and youth. One issue is the variability that is observed in motor performance both within and among individuals as they grow and develop. The second issue is the degree of stability that exists in the motor behavior of maturing children. An understanding of both variability and stability is necessary if parents and educators are to expedite the development of gross motor skills in boys and girls.

Variability in Motor Behavior

Variability or differences in motor behavior among children can be attributed to many influences. Among these are chronological age, gender, interest, motivation, capacity to learn, innate motor abilities, biological maturity, physical size, physique, body tissue composition, ethnic background, opportunity for practice, cultural support and encouragement, and mental or physical impairment due to injury, disease or genetic defects. While many of these influences are correlated (e.g. chronological age and biological maturity, cultural support and opportunity for practice) the relationships are not perfect. Therefore, differences in the performance of specific motor tasks will occur even when one or more of the influences cited above are held constant (e.g. age and gender).

Mean differences in the performance of selected motor skills as a function of age and gender were presented in previous sections of this chapter. Knowledge of the average skill performance of boys and girls at various age levels is helpful in establishing general expectations for group performance and in making comparisons between individuals and the group of reference. However, individuality in motor behavior is of greater importance because group means only reflect the collective change in the group. It is the behavior of the individual that must be changed in order for group behavior to change. Individual differences in motor behavior are present at any age level because all children do not develop biologically at the same rate; they are not reared in the same cultural environment; and, they do not possess the same genetic endowments. Parents and educators must be aware of these differences so that appropriate opportunities for skill learning and practice are provided to all children.

Individual differences exist throughout the human lifespan. They are already present in the neonate (Ames, 1966). For example, Apgar ratings (Apgar, 1953) of neonates obtained immediately after birth range anywhere from zero to 10.

Approximately 6% of the newborns are severely depressed (Apgar scores of 0-2), 24% are moderatley depressed (Apgar scores of 4-7) and 70% are in good to excellent condition (Apgar scores of 8-10). Apgar ratings are based on heart rate, respiratory effort, muscle tone, reflex irritability and color. Of these, muscle tone has the highest relationship with fine and gross motor coordination at 4 years of age (Edwards, 1968).

The extent of variability in motor behavior during infancy is well illustrated in Bayley's Scale for Infant Development (Bayley, 1969). For example, the mean age for walking without assistance is 11.7 months, but some infants walk alone as early as 9 months, whereas others do not walk alone until they are 17 months of age. Moreover, the average child can jump off a surface with both feet simultaneously at about 24 months, while others cannot do this until they are over 30 months old. Thus, the cumulative effect of various influences can result in a range of over 12 months for the development of specific motor skills during infancy.

Individual variation in performing motor skills continues to increase during early childhood. Examples of the extent of performance variation for young children is depicted in the B graphs of Figure 3. (The vertical bars represent 1 SD above and below the mean, with the bar for girls preceding that for the boys in each pair). Note that the dispersion of performance scores around the mean often greatly exceeds the average annual gains in performance. Thus, there is substantial overlap in performance from one age level to the next. For example, advanced 3-year-old boys may be able to jump farther or throw a tennis ball for greater distances than can poorly skilled or developmentally delayed 6-year-old boys. However, at the other extreme are the mature 6-year-old boys whose performance on skills greatly exceeds that of underdeveloped 3-year-old boys. There also is considerable performance overlap between boys and girls within the same age categories. This suggests that young boys and girls can be grouped together for participation in motor activities. However, even at these young ages, boys tend to show greater variability than girls and are the best performers on skills that require muscular strength and power (e.g. jumping and throwing). On the other hand, girls exhibit a greater range of performance on tasks demanding balance and coordination (e.g. one-foot balance and catching).

The magnitude of individual differences during middle and late childhood varies according to the nature of the task and whether or not boys and girls are grouped together for purposes of analyses. Longitudinal data from the motor performance study at Michigan State University presented in Figure 12 and 13 illustrate these facts (Haubenstricker & Ewing, 1985, April). Variability on the jump and reach (Figure 12), when boys and girls are examined separately, is relatively stable from age 8 through age 12 and then increases. However, when the performance variability of both gender groups is combined, there is a general increase in performance across the entire age span. This increase can be seen by visually comparing the top of the bar for males and the bottom of the bar for females at each age level across the age span presented. In contrast, on tasks where the opportunity for improvement diminishes with age (e.g. short dashes), within-gender variability declines, but combined gender variability remains relatively constant across age categories (Figure 13). The existence of significant gender differences during middle and late childhood, despite a substantial gender overlap in performance levels (Haubenstricker and Ewing, 1985, April), suggests that not all boys and girls will benefit equally when motor skills are taught coeducationally, particularly when the skills depend primarily on strength and power—nor will all boys and girls benefit equally when they are grouped by gender. The magnitude of within-gender and between-gender variation in skill performance indicates that ability grouping may be the most efficient way to present motor skill learning situations.

The impact of biological factors and cultural influences on the motor perfor-

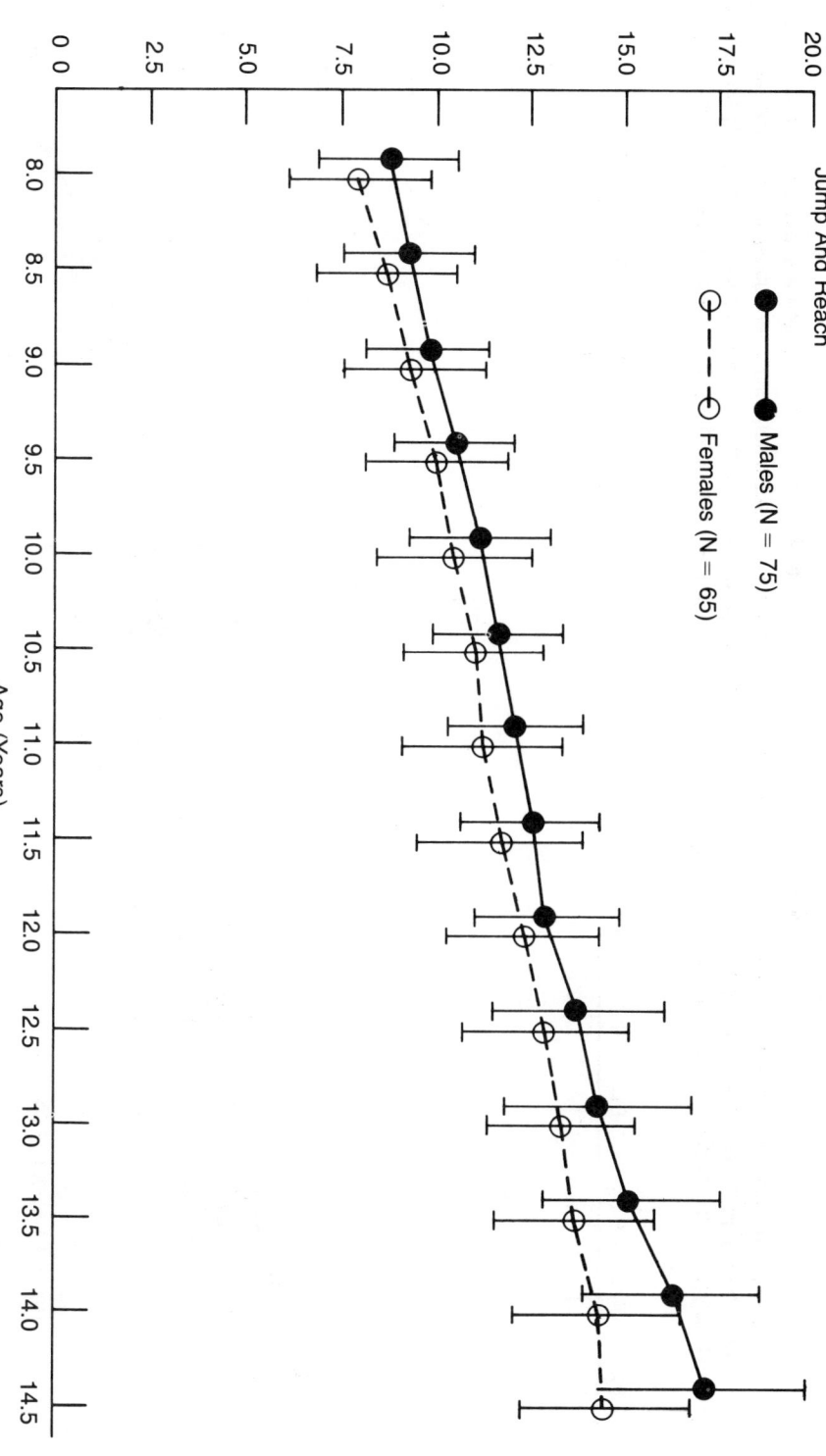

Fig. 12 Means and standard deviations for performance on the jump and reach (Motor Performance Study—Longitudinal data, Michigan State University). (From "Predicting motor performance from changes in body size and shape" by J. Haubenstricker & M. Ewing, April, 1985. Paper presented at the annual convention of the American Alliance of Health, Physical Education, Recreation and Dance, Atlanta, GA. Reprinted by permission of the authors).

Acquisition of Motor Skills 85

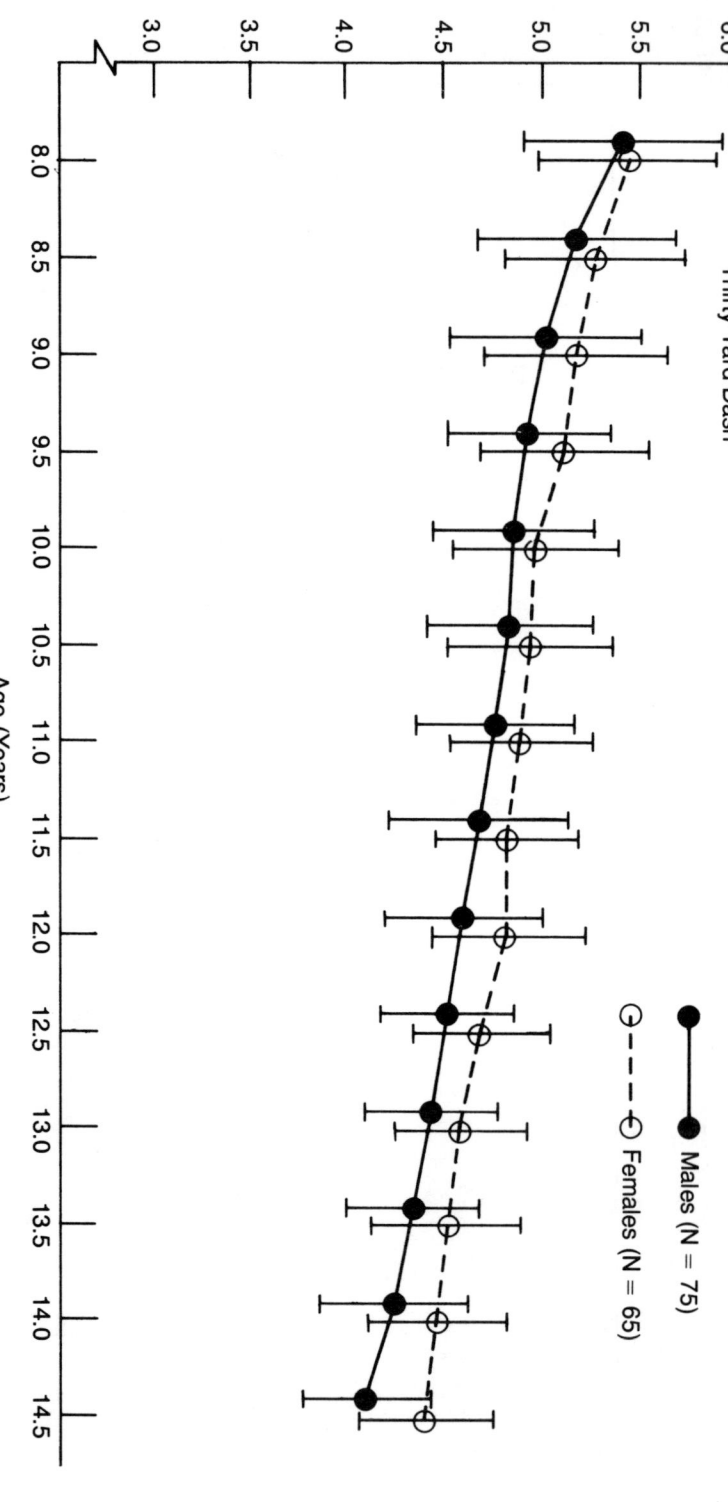

Fig. 13. Means and standard deviations for performance on the thirty yard dash (Motor Performance Study—Longitudinal data, Michigan State University). (From "Predicting motor performance from changes in body size and shape" by M. Haubenstricker & M. Ewing, April, 1985. Paper presented at the annual convention of the American Alliance of Health, Physical Education, Recreation and Dance, Atlanta, GA. Reprinted by permission of the authors).

mance of children has been discussed elsewhere in this book and therefore will not be considered in detail here. However, each factor or influence can contribute to variability in motor behavior. Generally, individuals subjected to the extremes of these variables are influenced the most, either favorably or unfavorably. For example, children who are biologically more mature, more muscular, taller and stronger characteristically perform motor skills better than late maturing, obese, shorter and weaker children (Malina & Rarick, 1973). Similarly, children who are encouraged by parents to learn motor skills, who possess the necessary attributes to learn (interest, motivation, attention, motor abilities, etc.), and who receive the opportunity to practice, obviously should be more skillful than children who receive no encouragement, who are deficient in the necessary attributes, and who do not have the opportunity to practice motor skills (Schmidt, 1982). The existence of ethnic differences in motor performance during the elementary and middle school years also contributes to this variability (Malina, 1973). Finally, the mentally impaired (Rarick, 1973a) and the learning disabled (Haubenstricker et al., 1981, April) consistently perform below the level of their normal counterparts.

Intraindividual variability, the degree to which an individual's performance on a task varies from trial to trial, is another dimension of motor behavior that is subject to numerous influences. Espenschade and Eckert (1980) have classified these influences into two categories: maturational and learning. On tasks that measure basic abilities which are controlled primarily by maturation (e.g. simple reaction time), individual performance variability occurs relative to the degree of maturation (Eckert & Eichorn, 1977) so that the ratio of variability to the mean is nearly constant across age cateogories. In other words, both the average performance of the individual and the amount of variability about that mean decrease (or increase) proportionately as age advances.

On tasks where a learning component is involved, intraindividual variability should decrease (or increase) beyond expectations based on maturational influences (Eckert, 1974). Indeed, one of the characteristics of skilled behavior is consistency in performance (i.e. reduced variability from trial-to-trial). Bruner (1973) regarded reduction in variability, greater anticipation and increased economy of effort as the hallmarks of skill acquisition. The amount of variability that an individual exhibits is also related to the complexity of motor task. Variability is likely to be greater in complex tasks than in simple tasks (Eckert, 1974).

Increased consistency or reduced intraindividual variability is desirable in motor behavior when the serial order of its movement components is correct and appropriately timed. (One also can become more consistent in performing a skill incorrectly.) Gentile (1972) referred to this aspect of skill acquisition as fixation. It is the phase of skill learning where appropriate movement patterns are assembled, integrated and performed in a relatively stable or constant environment. However, another phase, of skill acquisition involves diversification. In this phase the individual must learn to adapt or vary the skill to different situations of increasing complexity. This process may involve relatively minor adjustments, such as a diver adapting to a strange diving board or a golfer adjusting to the presence of dew on the golf green. In contrast, a task may require major adjustments, such as the transfer of a skill from a simple practice drill to an intensely competitive game. In this sense, increased individual variability is desirable, because flexibility or adaptability (i.e. the ability to diversify a skill to meet new demands) also is a characteristic of skilled performance (Sage, 1984). Unfortunately, not all children can learn to fixate and diversify motor skills to the same degree or at the same rate.

Summary. Variability in motor behavior is present at birth and continues through the childhood years. It is influenced by both maturational and environmental factors. Variability generally increases among children as they mature, but may decrease as maturational limits are reached or opportunities for improvement on a specific skill diminish. Within group variability on a skill generally increases when gender groups are combined. Intraindividual variability decreases as basic skills are learned; however, adaptability to new situations should increase with age and experience.

Parents, teachers, and coaches who seek to change the motor behavior of children should understand the constructs of intraindividual and interindividual variability. Children learn motor skills at different rates and to varying degrees of consistency and efficiency. There is considerable overlap in skill performance between adjacent age categories and between gender groups at given age levels. These, coupled with the existence of gender differences across age levels and extreme performance differences within gender groups at specific ages, signal the need for individualized learning opportunities for children. In the school setting, learning objectives, instructional strategies and organizational procedures should reflect the individuality of motor development in children.

Stability in Motor Behavior

Stability in motor behavior is defined as consistency in performance over a period of time. The term does not require that the performance scores of children must remain constant, because performance scores on motor skills are expected to improve as children advance in age. Rather, stability refers to the maintenance of one's relative position on a performance continuum within a group when serial measurements are taken over a period of years. For example, is the fastest 6-year-old runner still the fastest runner at 9 years? Does the slowest runner remain the slowest runner across successive years?

Stability is related to prediction. If performance on a motor skill is stable, then the accuracy of predicting a child's future performance on that skill is increased. However, if performance is unstable, there is little chance of correctly predicting future performance. The stability or instability of motor behavior has implications for parents and educators because unstable skills require a different set of expectations and strategies than skills that are stable.

How consistent must performance be in order for it to be stable? Can performance be stable, but not highly predictable? Bloom (1964) established a correlation coefficient of +.50 for assessment scores obtained at an interval of at least one year as the minimum requirement for a characteristic to be stable (e.g. performance on a specific skill). A coefficient of this magnitude may be useful for general group comparisons on skill performance, but it is of little value in predicting individual performance. Coefficients of +.90 or higher are required to make reasonably accurate predictions of individual performances on a selected skill.

The determination of stability in motor behavior requires longitudinal study because data on the same individuals must be obtained during the age span of interest. Unfortunately, longitudinal studies of motor skills are few in number. Moreover, the short duration of the studies and the small number of skills examined are additional limitations. Reviews on the stability of motor skills have recently been completed by Rarick (1973b), Branta, Haubenstricker and Seefeldt (1984), and Keogh and Sugden (1985).

The motor performance of children is not very stable, and therefore not very predictable across time. Coefficient of stability for various motor skills and fitness tasks are summarized in Tables 12 and 13. Although Bloom's criterion for stability is inadequate for predicting motor performance, it can be useful for comparing the relative stability of various motor skills. Also of interest is the consistency with which boys and girls, representing various population groups, perform on the motor skills.

Running. The running behavior of school age children is stable over an interval of at least two years (Table 12). For periods beyond two years, the available data are conflicting. Early reports by Espenschade (1940) and by Rarick and Smoll

Table 12
Coefficients of stability for basic motor skill performance in children and youth

Source	Boys 1	Boys 2	Boys 3	Boys 4	Boys 5	Boys 6	Girls 1	Girls 2	Girls 3	Girls 4	Girls 5	Girls 6
Run (Dash)												
Espenschade (1940) 13-16 yrs.	56 (50)	57 (45)	49 (46)				52 (55)	55 (55)	— (—)			
Glassow & Kruse (1960) Gr. 1-6							68 (82)	— (—)	74 (—)	84 (—)	70 (—)	
Rarick & Smoll (1967) 7-12 yrs.	78	69	46	42	38		93	91	78	83	92	
Branta et al. (1984) 5-10 yrs.	68	49	57	52	52		57	41	39	41	16	
8-14 yrs.	71	60	63	74	64	46	54	53	42	38	25	44
Standing Long Jump												
Espenschade (1940) 13-16 yrs.	68 (65)	57 (57)	72 (60)				58 (68)	56 (68)	68 (—)			
Glassow & Kruse (1960) Gr. 1-6							67 (79)	— (—)	67 (—)	61 (—)	74 (—)	
Ellis et al. (19) 10-16 yrs.	(81)	(73)	(63)	(54)	(47)	34						
Rarick & Smoll (1967) 7-12 yrs.	78	85	66	53	48		90	81	75	70	71	
Keogh (1969) 6-9 yrs.	75 (70)	57 (62)	60 (59)				67 (62)	44 (64)	70 (63)			
8-11 yrs.	78 (76)	87 (76)	73 (76)				50 (73)	62 (71)	59 (65)			
Branta et al. (1984) 5-10 yrs.	54	52	56	46	46		45	41	32	49	38	
8-14 yrs.	74	69	75	70	64	62	72	81	71	60	60	54
Jump and Reach												
Espenschade (1940) 13-16 yrs.	47 (54)	53 (46)	48 (46)				42 (50)	56 (48)	— (—)			
Branta et al (1984) 5-10 yrs.	62	36	42	37	43		61	40	37	22	31	
8-14 yrs	58	45	48	53	39	48	67	69	54	48	49	45
Distance Throw												
Espenschade (1940) 13-16 yrs.	81 (69)	67 (65)	75 (74)				81 (86)	77 (81)	84 (—)			
Keogh (1969) 6-9 yrs.	74 (78)	69 (74)	61 (71)				65 (59)	54 (40)	33 (25)			
8-11 yrs.	80 (85)	80 (81)	68 (76)				76 (73)	61 (69)	68 (69)			

Table 12 (continued)
Coefficients of stability for basic motor skill performance in children and youth

Source	Boys						Girls					
	1	2	3	4	5	6	1	2	3	4	5	6
Velocity Throw												
Glassow & Kruse (1960) Gr. 1-6							(72)	(—)	(—)	(—)	(—)	
Rarick & Smoll (1967) 7-12 yrs.	50	58	48	31	50		55	36	46	53	11	
Roberton et al. (1979) Gr. K-2	77	70					65	68				
	(77)	(—)					(69)	(—)				
Halverson et al. (1982) Gr. K-7	80	79	—	—	62ª	37ᵇ	92	95	—	—	85ª	84ᵇ
	(79)	(—)	(—)	(—)	(—)	(—)	(93)	(—)	(—)	(—)	(—)	(—)
Target Throw												
Espenschade (1940) 13-16 yrs.	46	25	—				50	39	—			
	(32)	(25)	(—)				(36)	(30)	(—)			

Note: All coefficients have been rounded to the nearest hundredth and decimals have been omitted. Coefficients without parentheses are individual values representing the relationship between performance at the first stage or grade listed and performance at successive age intervals (for Rarick & Smoll the comparisons are from age 12 forward). Coefficients within parentheses are composite means of two or more coefficients across the various age parings included in a study.

ªValue for Grade 2-7 interval.   ᵇValue for Grade 1-7 interval.

(1967) show the performance of boys to be unstable beyond two years. However, Branta et al. (1984) recently reported that the performance of boys running short dashes was stable for intervals of up to five years. Findings for females were the reverse of those reported for males. Although Glassow & Kruse (1960) and Rarick & Smoll (1967) reported that the running behavior of girls was stable over a period of five years, Branta and her associates discovered performance to be unstable after one or two years. The reason for this conflict between the two sets of data is not readily apparent because three of the studies involved midwestern children (Espenschade's study is the exception) and included approximately the same age groups.

Jumping. An assessment of stability in jumping horizontally and vertically can be made from available longitudinal data. Performance on the standing long jump was more stable for both boys and girls than was their performance in running short distances. Of the eight age groups for whom data are available (see Table 12), only the two youngest groups (Keogh, 1969; Branta et al. 1984) failed to show stability in jumping performance over a four year interval. Furthermore, there is little difference in the magnitude of the stability coefficients between the males and females. However, the coefficients are generally higher for older than for younger children. Thus, long jump performance from middle childhood to late childhood and early adolescence is more stable than it is from early childhood to the middle childhood years. In contrast to the standing long jump, performance on the vertical jump is quite unstable. Only the older female group of Branta et al. (1984) demonstrated stable jump and reach performance over a three year interval.

Throwing. The degree of stability in the throwing behavior of children and adolescents is related to the nature of the throwing skill. Performance on the throw for distance is quite stable for children, except for young girls (Keogh, 1969) and adolescents. The magnitude of the correlation coefficients also is quite high, indicating that more individuals will maintain their relative positions on this task over an extended number of years. Throwing velocity is less consistent than throwing for distance. Although most of the studies (Table 12) reported the throwing velocity of children to be stable over two years, there is less agreement concerning its stability over longer time intervals (Rarick & Smoll, 1967; Halverson et al., 1982). The limited data on throwing accuracy suggest that it is not a stable characteristic in children (Espenschade, 1940).

Motor Abilities. Longitudinal data on tasks used to assess basic motor abilities and fitness components provide opportunities to determine their relative stability. These tasks (presented in Table 13) include the Brace test (basic motor abilities), 50-foot hop (coordination and power), 30-yard agility run (agility and power), 400-foot shuttle run (agility and muscular endurance), flexed arm hang (strength and muscular endurance), timed sit-ups (strength and muscular endurance), and the sit-and-reach (flexibility).

Performance on the Brace test (a battery of individual tasks presumed to measure various innate abilities) is relatively stable over the age period of 13 to 16 years (Espenschade, 1940). In contrast, consistency in performing the 50-foot hop is much less than that for the Brace test. Many of the individual coefficients of stability fail to meet the +.50 criterion. However, the average coefficients (in parentheses) suggest that performance across certain age group combinations may be stable for intervals of up to three years.

Data from the 30-yard agility run and the 400-foot shuttle run indicate that older children are more stable in their performance on these tasks than younger children (Branta et al., 1984). Moreover, among the older children, the boys tended to perform with greater consistency and to maintain this stability over a longer period than girls, although the accuracy of predicting the future performance of either males or females on these tasks is low.

Children 8 years of age and older demonstrated stable performance on the flexed arm hang and on sit-ups for intervals of one to five years (Table 13). Boys were more predictable in their performance of these skills than girls (Branta et al., 1984). However, the performance of the younger group of children was not stable.

Measures of flexibility obtained on young children were stable for only one year (girls) or two years (boys). In contrast, flexibility scores obtained on 8-year-old children were still stable when correlated with measures taken from these same children six years later (Branta et al., 1984). The magnitude of the correlation coefficients was about the same for both males and females. Therefore, both boys and girls tended to hold their relative positions in their respective groups to about the same degree.

Summary. Stability in motor behavior is the consistency with which individuals perform specific motor skills over extended periods of time. Performance on motor tasks is less stable than other characteristics such as physical growth and strength (Rarick, 1973) because motor skills are more susceptible to environmental impact than physical growth and strength. The latter two are influenced more by genetic factors and therefore more resistant to environmental influences.

Performance on basic motor skills such as the dash, standing long jump and distance throw may be stable for three or more years. However, the peformance of children on other jumping and throwing tasks is stable for only one or two years. Future performance on these tasks cannot be predicted with accuracy.

Coefficients of stability for various motor ability and fitness tasks reveal consistency in performance for intervals of three to five years. Stable performance is more apt to occur during the middle and late childhood years than during early childhood.

Table 13
Coefficients of stability for motor ability & fitness skills in children and youth

	Time Interval (Years)											
	Boys						Girls					
Source	1	2	3	4	5	6	1	2	3	4	5	6
Brace Test												
Espenschade (1940)												
13-16 yrs.	70	50	74				75	66	62			
	(66)	(57)	(69)				(82)	(78)	(—)[a]			
Fifty-Foot Hop												
Keogh (1969)												
6-9 yrs.	49	50	42				43	47	52			
	(69)	(59)	(53)				(45)	(47)	(56)			
8-11 yrs.	52	52	32				42	39	45			
	(66)	(62)	(49)				(68)	(63)	(54)			
Thirty-Yard Agility Run												
Branta et al. (1984)												
5-10 yrs.	48	53	40	47	36		38	14	39	28	30	
8-14 yrs.	63	59	61	56	50	63	68	60	48	53	31	42
400-Foot Shuttle Run												
Branta et al. (1984)												
5-10 yrs.	59	47	27	40	24		51	37	40	35	46	
8-14 yrs.	71	56	64	70	51	70	59	52	53	47	31	53
Flexed Arm Hang												
Ellis et al. (1975)												
10-16 yrs.	(81)	(72)	(64)	(60)	(54)	54						
Branta et al. (1984)												
5-10 yrs.	70	39	48	39	34		48	35	34	35	24	
8-14 yrs.	90	81	76	76	68	52	70	65	60	64	52	44
Timed Sit-Ups												
Ellis et al. (1975)												
10-16 yrs.	(81)	(74)	(65)	(57)	(51)	40						
Sit and Reach												
Branta et al. (1984)												
5-10 yrs.	62	50	40	40	36		66	39	34	34	26	
8-14 yrs.	76	76	68	64	64	52	77	74	63	68	60	52

Note: All coefficients have been rounded to the nearest hundredth and decimals have been omitted. Coefficients without parentheses are individual values representing the relationship between performance at the first age listed and performance at successive age intervals. Coefficients in parentheses are composite means of two or more coefficients across the various pairings included in a study.

[a] No value reported for this interval.

Longitudinal data on motor performance support the following observations concerning the nature of stability and change (Rarick, 1973). First, the magnitude of the correlation coefficients decreases as the time interval between sets of data increases. Thus, the relative position of an individual within a group becomes more difficult to maintain as the number of years between measurements increased. Second, it is easier to predict from steady periods of growth than from rapid periods of growth. The middle and late childhood periods generally are defined as relatively stable periods for growth and development when compared to the early childhood years. The stability coefficients reported for middle and late childhood generally were of greater magnitude and extended across a greater interval of years than those obtained from younger children.

The results of these longitudinal studies carry several implications for parents, caretakers of children and educators in school settings. First, normally healthy children are not automatically predestined to succeed or fail in their attempts to acquire proficiency in specific motor skills, although some children may have more genetic potential to be successful than others. Thus, environmental factors are more influencial than genetic factors in determining the degree to which each child will achieve his or her potential for motor skill acquisition. Second, the lack of stability in motor skills provides an opportunity for change because the plasticity of a trait or characteristic is directly related to the amount of change it will tolerate. Because motor behavior during the childhood years is not sufficiently stable to permit its accurate prediction, the opportunity for initiating change, particularly during the early childhood years, is great. Thus the childhood years provide an excellent opportunity for children to acquire, correct and refine gross motor skills. Those concerned with the welfare of children have the responsibility to assist them in developing to their full potential. One method of enhancing the motor development of children is to encourage local school boards to provide sound, effective physical education programs, implemented by teachers who understand the immediate and long-term implications of efficient movement skills.

Summary

The reflexes and reactions of infancy are closely associated with the emerging movement skills of young children. Some reflexes persist throughout life in protective or supportive roles; some are extinquished or suppressed so that volitional actions may replace them, whereas others serve as the substrate for future movement tasks.

There is a well-defined order for the emergence and development of fundamental movement skills in infants and children, regardless of gender, race or culture. This genetically controlled order provides for the systematic evaluation of maturity and competence during infancy and early childhood.

The environments of infants and children have a profound effect on their development of movement skills. Genetic endowment determines the boundaries or potential for competence, but numerous environmental variables, including stimulation and opportunities to practice movement skills, determine to what degree the potential is realized.

The plasticity of motor behavior during childhood makes this an ideal time to promote change in the acquisition of new skills and in the refinement of those already present.

The well-documented levels or sequences in specific motor skills and the variability in their emergence illustrates the interplay between genetic and environmental influences on motor development.

Numerous instruments, in the form of scales, batteries, and tests, are available for the purpose of comparing individual progress on motor tasks against normative data. Parallel instruments, called criterion-referenced tests, permit comparisons of individual progress to some established sequence of behaviors. Thus, opportunities to compare individual progress to former status, and against the performance of peer groups, are available.

Movement skills and those requiring the manipulation and projection of objects are most efficiently learned between the ages of two and seven years, when the motivation to achieve and the opportunities to spend time in practice are available.

Although there are great similarities in motor proficiency within age groups, gender differences are present in early childhood and become more pronounced with age. Girls excel in tasks that require balance and agility, whereas boys excel in tasks that require muscular endurance and power. In qualitative and quantitative assessments of jumping, throwing, kicking and striking, boys outperformed girls during childhood, with differences becoming more distinct in adolescence.

Motorically adept children are more relaxed and eager to attempt new movement tasks. This cyclic process of attempting task and gaining competency builds a broad base of movement experiences, which enables individuals to experience the joy of moving efficiently and provides the healthful benefits of vigorous activity.

Variation in performing motor skills between children of the same chronological age increases as age advances. This increased variability reflects the greater influence of one's environment and the decreased influence of genetics on motor function as children become older.

The large intra- and interindividual variation in motor behavior that occurs during childhood suggests that the selection of learning objectives, instructional strategies and organized experiences must be structured to accommodate individuals, rather than groups of children.

Recent assessments of movement skills indicate that many school aged children do not achieve mature levels of performance, qualitatively, in the fundamental movement skills. Concomitantly, regression in some of these skills was noted in adolescence. These findings have implications for physical activity programs throughout the school age years.

References

American Alliance of Health, Physical Education, Recreation and Dance. (1976). *Youth fitness test manual* (rev. ed.). Reston, VA: AAHPERD Publications.

Ames, L.B. (1966). Individuality of motor development. *Journal of the American Physical Therapy Association, 46*, 121-127.

Apgar, V. (1953). A proposal for a new method of evaluation of the newborn infant. *Anesthesia and Analgesia, 32*, 260-267.

Astrand, P.O., Engstrom, L., Eriksson, B., Karlberg, P., Nylander, I., Saltin, B., & Thoren, C., (1963). Girl swimmers. *Acta Paediatrica*, (Supplement 147).

Atkinson, R. (1924). A motor efficiency study of 8,000 New York City high school boys. *American Physical Education Review, 29*, 56-59.

Atkinson, R. (1925). A study of athletic ability of high school girls. *American Physical Education Review, 30*, 389-399.

Bar-Or, O. (1975). Predicting athletic performance. *The Physician and Sports Medicine, 3*, 81-85.

Bayley, N. (1935). The development of motor abilities during the first three years. *Monographs of the Society for Research in Child Development, 1*, 1-26.

Bayley, N. (1936). *The California infant scale of motor development*. Berkeley: University of California Press.

Bayley, N. (1969). *Manual for the Bayley scales of infant development*. New York: The Psychological Corporation.

Beach, F.A., & Jaynes, J. (1954). Effects of early experience upon the behavior of animals. *Psychological Bulletin, 51*(3), 239-263.

Bernink, M., Erich, W., Peltenburg, A. Zonderland, M., & Huisveld, I. (1983). Body composition, biological maturation and socioeconomic status of young talented female swimmers and gymnasts. In A.P. Hollander, P. Huijing & G. de Groots (Eds.), *Biomechanics and medicine in swimming* (pp. 41-50). Champaign, IL: Human Kinetics Publishers.

Bliss, J. (1927). A study of progression based on age, sex, and individual differences in strength and skill. *American Physical Education Review, 32*, 11-21, 85-99.

Bloom, B.S. (1964). *Stability and change in human characteristics*. New York: Wiley.

Bobath, K. (1980). *A neurophysiological basis for the treatment of cerebral palsy*. Spastics International Medical Publications. London: William Heineman Medical Books Ltd.

Branta, C., Haubenstricker, J., & Seefeldt, V. (1984). Age changes in motor skills during childhood and adolescence. In R.L. Terjung (Ed.), *Exercise and sport sciences reviews* (Vol. 12, pp. 467-520). Lexington, MA: The Collamore Press.

Bruner, J.S. (1973). Organization of early skilled action. *Child Development, 44*, 1-11.

Bugyi, D., & Kausz, I. (1970). Radiographic determination of the skeletal age of young swimmers. *Journal of Sports Medicine and Physical Fitness, 10*, 269-270.

Clark, D.L., Kreutzberg, J.R., & Chee, F.K.W. (1977). Vestibular stimulation influence on motor development of infants. *Science, 196*, 1228-1229.

Clark, J.E., & Humphrey, J.H. (Eds). (1985). *Motor development: Current selected research* (Vol. 1). Princeton, NJ: Princeton Book Company.

Clark, J.E., & Phillips, S.J. (1985). A developmental sequence of the standing long jump. In J.E. Clark & J.H. Humphrey (Eds.), *Motor development: Current selected research* (Vol. 1), (pp. 76-85). Princeton, NJ: Princeton Book Company.

Clarke H.H. (1968). Characteristics of the young athlete: A longitudinal look. *Kinesiology Review, 3*, 33-42.

Clarke, H.H. (1971). *Physical and motor tests in the Medford boys' growth study*. Englewood Cliffs, NJ: Prentice-Hall.

Clarke, H.H., & Peterson, K. (1962). Differences in physical and motor traits between boys of advanced, normal and retarded maturity. *Research Quarterly, 33*, 13-25.

Corbin, C.B. (Ed.). (1980). *A textbook of motor development* (2nd ed.). Dubuque, IA: Wm. C. Brown.

Cowan, E.A., & Pratt, B.M. (1934). The hurdle jump as a developmental and diagnostic test of motor coordination for children from three to 12 years of age. *Child Development, 5*, 107-121.

Crampton, C.W. (1908). Physiological age—a fundamental principle. *American Physical Education Review, 13*, 1-12. Reprinted in *Child Development* (1944), *15*, 3-52.

Cummins, G., Garand, T., & Borysyk, L. (1972). Correlation of performance in track and field events to bone age. *Journal of Pediatrics, 80*, 970-973.

Cunningham, B.V. (1927). An experiment in measuring gross motor development of infants and young children. *Journal of Educational Psychology, 18*, 458-464.

Cunningham, D., Telford, P., & Swart, G. (1976). The cardiopulmonary capacities of young hockey players: Age 10. *Medicine and Science in Sports, 8*, 23-25.

Cureton, T.K. (1964). Improving the physical fitness of youth. *Monographs of the Society for Research in Child Development, 29*, 1-221.

Curtis, D.M. (1975). *Norms of an eleven year study of selected motor performance tests for Hawaiian children, five to 12 years of age*. Unpublished manuscript, Curriculum and Instruction Department, University of Hawaii at Manoa.

Deach, D. (1950). *Genetic development of motor skills in children two through six years of age*. Unpublished doctoral dissertation, University of Michigan, Ann Arbor.

Dennis, W. (1935). The effects of restricted practice on the reaching, sitting and standing of two infants. *Journal of Genetic Psychology, 47*, 17-32.

Dennis, W. (1938). Infant development under conditions of restricted practice and of minimum social stimulation: a preliminary report. *Journal of Genetic Psychology, 53*, 149-158.

Dennis, W., & Dennis, M.G. (1940). The effect of cradling practices upon the onset of walking in Hopi Indians. *Journal of Genetics Psychology, 56*, 77-86.

Dennis W., & Najarian. P. (1957). Infant development under environmental handicap. *Psychological Monographs: General and Applied, 71*(7), 1-13.

DeOreo, K.L. & Keogh, J. (1980). Performance of fundamental motor tasks. In C.B. Corbin (Ed.), *A textbook of motor development* (2nd ed.), (pp. 76-91). Dubuque, IA: Wm. C. Brown.

Dohrman, P. (1964). Throwing and kicking ability of 8-year-old boys and girls *Research Quarterly, 35,* 464-471.

DuRandt, R. (1985). Ball-catching proficiency among 4-, 6-, and 8-year-old girls. In J.E. Clark & J.H. Humphrey (Eds.), *Motor development: Current selected research* (Vol. 1), (pp. 35-43). Princeton, NJ: Princeton Book Company.

Dusenberry, L. (1952). A study of the effects of training in ball throwing by children ages three to seven. *Research Quarterly, 23,* 9-14.

Earls, N.F. (1975, March). *A three year study of changes in physical fitness, motor skills and physical education knowledge of elementary children.* Paper presented at the national convention of the American Association for Health, Physical Education and Recreation, Atlantic City, NJ.

Eckert, H.M. (1973). Age changes in motor skills. In G.L. Rarick (Ed.), *Physical activity: Human growth and development* (pp. 154-175). New York: Academic Press.

Eckert, H.M. (1974). Variability in skill acquisition. *Child Development, 45,* 487-489.

Eckert, H.M., & Eichorn, D.H. (1977). Developmental variability in reaction time. *Child Development, 48,* 452-458.

Edwards, N. (1968). The relationship between physical condition immediately after birth and mental and motor performance at age four. *Genetic Psychology Monographs, 78,* 257-289.

Ellis, J.D., Carron, .V., & Bailey, D.A. (1975). Physical performance in boys from ten through 16 years. *Human Biology, 47,* 263-281.

Espenschade, A. (1940). Motor performance in adolescence. *Monographs of the Society for Research in Child Development, 1,* 1-126.

Espenschade, A. (1960). Motor development. In W.R. Johnson (Ed.), *Science and medicine of exercise and sports* (pp. 419-439). New York: Harper and Row.

Espenschade, A., & Eckert, H.M. (1967), *Motor development.* Columbus, OH: Charles E. Merrill.

Espenschade, A., & Eckert, H.M. (1980). *Motor development* (2nd ed.). Columbus, OH: Charles E. Merrill.

Fiorentino, M.R. (1973). *Reflex testing methods for evaluating C.N.S. development* (2nd ed.). Springfield, IL: Charles C. Thomas.

Fleishman, E.A. (1964). *The structure and measurement of physical fitness.* Englewood Cliffs, NJ: Prentice-Hall.

Fortney, V.L. (1983). The kinematics and kinetics of the running pattern of 2-, 4-, and 6-year-old children. *Research Quarterly for Exercise and Sport, 54,* 126-135.

Frankenburg, W., & Dodds, J. (1967). The Denver developmental screening test. *Journal of Pediatrics, 71,* 181-191.

Gabbard, C., & Patterson P. (1981). Movement pattern analysis on the horizontal ladder among childen four to nine years. *Perceptual and Motor Skills, 52,* 937-939.

Gallahue, D.L. (1982). *Understanding motor development in children.* New York: Wiley.

Gentile, A.M. (1972). A working model of skill acquisition with application to teaching. *Quest, 17,* 3-32.

Gesell, A. (1928). *Infancy and human growth.* New York: Macmillan.

Gesell, A. (1940). *The first five years of life.* New York: Harper & Row.

Gesell, A., & Armatruda, C.S. (1941). *Developmental diagnosis.* New York: Harper and Row.

Gesell, A., & Thompson H. (1929). Learning and growth in identical infant twins: An experimental study of the method of co-twin control. *Genetic Psychology Monographs, 6,* 1-124.

Glassow, R., & Kruse, P. (1960). Motor performance of girls six to 14 years. *Research Quarterly, 31,* 426-433.

Goldberger, M., Gerney, P., & Chamberlain, J. (1982). The effects of three styles of teaching on the psychomotor performance and social development of fifth grade children. *Research Quarterly, 53,* 116-124.

Gutteridge, M. (1939). A study of motor achievements of young children. *Archives of Psychology, 244,* 1-178.

Hagberg, B.M. (1975). Pre-, peri-, and postnatal prevention of major neuropediatric handicaps. *Neuropediatrics, 6,* 331-338.

Hale, C. (1956). Prediction of baseball ability through an analysis of measures of strength and structure. *Research Quarterly, 27,* 276-284.

Halverson, H.M. (1931). An experimental study of prehension in infants by means of systematic cinema records. *Genetic Psychology Monographs, 10,* 107-286.

Halverson, L.E. (1966). Development of motor patterns in young children. *Quest, 6,* 44-53.

Halverson, L.E. & Roberton, M.A. (1979). The effects of instruction on overhand throwing development in children. In K. Newell & G. Roberts (Eds.), *Psychology of motor behavior and sport—1978* (pp. 258-269). Champaign, IL: Human Kinetics Publishers.

Halverson, L.E., Roberton, M.A., & Langendorfer, S. (1982). Development of the overarm throw: Movement and ball velocity changes by seventh grade. *Research Quarterly for Exercise and Sport, 53,* 198-205.

Halverson, L.E., Roberton, M.A., Safrit, M.J., & Roberts, T.W. (1977). Effect of guided practice on overhand-throw ball velocities of kindergarten children. *Research Quarterly, 48,* 311-318.

Halverson, L.E., & Williams, K. (1985). Developmental sequences for hopping over distance: A prelongitudinal screening. *Research Quarterly for Exercise and Sport, 56,* 37-44.

Hanson, M. (1965). *Motor performance testing of elementary school age children.* Unpublished doctoral dissertation, University of Washington, Seattle.

Hardin D., & Garcia, M. (1982). Diagnostic performance tests for elementary children—Grades 1 to 4. *Journal of Physical Education, Recreation and Dance, 53,* 48-49.

Hartman, D.M. (1943). The hurdle jump as a measure of the motor proficiency of young children. *Child Development, 14,* 201-211.

Haubenstricker, J., Branta, C., & Seefeldt, V. (1983, May). *Preliminary validation of developmental sequences of throwing and catching.* Paper presented at the international conference of the North American Society for the Psychology of Sport and Physical Activity, East Lansing, MI.

Haubenstricker, J., Branta, C., Ulrich, B., Brakora, L., & E-Lotfalian, A. (1984, February). *Quantitative and qualitative analysis of jumping behavior in young children.* Paper presented at the Midwest District convention of the American Alliance of Health, Physical Education, Recreation and Dance, Indianapolis, IN.

Haubenstricker, J., & Ewing, M. (1985, April). *Predicting motor performance from changes in body size and shape.* Paper presented at the national convention of the American Alliance of Health, Physical Education, Recreation and Dance, Atlanta, GA.

Haubenstricker, J., & Seefeldt, V. (1974, March). *Sequential progression in fundamental motor skills of children with learning disabilities.* Paper presented at the international conference of the Association for Children with Learning Disabilities, Houston, TX.

Haubenstricker, J., & Seefeldt, V. (1976). *A developmental sequence for skipping.* Unpublished manuscript, Michigan State University.

Haubenstricker, J., Seefeldt, V., Fountain, C., & Sapp, M. (1981, March). *Prelimi-

nary validation of a developmental sequence for kicking. Paper presented at the Midwest District convention of the American Alliance of Health, Physical Education, Recreation and Dance, Chicago, IL.

Haubenstricker, J., Seefeldt, V., Fountain, C., & Sapp. M. (1981, April). *The efficiency of the Bruininks-Oseretsky Test of Motor Proficiency in discriminating between normal children and those with gross motor dysfunction.* Paper presented at the national convention of the American Alliance of Health, Physical Education, Recreation and Dance, Boston, MA.

Hellebrandt, F.A., Rarick, G.L., Glassow, R., & Carns, M.L. (1961). Physiological analysis of basic motor skills. *American Journal of Physical Medicine, 40,* 14-25.

Hicks, J.A. (1930). The acquisition of motor skill in young children. *Child Development, 1,* 90-105.

Hicks, J.A., & Ralph, D.W. (1931). The effects of practice in tracing the Porteus diamond maze. *Child Development, 2,* 156-158.

Hilgard, J.R. (1932). Learning and maturation in preschool children. *Journal of Genetic Psychology, 41,* 36-56.

Hooker, D. (1944). *The origin of overt behavior.* Ann Arbor, MI: University of Michigan Press.

Howell, R., & Seefeldt, V. (1980, April). *Stability and predictability of motor performance in children and youth.* Paper presented at the national convention of the American Alliance of Health, Physical Education, Recreation and Dance, Detroit, MI.

Illingworth, R.S. (1970). *The development of the infant and young child: Normal and abnormal* (4th ed.). Baltimore: Williams and Wilkins.

Jenkins, L.A. (1930). *A comparison study of motor achievements of children, five, six and seven years of age.* Contributions to Education No. 414. New York: Teachers College, Columbia University.

Johnson, R.D. (1962). Measurement of achievement in fundamental skills of elementary school children. *Research Quarterly, 33,* 94-103.

Jones, H. (1949). *Motor performance and growth.* Berkeley, CA: University of California Press.

Kanetz, M., & Bar-Or, O. (1974). Relationship between anthropometric, developmental and physiological parameters and achievement in swimming in 10- to 12-year-old boys. *Israel Journal of Medical Sciences, 10,* 289 (abstract).

Keogh, J. (1965). *Motor performance of elementary school children.* (USPHS Grants MH 08319-01 and HD 01059). Department of Physical Education, University of California, Los Angeles.

Keogh, J. (1969). *Changes in motor performance during early school years.* Technical Report 2-69 (USPHS Grant HD 01059). Department of Physical Education, University of California, Los Angeles.

Keogh, J., & Sugden, D. (1985). *Motor skill development.* New York: Macmillan.

Kotulan, J., Reznickova, M., & Placheta, Z. (1980). Exercise and growth. In Z. Placheta (Ed.), *Youth and physical activity* (pp. 61-117). Brno: J.E. Purkyne University Medical Faculty.

Krogman, W. (1959). Maturation age of 55 boys in the Little League world series, 1957. *Research Quarterly, 30,* 54-56.

Latchaw, M. (1954). Measuring selected motor skills in fourth, fifth and sixth grades. *Research Quarterly, 25,* 439-449.

Lipsitt, L.P., & Kaye, H. (1964). Conditioned sucking in the human newborn. *Psychonomic Science, 1,* 29-30.

Malina, R.M. (1973). Ethnic and cultural factors in the development of motor abilities and strength in American children. In G.L. Rarick (Ed.), *Physical activity: Human growth and development* (pp. 333-363). New York: Academic Press.

Malina, R.M. (1975). *Growth and development: The first twenty years in man.* Minneapolis: Burgess.

Malina, R.M. (1982). Physical growth and maturity characteristics of young athletes. In R. Magill, M. Ash, & F. Smoll (Eds.), *Children and sport* (2nd ed.), (pp. 73-96). Champaign, IL: Human Kinetics Publishers.

Malina, R.M. (1983). Menarche in athletes: A synthesis and hypothesis. *Annals of Human Biology, 10,* 1-24.

Malina, R.M., & Rarick, G.L. (1973). Growth, physique, and motor performance. In G.L. Rarick (Ed.), *Physical activity: Human growth and development* (pp. 125-153). New York: Academic Press.

McCaskill, C.L., & Wellman, B.L. (1938). A study of common motor achievements at the preschool ages. *Child Development, 9,* 141-150.

McClenaghan, B.A., & Gallahue, D.L. (1978). *Fundamental movement: A developmental and remedial approach.* Philadelphia: W.B. Saunders.

McCraw, L.W., & Tolbert, J.W. (1953). Sociometric status and athletic ability of junior high boys. *Research Quarterly, 23,* 72-80.

McCraw, M.B. (1935). *A study of Johnny and Jimmy.* New York: Appleton-Century.

McGraw, M.B. (1939). Later development of children specifically trained during infancy: Johnny and Jimmy at school age. *Child Development, 10,* 1-19.

McGraw, M.B. (1940). Neuromuscular development of the human infant as exemplified in the achievement of erect locomotion. *Journal of Pediatrics, 17,* 747-771.

McGraw, M.B. (1954). Maturation of behavior. In L. Carmichael (Ed.), *Manual of Psychology.* New York: Wiley.

McGraw, M.B. (1963). *Neuromuscular maturation of the human infant.* New York: Hafner. (Originally published in 1943).

Michigan Study on Youth Sports. (1976). *Joint legislative study on youth sports programs: Phase I.* Report to the Joint Legislative Study Committee on Youth Sports Programs, State of Michigan, Lansing.

Milani-Comparetti, A., & Gidoni, E.A. (1967). Pattern analysis of motor development and its disorders. *Developmental Medicine and Child Neurology, 9,* 625-630.

Miller, J.L. (1957). Effect of instruction on development of throwing for accuracy of first grade children. *Research Quarterly, 28,* 132-137.

Miller, S. (1978). *The facilitation of fundamental motor skill learning in young children.* Unpublished doctoral dissertation, Michigan State University, East Lansing.

Milne, C., Seefeldt, V., & Reuschlein, P. (1976). Relationship between grade, sex, race, and motor performance in young children. *Research Quarterly, 47,* 726-730.

Mirenva, A.N. (1935). Psychomotor education and the general development of preschool children: Experiments with twin controls: *Journal of Genetic psychchology, 46,* 433-454.

Morris, A.M., Williams, J.M., Atwater, A.E., & Wilmore, J.H. (1982). Age and sex differences in motor performance of three through 6-year-old children. *Research Quarterly for Exercise and Sport, 53,* 214-221.

Poe, A. (1970). *Development of vertical jumping skill in children.* Unpublished manuscript, University of Wisconsin, Madison.

Poe, A. (1976). Description of the movement characteristics of 2-year-old children performing the jump and reach. *Research Quarterly, 47,* 260-268.

Rarick, G.L. (1964). Research evidence on the values of physical education. *Theory Into Practice, 3,* 108-111.

Rarick. G.L. (1973a). Motor performance of mentally retarded children. In G. L. Rarick (Ed.), *Physical activity: Human growth and development* (pp. 225-256). New York: Academic Press.

Rarick, G.L. (1973b). Stability and change in motor abilities. In G.L. Rarick (Ed.), *Physical activity: Human growth and development* (pp. 201-224). New York: Academic Press.

Rarick, G.L., & Oyster, N. (1964). Physical maturity, muscular strength and motor performance of young school age children. *Research Quarterly, 35,* 522-531.

Rarick, G.L., & Smoll, F.L. (1967). Stability of growth in strength and motor performance from childhood to adolescence. *Human Biology, 39,* 295-306.

Reuschlein, P., & Haubenstricker, J. (Eds.). *1984-1985 Physical education interpretive report: Grades 4, 7 and 10.* Michigan Educational Assessment Program, State Board of Education, Michigan Department of Education, Lansing.

Reuschlein, P., & Vogel, P. (1985). Motor performance and physical fitness status of regular and special education students. In J.E. Clark & J.H. Humphrey (Eds.) *Motor development: Current selected research* (Vol. 1), (pp. 147-165). Princeton, NJ: Princeton Book Company.

Richards, T.W. & Newberry, H. (1938). Studies in fetal behavior: III. Can performance on test items at six months postnatally be predicted on the basis of fetal activity? *Child Development, 9,* 79-86.

Ridenour, M.V. (Ed.). (1978). *Motor development: Issues and applications.* Princeton, NJ: Princeton Book Company.

Roberton, M.A. (1977). Stability of stage categorization across trials: Implications for the stage theory of overarm throw development. *Journal of Human Movement, 3,* 49-59.

Roberton, M.A. (1978). Stages in motor development. In M.V. Ridenour (Ed.), *Motor development: Issues and applications* (pp. 63-81). Princeton, NJ: Princeton Book Company.

Roberton, M.A. (1984). Changing motor patterns during childhood. In J.R. Thomas (Ed.), *Motor development during childhood and adolescence* (pp. 48-90). Minneapolis: Burgess.

Roberton, M.A., & Halverson, L.E. (1977). The developing child—His changing movement. In B.J. Logston et al. (Eds.), *Physical education for children: A focus on the teaching process* (pp. 24-67). Philadelphia: Lea & Febiger.

Roberton, M.A., & Halverson, L.E. (1984). *Developing children—Their changing movement: A guide for teachers.* Philadelphia: Lea & Febiger.

Roberton, M.A., Halverson, L.E., Langendorfer, S., & Williams, K. (1979). Longitudinal changes in children's overarm throw ball velocities. *Research Quarterly, 50,* 256-264.

Rochelle, R., Kelleher, M., & Thornton, R. (1961). Relationship of maturation age to incidence of injury in tackle football. *Research Quarterly, 32,* 78-82.

Rotch, T. (1908). Chronologic and anatomic age in early life. *Journal of the American Medical Association, 51,* 1197-1205.

Sage, G.H. (1984). *Motor learning and control: A neuropsychological approach.* Dubuque, IA: Wm. C. Brown.

Sapp, M. (1980). *Developmental sequence of galloping.* Unpublished manuscript, Michigan State University, East Lansing.

Schmidt, R.A. (1982). *Motor control and learning: A behavioral emphasis.* Champaign, IL: Human Kinetics publishers.

Seefeldt, V. (1972, March). *Developmental sequence of catching skill.* Paper presented at the national convention of the American Association for Health, Physical Education and Recreation, Houston, TX.

Seefeldt, V. (1979). Developmental motor patterns: Implications for elementary school physical education. In C. Nadeau, W. Holliwell, K. Newell, & G. Roberts (Eds.), *Psychology of motor behavior and sport—1979* (pp. 314-323). Champaign, IL: Human Kinetics Publishers.

Seefeldt, V., & Haubenstricker, J. (1974). *A developmental sequence for kicking.* Unpublished manuscript, Michigan State University, East Lansing.

Seefeldt, V., & Haubenstricker, J. (1976a). *A developmental sequence for hopping.* Unpublished manuscript, Michigan State University, East Lansing.

Seefeldt, V., & Haubenstricker, J. (1976b). *A developmental sequence for punting.*

Unpublished manuscript, Michigan State University, East Lansing.

Seefeldt, V., & Haubenstricker, J. (1976c). *A developmental sequence for striking*. Unpublished manuscript, Michigan State University, East Lansing.

Seefeldt, V., & Haubenstricker, J. (1976d). *A developmental sequence for throwing* (rev. ed.). Unpublished manuscript, Michigan State University, East Lansing.

Seefeldt, V., Reuschlein, P., & Vogel, P. (1972, March). *Sequencing motor skills within the physical education curriculum*. Paper presented at the national convention of the American Association for Health, Physical Education and Recreation, Houston, TX.

Seils, L.G. (1951). The relationship between measures of physical growth and gross motor performance of primary-grade school children. *Research Quarterly, 22*, 244-260.

Shirley, M. (1931). *The first two years: A study of twenty-five babies, I, Postural and locomotor development*. Minneapolis: University of Minnesota Press.

Sinclair, C.B. (1971). *Movement and movement patterns of early childhood*. Richmond, VA: State Department of Education.

Swartz, D., & Allen, M. (1975). Residual reflex patterns as a basis for diagnosing stroke faults. In J.P. Clarys & L. Levillie (Eds.), *Swimming II* (pp. 310-313). Baltimore: University Park Press.

Thomas, J.R. (Ed.). (1984). *Motor development during childhood and adolescence*. Minneapolis: Burgess.

Thompson, G., Blanksby, B., & Doran, G. (1974). Maturity and performance in age group competitive swimmers. *Australian Journal of Physical Education, 64*, 21-25.

Toole, T., & Arink, E.A. (1982). Movement education: Its effect on motor skill performance. *Research Quarterly, 53*, 156-162.

Touwen, B.C.L. (1971). A study on the development of some motor phenomena in infancy. *Developmental Medicine and Child Neurology, 13*, 435-446.

Twitchell, T.E. (1965). The automatic grasping responses of infants. *Neuropsychologia, 3*, 247-259.

Vilchkovsky, E.S. (1972). Motor development in pre-school and school age children. *Theory and Practice of Physical Culture, 6*, 29-33.

Vincent, M. (1968). Motor performance of girls from 12 through 18 years of age. *Research Quarterly, 39*, 1094-1100.

Walters, C.E. (1965). Prediction of postnatal development from fetal activity. *Child Development, 36*, 801-808.

Werner, P. (1974). Education of selected movement patterns of preschool children. *Perceptual and Motor Skills, 39*, 795-798.

Whittle, H.D. (1961). Effects of elementary school physical education upon aspects of physical, motor, and personality development. *Research Quarterly, 32*, 249-260.

Wickstrom, R.L. (1970). *Fundamental motor patterns*. Philadelphia: Lea & Febiger.

Wickstrom, R.L. (1974). Rope jumping: A preliminary report on developmental form. *Research Abstracts—1974*. Washington, DC: American Association for Health, Physical Education and Recreation.

Wickstrom, R.L. (1977). *Fundamental motor patterns* (2nd ed.). Philadelphia: Lea & Febiger.

Wickstrom, R.L. (1983). *Fundamental motor patterns* (3rd ed.). Philadelphia: Lea & Febiger.

Wild, M. (1938). The behavior patterns of throwing and some observations concerning its course of development in children. *Research Quarterly, 9*, 20-24.

Williams, H.G. (1983). *Perceptual and motor development*. Englewood Cliffs, NJ: Prentice-Hall.

Williams, H.G., & Breihan, S.K. (1979). *Motor control tasks for young children*. Unpublished manuscript, University of Toledo.

Williams, H., Temple, I., Logston, B., Scott, S., & Clement, A. (1971). *An investigation of the perceputal-motoyoung children*. Unpublished manuscript. Bowling Green State University.

Williams, K. (1980). Developmental characteristics of a forward roll. *Research Quarterly for Exercise and sport, 51*, 703-713.

Zelazo, P. (1972). "Walking" in the newborn. *Science, 176*, 314-315.

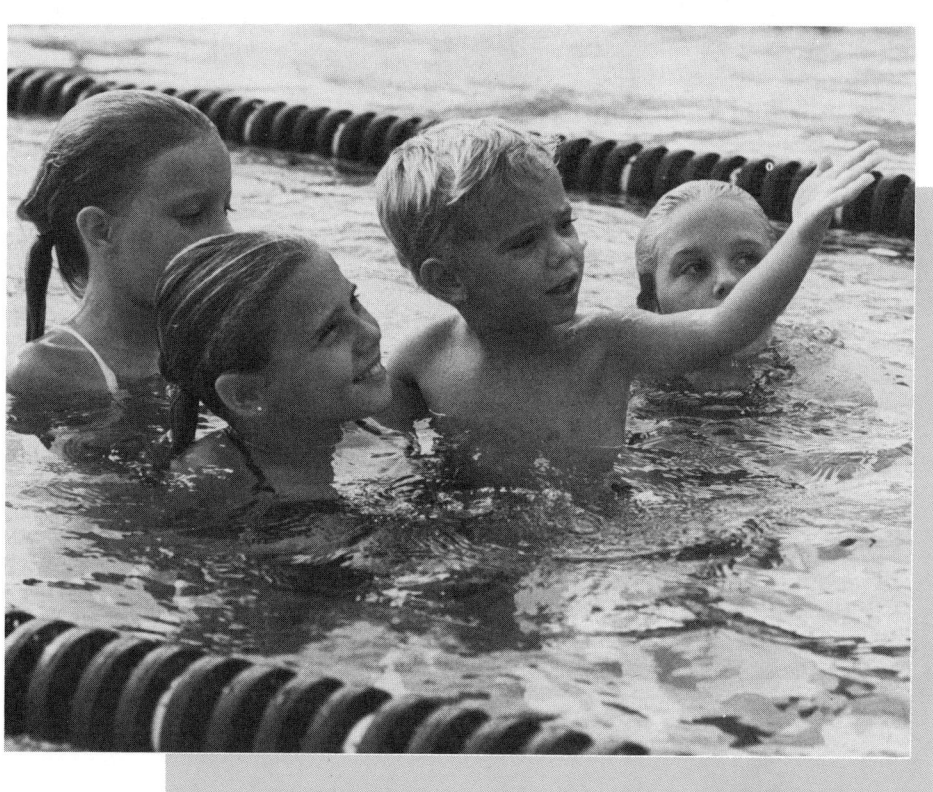

photo by Greg Merhar

CHAPTER THREE

The Development of Sensory-Motor Function in Young Children

Harriet G. Williams
The Motor Development/Motor Control Laboratory
Department of Physical Education
The University of South Carolina
Columbia, South Carolina

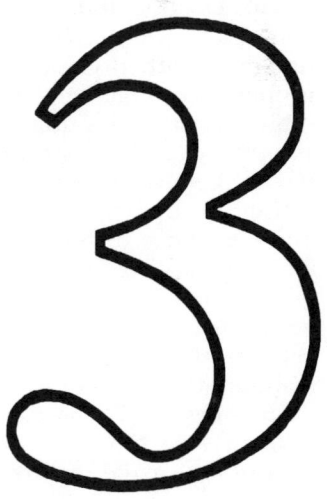

The concept of sensory-motor function is an old one. It implies that as refinement in various neural systems occurs, there is a concomitant change in associated sensory and motor processes and ultimately in the nature and quality of the overt motor behavior of the growing, developing organism. What do we know about the development of sensory-motor function in young children? To what extent are such changes attributable to experience or practice? How does the development of these functions differ, if at all, in children who are awkward or uncoordinated? These are questions to which there are, at present, no complete answers. The following discussion is intended to present a brief overview of the development of selected sensory-motor functions in young children and to help point the way to potential answers to such questions. For purposes of simplicity and limitations of space, the chapter will attempt to (a) provide a broad overview of the development of selected motor and/or neuromuscular functions in young children; (b) describe and explain what the role of sensory-motor experiences may be in the development of motor and cognitive functions in young children, and (c) show how neural development may be, in important ways, related to the sensory and motor experiences which the organism undergoes early in life.

Development of Motor Control in Young Children

Effective motor control in young children is, in part, a result of gaining control over the organization and execution of intricate patterns of peripheral muscle activity. To achieve such control requires that the child develop or acquire motor programs which, when activated, can consistently and systematically initiate and carry out the following: (a) selection of appropriate muscle groups to support the movement and the postural framework for the movement; (b) establishment of precise temporal and spatial parameters for contraction and relaxation of the selected muscle groups (agonists and antagonists alike); and (c) setting consistent and appropriate force parameters to guide production of muscular force. There is also agreement among many experts that motor skill development in both children and adults involves "learning" to progressively inhibit activity in muscle groups located in widespread parts of the body, and to channel activity to muscle groups essential to task performance (Herman, 1970; Hobart and Vorro, 1971; Payton and Kelley, 1972). Establishing motor programs which can execute these functions with precision and regularity is not something that occurs without proper encouragement and appropriate opportunity for practice and instruction.

Shambes (1976) studied a small number of 4- and 8-year-old children who were asked to assume a variety of familiar and unfamiliar balance positions. Evidence from this study indicated that although the overt body positions assumed by the two age groups were often the same, younger children tended to use both a larger number and a different aggregation of muscle groups than older children to maintain balance. Younger children also generated more force in active muscle groups than did older children. When children assumed well practiced or familiar positions (e.g. the upright standing position), there was little or no difference between the two groups in either the muscles used or in the force produced to maintain the position.

Shambes' (1976) work was elaborated upon and, in general, supported by Williams et al. (1983). Motor function involved in postural control in thirty-two 4-, 6-, and 8-year-old children was studied using electromyographic (EMG) procedures. Overall, postural responses of younger children were characterized by greater and more widespread EMG activity in muscle groups involved in maintaining posture. Six-year-old children showed more consistent and much less widespread EMG activity than 4-year-old children. Selection and use of muscle groups for balance maintenance were similar in children 6 and 8 years old. For both of these age groups, observed EMG activity was limited to a small number of muscle groups and the amount of EMG activity was dramatically decreased. It appears that observable differences may exist in the muscle selection and force production parameters of motor programs used by children of different ages to perform familiar and unfamiliar motor tasks involving balance. Such differences are less obvious after 6 years of age and almost non-existent when the task to be performed is a familiar or practiced one.

Woollacott (1983) has also identified some important differences in motor functions of children and adults as they pertain to maintaining balance. Consider a situation in which an individual is asked to stand on a moveable platform; visualize the platform being moved forward unexpectedly. The overt response of adults to this perturbation of balance is the swaying of the body in a backward direction. The initial neuromuscular response of the adult is the onset of activity in the distal agonist (tibialis anterior muscle), followed quickly by onset of activity in the proximal agonist (quadriceps muscle). The secondary neuromuscular response (when there is one and such responses occur only occasionally in adults) is onset of activity in the distal antagonist (gastrocnemius) followed by onset of activity in the proximal antagonist (hamstrings). The activity of agonist and antagonist muscle groups is always in a distal to proximal direction. In adults, the distal musculature is activated approximately 100 msec after the postural perturbation, while onset of activity in the proximal musculature occurs some 10 msec later. Adults also show fixed relationships between the distal and proximal musculature in both the latency of onset of EMG activity and the amplitude of EMG activity. In other words, there is an important invariant linkage (in terms of timing and force production parameters) between the two agonist muscles involved in counteracting induced backward body sway in adults.

Young children's reactions to such disturbances of balance are similar to adults ONLY in that the distal musculature is activated prior to the proximal musculature. In contrast to adults, children under 7 years of age tend consistently to activate both agonist and antagonist muscle groups to counteract the postural sway. Young children also tend to be more variable in the latency of onset of both distal and proximal muscle activity; in addition the mean latency for the onset of activity in the proximal musculature is 58 msec (compared to 10 msec for adults). The fixed time and force relationships between distal and proximal musculature seen in adults are less obvious and often non-existent in young children. Children 7 to 10 years of age, however, show adult-like responses to these perturbations of posture. It is interesting to note, as Woollacott (1983) has done, that these adult-like responses occur at a time when the cerebral cortex is nearing maturation.

How much of these differences between younger and older children and adults is a result of early sensory-motor experience is of course a moot question. There is some evidence to suggest that children must learn to integrate information from the major sensory systems in order to produce the more refined motor functions needed to regulate posture and movement appropriately. Forssberg and Nashner (1982) studied young children's ability to modify or attenuate certain postural responses when such responses were no longer appropriate. Children under 7 years were unable to modify or adapt such responses with only brief practice or experience (five trials); older children adapted quickly. Shumway-Cook and Woolacott (1983) reported that when young children were given more opportunity to experience or practice (e.g. 10-15 trials), they were also capable of adapting or modifying these responses. These observations suggest that one potentially important outcome of early sensory-motor experience may be an increased ability on the part of the child to fine-tune the processes involved in suppressing inappropriate neuromuscular responses involved in posture and movement control. Thus, from a practical point of view, environmental experience in the form of play or physical activity may be important for the young child in that it provides him/her with the opportunity to sort out which sensory information is relevant to task performance as well as with the opportunity to learn how to use that information to produce appropriate responses and suppress inappropriate ones.

Young children can also learn, with practice, to voluntarily control activity in single motor units (Simard, 1969). Children 3-12 years old were trained to use visual, auditory, and proprioceptive feedback to regulate the firing patterns of single motor units in the rhomboid muscle. Children of all ages learned to regulate such activity for a period of at least 10 minutes. With continued practice, most children were able to transfer control of such activity to other motor units within the same muscle as well as to motor units in other muscle groups. In general, children 8 years and older maintained more consistent control over motor unit activity than did younger children. Only children 7-9 years of age were able to learn to maintain control over activity in a single motor unit in the rhomboids and perform another movement simultaneously. These observations suggest that important improvements in certain motor functions, some of which are clearly experience-related, occur in children between 7 and 9 years of age.

All of the foregoing data suggest that both age and experience-related factors are important in the development of motor control functions in young children. Under normal circumstances, children need practice and experience to develop and refine the parameters of the motor programs involved in many aspects of motor skill performance. Programs of physical activity should include a variety of motor experiences to ensure the optimal development of such functions.

Vision and motor control. It is clear that early motor function in the form of postural control is dominated by the visual system. For example, infants 6-14 days old display postural reactions to an object moving on a collision course toward them (the 'looming' response) by raising the arms and withdrawing the head (Butterworth, 1982). If the object is not proceeding on a collision course, the child simply tracks the object and manifests no other response. Similar postural reactions to oncoming 'colliding' objects have been elicited in children with Down's Syndrome at 2 months of age. Lee and Aronson (1974) have also shown that young children who can stand independently react to erroneous visual feedback (feedback which indicates body sway is occurring when it is not) by swaying and falling in the opposite direction. Butterworth and Hicks (1977) reported a similar response in infants who can sit but who are not yet able to stand alone. Interestingly, adults can also be made to exhibit reactions similar to those of children when they are required to balance in an unfamiliar or in a very unstable position. These observations indicate that young infants carry out certain motor functions that involve postural reactions to selected aspects of the visual environment before they can stand or walk and before they have had much experience in interacting with their external world. This suggests that a potentially important and inherent linkage between visual and motor functions exists in young infants, a linkage that does not necessarily require previous experience or practice.

It has also been observed that children with Down's Syndrome who have just learned to stand show a greater sensitivity to 'distorted' visual feedback about body sway than do normal children of the same chronological age (Cicchetti and Stoufe, 1978). In addition, the intensity of these reactions decreases with experience (from 3-12 months) for both normal and developmentally delayed children. Thus, one of the important things that may occur as a result of experience or practice in the early years of growth and development is an opportunity for the child to "learn" (however brief or whatever form that learning may take) to use various forms of sensory information (e.g. to integrate visual, vestibular and proprioceptive information) to regulate motor functions such as those involved in balance.

The motorically awkward child. What do we know about the development of motor function in the awkward or uncoordinated child? Williams et al. (1983) observed that chronologically older children with mild motor development delays (clumsy children) displayed motor programs with muscle selection and force production parameters that were very similar to those seen in younger, motorically normal children. Other data (Williams et al., in press) indicate that motorically awkward children use trunk muscles (erector spinae) a much larger percentage of time during 30 seconds of quiet standing than they do lower leg muscles (gastrocnemius and tibialis anterior). In contrast, children with average or normal motor development use trunk and leg muscles for comparable percentages of time during quiet standing. Lesny et al. (1975) also reported that normal 10-year-old children display more symmetrical patterns of EMG activity in maintaining balance than do children with minimal brain damage. These latter children tend to exhibit flat EMGs in musculature of the lower extremities and high levels of EMG activity in upper extremity musculature. These data suggest that children with normal motor development use motor programs that distribute the load for muscular support (e.g. force production) in standing more evenly and consistently across both trunk and leg muscles, while motorically slow children tend to use motor programs that place a greater and more variable load for muscular support (e.g. force production) on trunk and upper extremity musculature.

Another set of studies has attempted to answer the question of how young children organize motor programs to regulate movement when they are asked to do two things at once. In other words, what happens when motorically normal and motorically awkward young children are asked to perform two motor-based tasks simultaneously? Williams et al. (1985) studied how young children organize motor programs to maintain a given body position or postural framework when they are asked simultaneously to carry-out a simple arm movement. The primary task of the child was to maintain balance in an upright standing position. The secondary task was to move the preferred arm through 90 degrees of shoulder abduction. The study involved 4-, 6-, 8-, and 10-year-old motorically normal and motorically awkward children and investigated the percentage of time EMG activity was present in selected leg and trunk muscles. Data from this study indicated that children with normal motor development tended to display patterns of leg muscle activity that were 'parallel' in nature; that is the duration of activity in the lower leg muscles (the gastrocnemius and tibialis anterior) was such that when duration of activity increased in one muscle it also increased in the other muscle and vice versa. Thus, cocontraction seemed to be the dominant mode of leg muscle control for normally developing children in maintaining a standing posture under these circumstances. In contrast, motorically awkward children tended to exhibit patterns of leg muscle activity that were reciprocal in nature. That is, when duration of activity in the gastrocnemius increased, duration of activity in the tibialis anterior decreased and vice versa. Thus, when motorically unskilled children performed a simple arm movement in the upright position, reciprocal inhibition tended to be the dominant mode of leg muscle control. Engelhorn (1983) has also reported that improvements in skill in performing an elbow flexion task tended to be accompanied by increased cocontraction of the biceps and triceps muscles.

Other evidence on children's performances under dual task conditions (children are asked to perform two tasks simultaneously) suggests that the strategies used by children with different levels of motor development to perform tasks under these conditions are quite distinct (Williams and Seymour, in press). Children were asked to perform a unimanual motor sequencing task (a series of six manipulative actions which involved a push, a pull, and turn of small levers) while they sang or recited a familiar rhyme or the alphabet. Seventy-three percent of 6- and 7-year-old children with normal motor development began and ended the two tasks together; they appeared to program the verbal and motor tasks to occur in concert with one another and to treat them as a single event. Children with poorer levels of motor development tended to use one of two strategies to perform under dual task conditions. The more common strategy was to start the two tasks together, to end the motor task first, and then to stop the verbalization. The other common strategy was to begin and end the motor task first and to 'sandwich' the verbalization between them. Motorically awkward children rarely if ever started and stopped the two tasks simultaneously. Awkward, uncoordinated children seemed to treat dual task situations as though they were comprised of two separate, independent events which were only loosely related in time and programmed them accordingly.

Other motor control functions that have commonly been found to differentiate between normal and motorically clumsy children are primitive postural reflexes and equilibrium and righting reflexes (Paine et al., 1964; Steinberg and Rendle-Short, 1977; Ayes, 1973). The development of postural reflexes in normal infants and infants with chronic brain syndromes was studied by Paine et al. (1964). Their data indicated that in comparison to normal infants, postural reflexes, in general, were more delayed in infants with neurological difficulties and that primitive reflexes persisted longer in these children. Normal motor development, including reaching and grasping behaviors, was also delayed in the latter group. Steinberg and Rendle-Short (1977) found that vestibular-based righting reactions were either inadequate or absent in children with minimal neurological dysfunction. Patterns of postural control typically become more refined with age; however, in children with motor development delays, such refinement is either lacking or is much slower in appearing (Williams et al., 1983; Rosenbloom and Horton, 1971). In general it has been shown that when development of higher motor function is interrupted, individuals lose some or all of their capacity to establish and use "effectively" motor programs for regulating posture and movement (Badke and Duncan, 1983; Harrison and Connolly, 1971). Data do indicate, however, that such individuals can, with the aid of augmented sensory-motor feedback, develop some aspects of motor programs and achieve more proficient posture and movement control.

Eye-hand coordination. The development and refinement of motor programs for control of gross body movement is also an important adjunct to the development of complex, coordinated movements of the arms and hands. As postural control increases, the hands of the child are more and more freed to be used in and to develop fine eye-hand coordination skills. Several behaviorally-based studies have shown that many functional eye-hand coordination skills are improved when appropriate postural support (in the form of artificial adaptive seating) is provided for the motorically involved child (Kamath, 1984; Bergen and Colangelo, 1982; Trefler et al., 1978).

With regard to the development of motor programs for control of eye-hand coordination, Bower (1979) has identified two phases of reaching/grasping behaviors in the young infant that provide some insight into the nature of such development. Phase 1, as Bower (1979) identifies it, involves a visually elicited but undifferentiated arm/hand movement in which reaching and grasping actions are not separated but are executed as a single unit. The reaching action is not visually controlled; the grasping action appears to be more visually guided. In Phase 2, these two components of eye-hand coordination are executed independently; the infant can reach but not grasp or can grasp without reaching. At this time the reaching action is visually guided, that is, it is or can be corrected by visual feedback; the grasping action is tactilely regulated. The former (Phase 1) is reminiscent of open-loop control, the latter (Phase 2) of closed-loop control. Phase 1 is characteristic of the first postnatal month; it disappears and then resurfaces at about 4 months; Phase 2 appears about the fifth postnatal month and persists throughout the first year. Thus, it appears that the older infant monitors and modifies ongoing motor programs for eye-hand coordination via visual feedback (perhaps because he/she is able to process and use visual information more efficiently than the younger infant). The younger infant either cannot or does not use visual feedback to any extent to regulate eye-hand coordination.

The nature of motor programs involved in eye-hand coordination in older children has been studied by Hay (1978) and Hay (1979). She reports that, like the young infant, eye-hand coordination movements in 5-year-old children are largely under open loop control; reaching and grasping movements consist of an initial ballastic movement followed by a sudden last minute "braking" at the end of the reaching action. At 7 years of age, children, like older infants, tend to use visual feedback to monitor or regulate motor programs involved in eye-hand coordination. At this age fine motor control is characterized by early "braking" of the initial ballistic reaching movement. Eye-hand coordination movements of 9-year-old children are characterized by a combination of both open and closed loop control. For example, in older children eye-hand coordination movements consist of an initial ballistic movement (open loop) followed by an early, smooth and often two-stage "braking" of the initial movement (closed loop). Hay (1979) suggests that the transition to closed loop control occurs in part because children 7 years and older are better able to integrate kinesthetic information derived from the movement of the hand through space with visual information available from both the moving hand and the target in space; this capacity to integrate visual and proprioceptive information enables older children to maintain more refined control over eye-hand coordination. Williams (1983) has reported similar observations on young children who are faced with judging when and how to intercept a moving object in space.

Data from both Hay (1979) and McCracken (1983) suggest that young children (under 7 years) do not use visual information as effectively as older children (9 years or above) in regulating motor programs for manipulative activity. In addition McCracken (1983) has reported that older boys (10 years of age) significantly improved their eye-hand coordination control with practice on a tapping task; young boys (6 years old) did not. It would appear that what may happen in the early development of eye-hand coordination is that children learn or develop the capacity to visually monitor motor programs for the control of manipulative activity and to integrate and use a number of different sources of sensory information to regulate the control of ongoing movements.

Although much of the information already reviewed has hinted at several possibilities for the role of experience in the development of sensory-motor function in young children, the results of some research on animals provides a slightly different perspective on the potential importance of 'experience' in such development. In 1974, Held and Bauer (1974) theorized that the young developing nervous system calibrated the motor programs used for control of posture and movement by comparing 'movement commands with sensory feedback from movement'. In other words, they suggested that the integration of visual and proprioceptive information associated with the same bodily movement provided the primary basis for the refinement of movement control. This implies that having the opportunity to integrate visual and proprioceptive information through contact with and/or movement in the environment and experiencing the specific movement-produced sensory stimulation created by that movement is a necessary ingredient for developing refined programs of motor control. Data from a subsequent study on monkeys supported this theoretical position. Indirectly Hein (1974) suggested that what occurs as the organism grows and develops is that he/she integrates visual and proprioceptive information produced by active movement and develops a body-centered map of external visual space. This map is then used by the organism to calibrate various parameters of the motor programs used in the regulation of posture, movement, and eye-hand coordination. Without active experience on the part of the young organism, these aspects of motor control are subject to less than optimal development.

Sensory-Motor Function and Cognitive Behavior

Appropriate levels of physical activity are universally recognized as important components of healthful living for adults. Likewise, there is little doubt that physical activity can and does contribute in important ways to the health and well-being of children (Goode, 1979). A growing body of evidence has accumulated that links physical activity and the concomitant experiences that go with it more and more strongly to a healthy, optimally functioning mind (and brain, as we have seen previously) and thus potentially to improved cognitive performance in young and old alike (Ramey and Haskins, 1981).

In 1964, the UNESCO Council supported a commitment to the equal development of intellectual, physical, moral and aesthetic capacities of children; they recommended that 1/6 to 1/3 of total school time available be given to physical activity (Bailey, 1976). The Canadian Medical Association and the U.S. Public Health Service (Green and Horton, 1982) both have stressed the need for increased time for participation in physical education. Volpe (1979) encouraged more time for physical activity to develop the adaptive potential of students. Adaptive behavior, as he defined it, constituted a fundamental process which children need in order to operate effectively as an agent in their own development, a part of which is cognitive development.

Early development of neuromuscular control and motor function seem to provide support for the early stages of learning (Shepard, 1983). For example, an important part of the early development and education of the preschool age child is the organization and refinement of crude movement responses into finely-tuned, coordinated movement patterns which can be used in a variety of ways to learn about and adapt to an everchanging and demanding environment. Barker and Wright (1958) suggested that in a single 24-hour period, young children may perform as many as 2000 movement responses which involve the use of or interaction with some 660 objects and which are an integral part of a wide variety of cognitive activities.

Experts in the field of perceptual-motor development have for a long time pointed to potentially significant relationships between early motor or neuromuscular development and cognitive growth in young children of pre- and primary school age (Chissom et al., 1972; Williams et al., 1978; Williams, 1983). Perceptual-motor development theory and research suggest that early sensory and motor experiences, physical activity, and cognitive growth go hand in hand. Although limited in scope and design, most research in this area indicates that basic motor skills (e.g. gross motor object and body projection skills and fine-motor skills involved in writing, drawing, and object manipulation, etc.) provide an important foundation for the development of more sophisticated perceptual and cognitive behaviors. Such relationships are clearly stronger in children younger than 7 years of age than in children who are older. In essence, evidence suggests that to function effectively in a cognitive mode, the young child must develop at least a minimal set of neuromuscular skills (e.g. Belka and Williams, 1978, 1979; Williams, 1983). Belka and Williams (1979) have also shown that cognitive performances of kindergarten age children can be predicted reasonably accurately from knowledge of the child's perceptual-motor development at pre-kindergarten ages.

Clearly, from a Piagetian point of view, the development of adequate psycho-motor abilities is a vital part of the total cycle of the child's cognitive growth and is particularly important in the early years of development (Piaget, 1963). Another factor to consider is that an important condition for learning, and thus for cognitive development, is an adequate level of arousal. Physical activity has been shown to have a strong and immediate effect on the level of arousal of the individual. Overall it would appear that for young children, participation in physical activity may indeed act to enhance emerging cognitive behavior.

From a more practical perspective, data from a study conducted in Trois-Rivieres, Quebec indicated that five additional hours of physical education activity per week positively affected language and math performance of public school primary level students. In addition to showing expected gains in maximal oxygen uptake, muscle strength and physical performance, these children also had consistently higher marks in classroom activities than did control students who did not participate in the additional physical activity. This improvement occurred in spite of the fact that classroom time was decreased by 13-14% (Sheppard, 1982).

Similarly a ten year study in Vanves, France (1951-1960) showed that increasing the time devoted to physical activity to 7-8 hours/week for elementary school children resulted not only in improved health, fitness and motor development, but also in enhanced academic performance, in increased independence of students and in decreased susceptibility to stress (Bailey, 1976). Bailey (1976) suggests that although physical activity did not make the students more intelligent, it may have helped to develop more keenly the "tools of intelligence." Bailey (1973), in a similar school-based study in Saskatoon, found that students who received additional hours of physical activity showed increases in concentration and decreases in disruptive behavior when compared to children in a control group.

Adequate self-esteem is also an important facet of mental health and can indirectly affect cognitive functioning. Physical activity may have some lasting effect on one's sense of self-worth and thus indirectly influence the cognitive performance of children. Self-efficacy, or a person's estimate of his ability to perform specific actions within highly specific circumstances, is enhanced through performance and experience (Coates et al., 1982). By increasing the child's capacity (from an energy point of view) to undertake physical and mental work, physical activity could increase the child's confidence in his/her ability to perform. Secondly, participation in physical activity tends to enhance the body image of the child and thus could have a positive effect on the child's attitude toward work and his potential for goal achievement. There is also considerable evidence to suggest that physically active individuals tend to respond less intensely to emotionally-laden stimuli (Raab and Krzywanek, 1966; Rivard et al., 1977). Such individuals tend to exhibit greater emotional stability and greater ability to cope with stress.

What are some of the physiological mechanisms by means of which physical activity and its concomitant sensory-motor stimulation might contribute to or provide support for the development of cognitive processes? There is considerable evidence from animal studies that an important element in early brain growth and development is sensory-motor stimulation. It is well documented that brains of sensory enriched (stimulated) animals demonstrate significant changes in anatomical and biochemical parameters that are believed to be indicative of a more efficiently functioning nervous system (e.g. Dobbing and Sands, 1973; Goldman, 1972; Greenough et al., 1976; Purpura, 1977; Rosenzweig and Bennett, 1972; Rosenzweig et al., 1972). (These data will be reviewed in more detail in another section.) If cognitive performance is in any way a reflection of optimal brain growth and development, then sensory-motor stimulation must be considered to be an important factor in at least the early development of the child's cognitive behavior. An important source of such stimulation for the young child is that provided through the child's involvement in movement and/or physical activity. When the child engages in physical activity at least two major sensory systems—vision and proprioception—are actively stimulated and thus sensory-motor experiences could contribute in significant ways to promoting neural development (Williams, 1979).

From another perspective, consider that, in general, individuals with cardiac insufficiency and/or those predisposed to cardiovascular disease (CVD) regardless of age, are slower in psychomotor and cognitive functions than those without such health problems (Abraham and Birren, 1973; Birren et al., 1963; Light, 1975; Wilke et al., 1976). Memory and intelligence also deteriorate more in hypertensive individuals than in normal individuals (Hamsher and Benton, 1978; Hartzog et al., 1978). Even individuals who are predisposed to CVD, but who do not show clinical symptoms of such, are slower in psychomotor and cognitive responses than controls (Abrahams and Birren, 1973).

Deterioration of the cardiovascular system reduces cerebral blood flow (CBF). There is little doubt that brain activity is affected by cerebral circulation. In addition, the relationship between electroencephalographic (EEG) activity, oxidative metabolism of brain tissues and CBF is also well documented (Ingvar, 1967; Ingvar and Lassen, 1975; Ingvar et al., 1976). Although total cerebral blood flow does not appear to be altered with activity, regional cerebral blood flow does shift according to metabolic demands of different regions (Halsey et al., 1979; Lassen et al., 1978). In other words, specific areas of the brain involved in the performance of an active task receive increased blood flow to support the work; other less active areas receive reduced blood flow. Increased CBF has been shown to occur following gross physical activity (e.g. treadmill running), manual activity and arousal reactions. Physical activity, in particular, has been shown to increase regional CBF in prefrontal, somatosensory and primary motor cortices in some cases as much as 30% (Lassen et al., 1978; Orgogoza and Larsen, 1979). Such evidence suggests a potential and important link among physical activity, sensory-motor stimulation and cognitive performance. Such data, however, do not provide an unequivocal case for causal links among these variables.

Glucose uptake and metabolism in the brain are also affected by physical activity. Glucose is important in brain function because it serves as the main fuel for energy metabolism in the mammalian brain. Sharp (1976) has clearly demonstrated that there are differences in glucose consumption in the brains of exercising versus resting animals and that there is a definite increase in glucose consumption in the brains of active animals. Consider then that if during physical activity different areas of the brain are regularly and systematically activated and as a result blood flow to these areas is increased and/or maintained for long periods of time, physical activity could act as an agent for developing and maintaining optimum vascularization of the brain, a condition which may be necessary to support processes involved in glucose production and utilization in the brain. If these latter processes are maintained at a high level, then the energy needed to support neural function is more likely to be available. Thus, it is possible that physical activity may be an important (if indirect) link in the chain of events that leads to optimal conditions for cognitive growth.

Sensory-Motor Experience and Brain Development

This section will explore the nature of the relationship between brain development and sensory-motor experience. By necessity, heavy emphasis will be placed on research on animals, since experimentation of this kind is difficult, if not impossible, to carry out with human beings and available data are indeed sparse. However, important lessons may be learned from work on animals.

There is believed to be a considerable amount of plasticity in the nervous system early in development, particularly of the cortical centers where higher order motor, perceptual and thought processes are based (Rosenzweig et al., 1972). Plasticity refers to the capacity of the nervous system to be changed or modified as a result of exposure to different kinds of stimulation. Modification of the nervous system has been shown, in many instances, to be directly related to the extent and kind of environmental stimulation experienced by the young, growing organism (Ferchmin and Eterovic, 1979; Rosenzweig and Bennett, 1972). Such environmental experiences may be very important to the development of a variety of human motor, perceptual and cognitive behaviors. The following discussion is not meant to suggest that a significant part of nervous system development is not maturationally and genetically based; rather, it is meant to examine the research which seems to indicate that environmental or sensory-motor stimulation of the growing nervous system may be vital to the growth and refinement of certain structural and functional characteristics of that system.

To fully understand the potential importance of early sensory-motor experiences in brain development, the nature of the changes which occur in the brain after sensory-motor stimulation must be identified. Let us look at the nature of such changes. The majority of studies on animals indicate that among the most important changes that occur in the brain as a result of sensory-motor or environmental stimulation are: an increase in weight and thickness of the cerebral cortex; an increase in the size of the cell bodies and nuclei of neurons; an increase in synaptic density; an increase in dendritic branching; and an increase in the amount of axon myelination (Davison and Dobbing, 1966; Mayers et al., 1971; Rosenzweig et al., 1972). All of these morphological changes are thought to contribute to more effective transmission, processing, and storing of information in the brain. Although admittedly all of these effects are small (e.g. when brains of enriched animals are compared to brains of impoverished animals, the differences described above are minimal), such effects have been consistently observed and have been reported to be present in animals in at least 16 different replications of Rosenzweig's original (1972) study.

For illustrative purposes this section will examine more closely what changes in dendritic branching and axon myelination might mean to the development of refined brain function. Normal and optimal neuronal functioning depend on the orderly development of synaptic and dendritic systems (Cragg, 1974). The number, distribution and functional types of synapses of different dendritic systems is essential to carrying out effective integrative and memory processes by the brain. The elaboration of dendritic systems is also significant to brain function, for dendrites provide more than 94% of the target sites for transmission and processing of information in the nervous system. Scheibel and Scheibel (1977) suggest that dendritic systems, in particular, provide sensitive indices to pathology of brain growth and that dendritic spine loss is often associated with profound, potentially irreversible changes in brain function. Dendritic spine loss, formation of nodules on dendritic spines, and curling or shrinkage of dendrites are conditions that typically accompany abnormal brain development. Purpura (1974) has reported that the brains of mentally retarded children have a reduced number of dendritic spines (called dendritic spine dysgenesis) and a bizarre curling of dendrites is often seen in children with Down's syndrome. For human beings, the period from 7 1/2 months prenatally to 6 months postnatally seems to be critical to development of synaptic and dendritic systems; however, dendritic branching appears to continue into at least the third decade of life. Early sensory-motor stimulation may play a significant role in the development of appropriate dendritic systems in the brain.

Most of the fast conducting pathways of the nervous system are myelinated; that is, during early growth, they develop a protein covering that aids and supports nerve impulse conduction. The nature and extent of such growth processes in the CNS can be estimated by assessing the amount and location of myelin present at different stages in development (Dekaban, 1970; Rorke and Riggs, 1969). The process of myelination begins during the prenatal period and continues into adolescence. Formation of myelin is very rapid during the last 2-3 fetal months and the first 4-5 postnatal years. In general, motor systems are myelinated in advance of sensory systems; the motor system is nearly complete in its myelination by two years of age (Yakolev and Lecours, 1967). Although the pattern of myelination in various sensory systems is complex, the somesthetic and/or proprioceptive systems appear to become myelinated in advance of the visual system, which appears to become myelinated in advance of the auditory system. The last parts of the nervous system to undergo myelination are those that are involved with complex memory and integrative functions. Such areas continue to be myelinated into (and perhaps beyond) the third decade of life. Sensory-motor stimulation may be one factor that affects the rate at which myelination of different parts of the nervous system occurs, and thus indirectly may affect the efficiency with which information is transmitted and processed by the brain.

The brain growth spurt is a period of rapid growth of the nervous system that begins during prenatal development (about 6 months) and continues into the postnatal years. During this time, dramatic changes occur in a wide variety of structural and functional characteristics of the brain (Dobbing, 1972; Dobbing and Sands, 1973). The most important of these changes are: rapid increase in myelination; significant growth of dendritic and synaptic systems; an increase in glial cell proliferation; and refinement of selected enzyme systems. The brain growth spurt is programmed to occur during a specific period of time, regardless of whether conditions are favorable for such growth (Dobbing and Sands, 1973; Dobbing and Smart, 1974). If unfavorable conditions do exist when the brain growth spurt occurs, optimum development of neural function may be permanently hindered. Common deficits have been observed when there is severe restriction of growth during this vulnerable period. These include: significant deficits in the quantity of myelin present in the brain; significant reduction in dendritic branching and formation of synaptic connections; permanent reduction in brain size; and permanent alteration of reflex ontogeny and thus of motor development (Dobbing, 1974, 1976; Dobbing et al., 1971; Dobbing and Smart, 1974). Note that these include some of the same characteristics that have been observed to be positively influenced by early sensory-motor stimulation.

Although in human beings the brain growth spurt begins about the 24th week of fetal life, the first two postnatal years seem to be very significant ones for promoting optimal development of brain function. This is a period of growth identified by Piaget (1963) as a crucial sensory-motor period, a time during which the child builds a basic repertoire of both manipulative and locomotor skills, learns to organize and use sensory information efficiently, and develops both goal-directed behavior and primitive notions of self, of time, and of space. Piaget (1963) suggests that these behaviors are developed in conjunction with and as a result of the child's own physical activity—his active movement in and exploration of the environment around him. This period of sensory-motor development provides the foundation for the development of imitation, symbolic play and language behaviors—all of which are important to the early cognitive functioning of the child. Thus, sensory-motor experience and physical activity may be important adjuncts to many aspects of both brain and behavioral development during these early years.

Also of importance to those of us concerned with learning processes, developmental play, and physical activity in children are data reported by Rosenzweig et al. (1972) from their work on the effects of enriched versus impoverished environmental experiences on neural development in young organisms. These data strongly indicate that environmental stimulation produces changes in the brain primarily if the organism exposed to the environmental stimulation *actively interacts* with that environment. In other words, observed changes in brain structure and function are more likely to occur if there is active physical exploration and/or manipulation of the environment by the organism. Thus, active physical or motor involvement on the part of the organism is an integral part of whatever process it is that is involved in producing the changes that accompany more refined neural function.

Although most CNS systems possess the capacity for modification, the visual system of young animals is particularly remarkable in its plasticity. The visual system will be used to show more specifically how sensory-motor experiences may contribute to neural development in the growing organism. For example, prior to any visual experience, large populations of visual cortex cells in the young cat show *no response* to visual input (Blakemore and Cooper, 1970; Blakemore and Mitchell, 1973). Furthermore, no cortical neurons recorded show even the vaguest preference for responding to different characteristics of visual stimuli (e.g. for responding to spatial orientation or to movement direction). Thus most inexperienced neurons of young animals are neither selective nor well-defined in their responses to visual stimualtion. In contrast, in normally reared adult cats, individual cortical cells are very sensitive to specific aspects of visual stimulation; they respond to the specific spatial orientation of the stimulus and to directional characteristics of stimuli that are moving in the environment. Interestingly, as the young cat has exposure to or experience with specific forms of environmental stimulation, visual cortex neurons quickly become conditioned to respond in very consistent ways to specific patterns of visual input. They rapidly develop sharply defined responses to a narrow range of specific spatial orientations of visual stimuli (e.g. vertical versus horizontal versus diagonal positions) and to various movement characterisitcs of these stimuli (Hirsch and Spinelli, 1971). Importantly, these responses are strongly biased toward the particular stimulus(i) to which the animal has been exposed. Thus, visual cortex cells become more defined in their responses to environmental stimuli to which they been systematically exposed. In fact, the more the cells are exposed to such stimuli, the more finely tuned their response to such stimuli becomes.

There is also some evidence to indicate that a wide range of adaptations to different forms of sensory stimulation or deprivation can and does occur (Blakemore and Cooper, 1970; Hirsch and Spinelli, 1971; Pettigrew et al., 1973). For example, most visual cortex cells respond to sensory input from both eyes; however, if artificial strabismus is created (one eye is deviated in its alignment with the other eye), and the animal views or experiences the visual environment under these circumstances, the end result is that cells in the visual cortex lose their binocularity and respond only to input from one eye. Input from the opposite eye is nonfunctional. The same situation holds true if the animal is exposed only to monocular stimulation, a condition in which the animal is permitted to use just one eye to see the visual world. In cases such as these, acuity, discrimination and many aspects of visuo-motor coordination which are common to normal animals are impaired in these animals. Only slight improvement in these behaviors occurs even after long periods of binocular stimulation. All of these data clearly suggest that environmental stimulation (experience) may be an important factor in determining both the kind and the range of stimuli to which the brain responds and the nature and precision of the response made to those stimuli. In this way sensory-motor stimulation which is an inherent part of motor skill development and physical activity may become an extremely important factor in promoting optimal growth and development of the nervous system of the young organism.

It should be noted that the neurophysiological changes observed in visual cortex cells do not always occur immediately after sensory experience. Rather, some passage of time may be required before some of the effects of sensory stimulation are observed. For example, Pettigrew and Garey (1974) and Garey and Pettigrew (1974) reported that after one hour of visual experience, 43.3% of a population of cells in the visual cortex of the cat were not immediately responsive to previously experienced visual stimulation. Another 28.3% of the cells responded only very broadly and to a wide variety of stimuli presented to either eye. During succeeding weeks (3 to 14 weeks), however, and without additional visual stimulation, the neurophysiological responses of these neurons changed gradually but dramatically. Approximately 54% of the cells studied subsequently showed adult-type responses and were driven optimally by the particular visual stimulus to which that eye had been exposed. Within this broad framework of time, there was also a more narrow or critical period of time (4-5 weeks) during which there was a peak in the development of the cell's response to sensory stimulation. Thus, there may be identifiable periods during which sensory-motor experiences are most important if they are to contribute to optimum development of underlying neural systems (Herschkowitz and Rossi, 1972). If information presently available on human neural development and information processing has any bearing at all on this issue, it would appear that perhaps the first six to ten years of life are significant ones for providing a wide range of sensory-motor experiences. However, such data need to be interpreted with the greatest of caution when making inferences about human development.

References

Abraham, J.P. & Birren, J.E. (1973). Reaction time as a function of age and behavioral predisposition to coronary heart disease. *Journal of Gerontology, 28,* 471-478.

Ayres, A.J. (1973). *Sensory integration and learning disorders.* Los Angeles: Western Psychological Services.

Badke, M.B. and Duncan, P.W. (1983). Patterns of rapid motor response during postural adjustments when standing in healthy subjects and hemiplegic patients. *Physical Therapy, 63,* 13-20.

Bailey, D. (1973). Inactivity and the Canadian child. In R.G. Goode and R. Volpe (Eds.), *The child and physical activity: Proceedings of a workshop for educting the growing child.* In Orban W.A.R. (Ed.), *Proceedings of the National Conference on Fitness and Health.* Ottawa: Department of National Health and Welfare, 13-22.

Bailey, D.A. (1976). The growing child and the need for physical activity. In J.G. Albinson & G.M. Andrew (Eds.), *Child in sport and physical activity.* Baltimore: University Park Press.

Bailey, D.A. (1973). Exercise, fitness, and physical education for the growing child. In Orban, W.A.R. (Ed.), *Proceedings of the National Conference on Fitness and Health.* Department of National Health and Welfare, 13-22.

Barker, R.G. and Wright, H.F. (1958). *Midwest and its children.* Evanston, Il: Row Peterson and Co.

Belka, D. and Williams, H.G. (1978). *Canonical relationships among perceptual-motor, perceputal and cognitive behaviors in young, normal children.* Unpublished paper, University of Toledo.

Belka, D. and Williams, H.G. (1979). Prediction of later cognitive behavior from early school perceputal-motor, perceptual and cognitive performances. *Perceptual and Motor Skills, 49,* 131-141.

Bergen, A.F. & Colangelo, C. (1982). *Positioning the client with central nervous system deficits: The wheelchair and other adapted equipment.* Valhalla, NY: Valhalla Rehabilitation Publications.

Birren, J.E., Carden, P.V. & Phillips, S.L. (1963). Reaction time as a function of the cardiac cycle in young adults. *Science, 140,* 195-196.

Blakemore, C. and G. Cooper (1978). Development of the brain depends on the visual environment. *Nature, 228,* 477-478.

Blakemore, C. & Mitchell, D. (1973). Environmental modification of the visual cortex and the neural basis of learning and memory. *Nature, 241,* 467-468.

Bower, T.G.R. (1979). *Human Development.* San Francisco: Freeman.

Butterworth, G. (1982). The origins of auditory-visual perception and visual proprioception in human development. In R. Walk and H. Pick (Eds.), *Intersensory Perception and Sensory Integration.* New York: Plenum Press.

Butterworth, G. & Hicks, L. (1977). Visual proprioception and postural stability in infancy: a developmental study. *Perception, 6,* 255-262.

Chissom, B.S., Thomas, J.F. & Biasiotto, J. (1972). Canonical validity of perceptual-motor skills for predicting an academic criterion. *Educational and Psychological Measurement. 32,* 1095-1098.

Cicchetti, D. & Stoufe, L.A. (1978). An organizational view of affect: Illustrations from the study of Down's Syndrome infants. In M. Lewis and I. Rosenblum (Eds.), *The development of affecxt.* New York: Plenum Press.

Coates, T.J., Petuson A.C. & Perry, C. 1982. Crossing the Barriers. In T.J. Coates, et al., *Promoting adolescent health: A dialogue in research and practice.* New York: Academic Press.

Cragg, B. Plasticity of synapses. (1974). *British Medical Bulletin, 30,* 141-144.

Davison A. & Dobbing, J. (1966). Myelination as a vulnerable period in brain development. *British Medical Bulletin, 22,* 40-49.

Dekaban, A. (1970). *Neurology of Early Childhood.* Baltimore, MD: Williams and Wilkins.

Dobbing, J. (1974). Human brain development and its vulnerability. Biologic and Clinical Aspects of Brain Development. *Mead Johnson Symposium on Perinatal and Developmental Medicine, 6,* 3-12.

Dobbing, J. (1976). Vulnerable periods in brain growth and somatic growth. In Roberts and Thomson (Eds), *The Biology of Human Fetal Growth.* New York: Halsted Press.

Dobbing, J. (1972). Vulnerable periods of brain development. In Elliot and Knight (Eds.), *Lipids, Malnutrition and the Developing Brain.* Amsterdam: Elsvier Publishers.

Dobbing, J., Hopewell, J., & Lynch, A. (1971). Vulnerability of developing brain: VII. Permanent deficits of neurons in cerebral and cerebellar cortex following early mild undernutrition. *Experimental Neurology, 32,* 439-477.

Dobbing, J. & Sands, J. (1973). Quantitative growth and development of human brain. *Archives of Diseases of Childhood, 48,* 757-767.

Dobbing, J. & Smart, J. (1974). Vulnerability of developing brain and behavior. *British Medical Bulletin, 30,* 164-168.

Engelhorn, R. (1983). Agonist and antagonist muscle EMG activity pattern changes with skill acquisition. *Research Quarterly for Exercise and Sport. 54,* 315-323.

Ferchmin, P. & Eterovic, V.A. (1979). Mechanism of brain growth by environmental stimulation. *Science, 205,* 522.

Forssberg, H. & Nashner L. (1982). Ontogenetic development of posture control in man: adaptation to altered support and visual conditions during stance. *Journal of Neuroscience, 2,* 545-552.

Garey, L. & Pettigrew, J. (1974). Ultrastructural changes in kitten visual cortex after environmental modification. *Brain Research, 66,* 165-172.

Goode, R.C. (1979). The child and physical activity. In R.G. Goode and R. Volpe (Eds.), The child and physical activity: Proceedings of a workshop for educational leaders. Toronto.

Goldman, P.S. (1972). Developmental determinants of cortical plasticity. *Acta Neurobiologaiae Experimentia, 32,* 495-511.

Green, L.W. & Horton, D. (1982). Adolescent health: Issues and challenges. In T.J. Coates, A.C. Peterson, and C. Perry (Eds.), *Promoting adolescent health: A dialogue on research and practice.* New York: Academic Press.

Greenough, W., Fass, B., & Devoogd, T. (1976). The influence of experience on recover following brain damage in rodents: hypothesis based on developmental research. In Walsh and Greenough, *Environments as Therapy for Brain Dysfunction* (pp. 10-50). New York: Plenum Press.

Halsey, J.J., Blauenstein, U.W., Wilson, E.M., & Willis, E.H. (1979). Regional

Hamsher, K. des., & Benton, A.L. (1978). Interactive effects of age and cerebral disease on cognitive performances. *Journal of Neurology, 217,* 195-200.

Harrison, A. & Connolly, K. (1971). The conscious control of fine levels of neuromuscular firing in spastic and normal subjects. *Developmental Medicine and Child Neurology, 13,* 762-771.

Hay, L. (1978). Accuracy of children on a open-loop pointing task. *Perceptual and Motor Skills. 47,* 1079-1082.

Hay, L. (1979). Spatial-temporal analysis of movements in children: motor programs versus feedback in the development of reaching. *Journal of Motor Behavior, 11,* 189-200.

Hein, A. (1974). Prerequisite for development of visually guided reaching in the kitten. *Brain Research, 71,* 259-263.

Held, R. & Bauer, J. (1974). Development of sensorially guided reaching in infant monkeys. *Brain Research, 71,* 265-271.

Herman, R. (1970). Electromyographic evidence of some control factors involved in the acquisition of skilled performance. *American Journal of Physical Medicine, 49,* 177-191.

Herschkowitz, N. & Rossi, E. (1972). Critical periods in brain development. In Elliot and Knight (Eds.), *Lipids, Malnutrition and the Developing Brain.* Amsterdam: Elsevier Publishers.

Hertzog, D., Schaie, W., & Gribben, K. (1978). Cardiovascular disease and changes in intellectual functioning from middle to old age. *Journal of Gerontology, 33,* 872-883.

Hirsch, H. & Spinelli, D. (1971). Modification of the distribution of receptive field orientation in cats by selective visual exposure during development. *Experimental Brain Research, 13,* 509-527.

Hobart, D.J. & Vorro, J. (1978). Kinematic and electromyographic differences between men and women during skill acquisition: A preliminary study. *Physical Therapy, 58,* 956-965.

Ingvar, D.H. (1967). Cerebral metabolism, cerebral blood flow and EEG. In Widen, L. (Ed.), *Recent Advances in Clinical Neurophysiology, Electroencephalography and Clinical Neurophysiology, Supplement 25,* 102-106.

Ingvar, D.H. & Lassen, N.A. (Eds.), (1975). *Brainwork, Alfred Benzon Symposium VIII,* Munksqaard Copenhagen.

Ingvar, D.H., Sjolund, B., & Ardo, A. (1976). Correlation between dominant EEG frequency, cerebral oxygen uptake and blood flow. *Encephalography and Clinical Neurophysiology, 41,* 268-276.

Kamath, D.G. (1984). The effects of the neck and trunk functional support on spasticityin cerebral palsy children. *Proceedings of the Second International Conference on Reabilitation Engineering,* Ottawa.

Lassen, N.A., Ingvar, D.H., & Shinhoj, E. (1978). Brain function and blood flow. *Scientific American, October,* 62-71.

Lee, D.N. & Aronson, E. (1974). Visual proprioceptive control of standing in human infants. *Percepiton and psychophysics, 15,* 529-532.

Lesny, I., Syrovathka, A., & Doubravsky, O. (1975). Postural polygraphy in children with minimal brain damage. *Electroencephalography and Clinical Neurophysiology, 39,* 440-441.

Light, K.C. (1975). Slowing of response time in young and middle aged hypertensive patients. *Experimental Aging Research, 1,* 209-227.

Mayers, K., Robertson, R., Rubel, E., & Thompson, R. (1971). Development of polysensory responses in association cortex of kitten. *Science, 171,* 1038-1040.

McCracken, H.D. (1983). Movement control in a reciprocal tapping task: A developmental study. *Journal of Motor Behavior, 15,* 262-279.

Orgogoza, J.M. & Larsen, B. (1979). Activation of the supplementary motor area during voluntary movement in man suggests that it works as a supramotor area. *Science, 206,* 847-850.

Paine, R.S., Brazelton, T.B., Donovan, D.E., Drorbaugh, J.E., Hubbell, J.P. & Sears, E.M., (1964). Evolution of postural reflexes in normal infants and in the presence of chronic brain syndromes. *Neurology, 14,* 1036-1048.

Payton, O.D. & Kelley, D.L. (1972). Electromyographic evidence of the acquisition of a motor skill: A pilot study. *Physical Therapy, 52,* 261-266.

Pettigrew, J. & Garey, L. (1974). Selective modification of single neuron properties in the visual coretex of kittens. *Brain Research, 66,* 160-164.

Pettigrew, J., Olson C. & Hirsch, H. (1973). Cortical effect of selective visual experience: degeneration or reorganization? *Brain Research, 51,* 345-351.

Piaget, J. (1963). *The Origins of Intelligence.* New York: W.W. Norton and Company, Inc.

Purpura, D. (1977). Factors contributing to abnormal neuronal development in cerebral cortex of human infant. In *Berenberg's Brain Fetal and Infant Development* (pp. 54-78). The Hague: Martinus Nijhoff Medical Division.

Purpura, D. (1974). Neuronal migration and dendritic differentiation: normal and aberrant development of human cerebral cortex. *Biologic and Clinical Aspects of Brain Development.* Mead Johnson Symposium on Perinatal and Developmental Medicine, *6,* 13-27.

Raab, W. & Krzywanek, H. (1966). Cardiac sympathetic tone and stress response to personality patterns and exercise habits. In Raab, W. (Ed.), *Prevention of Ischemic Heart Disease.* Springfield, IL: C.C. Thomas.

Ramey, C.T. & R. Haskins. (1981). The modification of intelligence through early experience. *Intelligénce, 5,* 5-19.

Rivard, G., Lavallee, H., Rajic, M., Shephard, R.J., Thinaudeau, P., Davignon, A. & Beaucage, C. (1977). Influence of competitive hockey on physical condition and psychological behavior of children. In Lavallee, H. and Shephard, R.J. (Eds), *Frontiers of Activity and Child Health* (pp. 335-354). Quebec: Pelican.

Rorke, L. & Riggs, H. (1969). *Myelination of the Brain in the Newborn.* Philadelphia: J.B. Lippincott Company.

Rosenbloom, L. & Horton, M.E., (1971). The maturation of fine prehension in young children. *Developmental Medicine and Child Neurology, 13,* 3-8.

Rosenzweig, M.R. & Bennett, E.L., & Diamond, M., (1972). Brain changes in response to experience. *Scientific American 226:* 22-29.

Scheibel, M. & Scheibel. A. (1977). Specific threats to brain development: dendritic changes. In Berenber (Ed.), *Brain Fetal and Infant Development* (pp. 302-315). The Hague: Martinus Nijhoff Medical Division.

Shambes, G.M. (1976) Static postural control in children. *American Journal of Physical Medicine, 55,* 221-252.

Sharp, F.R. (1976). Relative cerebral glucose uptake of neuronal perikarya and neuropil determined with 2-deoxyglucose in resting and swimming rats. *Brain Research, 110,* 127-139.

Shephard, R.J. (1982). *Physical Activity and Growth.* Chicago: Year Book Medical Publishers, Inc.

Shephard, R.J. (1983). Physical activity and the healthy mind. *Canadian Medical Association Journal, 128,* 525-530.

Shumway-Cook, A. & Woollacott, M. (1983). The development of postural control mechanisms in normal and in Down's Syndrome Children. *Neuroscience Abstracts.*

Simard, T. (1969). Fine sensorimotor control in healthy childrein: an electromyographic study. *Pediatrics, 43,* 1035-1041.

Steinberg, M. & Rendle-Short, J. (1977). Vestibular dysfunction in young children with minor neurological impairment. *Developmental Medicine and Child Neruol-*

ogy, *19,* 639-651.

Trefler, E., Hanks, S., Huggins, P., Chiarizzo, S. & Hobson, D., (1978). A modular seating system for cerebral palsied children. *Developmental Medicine and Child neurology, 20,* 199-204.

Volpe, R. (1979). Physical activity, intellectual and emotional development. In R.G. Goode and R. Volpe (Eds.), *The Child and Physical Activity,* Proceedings of a Workshop for Educational Leaders, Toronto.

Williams, H.G. (1979). Neurosensory development in young organisms. In F. Landry and W.A.R. Orban (Eds.), *Physical Activity and Human Well-Being.* Miami, FL: Symposia Specialists, 57-70.

Williams, H.G. (1983). *Perceptual and Motor Development.* Englewood Cliffs, NJ: Prentice Hall, Inc.

Williams, H.G., Fisher, J.M., & Tritschler, K.A., (1983). A descriptive analysis of static postural control in 4, 6 and 8 year old normal and motorically awkward children. *American Journal of Physical Medicine, 62,* 12-26.

Williams, H.G., Mcclenaghan, B., & Ward. D. Duration of muscle activity during standing in normally and slowly developing children. *American Journal of Physical Medicine, 64,* 171-189.

Willaims, H.G., & Seymour, C. Movement strategies in young normally and slowly developing children. *Child Development,* in press.

Willams, H.G., Temple, I. & Bateman, J., (1978). Perceptual-motor and cognitive learning in the young child. *Psychology of Motor Behavior and Sport II.* Champaign, IL: Human Kinetics Press.

Wilke, F.L. Eisdorfer, C., & Nowlin, J.B., (1976). Memory and blood pressure in the aged. *Experimental Aging Research, 2,* 2-16.

Woollacott, M.H. (1983). *Children's changing capacity to process information.* AAHPERD Symposium, Minneapolis, Minnesota.

Yakovlev, P. & Lecours, A., (1967). The myelogentic cycles of regional maturation of the brain. In: Minkowski (Ed.), *Regional Development of the Brain in Early Life,* Philadelphia: F.A. Davis Co.

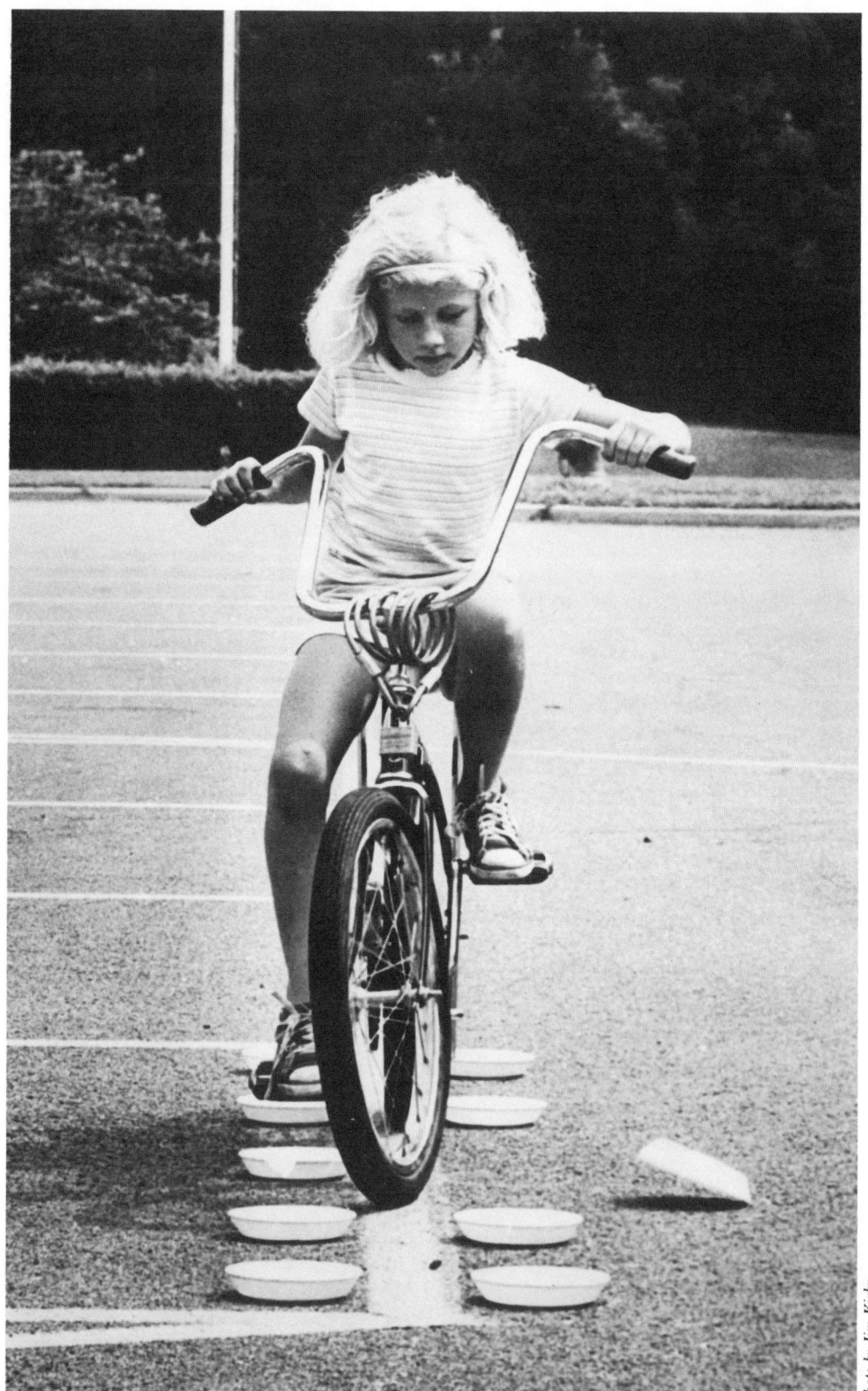

photo by Jim Kirby

CHAPTER FOUR

Memory Development and Motor Skill Acquisition

Jerry R. Thomas,
School of Health, Physical
Education, Recreation and Dance
Louisiana State University
Baton Rouge, Louisiana

Jere Dee Gallagher
Department of Health,
Physical and Recreation Education
University of Pittsburgh
Pittsburgh, Pennsylvania

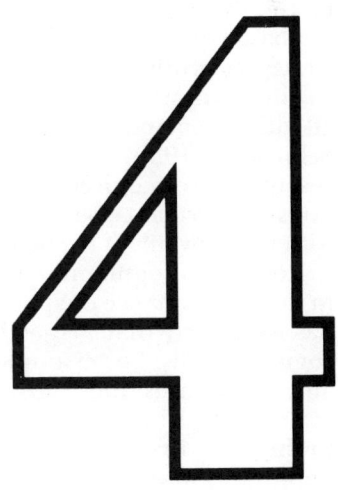

The purpose of this chapter is to review theory and research concerning the function of cognition in motor skill acquisition and performance. Of course, a short chapter cannot adequately cover the many years of research on this topic. Therefore, the approach taken here identifies the major mechanisms of memory and how they operate to influence skilled performance and learning. In particular, the information focuses on changes that occur across childhood and adolescence because these are the time periods during which most physical education and coaching instruction occurs.

Much of the literature on this topic is descriptive in nature. Theoretical models which explain the development of motor behavior have recently evolved and are incomplete at best. However, considerable advancement has occurred in the past 15 years. Thus, there is reason to be encouraged about the increased potential to not only describe motor behavior, but to predict its outcome and explain its control. The recent focus on understanding how movements are controlled—specifically, the description of the invariant and variant characteristics of movements—holds considerable promise for expanding our understanding of how the quality of movement can be influenced by instruction.

The chapter is organized to promote a general understanding of the process of skill acquisition and how developmental factors influence this process. First, the reader learns why cognitive processes are important in skill acquisition. This leads to the concept of the development of motor programs in memory, followed by a more specific model, Schema Theory, followed by developmental questions. Two important types of information are discussed within this framework—knowledge of results and modeling. This discussion is followed by an account of how memory and knowledge base development influence children's skill acquisition. The chapter concludes by presenting some of the factors that may be influenced during practice and motor performance.

Importance of Cognition in Motor Skill Acquisition

Cognition is important in motor skill learning and the performance of rapid movement tasks. Learning a motor skill involves internalizing the performance to reduce cognitive demands. The individual moves from the cognitive phase of learning (thinking, "What is the goal of the skill? What do I do to accomplish the task?") through the associative phase (thinking, "How do I adjust my stance to hit the baseball to left field?") to the autonomous phase (directing attention to the strategies involved).

Automation is important in learning a motor skill because it can reduce the attention demanded by the various decisions that an individual makes. Eberts and Schneider (1980) note that the benefits of automatic processing are that less resources are required, processing is faster, the task is less susceptible to distractions, performance becomes more accurate, and the internal structures associated with the movement become more economical and efficient.

Not only is cognition important in learning motor skills, but it is also important in the performance of sport skills in rapidly changing environments. Keel (1982) has suggested that fast-action sport skills are not perceptual-motor skills, but cognitive skills. For example, in a baseball game when there are runners on first and third bases and a ground ball is hit to the shortstop, the shortstop must evaluate the situation, the number of outs, the score, and quickly decide whether to throw to first, second, or home. Reaction to the start of a movement is less important, whereas the ability to anticipate and predict becomes critically important. In football, the ability of the linebacker to anticipate offensive plays allows sacking of the quarterback. Keel suggests that the "redundancy" inherent in a fast action skill is stored in memory and the skilled person has quick access to the *knowledge structures* that allow prediction and anticipation of events.

Whiting (1980) has stated that much of the research in motor control has ignored the influence of information processing capabilities. Motor skill acquisition and performance require the individual to attend to the environment in order to plan the correct movement, perform the movement while gathering information directed at success/failure of the movement, and then make the necessary changes for the next performance. Error information is used to modify the plan for subsequent performance. During information gathering and plan selection, cognition is important.

Plans for Movement

Planning a movement is necessary for the strategic control of the movement. A major characteristic is the generation of anticipatory signals (expected sensory consequences) that prepare the performer to accept certain kinds of information. These anticipatory signals are the basis on which the commands are organized, a major function being to serve as a referent for the interpretation of incoming feedback (Pribham, 1971, 1976).

Inherent in a movement plan is the intention to remember the movement. Developmentally, intention to remember does not exist until approximately 6 or 7 years of age (Apple et al., 1972; Kelso, Goodman, Stamm, & Hayes, 1979). A plan would consist of when and why one should intentionally store and retrieve information (Flavell & Wellman, 1977). An advantage of planning the movement is to reduce the demands placed on the individual. Thus, the mover can attend to higher order aspects of the skill during performance.

Two questions exist: "What is necessary to plan a movement?" and, "Do children plan along the same lines as adults?"

Motor Programs

Two popular theories of motor control have been motor programs and schema. Motor programs have been defined as abstract structures in memory which are prepared in advance of the movement. The motor program causes contraction and relaxation of specific muscles and causes the movement to occur without major involvement of feedback. Feedback, however, does operate at a very low level in the system to correct for minute errors in the way the program is being executed.

A major problem with the motor program theory involves storage. For each movement, a motor program would have to exist. This problem led researchers to the development of a generalized motor program. Schmidt (1982a) describes the essence of a generalized motor program as the presence of one program in memory to control a general category of skills (e.g., overhand throw for distance). The generalized program consists of two invariant features: phasing (relative timing) and relative force (relations among the forces used in various muscles participating in the action). In order to run the program, one or more parameters are selected in order to define the speed of the overall action, or forces used (type ball used, distance thrown, etc.). The parameters that have been researched with the generalized motor program are duration, force, space, and movement size.

Schema theory

Schmidt (1976, 1982b; Shapiro & Schmidt, 1982) developed a theory of motor learning that relies on the generalized motor program. Cognition is important in selecting the motor program and in the specification of the parameters in the program.

The theory does not account for selection of the generalized motor program, but once the program is selected there are four types of information that must be attended to and remembered: initial conditions, parameters used, movement outcome, and sensory consequences. This information is used to individualize the program (recall schema), and generate what is expected to occur (recognition schemas). The recall schema's major involvement is with response production.

The recall schema is defined as the relation between the past outcomes and response specifications. Functioning of the recall schema determines what set of specifications will achieve the desired outcome. By matching past response specifications to the new response specifications, the subject is able to prime the motor program.

As the performer uses the schema to generate responses specifications, he or she also generates the expected sensory consequences (desired outcome), which is the recognition schema. The recognition schema is then responsible for evaluation of the response-produced feedback.

Development of the ability to detect and correct errors is important. Schema theory explains this by the error labeling system. An abstraction of past sensory signals has been stored in comparison to the actual sensory consequences (based on knowledge of results). This comparison of anticipated and actual outcome is the error detection mechanism, which increases in strength from trial to trial. Once developed, the performer is able to attach labels to the errors and use subjective reinforcement to continue learning when knowledge of results has been withdrawn.

Both the recall and recognition schema are rules whose strengths are a positive function of the number of practice trials. Of importance during these trials is the variability of the practice. By practicing a wide range of desired outcomes, the individual becomes more adept at parameter selection and, perhaps, can select the parameters more quickly (Wallace & McGhee, 1979) from the knowledge base.

Development of a Plan

Once the mechanism and operation of a movement plan is established, the second question is, "Do young children plan movements?" The ability to construct a plan to remember appeared between 7 and 11 years of age when children were required to recall verbal information (Apple et al., 1972) and movements (Kelso et al., 1979). However, use of a strategy and plan selection does not appear until later in development (Gallagher & Thomas, 1981; Winther & Thomas, 1981b).

Of importance in the development of the recall schema are initial conditions, response-outcome information, and the parameters used when the program is executed. Stelmach (1982, p. 86) states that "observing the end result of a motor act is insufficient for making any type of statement about why it is successful or not." Therefore, some type of information concerning correctness of a movement is necessary. The two types of information discussed here are knowledge of results and a model's performance.

Knowledge of Results

The availability of information concerning one's performance is an important, if not essential, condition for increasing performance over trials on a motor task. Though often used interchangeably in the literature, feedback and knowledge of results (KR) are not synonymous. Schmidt (1975) categorized feedback as internal or external. The visual, auditory and proprioceptive systems are the vehicles for internal feedback, while external feedback is KR supplied by an outside source (information given by an observer) and yields information concerning errors. The difference between observation of the outcome (internal feedback) and KR is that with the observation data the individual must transform the data into error information.

KR can be classified as either quantitative or qualitative. Qualitative KR is general information (right, wrong; long, short). Quantitative KR includes magnitude of the error and has generally included direction (qualitative).

Time delay between completion of one trial on a task and initiation of the next trial is the interresponse interval. Closer inspection of this interval shows a division into the KR delay interval and post-KR interval. The KR delay interval is the time from completion of one response until KR is given. The post-KR interval is the period from the administration of KR until the start of the next trial. This has been described as the information processing interval.

Another variable associated with KR research is relative and absolute frequency of KR. Absolute frequency refers to the absolute number of times in a learning sequence that KR is provided to the learner. Relative frequency is defined as the number of KR trials, divided by the total number of trials given, and thus expressed as the proportion of trials for which KR was provided.

An oversight in many experiments on the variables influencing the effects of KR has been the failure to separate performance effects from learning effects. Performance effects are evident during acquisition trials (during which KR is given) while the relatively permanent or learning effects became apparent in trials after KR is withdrawn (when KR is not given).

Salmoni, Schmidt, and Walter (1984) have summarized the KR literature and have separated the effects of KR on performance and learning. They provide three general principles of KR and performance. Performance is increased by increasing the absolute and relative frequencies of KR and by KR precison. Interpolated activities in both KR delay and post-KR delay tend to degrade performance if either the activities or the learning task are demanding, and performance is strongly degraded by increased trials delay. Additionally, a post-KR delay that is too short can degrade performance.

Two major differences between the effects of KR on performance and learning deal with trials delay and relative frequency. Increasing the absolute and relative frequency of KR increases performance, but as the relative frequency decreases, learning increases. Additionally, trials delay enhances learning. Perhaps during this trials delay interval, the individual is forced to focus attention on other aspects of the movement important to retention that are ignored when KR is present on every trial.

From the two differing effects between performance and learning, a key question is, "What allows subjects to learn the task when they perform poorly during acquisition?" Salmoni et al. suggest that a trials delay forces the subject to attend directly to intrinsic feedback, rather than to rely on KR for guidance. Thus, the individual is forced to develop an error detection and correction mechanism to provide subjective reinforcement.

Other factors that are interrelated in their effects on the role of KR in performance and learning are contextual interference, error full learning, and practice variability. The effect of trials delay on the role of KR in performance and learning parallels the work on contextual interference (Salmoni et al., 1984). Many tasks require continual adjustments from one performance to the next (i.e., selection of motor program parameters, use of subjective reinforcement to modify parameters). Practicing the task with information about every trial or performing an open skill identically within a block of trials causes a detriment in performance. This is because the KR acts as guidance, or the requirement to choose one of several movements is not given. These findings also parallel those that have been noted from practice variability and error full learning: in order to adjust to a changing environment the learner must practice under a variety of circumstances and detect the relationship between the parameters selected and performance outcome.

Modeling

A second type of information available to the learner is observation of someone performing the task correctly (usually the teacher, but sometimes a peer). For this information to be of value in planning, the individual must be attentive to the modeled behavior and retain the modeled sequence of behavior. The major focus, developmentally, is if younger/older children are able to attend to and remember the task-appropriate cues. Here we need to determine whether learners merely try to copy the model, or if they match their performance to the models to detect errors. In the first situation, the model performs more of a "guidance" function than KR does and performance should deteriorate rapidly with the withdrawal of the model.

The effectiveness of a model for performance improvement has been investigated developmentally. Thomas, Pierce, and Ridsdale (1977) examined the effects of giving 7- and 9-year-old girls a model either at the beginning of the learning session, after they had already attempted the task, or without the model. Conclusions were that 9-year-olds could effectively use modeling cues regardless of when the model was given; the 7-year-olds, however, could use a model's performance only when the model was given before the practice.

Supporting and extending the work of Thomas et al. (1977), Weiss (1983) found that the effectiveness of a model depended on differences in cognitive development evident in children of different ages. The major factors in her study were a model vs. no model condition and verbal vs. no verbal label groups for 5- and 7-year-old children. Results indicated that several cognitive developmental factors (attention span, memory capacity, coding capabilities, and physical abilities) were necessary for a model to be effective in skill learning.

The modeling literature has used simple tasks and the learners were in the cognitive phases of learning (developing the general strategy to approach the task). For the Thomas et al. study, the learner used the model to determine which of the two strategies to use to balance on the stabilometer. The children in Weiss's study used the model to determine sequencing of skills that they could already perform individually. A future area of investigation should be later stages of learning and how a model can be used to refine parameter selection and error detection and correction.

Relationship of Motor Programs to the Control of Movement

The purpose of the generalized motor program is to allow the individual to switch attention from the control of movement to the higher order structures. During early skill learning, performance is characterized by slow, jerky movements because of the continuous necessity to use internal and external feedback. The unskilled person makes a movement, watches the consequences of that movement, makes a second movement, evaluates the results, and so on. With practice, however, sequencing and timing of the movement shift from direct visual control to an internal and more automatic form of control. As a result, performance appears to be rapid, smooth and coordinated.

To this point, the discussion has emphasized the importance of cognition in selecting a plan to move, selecting parameters for the generalized program, and in the evaluation of the movement. The control of movement appears to have three stages: stimulus identification, response selection, and response programming. During stimulus identification, one perceives the environment, and then selects the appropriate skill. During response programming, the appropriate parameters are selected, and the response is initiated. These stages account for characteristics in responding and clearly are memory dependent. Of importance is the question "Are young children's performances influenced by memory limitations?"

Cognition and Developmental Skill Acquisition

The study of movement development (Elliott & Connolly, 1974, p. 135) investigates "how the mover achieves increased sophistication in organization, execution and refinement of movement action plans." Many motor skills require a rapid response to external factors, in addition to rapid execution. Thus, the ability to make a quick decision is critical. During these skills, the young child not only performs more slowly, but if the speed requirements are increased, an inverse relationship of age and performance is noted (Chi, 1976; Gallagher & Thomas, 1980). Young children not only perform poorly with increased speed but also frequently select an inappropriate response (McCracken, 1983).

For adults, a rapid decision seems to be an automatic response. Automaticity of processing may be related to efficiency of speeded information processing (Keating & Bobbit, 1978; Mannis, Keating, & Morrison, 1980; Wickens, 1974). Posner and Schneider (1975) were concerned with the manner in which automatic and nonautomatic processes interact in the determination of performance of tasks requiring rapid response. Perhaps the issue is that increasing the speed of response causes a marked deterioration of children's performance.

Thus, for movement development, we need to determine how individuals learn to automate a response (motor program), and how they specify the parameters. Hasher and Zacks (1979) identified two sources as the origin of automatic processes: heredity and practice. The hereditary source suggests the nervous system is prewired for automaticity of response (e.g., reflexive behavior). Practice is repeated experience.

Atkinson and Schiffrin (1968, 1971) and Schiffrin and Schneider (1977) state that automation of response by practice is developed by effortful processes such as rehearsal and organization. Chi (1976) expanded the use of effortful or control processes into a developmental framework to suggest how effortful processes are learned. The next section deals with the development of these processes in a motor memory paradigm.

Memory Model

A general information processing model includes three stages: sensory store, short term store (STS), and long term store (LTS) (Atkinson & Schiffrin, 1968, 1971; Schiffrin & Schneider, 1977). Thomas, Thomas, and Gallagher (1981) and Thomas (1980) have hypothesized a developmental memory model that expands on STS and LTS. The individual must selectively attend to task-relevant cues in sensory store and then perceive the information. After perception, the information is moved into memory. Memory is divided into working memory and knowledge base. Familiarity with the information in knowledge base increases the amount of information that is moved into working memory. In working memory, control processes are used to either maintain information in working memory or move it to knowledge base.

Sensory store is thought to be a relatively complete copy of the physical stimulus containing the perceptual/kinesthetic array prior to processing. Information that is not processed within specific time limits is lost to the system. Sensory store is capable of storing large amounts of information for very brief periods of time. The developmental questions concerning sensory store are twofold. First, does the size of sensory store change with age? And second, is the information in sensory store available longer for older children and adults? The research from iconic (visual) and ecoic (auditory) sensory store suggest that the capacity and rate of decay is invariant with age when an array of seven geometric figures is displayed (Morrison, Holms & Haith, 1974; Sheingold, 1973), for spatial location of dot patterns (Finkel, 1973), and for sound (Frank & Rabinovitch, 1974; Seigel & Allik

1973). Preliminary data by Gallagher (1980, Exp. 1) shows similar findings for kinesthetic sensory store.

Perception is the attaching of a meaningful label to the information attended to in sensory store. With age, there is a shift in the hierarchy of the dominant sensory systems; an increase or improvement in intrasensory discrimination and an accompanying improvement in intersensory integration (Williams, 1983; Williams, this book). The shift in dominance of the sensory systems is from tactile-kinesthetic receptors to visual control of behavior. An increase in intrasensory discrimination is evident in the child's improved capacity for more refinded discrimination. Thomas and Thomas (1980) reported an increased sensitivity with age for detecting movement accuracy. They discovered an increase of roughly 100% in sensitivity level from 7 to 11 years and 50% from 11 years to adulthood.

Memory Strategy Usage

The importance of memory strategy usage can be seen in study by Gallagher (1980, Exp. 2). Essentially, children performed simple movements as efficiently as adults, but performance was impaired when complexity was increased. For example, when asked merely to recall a linear arm movement, 5-, 7-, 11-, and 19-year-old subjects were similar in recall accuracy. However, when series of three and five movements were presented, the younger children's performance deteriorated rapidly. The following discussion describes memory strategies the adults might have been using, which the children lacked.

Selective attention serves in the perceputal encoding (labeling) of task-appropriate cues and as a control process during recoding, grouping, and rehearsal. The developmental trend associated with this control process is from overexclusiveness to overinclusiveness to selective attention (Ross, 1976). Attention to limited cues, regardless of task appropriateness, describes the overexclusive child (up to 5-6 years of age). The child is unaware of most of the environment (incidental memory recall is low). The overexclusive child (between 6-7 years and 11-12 years) attends to the entire display without focusing on task-appropriate cues. Thus, the child constantly attends to irrelevant information which serves as distractors from task performance (incidental memory recall is high). At approximately 11 years of age, the child develops the abilty to selectively attend to task-appropriate cues and ignore irrelevant information.

Stratton (1978) reviewed basic research on selective attention to conclude that teachers should evaluate task requirements, environmental demands, and teacher input. During the performance of most motor skills, a wealth of task-irrelevant cues are available. Younger children acquire strategies of selective attention when higher levels of interference are imposed early in the learning situation and the child is cued to those that are task appropriate. This allows the child to develop a plan to deal with the irrelevant information. Note, however, the irrelevant information cannot reach a level which prevents learning of the primary task.

Labeling is one aspect of perception, and increasing the meaningfulness of the label improves performance. Winther and Thomas (1981a) investigated the developmental effects of labeling a movement and substantiated Chi's (1976) development of a labeling strategy. Younger children's (5-year-olds) performance improved when they were forced to label a movement with a meaningful label. Adult performance was hindered when forced to use an irrelevant label. Weiss (1983) expanded this to a more ecologically valid paradigm to find that younger children (5-year-olds) benefited more from a model when verbal labels were given by the model.

Rehearsal is important to maintain information in memory and transfer it to knowledge base. The importance of active rehearsal is demonstrated in a study by Gallagher and Thomas (1984). Given a series of eight movements, 5- and 7-

year-old children chose to rehearse on an instance-by-instance basis, while 11- and 19-year-old subjects grouped the movements for recall. When forced to rehearse in an adult fashion, the 5- and 7-year-old children's performance improved. Similar findings have been reported with mentally retarded children. Reid's (1980) subjects were mentally retarded children in the IQ range from 43-83, while Schroeder (1981) studied severely mentally retarded subjects to find that when taught a rehearsal strategy, the subjects were able to recall more effectively either a preselected movement or a series of movements.

Organization is a strategy used to combine information that is meaningful in order to reduce cognitive demands. Instead of thinking of separate pieces of information, the individual groups and recodes the information into one unit. Using a series of eight movements, and manipulating the degree of organization in the material, Gallagher and Thomas (1986) found that 5-year-old children were unable to increase performance regardless of organization strategy or input of information. The 7-year-old children were able to use organized input to facilitate recall, but the strategy failed to transfer to a new task. Eleven-year-old children's performance conformed to the predictions, with the exception of the unorganized input group. It was anticipated that the 11-year-old children used organized input and showed some transfer of strategy. However, they could not restructure the information or provide self-generated organization. Nineteen-year-old subjects organized the information regardless of input.

Integrating the studies on rehearsal and organization of input, Gallagher and Thomas (1986) indicated that forcing the use of the strategies was of greater importance to younger children but it had less effect on older children and adults. The older children and adults were using the strategies when not forced to do so, whereas the younger children were not. Even though the 5-year-old children were given the organizational cues, they failed to recall the movements in order (from short to long). Forcing rehearsal, on the other hand, aided recall of the 5-year-old children. The 7-year-old children used the organizational strategy to recall eight movements. The older children and adults in the self-determined strategy were similar in recall to the organizational strategy. They rehearsed spatially similar groups of movements.

Thus, younger children do not spontaneously use memory strategies. However, as Chi (1982) has suggested, this could be due to an inefficient knowledge base.

Knowledge Base Development

A child's knowledge base has been said to be deficient in at least three ways (Brown, 1982): the amount of information it contains, the organization and internal coherence of that information, and the number of available routes by which the information can be reached (familiarity). An impoverished knowledge base can influence speed of encoding, naming, recognition, and ease of search and retrieval. The issue becomes a problem, not only of an adequate use and control of the routes available to the system, but also of accessing and using the resources available (Brown, 1982; Brown & Campione, 1979). As mentioned previously, this is what Keel considers knowledge structures, which permit quick action via prediction and anticipation of the environment.

The failure of a child to use available resources has been demonstrated in developmental motor memory research. When learning a motor skill, young children appear to ignore certain relevant information. When using KR to learn a ballistic movement, children (8, 10, and 14 years old) chose to respond shortly after receiving KR, whereas the adults delayed their movements. The adults took significantly longer to initate the succeeding response after receiving KR and their performance was significantly better than that of lower age groups (Barclay & Newell, 1980). When forced to delay responding, the younger childen (7 and 11 years) reached parity to adults for a simple movement task (Gallagher & Thomas, 1980).

From another paradigm, when able to preselect a movement, older children and adults tended to select easily codable movement lengths (by the shoulder, chin, middle, etc.), whereas younger children did not select movements that were easily codable. However, when the children did code the movements in relation to their bodies, their movements were recalled similarly to those of adults (Gallagher & Thomas, 1981; Winther & Thomas, 1981b).

Because the knowledge base is globally deficient in young children does not mean that a child may not develop a rich knowledge base in a special area. The development of automatic use of memory strategies appears to be related to knowledge base. Chi (1982) has domonstrated that a 5-year-old used a regular retrieval order for four trials when remembering children in her class. She recalled using the seat position in a row, not the taxonomic categories used by adults (age, grade, and sex), but it was still a successful strategy. This suggests that the organization and internal coherence of that information was dissimilar to adults, yet was highly familiar and easily accessible for the younger child. A 4½-year-old demonstrated a sophisticated strategy when recalling familiar dinosaurs (Chi & Koeske, 1983). The child sorted on an abstract dimension, one which has been found by zoologists to be basic to classification of the dinosaurs. This sophisticated strategy is normally not evident until at least 9 years of age. For the less familiar dinosaurs, the child did not sort along these dimensions. This impressive performance can be attributed to the well organized and highly enriched representation that the child had of dinosaurs.

Chi's interpretation of the influence of knowledge base on strategy use is that it may not be a lack of a classification principle on the part of the child, but that the representation of the stimuli may not be organized in memory on the basis of conceptual dimensions, even though such dimensions may be present as attributes linked to each stimulus item. Experience (practice) may gradually alter the representation so that the relevant conceptual dimensions become more salient with increasing age. This explanation would predict that in certain situations, even young children may be as familiar with certain knowledge structures as adults. Such an explanation would still be consistent with the assumptions underlying the traditional interpretation, namely, that children do have knowledge of category membership and they do have the same membership composition for categories as older children and adults, albeit only the dominant ones.

Chi's study shows that a child's organizing principle can be abstract and taxonomic, if the stimulus material is overlearned. This enriched practice gives the child the opportunity to reorganize his or her semantic structure, so that the relevant conceptual dimensions become salient, and organization is then based on these dimensions. It thus appears from the psychological literature that, when the semantic network exists in memory, the child is able to use the more mature strategies automatically.

In the typical developmental movement paradigm, both adults and children are assumed naive. However, as Brown (1982) has suggested, the child, although perhaps an expert in one domain, is generally a "universal novice," whereas adults know how to become an expert in new domains; they are able to demonstrate transfer from a wide variety of past experiences.

These findings seem to have implications for sport skill development in children. The knowledge base is highly structured in many sport settings. In fact, the change in game performance over a sport season may be more knowledge base related than skill related. That is, a child's ability to anticipate possible outcomes and select appropriate responses is a major source of improved performance during the sport season. In effect, the child has developed a series of if/then rules which were weighted according to the probability of their occurrence during specific game situations. These if/then rules have been developed over practice sessions and previous game experiences and comprise an important part of the specific knowledge base. As the game situation dictates (fits the characteristics of the if/then rule), the rule is retrieved and readied for action. Since several rules may fit any given circumstance, these rules are weighted by their likelihood of occurrence. This total process is useful in reducing the processing load as the game progresses, as well as increasing the speed and quality of the child's response. Of course, increased sport skill is also important, but the relationship between sport knowledge base and sport performance has been much neglected.

Decision Making

Selection of a task-appropriate strategy is important in motor skill performance. A developmental difference appears to exist, with older children and adults approaching the task with a more efficient strategy. Kerr (1975) and Salmoni and Pascoe (1978) found that older children and adults were able to do a reciprocal tapping task with greater speed due to the strategy used to perform the task. The older children treated the task as one of a continuous nature, the young children regarded it as a series of discrete movements. The muscular response for older children was a more efficient horizontal movement with minimal arch between targets, while the younger children used movements with a high arch. McCracken (1983) also reported finding that older children had fewer eye movements and tended to focus on one target, while younger kids alternated their attention between the two targets. Similar findings have been reported using a gross body-location task. Thomas, Thomas, Lee, Testerman, and Ashy (1983) found that when subjects were required to jog along a track and reproduce the distance jogged, the older children used a counting strategy (number of steps) whereas the younger children just tried to remember the required distance.

Factors to Influence During Practice and Performance

The purpose of practice sessions is to automate motor skills in order to subsequently maximize performance. To develop a most efficient practice session, several factors must be considered: goals, plans, organization, cues, models, and KR.

The first major consideration in developing the practice session is to make contextual conditions as similar to those during performance as possible. With the wealth of task-irrelevant cues available, the child needs to be forced to attend to those that are task appropriate.

At the outset of the practice situation, the learner needs to understand the goal. Goal setting involves knowledge of the desired outcomes during practice. This allows for more efficient practice and aids the child in carryover to the next practice session.

Following goal setting the performer must select the most efficient plan for the movement. Young children should be forced to attend to program selection and parameterization. Models can play an important role in aiding the child in understanding the goal of the task and selection of the appropriate motor program. For peak efficiency of model performance, the model needs to appropriately label task relevant cues.

Organization relates to sequencing appropriate skill parts and forcing rehearsal to reduce demands of the task. Most complex motor skills have a specified organization structure and timing from one movement segment to the next is critical. Parts of the skill that are interrelated and dependent on each other for carrying out the movements must not be separated.

Knowledge of performance is critically important in the learning of motor skills. Young children tend to ignore knowledge of performance but when they do use it, they take longer to integrate the information for performance improvement. Since it is practically impossible for the teacher to provide knowledge of performance to a child on all trials, the child needs to develop an error detection and correction mechanism. Drawing from trials delay research, it seems plausible to conclude that the learner should not receive error information on every trial, but should be given summary information and then attempt to integrate this information for task improvement.

Considering that the knowledge base of the learner is important, practice sessions which provide possible alternatives for action and aid the child in weighing possible alternatives are essential to skillful sport performance. The teacher/coach is structuring the knowledge base and increasing the speed of decision making by providing situationally specific practice. Of course, practicing the physical skills themselves cannot be neglected. But being able to skillfully field and throw a ground ball in baseball is of little value unless the ball is thrown to the correct place.

Summary

Cognition is important in motor skill learning and performance. Developmentally, several factors are evident that restrict the performance of younger childen when compared to adults. These factors, however, seem to be modifiable if the environment is structured to make the child aware of the importance of cognition.

During the learning of motor skills the following factors need to be considered: plan formulation, memory strategies, knowledge base of the learner, and feedback. Developing a movement plan is important for strategic control. The plan is the basis on which the movement is organized. Young children need to be forced to develop a plan.

Since young children do not use the same memory strategies as adults, it is important for the teacher/coach to structure the environment to force selective attention, labeling, rehearsal, and organization. An impoverished knowledge base can influence speed of encoding, naming, recognition, and ease of search and retrieval. Since young children are universal novices, the teacher/coach needs to provide practices that allow the child to increase the salience of relevant conceputal dimension.

Feedback is very important during learning. During practice, information concerning correctness of performance becomes important. Principles of KR and learning indicate that giving summary information after practice on several trials might enhance learning. A different type of information concerning performance is a model of performance. The ability to use the information from a model increases if the task appropriate cues are labeled. For a young child, the model needs to be presented prior to performance.

When structuring the practice situation, the teacher should be concerned with the type skill (open, closed) and the environment. Contextual conditions should parallel those that are important during performance. For open skills, selection of appropriate response parameters is important. On the other hand, for closed skills the individual should repeatedly practice the same situation.

References

Apple, L.F., Cooper, R.G., McCarrell, N., Sims-Knight, J., Yussen, S.R., & Flavell, J.H. (1972). The development of the distinction between perceiving and memorizing. *Child Development, 43,* 1365-1381.

Atkinson, R.C., & Schiffrin, R.M. (1968). Human memory: A proposed system and its control processes. In K.W. Spence & J.T. Spence (Eds.), *The psychology of learning and motivation* (pp. 90-197). New York: Academic Press.

Atkinson, R.C., & Schiffrin, R.M. (1971, August). The control of short-term memory. *Scientific American*, 82-90.

Barclay, C., & Newell, K. (1980). Children's processing of information in motor skill acquisition. *Journal of Experimental Child Psychology, 30*, 98-108.

Brown, A. (1982). Learning and development: the problems of compatibility, access, and induction. *Human Development, 25*, 89-115.

Brown, A.L., & Campione, J.C. (1979). Inducing flexible thinking: A problem of access. In M. Friedman, S.D. Das, & N. O'Connor (Eds.), *Intelligence and learning* (pp. 85-530). New York: Plenum Press.

Chi, M.T.H. (1976). Short-term memory limitations in children: Capacity or processing deficits? *Memory and Cognition, 4*, 559-572.

Chi, M.T.H. (1982). Knowledge development and memory performance. In M. Friedman, J.P. Das, and N. O'Connor (Eds.), *Intelligence and learning* (pp. 221-230). New York: Plenum Press.

Chi, M.T.H., & Koeske, R.D. (1983). Network representation of a child's dinosaur knowledge. *Development Psychology, 19*, 29-39.

Eberts, R., & Schneider, W. (1980). *The automatic and controlled processing of temporal and spatial patterns* (Report No. 8003). Arlington, VA: Office of Naval Research.

Elliot, J.M. & Connolly, K.J. (1974). Hierarchical structure in skill development. In K.J. Connolly & J.S. Bruner (Eds.), *The growth of competence* (pp. 135-168). New York: Academic Press.

Finkel, D.L. (1973). A developmental comparison of the processing of two types of visual information. *Journal of Experimental Child Psychology, 16*, 250-266.

Flavell, J.H., & Wellman, H.M. (1977). Metamemory. In R.V. Kail & J.W. Hagen (Eds.), *Perspective on the development of memory and cognition* (pp. 3-34). Hillsdale, NJ: Lawrence Erlbaum Associates.

Frank, H.S., & Rabinovitch, M.J. (1974). Auditory short-term memory: Developmental changes in precategorical acoustic store. *Child Development, 45*, 522-526.

Gallagher, J.D. (1981). Adult-child motor performance differences: A developmental perspective of control processing deficits. (Doctoral dissertation, Louisiana State University, 1980). *Dissertation Abstracts International, 41*, 1474-A.

Gallagher, J.D., & Thomas J.R. (1980). Effects of varying post-KR intervals upon children's motor performance. *Journal of Motor Behavior, 12*, 41-56.

Gallagher, J.D., & Thomas, J.R. (1981, April). Developmental effects in preselected and constrained movements. Paper presented at AAHPERD Convention, Boston, Mass.

Gallagher, J.D. & Thomas, J.T. (1984). Rehearsal strategy effects on developmental differences for recall of a movement series. *Research Quarterly for Exercise and Sport, 55*, 123-128.

Gallagher, J.D. & Thomas, J.R. (1986). Developmental effects of grouping and recoding on learning a movement series. *Research Quarterly for Exercise and Sport, 57*, 117-127.

Hasker, L. & Zack, R. (1979). Automatic and effortful processes in memory. *Journal of Experimental Psychology: General, 108*, 356-388.

Keating, D.P., & Bobbitt, B. (1978). Individual and developmental differences in cognitive processing components of mental ability. *Child Development, 49*, 155-167.

Keel, S.W. (1982). Component analysis and conceptions of skill. In J.A.S. Kelso (Ed.), *Human motor behavior: An introduction* (pp. 143-160). Hillsdale, NJ: Lawrence Erlbaum Associates.

Kelso, J.A.S., Goodman, D., Stamm, C.L., & Hays, C. (1979). Movement coding and memory in retarded children. *American Journal of Mental Deficiency, 83*, 601-611.

Kerr, R. (1975). Movement control and maturation in elementary grade children. *Perceptual and Motor Skills, 41*, 151-154.

McCracken, H.D. (1983). Movement control in a reciprocal tapping task: developmental study. *Journal of Motor Behavior, 15,* 262-279.

Mannis, F.O., Keating, D.P., & Morrison, F.J. (1980). Developmental differences in the allocation of processing capacity. *Journal of Experimental Child Psychology, 29,* 159-169.

Morrison, F.J., Holmes, D.L., & Haith, M.M. (1974). A developmental study of the effect of familiarity on short-term visual memory. *Journal of Experimental Child Psychology, 18,* 412-425.

Posner, M.I., & Schneider, C.P. (1975). Attention and cognitive control. In R.L. Solso (Ed.), *Information processing and cognition: The Loyola Symposium* (pp. 55-86). Hillsdale, NJ: Erlbaum.

Pribham, K.H. (1971). *Languages in the brain.* Englewood Cliffs, NJ: Prentice Hall.

Pribham, K. (1976). Executive functions of the frontal lobes. In T. Pesiraju (Ed.), *Mechanisms in transmission of signals of conscious behavior* (pp. 303-322). Amsterdam: Elsevier.

Reid, G. (1980). The effects of memory strategy instruction in the short-term motor memory of the mentally retarded. *Journal of Motor Behavior, 12,* 221-228.

Ross, A. (1976). *Psychological aspects of learning disabilities and reading disorders.* New York: McGraw-Hill Book Co.

Salmoni, A., & Pascoe, C. (1978). Fitts reciprocal tapping task: A developmental study. In G. Roberts & K. Newell (Eds.), *Psychology of motor behavior and sport* (pp. 288-294). Champaign, IL: Human Kinetics.

Salmoni, A.W., Schmidt, R.A., & Walter, C.B. (1984). Knowledge of results and motor learning: A review and critical reappraisal. *Psychological Bulletin, 95,* 355-386.

Schiffrin, R.M., & Schneider, W. (1977). Controlled and automatic human information processing: II. Perceptural learning, automatic attending, and a general theory. *Psychological Review, 84,* 127-190.

Schmidt, R.A. (1975). A schema theory of discrete motor skill learning. *Psychological Review, 82,* 225-260.

Schmidt, R.A. (1976). The schema as a solution to some persistent problems in motor learning theory. In G.E. Stelmach (Ed.), *Motor control: Issues and trends* (pp. 41-66). New York: Academic Press.

Schmidt, R.A. (1982a). More on motor programs. In J.A.S. Kelso (Ed.), *Human motor behavior: An introduction* (pp. 189-218). Hillsdale, NJ: Lawrence Erlbaum Associates.

Schmidt, R.A. (1982b). The schema concept. In J.A.S. Kelso (Ed.), *Human motor behavior: An introduction* (pp. 219-235). Hillsdale, NJ: Lawrence Erlbaum Associates.

Schroeder, R.K. (1982). The effects of rehearsal on information processing efficiency of severely/profoundly retarded and normal individuals. (Doctoral dissertation, Louisiana State University, 1981). *Dissertation Abstracts International, 42,* 1102-A.

Shapiro, D.C., & Schmidt, R.A. (1982). In J.A.S. Kelso & J.E. Clark (Eds.), *The development of movement control and co-ordination* (pp. 113-150). New York: John Wiley & Sons, Ltd.

Sheingold, K. (1973). Developmental differences in intake and storage of visual information. *Journal of Experimental Child Psychology, 16,* 1-11.

Siegel, A.W., & Allik, J.P. (1973). A developmental study of visual and auditory short-term memory. *Journal of Verbal Learning and Verbal Behavior, 12,* 409-418.

Stelmach, G.E. (1982). Information processing framework for understanding human motor behavior. In J.A.S. Kelso (Ed.), *Human motor behavior: An introduction* (pp. 63-91). Hillsdale, NJ: Lawrence Erlbaum Associates.

Stratton, R. (1978). Information processing deficits in children's motor performance: Implications for instruction. *Motor Skills: Theory into Practice, 3,* 49-55.

Thomas J.R. (1980). Acquisition of motor skills: Information processing differences between children and adults. *Research Quarterly for Exercise and Sport, 51,* 158-173.

Thomas, J.R., Pierce, C., Ridsdale, S. (1977). Age differences in children's ability to model motor behavior. *Research Quarterly for Exercise and Sport, 48,* 592-297.

Thomas, J.R., Thomas, K.T., & Gallagher, J.D. (1981). Introduction: children's processing of information in physical activity and sport. In A. Morris (Ed.), *Motor development: Theory into practice* (pp. 1-6). Newton, CT: Motor Skills: Theory into Practice 3.

Thomas, J.R., Thomas, K.T., Lee, A.M., Lesterman, E., & Ashy, M. (1983). Age differences in use of strategy for recall of movement in a large scale environment. *Research Quarterly for Exercise and Sport, 54,* 264-272.

Thomas, K.T., & Thomas, J.R. (1980, October). *Developmental differences: The measurement of difference thresholds for movement location.* Paper presented at Computer Workshop and Measurement Symposium, Rice University, Houston, Texas.

Wallace, S.A., & McGhee, R.C. (1979). The independence of recall and recognition in motor learning. *Journal of Motor Behavior, 11,* 141-151.

Weiss, M.R. (1983). Modeling and motor performance: A developmental perspective. *Research Quarterly for Exercise and Sport, 54,* 190-197.

Whiting, H.T.A. (1980). Dimensions of control in motor learning. In G.E. Stelmach & J. Requin (Eds.), *Tutorials in motor behavior* (pp. 537-550). Holland: North-Holland Publishing Co.

Wickens, C.D. (1974). Temporal limits of human information processing: A developmental study. *Psychological Bulletin, 81,* 739-755.

Williams, H. (1983). *Perceptual and motor development.* Englewood Cliffs, NJ: Prentice-Hall, Inc.

Winther, K.T., & Thomas, J.R. (1981a). Developmental differences in children's labeling of movement. *Journal of Motor Behavior, 13,* 77-90.

Winther, K.T., & Thomas, J.R. (1981b, April). Knowledge of movement response mode: Effects of development. Paper presented at AAHPERD Convention, Boston, Mass.

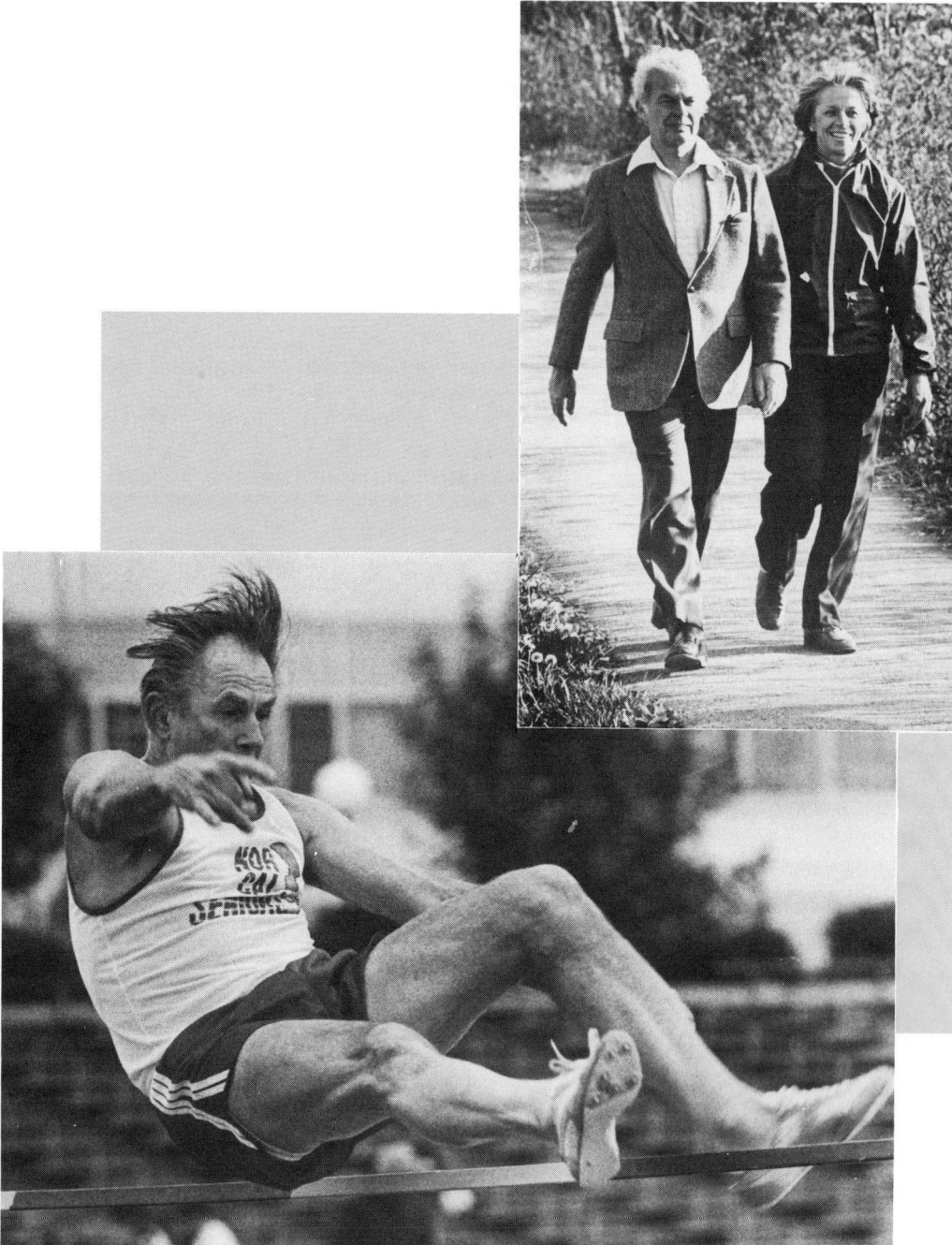

photo by Jim Kirby

CHAPTER FIVE

Physical Activity and the Prevention of Premature Aging

Waneen Wyrick Spirduso
Department of Physical and Health Education
The University of Texas
Austin, Texas

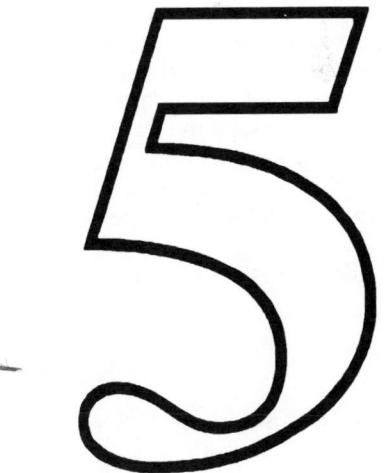

Aging is inevitable. It begins happening to everyone from the moment of birth. Yet, few individuals focus any attention at all on it until they approach middle age. When the physical signs begin to appear, the process becomes relevant.

Society has only recently shown interest in the process of aging, and this interest has probably been motivated by the realization on the part of those in leadership capacities that the "greying of America" has brought with it a staggering financial cost. In 1900, only four percent of the population of the United States was 65 or older. In 1980 that percentage had risen to 11% (Soldo, 1980). By the year 2000, 32 million people will be 65 or older, and by the year 2030, it is anticipated that 17-20% of our population will be 65 or older (National Institutes of Health, 1983). In 1900 there were 123,000 Americans 85 or older; today, there are about 2.5 million. By the year 2050, it is estimated that more than 16 million people (five percent of our poulation), will be over 85. Today, those 11% of our population over 65 account for 29% of our health care costs, or three times the cost of those individuals under 65 years of age. In addition, this is a very large segment of our population to be non-productive, yet receiving medical care. The spector of the "baby boomers" entering retirement (in 2010) is enough to frighten the most optimistic civic planners. In the past the emphasis has been on medical treatment and delivery of services to the aged and the physically debilitated. Many enlightened people in leadership roles are coming to realize that the cost of lifestyle interventions that will postpone the disease processes and debilitation that sometimes accompany old age are far more cost effective than treatment.

Some aging effects can be postponed; others cannot (Fries & Crapo, 1981). Some unchangeable effects of aging are arterial wall rigidity, cataract formation, graying of hair, thinning of hair, kidney reserve, and elasticity of skin. Many of the ravaging effects of aging are modifiable, however. For example, some aging effects on skin can be postponed by avoiding sun exposure. Osteoporosis, or bone loss, can be modified by diet and exercise. Intellectual functioning and sociability can be maintained with practice. To a large extent, optimum functioning in adult years and old age is a matter of personal choice of lifestyle.

Exercise is a lifestyle intervention that is inexpensive, yet has the potential to provide substantial benefits to the well-being of all adults. Generally believed and much publicized in popular literature are several health benefits of exercise: (a) a stronger heart and open blood vessels; (b) regulated metabolic functions, such as control of blood sugar; (c) controlled anxiety or depression; (d) a bolstered immune defense; and (e) stronger bone and muscle (Simon, 1985). These benefits are discussed in chapters 1, 6, 7, 9, 10 and 11 of this book; the focus of this chapter will be on the special contributions that chronic physical activity can make to the aging motor system. Effects of exercise on aging muscular, strength, endurance, and psychomotor performance will be reviewed. Mechanisms by which these effects might occur are summarized. The chapter concludes with a discussion of biological versus chronological age, longevity, and quality of life.

Spontaneous Physical Activity

It is a common observation that as individuals age, the amount of physical activity, in both work and leisure, declines. Physical activity drops precipitously in off-job activity beginning at age 20, and a big change in the amount of voluntary activity begins in the years 40-49 (for an excellent review of the decline of physical activity in human beings and proposed factors accounting for this decline, see Ostrow, 1984). Not only does participation in physical activity decline, but the selection of activities requiring more vigorous expenditure of energy also is substantially less among older individuals. Vigorous activity such as jogging or bicycling is chosen by about 19-28% of the population who are 22-29 years of age, but by only 1-4% of those over the age of 60. The percentage is even lower when males are excluded from the sample.

In fact, regular sport involvement is inversely related to age. Many factors have been proposed as contributing to this change in physical activity pattern. Boothby, Tungatt, and Townsend (1981) describe these as declining physical ability, loss of interest, social constraints and commitments, limited access to facilities, and dissolution of social contacts and orks.

As Winer (1979) describes in more detail, many individuals have a psychologically difficult time dealing with their deteriorating physical abilities. Some have been accustomed to being very good in sport in their youth. They took great pride in their physical capabilities. With age, they must become satisfied with outstanding performances within their age groups, then with a good effort that doesn't necessarily result in a good performance, and finally with just being active. For many, these changes are not acceptable, and withdrawal from activity preserves them from constant reminders of faded abilities.

Age role expectations serve as powerful social constraints to physical activity in the elderly. The older individuals become, the less others expect them to be active. Riley and Waring (1978) describe the phenomenon of age stratification, in which a society assigns people to opportunities and responsibilities based on chronological age. Certain behaviors are appropriate for some ages, but not for others. College students, for example, view vigorous activities such as basketball as being more and more inappropriate as individuals age (Ostrow, 1984). Consequently, many older individuals internalize the expectation that relatively little exercise is appropriate for their age group. They come to believe that their need for exercise diminishes with age and eventually disappears, that their own physical capacities are less than they are, that light, sporadic exercise is not of much benefit, and that the risks involved in vigorous exercise after middle age are greater than they really are.

Exacerbating the tendency to withdraw from physical activity is the fact that older individuals many times have limited access to physical activity facilities. Gathering places for senior citizens rarely have gymnasia. The very old eventually lose their mobility when they lose the capacity to drive automobiles to their destinations. They become dependent on others to transport them to their chosen activities, and if the individuals who are their source of transportation have a negative attitude regarding physical activity, then daily systematic exercise may become difficult to accomplish.

Older individuals begin to lose their social contacts and networks. Friends and relatives die or move away. The social enjoyment of walking, swimming, cycling, or jogging with a friend or friends, which young people enjoy so much, is more difficult to obtain. Most 80-year-old people don't have many friends their age. Their peer network is considerably depleted. Thus, the social reinforcement of physical activity is dulled.

Even though many complex factors have been proposed as reasons why the incidence of physical activity decreases with age—educational level, occupation, income, geographical area, attitudes toward exercise—it is interesting to note that spontaneous physical activity also declines in animals. Common observations of domesticated pets such as dogs and cats offer evidence that as these animals age they become less active. Older wild animals travel less and are less physically active. Male rats in laboratory cages that contain running wheels regress from running almost 5 miles each night when they are young to running only about half a mile when they are old (Goodrick, 1980). In fact, spontaneous motor activity, as assessed by the Animex Activity Meter, is used as a biological age marker for the rat (Hofecker, Skalicky, Kment, & Niedermüller, 1980).

From observations of both humans and animals, then, spontaneous physical activity declines with age. Thus the benefits that accrue from exercise and regular participation in physical activity are increasingly lost to the aging, yet the evidence suggests that the benefits of physical activity may be even more important as age increases. In fact, it is hard to imagine a group for which chronic exercise is more important in terms of enhancing the quality of life.

Strength

From the perspective that spontaneous physical activity decreases with age, it is not surprising that strength, muscle mass, and many other parameters of muscle physiology also decline with increased age. One of the challenging aging research questions of the future will be to determine whether decreased physical activity precedes muscular decline, whether changes in the neuromuscular system precipitate decreases in physical activity, or whether both of these factors interact and occur in parallel. At any rate, it is clear that decreases of strength and atrophy of muscle occur in aged individuals (Astrand & Rodahl, 1970; Hettinger, 1961). Studies conducted during the past century support the observation that strength declines from about age 30, that there is a greater decline in proximal muscles of the lower extremity, and that the maximum strength in women is reached sooner and declines earlier (Asmussen & Heeboll-Neilsen, 1962).

Maximum isometric muscular force that can be exerted declines with age (see Larsson, 1982, for a table of strength losses from age 20-69). Dynamic strength, as measured by isokinetic devices, reveals the greatest strength losses, particularly at high speeds of contraction (Larsson, Grimby, & Karlsson, 1979). While absolute tension level is impaired, the rate of relative tension development is the same in young and old individuals. The rate of relative tension is unimpaired and related to fast twitch fiber size, while absolute tension level is impaired and unrelated to fast twitch fiber size in the aged (see Clarkson, Kroll, & Melchionda, 1981, for clarification of these statements). Endocrine influences, such as changes in male sex hormone, thyroid, corticosteroids, and insulin also probably contribute to deterioration of muscle function in aging.

Very little research has been conducted to determine the effects of strength training on older individuals, for strength training studies are difficult to conduct in aged samples. To estimate the highest levels of aerobic capacity attainable in aged individuals, one needs only to read the long distance record times of Masters participants, based on thousands of older men and women who participate in endurance events such as jogging, swimming, cycling, and walking. Determining, on the same observational basis, what the maximum strength performances might be is quite speculative, as comparatively few older individuals participate on a regular basis in strength or power type events such as weight lifting, pole vaulting, or discus throwing. The numbers of individuals who participate in Masters competitions in these power and strength events is small. A substantially smaller pool of competitors enter events requiring explosive contraction and power production. The fact that there are such smaller numbers in these events makes it difficult even to know what the limits and distribution of human performance are in these types of activities. Consequently, when researchers study weight training in older samples, they are confronted with a sample of individuals who have done almost no weight work; subjects are untrained, questionably motivated, and may have some concerns about the health risks involved in the training. In addition, heavy resistive exercise is generally contraindicated by the medical profession for individuals over the age of 60. Certainly caution must be exercised by aged persons involved in weight training.

In spite of the problems which contribute to the disinclination of researchers to study weight training in older populations, a few researchers have reported that work-induced muscle hypertrophy does occur in aged humans (Tomanek & Wood, 1970) and in aged animals (Goldspink & Howells, 1974). The absolute amount of hypertrophy is not as great in the old as in the young, but it is present. Moritani and deVries (1980) corroborated the report that old individuals produce similar and significant percent increases in strength after eight weeks of progressive strength training. In addition, they suggested that the strength gains in the old and the young were made through different mechanisms. By using a controversial concept of "efficiency of electrical activity" (deVries, 1968), they concluded that the increases in strength seen in the young subjects were attributed to hypertrophy of muscle fibers, whereas the increases in strength in the old subjects were due to neural factors that increased maximal muscle activation level.

Even though the absolute strength gains that can be made through weight training are less in the old than the young, the records from the American Masters competitions in weight lifting indicate that weight lifting performances reveal that an incredible display of strength through systematic weight training can be accomplished by older indviduals. Whether this is the attainment of strength or the maintenance of strength is not known, as longitudinal records of strength performance in Masters weight lifters have not been reported. The weight lifting loss in bench pressing records is approximately 20% per decade, but a 74-year-old Bulgarian weight lifter recently bench pressed 341 pounds. Another Bulgarian lifted 242 pounds in the dead lift category. Thus, amazingly high levels of strength can be produced even at very old ages. There is, however, a greater absolute loss of strength, especially in the performances requiring the heaviest production of strength or power, in the old than in the young. It should also be remembered that the higher the age category the fewer the participants within each category. Thus, there is a greater probability that one or two extraordinary individuals may bias the averages for a specific age group.

Endurance

Muscular endurance, that is, the capacity to produce less than maximal muscular force repetitively, also declines with aging. Muscle tissue atrophies, the lower limbs being more affected than the upper limbs. The severe decrease in muscle mass may be due to a decrease in the number of muscle fibers, the size of the fibers, or both. Larsson (1982) suggests that both the neural and muscular alterations that are seen in age-related muscular atrophy may be due more to some secondary factors, such as nutritional deficiencies, disuse, denervating processes, and endocrine alterations, that many times accompany aging, than to primary factors of age deterioration.

If muscular training continues, endurance is more easily retained than strength production as aging progresses. For example, the relative decline for grip strength endurance is less than for grip force production. In fact, when endurance is expressed as a percent of maximum isometric strength held over as long a time as possible, grip strength endurance can be maintained or even improved up to the eighth decade (Aniansson, Grimby, Hedberg, Rundgren, & Sperling, 1978; Larsson & Karlsson, 1978; Petrofsky & Lind, 1975 a, b). Relative dynamic endurance of knee extensor muscles was preserved or slightly improved up to age 65 (Larsson & Karlsson, 1978). One of the reasons why endurance may be retained better than strength is that the percentage of slow oxidative fibers, Type I red fibers, which are essential for endurance performances, is proportionately greater relative to Type II fibers in older individuals (Costill et al., 1976; Gollnick, Armstrong, Saubert, Piehl, & Saltin, 1972). That is, the relative number of fast contracting glycolytic fibers (Type II) declines linearly from the third to the seventh decade (Larsson et al., 1978). Larsson (1982) found that age-related Type II muscle fiber atrophy was attenuated after four months of intense strength training conducted twice a week. Both a change in fiber type ratio and/or a change in cross sectional area may be expressed as atrophy, but Larsson's (1982) results suggest that one of the results of muscular training in the aged may be an alteration of the fiber type ratio.

The fact that older individuals can maintain some muscular endurance with training may be one of the reasons why older individuals seem to gravitate toward endurance types of sports and activities for their exercise or leisure physical activity. Many runners, cyclists, and swimmers who enjoy competing in these events switch from the short, power requiring distances to the longer, endurance demanding events (Kavanagh & Shepherd, 1977). Because muscular endurance can be maintained well, their performances in these events are largely limited by the age related effects on their aerobic endurance.

Cardiovascular Integrity

Limitations on maximum force and short term motor responses reside in the neuromuscular system, but when the motor system is called upon over a longer period of time, the integrity and function not only of muscular endurance, but of the cardiorespiratory system, contributes major limitations in the overall work that can be done. Age-related cardiovascular changes, such as a decrease in oxygen consumption, cardiac output, maximum heart rate, maximum systemic arterial-venous oxygen difference, exercising blood flow, and an increase in resting blood pressure with age have been the major focus of research in the physical capacities of the age for many years (for review, see Skinner, Tipton, & Vailas, 1982; Ostrow, 1984).

Maximum oxygen consumption is the best indicator of cardiovascular integrity, encompassing such factors as maximum heart rate, maximum stroke volume, maximum blood flow through the musculature, and maximal systematic arterial-venous oxygen difference. As a basis of comparison across body size, maximum oxygen consumption is expressed as ml of oxygen/kg of body weight. It thus takes into account changes in body fat, which as emphasized earlier, increases as individuals age and grow more sedentary. Master athletes have significantly lower body fat than sedentry individuals their own age and gender (Heath, Hagberg, Ehsani, & Holloszy, 1981; Shepherd & Kavanagh, 1978). If the activity level of the subjects is considered, experimenters can come closer to disassociating the effects of disuse, which are the result of a sedentry life style, from normal physiological deterioration that occurs with aging. Unfortunately there are very few studies where activity level has been controlled.

When the functional capacity of older individuals who have maintained their training is analyzed, particularly when the activity has been initiated early in life, the comparison is striking. Impressive aerobic performances, which rely on a healthy and efficient cardiovascular system, have been recorded in quite old individuals who have continued to train their entire lives. In fact, in athletes who continue to train, pronounced age-related decrements do not occur until after age 60 (Pollock, Miller, & Wilmore, 1974). Cardiovascular function superior to that of average men was maintained by male champion runners up until the age of 57 when the longitudinal observations were terminated (Robinson, Dill, Robinson, Tzankiff, & Wagner, 1976).

In an extensive review, Ostrow (1984) concluded that regular systematic aerobic exercise also improves the cardiovascular efficiency of older adults who are not athletes. In older adults of both genders, consistent submaximal exercise can increase maximal oxygen consumption, stroke volume, recovery heart rate, post-exercise blood lactate levels, oxygen pulse, and decrease systolic blood pressure. Although it is very difficult to compare the results of studies, Hodgson and Buskirk (1977) concluded from their analysis of 11 cross sectional studies of training effects that 60-year-old individuals can increase their maximal oxygen consumption through training almost as much as 30-year-olds, although the absolute levels of oxygen consumption are not as great. A recent study (Heath et al., 1981) demonstrated that when a similar training stimulus was maintained in young and old Master athletes, the O_2 pulse (stroke volume × artero-venous oxygen difference) was the same. That is, the ability to deliver oxygen and utilize oxygen per beat of the heart was maintained through training. Starnes, Beyer, and Edington (1983) recently demonstrated that old rats that trained regularly had significantly greater cardiac outputs and coronary blood flow than their sedentary age-matched controls when their hearts were stimulated to work a high workload. These findings, taken together, indicate that the main decrement that occurs in aging that limits maximum aerobic capacity of the older athletes is maximum heart rate. No matter how much older individuals may train, they cannot attain as high a maximum heart rate as they could when they were younger. The inability to achieve as high a maximum heart rate in older individuals appears to be related to a prolonged excitation-contraction cycle (Lakatta & Yin, 1982).

Within the perspective that older, well-conditioned individuals cannot function at levels that are absolutely as high as those of younger individuals, older, well-conditioned individuals can nonetheless function very well, and certainly at the level of younger, less well-conditioned individuals. The effects of exercise on the functional capacity of the cardiovascular system of adults is impressive and has many social and economic implications. This subject is treated in more detail in Chapter 10, where it is placed within the context of the overall discussion of the cardiorespiratory adaptations to chronic endurance exercise.

Even though relative muscular endurance and all but maximum heart rate can be maintained with training, absolute endurance does decline as individuals age. In the elite competitors' Masters records, the decline in endurance is steeper in those events that involve longer distances. For example, the percent loss in 70-year-olds from age 40 is greatest in the 10,000 meter event (approximately 45%), next greatest in the 1500 meter event (approximately 33%) and least in the 100 meter event (10%). Of course, the same sampling problems exist with these comparisons that were mentioned in the analysis of strength performances in the oldest categories. Fewer very old individuals run marathons compared to 10,000 meter races; therefore, the older categories in the longest distances are more susceptible to sampling bias and less representative of what older individuals might be capable of doing. Although the performances decline more in long distances than in short ones, it nevertheless remains significant that a well-trained 70-year-old champion can run a marathon 70% as fast as a world class young runner. The record for men over 70 is 3.73 meters per second, compared to the world record of 5.45 meters/sec, or a 32% decrease in velocity from the third decade to the eighth decade (Moore, 1975).

Psychomotor Performance

The decline of spontaneous physical activity, muscular strength, and endurance with age are common observations by even the most casual observers. Yet the decline in psychomotor behaviors with age is not so readily noticed, particularly if the behaviors can be accomplished with no speed requirement. In most states, for example, authorities assume that the complex sensorimotor integration and intricacies of rapid judgement necessary to maneuver an automobile successfully do not deteriorate enough with age to warrant screening driving abilities each year after the age of 65. Automobile driving and many other functional behaviors are so complex as to be difficult to test, but the process of understanding such complex motor tasks has been undertaken by analyzing simpler psychomotor tasks that represent different components of these more complex tasks. The psychomotor tasks studied are those requiring motor behaviors where the primary determinant for successful completion of the task is the motor behavior itself, rather than verbal or cognitive elements of the task. The behaviors focused on in this section are tasks that require extremely rapid movements in order to achieve a goal.

Performance is slower in aged individuals on psychomotor tasks such as the digit symbol substitution test (Weschler, 1958), tapping in place (Katzman & Terry, 1982), tapping two targets alternately (Welford, 1977), and moving a lever from side to side (Birren, Woods, & Williams, 1979). Even simple motor tasks such as crossing off symbols, copying, and tracing are slower (Birren et al., 1979; Storandt, 1976; Welford, 1977). These tasks all require speed of information processing and motor programming.

Particularly dramatic is the decline in response speed that occurs in little-practiced simple and choice reaction time (Birren et al., 1979) and in performance on tasks that require the coordination of two movements simultaneously (Rabbitt & Rogers, 1965). In fact, the more complex the choice reaction time task, the greater the reactivity deficits that are seen in the elderly (Cerella, Poon, & Williams, 1980). Choice reaction time paradigms that require spatial or symbolic transformations produce slower reaction times than those requiring no transformations. Even slower are the reaction times of the aged to stimuli displays involving both spatial and symbolic transformations.

Birren et al. (1979) have suggested that a "general speed factor" linearly declines with passing decades, the result of an aging central nervous system that is manifested in slower behavioral interactions with environmental stimuli. Yet, slowing of psychomotor capacity doesn't seem to be universal; the slowing seems greatly attenuated in some people. Health status also seems to have an effect (Milligan, Powell, Harley, & Furchtgott, 1984). In fact, psychomotor speed seems to be maintained in individuals who are physically active, exercising several days a week. Many investigators have found that older individuals who exercise consistently are faster in measures of simple and choice reaction time (Hart, 1981; Sherwood & Selder, 1979; Spirduso, 1975; Spirduso & Clifford, 1978). Spirduso, Osborne, MacCrae, and Gilliam (1985) compared different types of psychomotor tasks in physically trained women over 50 years of age to sedentary women of similar ages. The tasks placing a premium on speed of response were performed significantly faster by the exercised women: simple and choice reaction time, and stationary tapping. No differences existed between the exercised and sedentary groups on tasks requiring higher forms of information processing: trailmaking, digit symbol substitution, and tapping between targets. Dustman et al. (1984), however, found that older individuals who were aerobically trained for 4 months were significantly faster at the conclusion of the training in several types of perceptual and psychomotor tasks: simple reaction time, critical flicker fusion, digit symbol substitution, and Stroop tests. Neither control group—the aged control subjects, nor the aged strength-training subjects in the Dustman et al. (1984) study—were significantly faster at the conclusion of the study. Only those subjects who had aerobically exercised displayed exercise effects on psychomotor performance. Dustman et al. (1984) might have observed differences that result from relatively acute exercise-induced adaptive overshoot in some system that dissipates over a more extended period of time as the body chronically adapts to the increased exercise load. Since Dustman et al. (1984) also found exercise group differences in other measures of cognitive functioning such as mental flexibility and visuomotor speed, this supports their finding of differences in the digit symbol substitution test. Others have also reported effects of a short-term exercise program on another measure of cognitive function, crystalized intelligence (Elsayed, Ismail, & Young, 1980; Powell, & Pohndorf, 1971). The significance of these findings lies in the observation that the physically active individuals were performing psychomotor tasks requiring almost no strength or endurance to perform the task. Reaction time tasks, digit symbol, and stationary tapping tasks require very small movements of the fingers, so increases in muscular strength and endurance of the leg musculature resulting from running are not likely to affect these psychomotor performances. Rather, general cardiovascular endurance seems to have some type of "tuning", or selective arousal effect on central nervous system function.

The reverse effect is seen in individuals who have cardiovascular pathologies. Reaction time, for example, is slowest in the cerebrovascular diseased, and in patients who have transient ischemic attacks and strokes (Speith, 1965). It is next slowest in brain damaged (Benton, 1977; Hicks & Birren, 1970; Light, 1978; Miller, 1970) and untreated hypertensive patients (Speith, 1965). Reaction time is also slower than normal in those with coronary heart disease (Botwinick & Storandt, 1974; Hertzog, Schaie, & Gribbin, 1978; Speith, 1964, 1965). In fact, Ferris, Crook, Sathananthan, and Gershon (1976) reported that disjunctive reaction time predicted disease-related mental decline with 86% accuracy. Tapping speed was also slower in those with cardiovascular disease and hypertension (Enzer, Simonson, & Blankenstein, 1942).

While the mechanisms operative in retarding age-related psychomotor slowing in healthy, physically active individuals are probably quite different from those impaired in aged, cardiovascularly diseased patients, nevertheless certain observations can be made. The strongest relationship of physical fitness to psychomotor performance appears to be in psychomotor speed factors, primarily in simple responses. While simple reaction time and more complex reaction time have both been reported to be faster in exercised older individuals, the exercised/sedentary differences seen in choice reaction time are not greater than those seen in simple reaction time. The physically active women in Spirduso's study were 14msec faster than the sedentary women in choice reaction time, but they were 20 msec faster in simple reaction time. Hick's law, $CRT = a + b (\log_2 (N))$ expresses the relationship between reaction time and the number of choices to be made. N is the number of stimulus-response alternatives, a (constant) is the overall speed of the perceptual and motor system exclusive of decision making time, and b (slope) is the speed of decision making. If Hick's law accurately reflects the relationship between response speed and environmental stimuli, and no additional differences exist between exercised and sedentary individuals on choice reaction time, then the major effect of chronic exercise on psychomotor speed must be on the general overall speed of the perceptual and motor system. The fact that Spirduso's exercised subjects were not significantly faster on tasks placing a premium on scanning, accuracy, and decision making (trail-making, digit symbol substitution) supports this notion. Birren, et al. (1979) suggested that increased sympathetic activity in hypertensive patients may lead to relative inhibition of the central nervous system with regard to facilitating perceptual and motor responses. Conversely, the vagal, parasympathetic tone present in the highly physically conditioned individual may produce a highly facilitated central nervous system response. DeVries (1970) suggested long ago that physically active individuals may be able to maintain a higher arousal level under certain conditions, and Batkin (1981) suggested that "some efficient integration of autonomic activity with speed of behavior appears to exist in well functioning individuals." The evidence seems to support the notion that many of the effects of aging such as physical endurance, cardiac reserve, pulmonary reserve, physical strength, serum cholesterol, and systolic blood pressure, are modifiable by chronic exercise, and that some of these may well influence some types of mental processing by acting upon the central nervous system. In addition, the neuroendocrine responses that occur in response to exercise may well have a direct effect on some neurotransmitter systems, such as the dopaminergic system, that have been strongly related to the functioning of the motor system (Gilliam et al., 1984; Gilliam, 1985).

Mechanisms by Which Physical Activity may Influence the Aging Motor System

Systematic and consistent physical activity requiring aerobic and strength challenges clearly produces a functional capacity that is much greater than that observed in sedentary individuals. The enhanced functional capacity appears to extend to central as well as peripheral functioning, so that the decline in some types of psychomotor performance as well as cardiovascular, respiratory, and muscular capacity is also attenuated. The search for mechanisms by which exercise might prolong the integrity of the motor system is in its infancy, particularly with regard to the mechanisms by which physical activity might influence psychomotor efficiency. Several lines of research related to the effects of exercise have been pursued, including the trophic effects of muscular activity on the neuromuscular system, the morphological changes in brain that accompany motor activity, movement-related alterations in regional blood flow in the brain, and neuroendocrine adaptations to physical activity. Each of these topics is treated more thoroughly in Spirduso (1982), but a summary is provided here.

The loss of motor neurons, and consequently, motor units with age is striking. Less than half of the motor units present in youth remain in the aged individual (Brown, 1972).

The decrease in motor activity that is seen in old animals and human beings in many ways simulates the disuse paradigms that have been implemented in laboratories by physical activity constraints such as casting limbs, reducing living space, or suspending animals so that only certain limbs are functional. As anyone who has observed the atrophy and limited movement of a limb removed from a cast can attest, disuse is extremely detrimental to the neuromuscular system. Disuse is associated with a reduction in the quantity of neuronal firing and a decrease in the frequency of discharge of those neurons that remain active (Smith & Dugal, 1965). Nerve cells have a trophic influence on the muscle fibers they innervate; similarly, muscular contraction has a trophic influence on its innervating neuron and associated interneurons (Eccles, 1973). Proteins from an extract of rat skeletal muscle have been shown to promote neuritic outgrowth and increase neuronal cholinergic activity when added to cultures of dissociated ventral spinal cord from fetal rats (Smith & Appel, 1983). Others have shown that the addition of muscle extract enhances the survival of motoneurons in dissociated cell cultures. Muscle properties and integrity may influence the effectiveness of synaptic terminals by transferring chemicals from the postsynaptic cells to the presynaptic terminals (Atwood & Bittner, 1971). Long ago Vogt and Vogt (1946) proposed that frequent firing of action potentials postpones nerve cell aging. Although Eccles (1973) traced the trophic effect of muscular contraction into the central nervous system only so far as its innervating neuron and immediate central connections, the trophic exchange of muscular activity could include to some degree the entire multilevel neuronal network contributing to the movement. Daily endurance training was shown to prevent the attrition of both slow and fast twitch fibers (Faulkner, Maxwell, & Lieberman, 1971), suggesting that individuals who exercise daily may more successfully maintains the capacity to recruit fast twitch fibers. Gutmann and Hanzlikova (1972), however, recognized that inactivity does not alone account for the muscular atrophy seen in aging; that there appears to be a basic disturbance of neuronal metabolism with age. Confirming this, Farrar, Martin, & Ardies (1981) found no difference in the mass of the gastrocnemius-plantaris muscles of young and old exercised rats when they were compared to sedentary rats. But Gutmann and Hanzlikova (1972) were early proponents of the idea that the decreasing amounts of neural activity that occur in an aging system might influence its retention of neurosecretory trophic exchange, which in turn would accelerate the decrease in neural activity.

Exercise may have other effects that are beneficial to muscle contractility. By stimulating blood flow, exercise may enhance contractility and permeability of blood vessels, thus preventing local ischemia (Samorajski, 1976). A healthy circulation stabilizes temperature in the extremities, which in turn maintains functions such as normal nerve conduction velocity and spinal reflex loops.

Many investigators have shown that morphological brain changes, such as changes in neuronal cell structure, number, and density parallel motor activity in animals. That is, when older animals are provided with motor challenges or reared in enriched environments that facilitate and promote physical activity, dramatic changes in several morphological markers are seen. Even in young animals forced to learn a task that activates one limb more than the other, substantial changes are seen in neuronal characteristics of the cortical hemisphere contralateral to the practiced limb. Whole brain weights have been reported to be lower in inactive animals when compared to active ones (Pysh & Weiss, 1979). The brain is a very plastic organ, and evidence is accumulating that physical activity, or the lack thereof, can have a profound effect on its structure as well as its function.

Another mechanism by which exercise may contribute to the maintenance of central nervous system control of the motor system is by enhancing the blood flow to the brain region associated with the ideation or activation of movement patterns. Frequent blood flow to an area ensures that metabolic needs are satisfied, supports activation of the area, and perhaps serves a trophic function. Many investigators have shown that regional cerebral blood flow alterations are associated not only with an actual movement, but with ideation that is associated with movement. The long term effect that gross body exercise, or even specific discrete movements, might have upon regional blood flow alterations is not known at this time. It is, however, an area that is under investigation.

The response of the neuroendocrine system to exercise may include some tuning or enhancement of neuroendocrine adaptations to exercise stress. Exercise might maintain a generalized neuroendocrine adaptability that in turn facilitates the regulation and control of many enzymatic responses to task demands. Landfield, Lindsey, and Lynch (1978) have proposed a neuroendocrine theory of aging, which suggests that the neuroendocrine system accelerates aging through hormonal actions on target brain cells. Yet, many investigators have shown that chronic exercise substantially alters hormonal response. For example, aging degrades glucose tolerance, or the ability to dispose of administered glucose efficiently (Andres & Tobin, 1977), but physical conditioning appears to fine-tune the system's response to glucose. Chronic exercise might maintain some hormonal regulatory systems, consequently controlling key enzymatic functions that influence nervous system integrity.

A final mechanism that seems very promising is the effect of physical activity on key neurotransmitters in the central nervous system. The catecholamine system, particularly the nigrostriatal dopamine system, decreases in both neurotransmitter levels and receptor numbers with age (McGeer & McGeer, 1976). In fact, it is the decline of this system, acutely in the case of Parkinson's disease, and more gradually in the case of aging, that has been closely associated to many aspects of motor system deterioration. Until recently, little thought had been given to the possibility that chronic exercise might influence neurotransmitter receptor numbers or function, thus impacting some aspects of brain function. Some early evidence by Brown et al. (1979) suggests that whole brain resting catecholamines of chronically exercising animals were higher than sedentary animals. Others have reported acute effects of exercise on serotonin levels, and norephinepherine as well as dopamine. More recently, Gilliam et al. (1984), in studying the characteristics of an analogue of the neurotransmitter dopamine, found evidence that chronic exercise changed some of the characteristics of the neurotransmitter, and these changes were in the direction opposite to the changes associated with aging.

Conversely, higher catecholamine activity has been seen in hyperactive rats than in hypoactive rats, which suggests that catecholamine levels may not only respond to acute bouts of exercise, but may influence activity levels within a species.

Thus, several mechanisms of the neuromuscular apparatus appear to be influenced by chronic physical activity. These influences may postpone early deterioration of central nervous system control and consequently of neuromuscular function.

Biological Age

The discussions to this point have stressed the fact that dramatic changes can be made in the age-related deterioration curves of strength, endurance, cardiovascular integrity, and psychomotor functioning when these systems are continually challenged throughout life. The difference between individuals who stop using their bodies and those who exercise daily is substantial. When these differences are added to genetic and environmentally shaped differences already existing in our population, the interaction produces an even wider distribution of capabilities in the older adults that is seen in young adults. The variability of the way individuals age has been expressed as biological age versus chronological age. Biological age is a familiar concept in child development, where there are obvious differentiating landmarks such as skeletal, dental, and sexual maturation changes. Yet it has become clear that biological age is also drastically different from chronological age in some adults. The landmarks are not as obvious.

Several investigators have developed test batteries designed to measure biological age and to determine whether biological age, more than chronological age, is predictive of function and longevity in older populations. Borkan and Norris (1980), for example, combined a large number of age-related parameters in a multiple regression equation and predicted biological age from the relationship of scores on these parameters to chronological age. The test items in their biological age test battery included only the variables that had a clear directional trend with aging, shown both cross-sectionally and longitudinally. In order to be included, the cross sectional score on a particular parameter had to be the result of a change over time, not a result of genetic endowment, measurement error, or daily fluctuation. The variables in their test battery covered a wide range of physical functions. Biological age was computed by a) regressing the data linearly on age, b) subtracting individual scores from the scores predicted by the regression equation (a procedure which yielded a residual score), c) standardizing the residual scores using a Z transformation, and d) converting the data so that positive standard scores always denoted biologically older individuals. Thus, if an individual had a positive biological age score, he was viewed as responding on a test in a manner characteristic of men older than himself. Conversely, if he had a negative biological age score, his response was more like men younger than himself. They found that individuals who "looked older" than their age also were biologically older on this test battery, and that the biological age of the subjects who died during their longitudinal study was higher than that of the surviving subjects. The parameters that significantly predicted death were forced expiratory volume, vital capacity, systolic blood pressure, albumin levels, globulin, tapping performance, simple and choice reaction time, and foot reaction time. Several other investigators have constructed biological age batteries and have found them to be predictive of function and longevity. Another example is that of Botwinick, West, and Storandt (1978), who found that three psychomotor tasks, two learning and memory tests, two personality sub-tests, and a self-report health rating significantly differentiated between a group that survived and a group that died subsequent to their investigation. Common to many of these biological age test batteries is the significant contribution made by performance on psychomotor tests. To some extent psychomotor tasks requiring speed may be considered a behavioral window through which the central nervous system's integrity may be viewed.

When older individuals train intensely and improve their cardiovascular-respiratory and neuromuscular function dramatically, thus attaining values (biological age scores) that are better than those of individuals who are much younger, there are many who would describe them as being physiologically or biologically younger than their sedentary counterparts. However, this implies that the aging process has slowed down, or that the rate of aging has changed. In fact, there is no evidence that the rate of aging can be changed in humans. Skinner et al. (1982, p. 431) explain that "The fact that well-trained men of 60 years have the same functional capacities as those of 40-year-old men does not mean that they are 20 years younger. Since they have lived for 60 years, they have had many more physiological changes in the various systems within their bodies than the 40-year-old population. Therefore, they are 60-year-old men who are in better condition than other men of their age." Nevertheless, they have the functional capacity of individuals 20 years younger. Even if their level of health and fitness does not contribute to a prolonged life, it contributes substantially to a higher quality of life in the waning years prior to death.

Longevity

No discussion of the contributions of physical activity to human well-being would be complete without addressing the question of whether chronic exercise results, ultimately, in a longer life. It has always seemed as though daily exercise should make people live longer. It may do so by interacting with secondary causes of aging, as it is generally incompatible with smoking, obesity, and high blood pressure. It has also been thought by many researchers to be related to a decreased incidence of heart disease. The belief that physically fit humans live longer has proven, until relatively recently, to be stubbornly resistent to scientific verification.

Early attempts to determine whether physical activity would increase longevity involved comparing the longevity of athletes with nonathletes, on the assumption that athletes were more physically active than nonathletes. Stephens, Van Huss, Olson, and Montoye (1984) reviewed many studies dealing with this comparison, as well as the comparison of athletes with appropriate control groups. Their conclusion is that athletes do live longer than the general population, but that there are so many problems associated with this type of comparison as to render it useless. Athletes may differ from nonathletes in many ways other than the extent of physical activity: their physical ability, educational level, body type, and vocational and avocational physical demands, to name a few. Athletes as a group are not even homogeneous, varying in length of athletic participation, intensity of training, and the physical demands of the sport. When all of these factors were considered, Stephens et al. (1984) could not come to a definite answer regarding the longevity of athletes compared to nonathletes. Polednak (1979) also concluded, after analyzing several studies of athlete's longevity, that no clear evidence existed to support the notion that athletes live longer. In some of the studies reviewed, nonathletic control groups lived longer than athletes. Paffenbarger et al. (1984), by carefully controlling for factors such as smoking, obesity, weight gain, and hypertension, observed that a relationship exists between exercise and longevity in athletes, but that it is related to the amount of habitual post-college exercise, not to their athletic status.

Hayflick (1982) makes the observation that "lumberjacks and stevedores do not live longer than taxidrivers and businessmen." However, in human studies—particularly early ones—several factors have been confounded: type and extent of exercise, socioeconomics, athletic status, educational level, and the ratio and amount of on-work to off-work physical activity. Rose and Cohen (1977) statistically isolated these factors in a careful and systematic study of 2000 males of various ages, using careful controls for the secular effect, disease, smoking, familial factors, and health habits. They found that men with light-work occupations, but heavy off-work exercise patterns live 3.8 years longer than men with light-work on and off the job. Men with heavy off-work physical activity in both their 20's and 40's lived 4.6 years longer than men with light work on and off the job.

Men with heavy off-work exercise in both their 20's and 40's lived 7.1 years longer than those who exercised extensively in their 20's, but dropped to light exercise in their 40's. The best predictor of long life in this study, other than number of illnesses, smoking behavior, anxiety level, place of residence (rural or urban) and occupational level, was off-work physical activity in the years 40-49. Very recently, in a widely publicized epidemiological study, Paffenbarger et al. (1986) reported that evidence from a study of the life style characteristics of 16,936 Harvard alumni revealed a 1-2 year extension of life attributed to adequate exercise. Rates of death were substantially lower in alumni who expended 2000 or more kcal during exercise weekly. "With or without consideration of hypertension, cigarette smoking, extremes or gains in body weight, or early parental death, alumni mortality rates were significantly lower among the physically active."

Studies of the effect of exercise on longevity in animals, in which better diet, environmental, and genetic controls were employed, have been more supportive of the notion that exercise prolongs life. In five out of six studies, exercised rats lived longer than sedentary rates, and the exercise was not very great in some cases (Drori & Folman, 1976; Edington, Cosmas, & McCafferty, 1972; Goodrick, 1974; Goodrick, 1980; Retzlaff, Fontaine, & Futura, 1966; Sperling, Looslie, & McCoy, 1978). The lone investigator who failed to find exercise effects used only 7 rats, 4 runners and 3 controls (Slonaker, 1912). This study was primarily observational in nature.

The term longevity can mean at least two things. One meaning is that life expectancy is increased; that is, the extent to which individuals can *expect* to live, barring illness or accidents, to the mean age that human beings attain, about 85 ± 5 years (Fries & Crapo, 1981). Another way in which the term longevity is used is to mean the life span of a species; that is, the *maximum* attainable age for a given species. The evidence that exercise can contribute to extending the life span in animals is very weak; for human beings it is nonexistent. Research findings are, however, suggestive that a lifestyle of vigorous activity can increase life expectancy. Other beneficial health habits such as nonsmoking, weight control, good nutrition, medical attention, ample sleep, and moderate alcohol consumption are also practiced by chronic exercisers, and it is probable that the cumulative beneficial effect of all of these contributes to enabling these individuals to fulfill their life expectancy.

Summary

The proportion of Americans 65 or older is growing greater with each decade. It is estimated that by 2030, 17-20% of our population will be 65 or older.

As individuals age, their spontaneous physical activity decreases; this is true even more for women than for men. In fact, regular sports involvement is inversely related to age.

Some of the factors responsible for the declining physical activity of older individuals are a) declining physical abilities, b) loss of interest, c) social constraints, d) limited access to facilities, and e) a dissolution of social contacts and networks.

Exercise is a lifestyle intervention, which by preventing some disease processes and postponing some of the debilitation that accompanies old age, is more cost effective than medical treatment and services.

Maximum isometric and dynamic muscular force decline with age; dynamic strength decreases more than isometric strength. Although there is a greater absolute loss of strength in the old than in the young, the rate of relative tension development is the same.

Strength training, although viewed by some to be contraindicated for older individuals, does produce muscle hypertrophy in the aged. Older individuals can produce similar and significant percent increases in strength after at least eight weeks of strength training. The performances in Masters weight lifting contests reveal that individuals in their late 60's and 70's can lift great amounts of weight. Caution should be exercised by older individuals who train with weights.

Absolute endurance declines with age, but with training relative endurance can be maintained. When endurance is expressed as a percent of maximum isometric strength held over as long a time as possible, grip strength endurance can be maintained or even improved up to the eighth decade.

Because psychomotor behaviors are heavily dependent upon central nervous system integrity, evidence that health and physical fitness are related to psychomotor peformance suggests that a lifestyle of exercise may maintain optimum brain function in some types of behavior.

Consistent submaximal exercise can increase, in older adults of both genders, maximal oxygen consumption, stroke volume, recovery heart rate, post-exercise blood lactate levels, oxygen pulse, and can decrease systolic blood pressure. Older, well-conditioned individuals can function aerobically as well as or better than many less well trained individuals.

Several mechanisms have the potential to explain how health and physical fitness might influence central nervous system function: muscle contraction enhances the health of its innervating neurons and neuronal networks; movements appear to produce changes in the structure of neurons in related parts of the brain; blood flow, providing nutrients to support the increased metabolism in these associated regions also increases as the movements begin and continue; and neurotransmitter function appears to be influenced by exercise.

Biological age is a term used to express functional capacity relative to chronological age. An individual whose physical and mental functional capacities are more similar to younger individuals than to his/her chronological peers is said to have a younger biological age. This does not imply that the individual rate of aging has changed, or that the individual is in fact "biologically younger," but that he/she functions as a much younger person.

The evidence that consistent lifelong exercise will lengthen the life span of human beings is very weak, if non-existent. The evidence is compelling, however, that exercise and other beneficial health habits such as nonsmoking, weight control, good nutrition, medical attention, ample sleep, and moderate alcohol consumption, which are also usually practiced by chronic exercisers, provide a cumulative beneficial effect of all of these that may enable these individuals to fulfill their life expectancy.

References

Andres, R. & Tobin, J.D. (1977). Endocrine systems. In C.E. Finch & L. Hayflick (Eds.), *Handbook of the biology of aging* (pp. 357-378). New York: Van Nostrand Reinhold Co.

Aniansson, A., Grimby, G., Hedberg, M., Rundgren, A., & Sperling, L. (1978). Muscle function in old age. *Scandinavian Journal of Rehabilitation and Medicine Supplement., 6,* 43-49.

Asmussen, E. & Heeboll-Nielsen, K. (1962). Isometric muscle strength of adult men and women. In E. Asmussen, A. Fredsted, & E. Ryge (Eds.), *Community*

Testing Observation Institute Danish National Association Infantile Paralysis., 11, 1-43.

Astrand, P.O. & Rodahl, K. (1970). *Textbook of work physiology.* New York: McGraw-Hill Book Co.

Atwood, H.L. & Bittner, G.D. (1971). Matching of excitatory and inhibitory inputs to crustacean muscle fibers. *Journal of Neurophysiology, 34,* 157-170.

Batkin, S. (1981). *Aging and the nervous system.* Communication to the XIII International Congress of Gerontology, Hamburg, Germany.

Benton, A.L. (1977). Interactive effects of age and brain disease on reaction time. *Archives of Neurology, 34,* 369-370.

Birren, J.E., Woods, A.M., & Williams, M.V. (1979). Speed of behavior as an indicator of age changes and the integrity of the nervous system. In F. Hoffmeister and C. Muller (Eds.), *Brain function in Old Age* (pp. 10-44). Berlin: Springer-Verlag.

Borkin, G.A. & Norris, A.H. (1980). Assessment of biological age using a profile of physical parameters. *Journal of Gerontology, 35,* 177-184.

Boothby, J., Tungatt, J.F. & Townsend, A.R. (1981). Ceasing participation in sports activity: Reported reasons and their implications. *Journal of Leisure Research, 13,* 1-14.

Botwinick, J. & Storandt, M. (1974). Speed functions, vocabulary ability and age. *Perceptual Motor Skills, 36,* 1128.

Botwinick, J., West, R., & Storandt, M. (1978). Predicting death from behavioral test performance. *Journal of Gerontology, 33,* 755-762.

Brown, B.S., Payne, T., Kim, C., Moore, G., Krebs, P. & Martin, W. (1979). Chronic response of rat brain norepinephrine and serotonin levels to endurance training. *Journal of Applied Physiology, 46,* 12-23.

Brown, W.F. (1972). A method for estimating the number of motor units in thenar muscles and the changes in motor unit count with aging. *Journal of Neurology and Neurosurgical Psychiatry, 35,* 845-852.

Cerella, J., Poon, L.W., Williams, D.M. (1980). Age and the complexity hypothesis. In L.W. Poon (Ed.), *Aging in the 1980's* (pp. 332-340). Washington, DC: American Psychological Association.

National adult physical fitness survey. (1974). In H.H. Clarke (Ed.), *Physical Fitness Research Digest, 4,* 1-27.

Clarkson, P., Kroll, W., & Melchionda, A.M. (1981). Age, isometric strength, rate of tension development and fiber type composition. *Journal of Gerontology, 36,* 648-653.

Costill, D.L., Daniels, J., Evans, W., Fink, W., Krahenbul, G., & Saltin, B. (1976) Skeletal muscle enzymes and fiber compositions in male and female track athletes. *Journal of Applied Physiology, 40,* 149-154.

deVries, H.A. (1968). Efficiency of electrical activity as a physiological measure of the functional state of muscle tissue. *American Journal of Physical Medicine, 47,* 10-22.

deVries, H.A. (1970). Physiological effects of an exercise training regimen upon men 52 to 88. *Journal of Gerontology, 25,* 325-336.

Dustman, R.E., Ruhling, R.O., Russell, E.M., Shearer, D.E., Bonekat, W., Shigeoka, J.W., Wood, J.S., & Bradford, D.C. (1984). Aerobic exercise training and improved neuropsychological function of older individuals. *Neurobiology of Aging, 5,* 35-42.

Drinkwater, B.L., Horvath, S.M., & Wells, C.L. (1975). Aerobic power of females, ages 10 to 68. *Journal of Gerontology, 30,* 385-394.

Drori, D. & Folman, Y. (1976) Environmental effects of longevity in the male rat: Exercise, mating, castration, and restricted feeding. *Experimental Gerontology, 11,* 25-32.

Eccles, J.C. (1973) Tropic influences in the mammalian central nervous system. In M. Rockstein (Ed.), *Development and Aging in the Nervous System* (pp. 89-104).

New York: Academic Press.

Edington, D., Cosmas, A.C., & McCafferty, W.B. (1972). Exercise and longevity: Evidence for a threshold age. *Journal of Gerontology, 27,* 341-343.

Elsayed, M., Ismail, A.H., & Young, R.J. (1980). Intellectual differences of adult men related to age and physical fitness before and after an exercise program. *Journal of Gerontology, 35,* 383-387.

Enzer, N., Simonson, E., & Blankstein, S.S. (1942). Fatigue of patients with circulatory insufficiency, investigated by means of fusion frequency of flicker. *Annals of International Medicine, 16,* 701-707.

Farrar, R.P., Martin, T.P., & Ardies, C.M. (1981). The interaction of aging and endurance exercise upon the mitochondrial function of skeletal muscle. *Journal of Gerontology, 36,* 642-647.

Ferris, S., Crook, T., Sathananthan, G., & Gershon, S. (1976). Reaction time as a diagnostic measure in senility. *Journal of the American Geriatrics Society, 24,* 529-533.

Fries, J.F. & Crapo, L.M. (1981). *Vitality and aging.* San Francisco: W.H. Freeman.

Gilliam, P.E. (1985). The effects of age on reactive capacity and nigrostriatal dopamine function (Doctoral dissertation, University of Texas, 1985). *Dissertation Abstracts International.*

Gilliam, P.E., Spirduso, W.W., Martin, T.P., Walters, T.J., Wilcox, R.E. & Farrar, R.P. (1984). The effects of exercise training on (3H)-spiperone binding in rat striatum. *Pharmacology, Biochemistry, and Behavior, 20,* 863-867.

Goldspink, G. & Howells, K.F. (1974). Work-induced hypertrophy in exercised normal muscles of different ages and the reversibility of hypertrophy after cessation of exercise. *Journal of Physiology, 239,* 179-193.

Gollnick, P.D., Armstrong, R.B., Saubert, C.W., Piehl, K., & Saltin, B. (1972). Enzyme activity and fiber composition in skeletal muscle of untrained and trained men. *Journal of Applied Physiology, 33,* 312-319.

Goodrick, C.L. (1974). Effects of long-term voluntary wheel exercise on male and female Wistar rats. *Gerontology, 26,* 22-33.

Goodrick, C.L. (1980). The effects of exercise on longevity and behavior of hybrid mice which differ in coat color. *Journal of Gerontology, 29,* 129-133.

Gutmann, E. & Hanzlikova, V. (1972). *Age changes in the neuromuscular system.* Bristol, England: Scientechnica.

Hart, B.A. (1981). The effect of age and habitual activity on the fractionated components of resisted and unresisted response time. *Medicine and Science in Sports and Exercise, 13,* 78.

Hayflick, L. (1982). On slowing old age. *Executive Health, 18,* 4.

Heath, G., Hagberg, J., Ehsani, A., & Holloszy, J. (1981). A physiological comparison of young and older endurance athletes. *Journal of Applied Physiology, 51,* 634-640.

Hertzog, C., Schaie, K.W., & Gribbin, K. (1978). Cardiovascular disease and changes in intellectual functioning from middle to old age. *Journal of Gerontology, 33,* 872-883.

Hettinger, T. (1961). *Physiology of strength.* Springfield, IL: C.C. Thomas Publishers.

Hicks, L.H. & Birren, J.E. (1970). Aging, brain damage, and psychomotor slowing. *Psychological Bulletin, 74,* 377-396.

Hodgson, J.L. & Buskirk, E.R. (1977). Physical fitness and age, with emphasis on cardiovascular function in the elderly. *Journal of the American Geriatrics Society, 25,* 385-392.

Hofecker, G., Kalicky, M., Kment, A., & Niedermüller, H. (1980). Models of the biological age of the rat. I. A factor model of age parameters. *Mechanisms of aging and development, 14,* 345-359.

Katzman, R. & Terry, R. (1982). Normal aging of the nervous system. In R.

Katzman & R. Terry (Eds.), *The Neurology of Aging*. Philadelphia: F.A. Davis.

Kavanagh, T. & Shephard, R.J. (1977). The effects of continued training on the aging process. *Annals of New York Academy of Sciences*, 656-670.

Lakatta, E.G. & Yin, F.C.P. (1982). Myocardial aging: Functional alterations and related cellular mechanisms. *American Journal of Physiology, 242*, H927-H941.

Landfield, P.W., Lindsey, J.D., & Lynch, G. (1978). Apparent acceleration of brain aging pathology by prolonged administration of glucocorticoids. *Society for Neuroscience Abstracts, 4*, 350.

Larsson, L. (1982). Aging in mammalian skeletal muscle. In J. Mortimer, F.J. Pirozzolo, & G.J. Maletta (Eds.), *The aging motor system*. New York: Praeger Scientific.

Larsson, L., Grimby, G., & Karlsson, J. (1979). Muscle strength and speed of movement in relation to age and muscle morphology. *Journal of Applied Physiology, 46*, 451-456.

Larsson, L. & Karlsson, J. (1978). Isometric and dynamic endurance as a function of age and skeletal muscle characteristics. *Acta Physiologica Scandinavica, 104*, 129-136.

Light, K. (1978). Effects of mild cardiovascular and cerebrovascular disorders on serial reaction time performance. *Experimental Aging Research, 4*, 3-22.

McGeer, P.L. & McGeer, E.G. (1976). Enzymes associated with the metabolism of catecholamines, acetylcholine, and gamma-aminobutyric acid in human controls and patients with Parkinson's disease and Huntington's chorea. *Journal of Neurochemistry, 26*, 65-76.

Miller, E. (1970). Simple and choice reaction time following severe head injury. *Cortex, 6*, 121-12f

Milligan, W.L., Powell, D.A., Harley, C. & Furchtgott, E. (1984). A comparison of physical health and psychosocial variables as predictors of reaction time and serial learning performance in elderly men. *Journal of Gerontology, 39*, 709-710.

Moore, D.H. (1975). A study of age group track and field records to relate age and running speed. *Nature, 253*, 264-265.

Montoye, H.J. (1975). *Physical activity-health: An epidemiologic study of an entire community*. Englewood Cliffs, N.J., Prentice-Hall.

Moritani, T. & deVries, H.A. (1980). Potential for gross muscle hypertrophy in older men. *Journal of Gerontology, 35*, 672-682.

National Institute of Health. (1983). *Special Report on Aging* (Publication No. 83-2489). Washington, DC: U.S. Government Printing Office.

Ostrow, A. (1984). *Physical activity in the older adult*. Princeton, NJ: Princeton Book Company.

Paffenbarger, R.S., Jr., Hyde, R.T., Wing, A.L., & Steinmetz, C.H. (1984). A Natural history of athleticism and cardiovascular health. *Journal of the American Medical Association, 252*, 491-495.

Paffenbarger, R.S., Jr., Hyde, R.T., Wing, A.L., & Hsieh, C. (1986). Physical activity, all-cause mortality, and longevity of college alumni. *New England Journal of Medicine, 314*, 605-613.

Petrofsky, J.S. & Lind, A.R. (1975a). Aging isometric strength and endurance and cardiovascular responses to static effort. *Journal of Applied Physiology, 38*, 91-95.

Petrofsky, J.S. & Lind, A.R. (1975b). Isometric strength, endurance, and the blood pressure and heart rate responses during isometric exercise in healthy men and women, with special reference to age and body fat content. *Pflugers Archives, 360*, 49-61.

Polednak, A.P. (1979). *The longevity of athletes*. Springfield, IL: Charles C. Thomas.

Pollock, M.L., Miller, H.S. & Wilmore, J. (1974). Physiological characteristics of champion American track athletes 40 to 75 years of age. *Journal of Gerontology, 29*, 645-649.

Powell, R.R. & Pohndorf, R.H. (1971). Comparison of adult exercisers and non-exercisers on fluid intelligence and selected physiological variables. *Research Quarterly, 42,* 70-77.

Pysh, J.J. & Weiss, G.M. (1979). Exercise during development induces an increase in Purkinje cell dendritic tree size. *Science, 206,* 230-231.

Rabbitt, P. & Rogers, M. (1965). Age and choice between responses in a self-paced repetitive task. *Ergonomics, 8,* 435-444.

Retzlaff, E., Fontaine, J. & Futura, W. (1966). Effect of daily exercise on lifespan of albino rats. *Geriatrics, 21,* 171.

Reigel, P.S. (1981). Athletic records and human endurance. *American Scientist, 69,* 285-290.

Riley, M.W. & Waring, J. (1978). Most of the problems of aging are not biological, but social. In R. Gross, B. Gross, and S. Seidman (Eds.), *The new old: struggling for decent aging.* Garden City, N.Y.: Anchor Press.

Robinson, S., Dill, D.B., Robinson, R.D., Tzankoff, S.P. & Wagner, J.A. (1976). Physiological aging of champion runners. *Journal of Applied Physiology, 41,* 46-51.

Rose, C.L. & Cohen, M.L. (1977). Relative importance of physical activity for longevity. *Annals of the New York Academy of Sciences, 310,* 671-702.

Samorajski, T. (1976). How the human body responds to aging. *Journal of the American Geriatric Society, 24,* 4-11.

Shepherd, R.J. & Kavanagh, T. (1978). The effects of training on the aging process. *Physician and Sports Medicine, 6,* 33-40.

Sherwood, D.E. & Selder, D.J. (1979). Cardiovascular health, reaction time, and aging. *Medicine and Science in Exercise and Sport, 11,* 186-189.

Simon, H. (1985). Exercise and well being. *Harvard Medical School Health Letter, 10,* 3-4.

Skinner, J.S., Tipton, C.M. & Vailas, A.C. (1982). Exercise, physical training, and the aging process. In A. Vijdik (Ed.), *Lectures in Gerontology* (pp. 407-439). New York: Academic Press.

Slonaker, J. (1912). The normal activity of the albino rat from birth to natural death, its rate of growth and the duration of life. *Journal of Animal Behavior, 2,* 20-42.

Smith, E.L. (1981). The interaction of nature and nurture. In E.L. Smith and R.C. Serfass (Eds.), *Exercise and aging* (pp. 11-18). Hillside, NJ: Enslow.

Smith, R.G., & Appel, S.H. (1983). Extracts of skeletal muscle increase neurite outgrowth and cholinergic activity of fetal rat spinal motor neurons. *Science, 219,* 1079-1080.

Smith, L.C. & Dugall, L.D. (1965). Age and spontaneous running activity of old male rats. *Canadian Journal of Applied Physiology and Pharmacology, 43,* 852-856.

Soldo, B.J. (1980) America's elderly in the 1980's. *Population Bulletin, 35,* 3-48.

Speith, W. (1964). Cardiovascular health status, age, and psychological performance. *Journal of Gerontology, 19,* 277-284.

Speith, W. (1965). Slowness of task performance and cardiovascular diseases. In A.R. Welford & J.E. Birren (Eds.), *Behavior, aging and the nervous system* (pp. 366-400). Springfield, IL: Charles C. Thomas.

Sperling, G.A., Looslie, J.K. & McCay, C.M. (1978). Effects of sulfamerazine and exercise on life span of rats and hamsters. *Gerontology, 24,* 220-224.

Spirduso, W.W. (1975). Reaction and movement time as a function of age and physical activity level. *Journal of Gerontology, 30,* 435.

Spirduso, W.W. (1982). Effects of physiological fitness on the aging motor system. In Mortimer, J., Pirozzolo, F.J., & Maletta, G.J. (Eds.), *The Aging Motor System.* New York: Praeger Scientific.

Spirduso, W.W. & Clifford, P. (1978). Replication of age and physical activity effects on reaction and movement time. *Journal of Gerontology, 33,* 26-30.

Spirduso, W.W., Osborne, L., MacCrae, H. & Gilliam, P. (1985). *Physical fitness and psychomotor task performance in elderly women.* Unpublished manuscript.

Starnes, J.W., Beyer, R.E. & Edington, D.W. (1983). Myocardial adaptations to endurance exercise in aged rats. *American Journal of Physiology, 245,* H560-H566.

Stephens, K.E., Van Huss, W.D., Olson, H.W. & Montoye, H.J. (1984). The longevity, morbidity, and physical fitness of former athletes: An update. *The Academy Papers, 17,* 101-119.

Stones, M.J. & Kozma, A. (1982). Cross-sectional, longitudinal, and secular age trends in athletic performances. *Experimental Aging Research, 8,* 185-188.

Storandt, M. (1976). Speed and coding effects in relation to age and ability level. *Developmental Psychology, 12,* 177-178.

Swanson, M.B. (1976). *Physical activity attitudes of senior citizens.* Unpublished master's thesis, University of Montana.

Tomanek, R.J. & Wood, Y.K. (1970). Compensatory hypertrophy of the plantaris muscle in relation to age. *Journal of Gerontology, 25,* 23-29.

Vogt, C. & Vogt, O. (1946). Aging of nerve cells. *Nature, 58,* 304.

Welford, A.T. (1977). Serial reaction times, continuity of task, single-channel effects, and age. In S. Dornic (Ed.), *Attention and Performance VI.* Hillsdale, NJ: Lawrence Erlbaum.

Weschler, D. (1958). *The measurement and appraisal of adult intelligence.* Baltimore: Williams and Wilkins.

Winer, F. (1979). The elderly jock and how he got that way. In J.H. Goldstein (Ed.), *Sports, games, and play: Social and psychological view points.* Hillsdale, NJ: Lawrence Erlbaum.

Section II

BIOLOGICAL PERSPECTIVE

- Physical Activity and Body Composition
- Neuromuscular Adaptations to High-Resistance Exercise
- Menstruation, Pregnancy, and Menopause
- Nutrition and Ergogenic Aids
- Cardiorespiratory Adaptations to Chronic Endurance Exercise

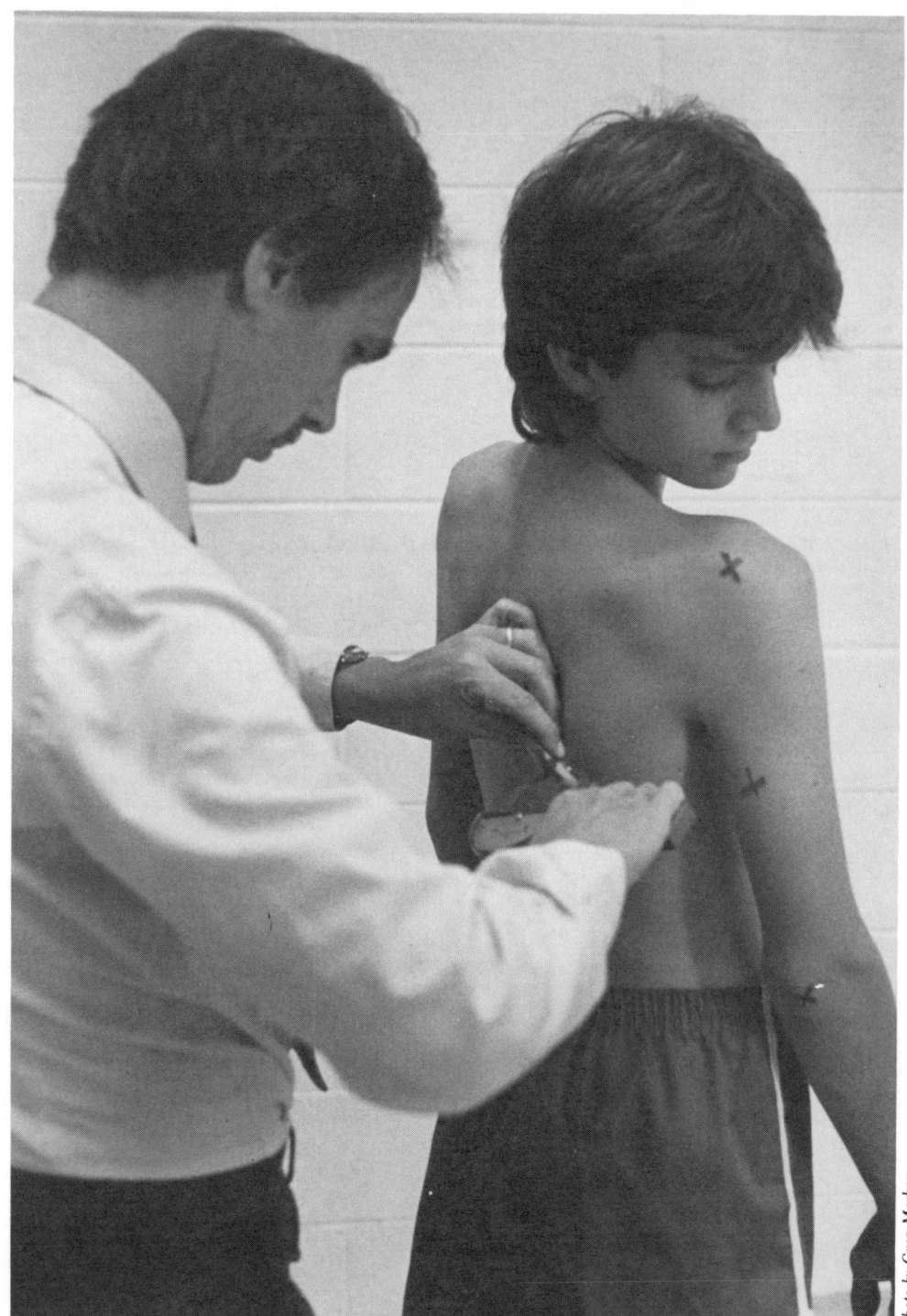

photo by Greg Merhar

CHAPTER SIX

Physical Activity and Body Composition

Pat Eisenman
College of Health
The University of Utah
Salt Lake City, Utah

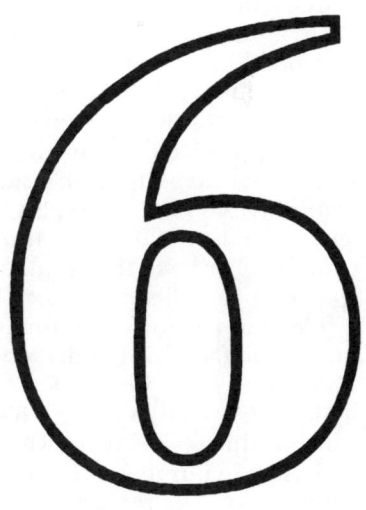

Interest in the role of exercise and physical activity in weight control and the treatment of obesity has been on the rise. Disenchantment with the long term prognosis for dietary weight control strategies and expanded awareness of the potential influences on body composition are two of the more obvious reasons for this resurgence of interest in physical activity as a method for regulating body weight.

The precise interactions between physical activity and body composition are not known; however, considerable efforts have already gone into elucidating such interactions, and the research is accelerating as expanding technologies facilitate new approaches for research. The purpose of this chapter will be to present what is currently known about the influence of the intensity, frequency, duration and type of activity on the body weight and its composition. Interpretation of the literature concerning exercise and body composition depends on an understanding of the underlying assumptions and potential limitations of the techniques used in the assessment of body composition. Therefore, attention will be focused first on examining the assumptions and limitations of these assessment procedures.

Measurement of Body Composition

The human body is composed of four basic chemical constituents: water, protein, mineral, and fat (Brozek, 1966). Direct information about the relative contribution of these constituents to the body mass has been derived from the biochemical analyses of cadavers. Despite an inadequate number of cadaver studies, such data provide the theoretical basis for the indirect methods which are utilized for the *in vivo* estimation of body composition.

Typically, the indirect methods have employed a two compartment model. Body weight is partitioned into a fat and fat-free component. One component is measured directly and the other is determined by subtraction. Body density assessment procedures predict the fat weight and subtract this weight from the total body weight to estimate the fat-free weight (FFW). Unfortunately, the limitations inherent in the utilization of the assessment procedures are frequently disregarded. The resulting overestimations or underestimations of fat weight can in turn detract from the examination of relationships between physical activity and body composition. Studies on children are particularly illustrative of this point. Wilmore and McNamara (1974) have reported that hydrostatic weighing frequently results in estimated percent fat values for boys 8-12 years of age that would appear to be an overestimation of actual values on the basis of comparison with visual inspection and skinfold data. Similarly, when underwater weighing young wrestlers we have also begun using Tanner stages to identify maturational level (Tanner, 1962). For those wrestlers in the beginning stages of maturation (Tanner 2 or less), the resultant percent fat estimations are typically over 20%, in spite of a very "lean" physical appearance for many of the young wrestlers.

These apparent overestimations of the fat weight in children are thought to be due to the fact that children do not possess the same bone density and total body water content as do adults. Consequently, the true density of the fat-free component of their body weight is less than the fat-free density assumed in the equation which estimates fat from whole body density (Wilmore, 1983a).

Because a number of different procedures have been employed to predict body composition, the remainder of this section will briefly examine these procedures. A synopsis of the underlying assumptions and potential limitations for a given procedure will also be presented.

Body Density Assessment

Body density (mass/unit volume) is determined by hydrostatic weighing, or air, helium, or water displacement. Of these, hydrostatic weighing is the more widely used method. Archimedes' principle is utilized to measure body density, then this density determination must be converted to a percent fat value. The two most frequently used formulae are:

1. % Fat $= \left(\dfrac{4.570}{\text{density}}\right) - 4.142$ (Brozek, Grande, Anderson and Keys, 1963)

2. % Fat $= \left(\dfrac{4.950}{\text{density}}\right) - 4.500$ (Siri, 1956)

Both of these fomulae are predicated upon assumptions made about adults. They assume that the densities of fat (0.09 gm/cc) and the fat (1.10 gm/cc) weight are known and constant between individuals. They further assume that the density of the individual tissues of the fat-free component, for example, bone and muscle, are constant within an individual so that the proportional contribution to the density of the fat-free component remains constant. A final assumption is that all adults are identical in composition except for variability in the quantity of fat weight (Wilmore, 1983a).

The density of human body fat is relatively constant within and between individuals despite variability of age, sex, or location within the body. The density of the fat-free or lean component is much more variable. As children mature, the mineral content of their bones increases, thus altering the density of their bones, conversely, as we age, bone mineral content is lost and so older populations will have lower bone densities than younger groups of adults. Recent cadaver studies have confirmed that there is considerable variability in both the densities and proportions of the lean tisues for adults of similar ages.

Gamma Ray Spectrometry

Most of the potassium which is present in the body is in the cells, particularly the muscle cells (Forbes & Lewis, 1956; Forbes, Gallup and Hursh, 1961). About 0.012% of the potassium in man is in the form of K40, a naturally occurring radioisotope (Behnke & Wilmore, 1974). Thus, the concentration of K40 in the body may be measured via a gamma ray detector. By assuming that there is a constant proportion of potassium in the FFW, the FFW may be predicted. In actuality, three different formulae are utilized, because potassium content varies with gender and age. There are separate formulae for males over 18 years of age, females over 18 years of age and children under 13 years of age (Malina, 1980).

Because it is not known when adult concentrations of potassium in lean tissue are attained and gamma ray spectrometry predicts only the muscle mass, care should be taken in interpretating the results of studies which measure K40 concentrations (Malina, 1980).

Total Body Water Determinations

A number of different procedures have been developed to measure total body water (Behnke & Wilmore, 1974; Lukaski and Johnson, 1985). The prediction of body composition is made by assuming that about 72 to 73% of the FFW in normally hydrated individuals is water.

There is, however, considerable debate as to what the actual percentage of the FFW is water (Presta et al., 1983). It is not clear when adult hydration of the lean tissues is attained. There is also a systematic loss of hydration associated with aging. In addition, these total body water techniques are difficult to administer and so their use in the exercise literature is limited.

Anthropometric Estimates of FFW and Fat

The need for field procedures to assess body composition has prompted the development of anthropometric methods for estimating body composition.

Brozek and Keys (1951) were the first to publish regression equations for the estimation of body density from anthropometric measurements. Since that time numerous other prediction equations have become available. Some of these equations utilize skinfold measurements to predict body density, while others involve a series of skeletal widths, limb lengths, and or limb circumferences. The large number of available equations reflects population specificity—that is, an equation is specific to the population from which it was derived.

Many of these original equations used a linear regression model, while more recent research suggests that the data are curvi-linear—small skinfold thicknesses are associated with relatively small fat percentages, while larger skinfolds are associated with disproportionately larger fat percentages (Durnin & Wormersley, 1974). Studies by Jackson and Pollock (1978) and Jackson, Pollock, and Ward (1980) have employed quadratic regression analysis, resulting in generalized equations that are independent of age and body composition.

Most of these anthropometric equations use body density determinations as the criterion measure for the development of the prediction equations. Inaccuracies in the underlying assumptions relative to the population being studied would also detract from the accuracy of the resultant prediction equations.

Even if anthropometric prediction equations are appropriate for assessing body composition prior to the initiation of an activity program, they may not be appropriate for evaluating changes in the total fat content of the body. Moody, Wilmore, and Girandolo (1972) as well and Zuti and Golding (1976) have noted that decreases in skinfolds do not parallel alterations in body density as determined by hydrostatic weighing. Sinning (1974), however, has reported success in using skinfold predictions to evaluate body composition changes for wrestlers during their season. Obviously, there is a need for more information about the influence of exercise on the internal, as well as the subcutaneous, fat for individuals of varying initial fat levels.

Overview of Body Composition Measurement

It has become increasingly evident that the laboratory techniques that have been utilized for measuring body density are not appropriate for all segments of the population (Lohman, 1981). Any examination of the existing literature on the effects of exercise on body composition needs to consider the body composition techniques employed and any possible violations of the assumptions for that particular technique.

The limitations of a two component model (Lohman, 1983) are also becoming obvious; consequently, some investigators have opted for three or four component models for body weight (Sjostrom, 1980). This will require the application of more and more sophisticated measurement procedures. The utilization of techniques and procedures such as ultrasound (Volz & Ostrove, 1984) and computed tomography (Borkan et al., 1982) to examine changes or alterations in tissues in specific regions of the body should also enhance our future understanding of body composition and provide additional information relative to the influence of physical activity on body composition.

In spite of previous limitations in techniques, considerable knowledge about the impact of activity on body composition is available.

The Growth Years

Identifying the influence of regular physical activity on the body composition of children and adolescents is very difficult because body composition, as well as height and weight, change as growth and maturation occur (for a detailed account of these growth related changes see chapter 1, by R. Malina). This normal interaction between growth, maturation, and alterations in body composition complicates the task of differentiating between the effects of these growth related changes.

The research examining the influence of physical activity on the developing body composition of rats and other animals is much more extensive than the available studies on growing children (Wilmore, 1983b). While it is possible to use animals and design studies which rigorously control dietary intake, activity frequency, intensity and duration, such control is just not possible nor ethical with human subjects. Consequently, a variety of different approaches have been conceived to examine the association between physical activity and body composition in growing children.

Body Composition and Activity

A typical strategy has been to compare activity level at the time of the study with the child's current body composition. This approach has yielded inconsistent results across studies (Forbes, 1978). Some have reported that leaner children are more active (Forbes, 1975; Abraham & Nordsieck, 1971). Others have not observed a significant relationship (Johnson, Burke, and Mayer, 1956). Even in those studies where there appeared to be a relationship between fatness and lack of activity, it is unclear whether the lack of activity is a cause or an effect of the fatness (Leighton, Shapiro, Crawford, and Huenemann, 1981).

In order to address this issue, Leighton et al. (1981) modified the simple cross-sectional design and utilized longitudinal activity records to determine past and present activity patterns and their relation to current body composition parameters. Their subjects were all within a month of 8.75 years of age, minimizing the heterogeneity of developmental levels which confounds many studies of children. For the girls in this study, there was no relationship between current percent fat and past activity indicators. However, there were small but significant relationships between fatness and past activity for the boys. Leighton's group also noted that the fatter children at one age were not necessarily the fatter children at another age. Seemingly, the development of relative leaness/fatness is a gradual process and fatness may be more related to past activity levels than current activity.

Most studies, however, have not viewed activity patterns over an extended time period. Brownell and Kaye (1982) designed a program for obese children. As a result of participating in a 10-week school-based behavior modification, nutrition education, and physical activity program, 95% of the children lost fat weight and reversed the steady weight gain pattern which they had demonstrated in the three years before the intervention period. The children in the control group continued to gain weight, leading Brownell and Kaye to conclude that increased physical activity, nutritional information, and psychological support can decrease the degree of fatness in overweight children. They further noted that participation in non-competitive activities, rather than competitive physical activities, was important for the weight loss process. Other researchers (Coates and Thoresen, 1978; Epstein, Wing, Steranchak, Dickson, and Michelson, 1980) have also reported that behavior modification, nutrition education, and increased physical activity can interact to decrease obesity in clinical settings. But the long-term efficacy of such programs on the body compositon of obese children has not been established.

Trained vs. Untrained

The long-term effects of physical activity on the body composition of normal weight children and adolescents is poorly documented, but several investigators have evaluated the body composition of various groups of young athletes. Comparing the body composition and somatotype characteristics of Junior Olympic athletes with similar aged but non-athletic peers, Thorland et al. (1981) reported that all of the male Junior Olympians, with the exception of the throwers, had lower percent fat values than their non-athlete peers. Comparisons for the female athletes revealed that except for the gymnasts, they had higher lean body masses than their non-athlete peers. Only the female throwers approached the percent fat values characteristic of the non-athletic girl.

Several investigators (Katch and Michael, 1971; Parizkova, 1977) have observed that young athletes tend to have less body fat than their non-athlete counterparts. It is possible, however, that the relative leaness of young athletes is a reflection of selection rather than the specific result of training. Davies, Barnes, and Godfrey (1972) have demonstrated that maximal exercise performance in children is related to the amount of muscle which can be brought into use. Consequently, those young performers who have relatively lower fat weights should have higher performance potentials. Although longitudinal studies, with appropriate control subjects, are needed to discern the relative contribution of training and genetics to the body composition of young athletes (Malina, 1983), there are some data to suggest that regular physical activity does influence the body composition of normal weight children.

Parizkova (1977) followed boys engaging in three different levels of physical training over a seven year period. Initially all of the boys had similar anthropometric characteristics and relative leaness/fatness. During the study one group trained regularly for six intensive hours per week. Another group trained, but not on a regular basis (particpated in school sports for about four hours of organized exercise per week). The third group was considered to be untrained because they particpated in only 2.5 hours of activity per week including school physical education. As the study progressed, the high intensity training group was observed to have significantly more lean body mass and less fat than either of the other two groups of boys.

In another longitudinal study extending over 30 months, Parizkova (1977) evaluated the effect of different intensities of physical training on skinfold thicknesses of girls ages 14 and 15 years. Physical inactivity was associated with increased skinfold thicknesses, but these skinfolds were reduced when physical training was introduced. Furthermore, the greatest reductions in skinfold thickness were noted during the most intense training periods and changes in skinfold thicknesses paralleled changes in body density measurements. Caloric intake decreased during the periods of decreased training or physical inactivity, so the increases in fat deposition during lower activity periods cannot be entirely attributed to imbalances in caloric intake and expenditure. Rather, adaptions to physical training seem to evoke metabolic alterations which facilitate the utilization of free fatty acids and minimize the deposition of fat (Oscai, 1973).

Socio-psychological Development

In addition to demonstrating that physical activity can decrease the relative fatness during the growth years, research also suggests that excessive body fat detracts from the performance capacities and overall fitness of children. Since the participation in and the mastery of movement behaviors is perhaps the child's most prominent means of self expression (Singer, 1973), any factor which detracts from performance potentials should be viewed as a negative factor relative to a child's development. The psychological and sociological stigmas of moderate obesity may well be as destructive as the physiological ramifications (Brownell, 1982).

Summary

Physical activity can have a profound effect on the body composition during the growth years. Both boys and girls who engage in regular physical activity tend to have less body fat than their more sedentary peers. This relative leanness is related to the duration and intensity of the training. Less body fat is deposited during periods of intense training due to the increased caloric expenditure and metabolic adaptations which favor the utilization of free fatty acids. Genetics is also an important variable which facilitates the establishment of the low body fats achieved by some athletes.

The life-long impact of regular physical activity during the growth years is yet to be determined, but the reversibility of skinfold thicknesses with fluctuations in the training intensities of children indicates that the impact of exercise on fat deposition is dependent upon continual participation. The life-long impact of regular physical activity on lean body mass is also unknown. While some physically active children do have greater lean body masses than non-active children, it is not known whether these differences carry over into adulthood. Furthermore, the indirect body composition techniques currently utilized are based on models derived from adults and may not accurately portray the absolute magnitude of a child's lean body mass. Also, the two compartment model of body composition does not allow for the evaluation of changes in the various lean tissues, that is, muscle mass and bone mass. Considerably more research will be necessary to futher elucidate the effect of regular physical activity on body composition during the growth years.

Adults

Athletes vs. Non-athletes

One of the most striking physical differences between athletes and sedentary adults is the difference in fat weight. Although there is considerable variability in body composition among the different types of athletes, generally speaking athletes have lower fat percentages than do non-athletes (Upton, Hagan, Rosentswieg, & Gettman, 1983). Athletes must move their body mass quickly and efficiently to be successful in most sports, consequently, it is becoming increasingly evident that there is an optimal or desirable body composition for various groups of athletes (for a comprehensive summary of body composition values for both male and female athletes see Wilmore, 1982).

Generally speaking, differences in lean body mass between athletes and non-athletes does not appear to be as consistent as are the differences in fat percentages. Upton and associates (1983) compared the lean body masses of middle-aged women distance runners and sendentary women and observed that both groups of women had similar lean body masses. The sedentary women were heavier than the runners, but the extra weight was fat weight. On the other hand, Katch, Katch, and Behnke (1980) have reported that female athletes who participate in certain types of sports will have low fat weights and greater than average lean body masses. Similar observations have been made on female athletes. Male runners tend to have low fat weights and more normal lean body weights for their stature, while many football players have lean body masses which are considerably larger than the typical male (Wilmore and Haskell, 1972).

Certainly, these types of cross-sectional studies support the premise that participation in the physical activity required in training for sports can help to decrease fat stores; however, it is still possible that genetics plays a role. Perhaps those individuals whose genetic make-up allows them to achieve low fat weights have a performance advantage and are more likely to become successful athletes. Longitudinal studies are needed to resolve this issue. Such longitudinal studies are also necessary to determine if chronic physical activity can result in greater than normal increases in the various components of the fat free weight. Certainly, an increased muscle mass may be important for the development of certain sport skills, but implications for health and physical well-being may be even more compelling.

For example, one of the important determinants of daily caloric expenditure is the muscle mass (Webb, 1981). If exercise can be used to increase muscle mass in early adulthood and prevent some of the lean tissue losses typically associated with aging, perhaps the onset of obesity in adults could be curtailed.

Bone, as well as muscle mass, seems to respond to certain types of physical activty by increasing its density and thus the total bone mass (Oyster, Morton and Linnell, 1984). Although bone metabolism does not influence metabolic rate as greatly as does muscle mass, an increased bone density could be a significant deterent to age-related osteoporosis, particularly in women (Brewer, Meyer, Keele, Upton and Hagan, 1983). Skeletal fracture associated with osteoporosis is a serious and costly health problem, and so the preliminary research on the utilization of diet and exercise as a preventive strategy is promising (Avioli, 1983).

In spite of the potential for the mechanical stresses associated with exercise to prevent the reabsorption of bone, there is some concern that certain types or intensities of physical activity may interact with other factors and have a negative impact on bone density. More specifically Lindberg, et al. (1984) have documented that young, female distance runners who are amenorrheic have lower bone densities than their more sedentary, eumenorrheic peers. The mechanism for the reduced bone mass is thought to be attributed to estrogen deficiencies associated with the amenorrhea. However, the observation that amenorrheic rowers do not seem to have a reduced bone mass suggests that mechanical stresses other than just weight-bearing may be able to offset depressed estrogen levels (Drinkwater, et al., 1984). Certainly the role of dietary calcium and protein and exercise also warrants research. Longitudinal studies which compare men and women involved in varying intensities of training with their sendentary counterparts would be the ideal way to examine the influence of activity on components of the lean body mass.

In spite of the paucity of long term studies, there are numerous short term studies which examine the effects of various types of exercise on body weight and body composition in adults. The preponderance of this literature is limited to examining alterations in the relative contribution of fat to the body weight. The results of this research indicate that adults who participate in regular physical activity can expect to lose fat weight, but there is a great deal of variety in the specific reports. Moody (1972) reported that the mean percent fat for a group of young women decreased from 38.6% to 28.5% as a result of a walking-jogging program. Conversely, in following a group of men 28 to 39 years of age, Pollack, Cureton, and Greninger (1969) noted that after 20 weeks of a walk-jog program the percent fat values went from 18.0 to 18.9%. Upon reviewing 55 exercise and weight control studies, Wilmore (1983a) concluded that exercise training results in moderate losses in total body weight, moderate to large losses in body fat, and small to moderate increases in lean body mass.

Duration, Intensity, and Frequency

There are a number of factors contributing to the disparity in the results of these studies. According to Moody (1972), a minimum of 30 minutes of continuous activity is necessary for an exercise program to be efficacious with respect to weight control. The intensity of the activity is also important. If the exercise is too intense, the utilization of free fatty acids is limited and muscular fatique is likely to terminate the exercise session before a significant degree of fat lipolysis has taken place (Katch and McArdle, 1977). Optimal stimulation of lipolysis is a function of the duration of the training program, as well as the exercise intensity. In asessing the effect of physical fitness on adipocyte lipolysis, Despres et al. (1984b) observed that basal lipolysis and epinephrine-stimualted lipolysis are significantly higher in trained subjects than sedentary subjects. More specifically, the subjects who were trained marathon runners demonstrated basal lipolysis similar to the subjects who had been in a vigorous 4-month fitness program; however, the 4-month training group did have a greater epinepherine-stimulated lipolysis than the marathon group. Others have shown that there is an increase in fat mobilization and an increase in the oxidation of fat by muscles during exercise in trained subjects (Evans, Bennett, Costill, & Fink, 1979). These metabolic adaptations are thought to help spare glycogen stores and increase endurance. They are also fundamental to the utilization of exercise as a strategy for controlling fat weight by metabolising the free fatty acids associated with increased atherosclerotic risk (Sutherland, Woodhouse , and Heyworth, 1981). It is also encouraging that four months of aerobic training appears to be sufficient to induce maximal adaptation of epinephrine-stimulated lipolysis in male subjects (Despres et al., 1984b).

Gender of Subjects

It was necessary to stipulate the gender of the subjects in the preceeding sentence because some researchers have suggested that gender influences some of the metabolic adaptations induced in lipocytes by exercise. Despres et al. (1984a) have reported that fat cells in women are less sensitive to training adaptations than the fat cells in men. Upon particpating in comparable exercise programs, there were significant differences in fat morphology between groups of male and female subjects. While the men lowered their adiposity, the women did not. Furthermore, the women experienced only a 46% increase in epinephrine-stimulated lipolysis as compared to a 66% increase in men. The gender difference in responsiveness to epinephrine-stimulated lipolysis seems to suggest that the training stimulus required to induce a significant weight loss in women is greater than in men.

The mechanism for this difference in training-induced weight loss is not known, but recent data suggest that the gonadal steroids may be involved in the explanation. Wade and Gray (1979) have hypothesized that the gonadal steroids have a role in the control of food intake and fat deposition. Others have suggested that these hormones may be involved in the regulation of lipolysis, lipogenesis, and adipose-tissue lipoprotein lipase activity (Kim and Kalkhoff, 1975).

Genetics

It is also possible that heredity influences training-induced adaptations of the adipocytes. Several studies have documented the genetic component in body fatness with their high parent-child and sib-sib correlations for body fatness (Osborne and deGeorge, 1959; Brook, Huntley, and Slack, 1975). Furthermore, these researchers have noted that biological relatives exhibit similar degrees of fatness when there is statistical control over food consumption, caloric expenditure, and socioeconomic indicators (Bouchard et al., 1982). The results of Despres et al. (1983) are also in accordance with the overall theme that there is a genetic basis to adipocyte adaptations to exercise. Following the training of 15 pairs of monozygotic twins, they note that the magnitude of increase in stimulated adipose tissue lipolysis over pretraining values was quite similar within twin pairs, but differed markedly between pairs. Certainly more work is needed to clarify the mechanisms and the locus of this genetic-training interaction phenomenon.

Age and Initial Fat Percentage

Age and initial fat levels are two other factors which seem to influence the variability of outcome in exercise and weight control studies. White and Young (1978), in a study which compared the effects of a 12-week exercise program on body composition variables in nonobese young and middle-age females, noted that the younger group (21-32 years of age) did not change significantly on any of the skinfolds or their predicted percent body fat. In contrast, the middle-aged group experienced a significant increase in body density due to a significant decrease in their supra-iliac skinfold thickness. While not obese, the older group had a relatively higher initial fat percentage than the younger group.

Similarly, the subjects of Franklin et al. (1979) did not differ in age, but one group was obese (over 30% fat) and the other group of women were lean to normal. Following a 12-week (4 days/week) physical conditioning program, body weights remained unchanged for the normal group while the obese group lost weight. Both groups experienced a significant decrease in skinfold thicknesses, but with a greater reduction in the obese group. Fatness decreased slightly in the normal group and substantially more in the obese group, while fat free weight remained unchanged for both groups. Bjorntorp (1980) speculates that the magnitude of the weight loss due to physical training is dependent upon the potential of adipose tissue to decrease to a specific fat cell size. In other words, individuals with large fat cells have the potential for more fat loss than do individuals with a large number of fat cells.

Thermic Effects

It is also possible that such factors as age and relative fatness may interact with the thermic effect of food and exercise, influencing the fat metabolism responses of subjects to exercise (Segal and Gutin, 1983). Impaired thermogenesis, which is a decreased ability to dissipate heat by varying the metabolic rate, has been proposed as a possible physiological mechanism underlying the etiology, persistence, and proneness to obesity (James and Trayhurn, 1981; Jung, Shetty, and James, 1979).

Typically, thermogenic responses are stimulated by specific stimuli, such as changes in ambient temperature, the acute ingestion of food, chronic overfeeding, physical exercise, certain hormones, or a combination of these factors. Upon comparing the thermogenic responses of 10 lean and 10 moderately obese women to food, exercise, and food plus exercise, Segal and Gutin (1983) observed that exercise potentiates the thermic effect of the food for the lean women but not for the obese women. This reduced response to the combined stimulus of food plus exercise may constitute a subtle metabolic factor contributing to obesity.

In addition, dynamic interactions between dietary intake and exercise may account for some of the disparity in results in the weight control literature (Apfelbaum, Bostsarron, and Lacatis, 1971). If subjects were to alter their caloric intake, the pattern of their eating throughout the day, or even the relative composition of the calories they consume, these factors might influence the thermogenic responses of the subject and thwart or potentiate the fat mobilization processes. It is known that very active persons eat more food than their sedentary counterparts (Medical News, 1983; Baecke, Van Stavern, and Burema, 1983). If obese, beginning exercises were to decrease their energy intake, some of the thermic effect of the exercise may be negated. Another factor influencing the relatively poor weight losses that are sometimes experienced by beginning exercisers trying to lose weight might be the fact that exercise increases muscle glycogen stores. Perhaps the exercise-induced increases in muscle glycogen may have negated the expected weight loss during an exercise program (Warwick and Garrow, 1981).

Assessment Procedures

Still another variable which deserves some attention relative to the interpretation of exercise and body composition studies is the body composition evaluation procedure itself. Body weight alone is not sensitive to changes in composition, and even some of the indirect measures of body composition may not be sensitive to shifts in muscle glycogen or changes in the density of the various lean tissues themselves. For example, Zuti and Golding (1976) have reported that skinfold changes associated with weight loss do not parallel changes in body density as determined by hydrostatic weighing. Furthermore, researchers (Oyster et al., 1984; Brewer, Meyer, Keele, Upton and Hagan, 1983) who have studied the effects of physical activity upon aged individuals have noted that bone density changes may be induced with physical activity. Since most existing body composition prediction procedures assume a constant lean tissue density, the resultant body density predictions may not accurately reflect actual body composition changes.

Spot Reduction

Total body composition predictions all fail to provide information about alterations in specific fat deposits. The public has long believed that the fat deposits in the immediate areas of an exercising muscle will diminish in size if those specific muscles are used in calisthenics and other strengthening activities. This concept has been referred to as spot reduction and is of considerable interest, paticularly to women who are dissatisfied with their fat distribution rather than the total content of their fat. Shade, Hellebrandt, Waterland and Carns (1962) and Gwinup, Chelvam, and Steinberg (1971) have refuted the concept of spot reduction; however, there are contradictory results in the literature. Simko, Merrifield, and Stouffer (1974) had 11 female college students complete a regimen of isometric and isokinetic exercises with the knee-extensors and the knee flexors. After 9 weeks of exercise they reported that the skinfolds over the exercising thigh muscles decreased significantly, but there were no changes in skinfold thicknesses at four other sites. The control group of five women did not experience changes in any of their skinfold thicknesses, leading the researchers to speculate that the fatty acids required for the metabolism of exercising muscle may originate from the fat deposit nearest to the muscles. Since adipocyte lipolysis is mediated by hormonal action it is difficult to explain why the fat deposit closest to the working muscle would be the most likely source for lipolysis. Krothiewski et al. (1979) proposed a plausible alternative hypothesis. As a result of having 10 middle age women participate in a five-week program of one-leg exercise, a decrease in the subcutaneous tissue in the exercising leg as measured by ultrasound and skinfold calipers was noted. This decrease in the thickness of the subcutaneous fat was not associated with a significant decrease in fat cell size and there was no decrease in the subcutaneous fat in the nonexercising leg. Also, muscle size increased in only the exercising leg, leading these researchers to hypothesize that the decreased fat thickness was due to geometircal factors secondary to hypertrophy of the underlying muscle rather than local emptying of the fat deposit over the exercising muscle.

Summary

Certainly, developing research technologies such as ultrasound should further enhance our understanding of underlying physiological and biophysical mechanisms involved in responses to chronic physical activity. Such information will be valuable in structuring physical activity experiences to enable adults to better achieve muscle masses, bone masses and fat weights that are associated with optimal health. Although much research will be required before the full potential of physical activity is realized, the existing research literature supports the premise that appropriate physical activities can and do have a positive influence on body composition. More specifically, for optimal weight loss (Franklin, 1984b; ACSM, 1979), exercise training should be of a moderate intensity (e.g. 60-70% of maximal heart rate) and long duration (at least 30 minutes). During this type of mild-to-moderate intensity aerobic exercise, blood lactate remains low, allowing individuals to utilize free fatty acids as a fuel source and to prolong the duration of the activity. This exercise intensity also helps to prevent orthopedic traumas which are more prevalent with high intensity, anaerobic exercise, particularly if it is weight bearing. In addition, the exercise program should be performed for a minimum of three days per week for at least three months (Bjorntorp, 1978).

The preferred types of physical activity for fat loss employ large muscle groups, are performed continuously, and are rhythmical and aerobic in nature, such as jogging, running, bicycling, cross country skiing, and swimming. Sustained compliance and not the mode of activity is the important factor in programs designed to reduce body fat. In addition, systematically increasing the physical activity component in daily living (walking up more stairs, etc.) is advantageous.

Although anaerobic activities, with their increased lactic acid levels, do not appear to be as effective as aerobic exercise in weight reduction program (Girandola, 1976), select anaerobic activities (e.g., weight lifting and other resistive exercises) may effect increases in lean body mass, resulting in increased resting metabolic rates and promote muscle tone, thereby reducing girth measures.

Unfortunately, there is a paucity of longitudinal research examining the effects of exercise on body composition in adults. Compliance in those long term projects is also discouraging. But the potential for exercise as an important determinant of body composition in the adult should stimulate renewed efforts at designing improved motivational strategies (Franklin, 1984b) and the application of technology to further our understanding of exercise-body composition interactions.

Exercise in the Treatment of Obesity

Obesity has become a serious health problem in the United States. In a northern Manhattan study of more than 700 youngsters three to five years of age, the incidence of obesity was over 13% (Ginsberg-Fellner and Carmel, 1974). It has been estimated that nearly 12% of prepubertal children and 16% of adolescents are obese. While clearly identifiable physical problems are rarely present in the pediatric age group, the dangers of obesity increase with age (Hammer, 1975). Generally speaking, men and women with excessive amounts of fat weight have an increased likelihood of dying at a younger age than people with more normal fat weights (Lucas, 1984). More specifically, obesity has been related to non-insulin dependent diabetes, hyperlipideamia, hypertension, surgical risk, renal problems, degenerative joint disease, and complications during pregnancy. Consequently, weight reduction is frequently prescribed as part of the medical treatment for many cardiorespiratory, metabolic, and musculo-skeletal conditions (Franklin and Rubenfire, 1980).

In the past, the basis of these weight reduction prescriptions has been the restriction of caloric intake. Certainly, if one applies the law of conservation of energy to the body's metabolism, body weight is the end result of energy consumption versus energy expenditure. Unfortunately, this simple expression of the energy balance equation does not consider the myriad of factors which influence the transfer of energy within the body. While it is true that some obese persons eat significantly more than lean individuals, studies have verified that many obese people eat less than their leaner counterparts (Kannel and Corgon, 1975). It has also been documented that metabolic rates decrease, by as much as 25% in two weeks, with restrictions in caloric consumption (Thompson, Jarvie, Lahey, and Cureton, 1982). These factors, along with psychological and social factors, probably account for the poor record of obesity treatments which rely chiefly on caloric restriction, with long term success being achieved in as few as 5% and probably no more than 20% of all cases (MacKeen, Franklin, Nicholas, and Buskirk, 1983).

While there are also difficulties in effecting long-term compliance with exercise programs, the introduction of regular physical activity into the treatment of obesity has some unique advantages. There are numerous physical and psychological adaptations to regular exercise, including changes in the circulatory and muscular systems which have been presented in chapters 5, 8, 10 and 11. In addition, regular physical activity seems to hold particular promise as a strategy for the treatment of obesity because exercise may (a) increase energy expenditure, (b) suppress appetite, (c) increase basal metabolism, (d) stimulate fat loss, and (e) minimize loss of lean tissue (Brownell, 1982; Thompson et al., 1982). There are some data to substantiate the theory that exercise leads to appetite suppression and a decreased caloric intake in the obese. However, other researchers have not found this to be the case. In one study, 14 middle-aged men participated in a running program for two years. No specific instructions about dieting were given to these subjects, and in fact, during the course of the first six months of the study they actually increased their caloric consumption. In addition to increasing their daily caloric intake by about 15% these runners also increased their consumption of carbohydrates from 230 grams/day to 304 grams/day. In spite of consuming more calories than usual, these runners were also becoming leaner. Their body fat dropped from an initial value of 21.6% to 20% at six months and to 18% at two years. Although these subjects were running an average of 12 miles a week, this exercise alone is not sufficient to account for the total fat loss that was experienced (Medical News, 1983).

Unfortunately, exercise critics totally disregard reports of this nature. Instead, they discount the impact that physical activity can make upon weight control by pointing out that it takes 36 hours of walking to expend enough calories to utilize a pound of fat. It is, however, inappropriate to imply that the impact of exercise on weight control depends on a single bout of exercise. Rather, the calorie-expending effects of exercise are cumulative. If the 36 hours of walking is divided into a 30 minute period each day, this would account for approximately five pounds of fat per year. Because extra fat pounds are typically acquired over a period of months, it is unrealistic to expect that they be lost rapidly.

The potential for the impact of exercise on the body's fat stores is even more profound, given the post-exercise metabolic rate or thermic effect of exercise (Newsholme, 1980). In other words, as a result of exercising, the body's metabolism is elevated and remains elevated for up to six hours following the activty bout. This elevation in metabolism can account for about 50 to 60 extra calories. Over the course of several weeks of regular physical activity this increased rate of expenditure would be cumulative. Moderate exercise has also been shown to potentiate the thermic effect of food, providing still another mechanism for increased energy expenditure (Segal and Gutin, 1983). Finally, if resistive exercise is utilized to increase the body's muscle mass, this would increase daily energy expenditure because energy expenditure has been found to vary with the fat-free mass (Webb, 1981). These exercise-related influences on energy expenditure contrast sharply with the effects of caloric restriction on energy expenditure. Caloric restriction results in a 15% to 30% decrease in basal metabolic rate in both lean and obese subjects (Thompson et al., 1982). Decreases in BMR can reach 20% in as little as two weeks and are measureable within 48 hours of initiation of caloric restriction. Conceivably, this increase in metabolic efficiency is a protective mechanism, but it serves to thwart weight loss. Furthermore, repeated episodes of dieting or caloric restriction may result in ever increasing body fat percentages, because the metabolic rate returns to normal more slowly than the dieter's eating habits. Consequently "extra" calories are stored as fat. There is some evidence that exercise can help offset or counteract the tendency for a decrease in metabolic rate which usually accompanies caloric restriction (Thompson et al., 1982). Weight loss, achieved through dieting alone, is approximately 75% fat and 25% lean tissue. When diet and exercise are combined, the loss of lean tissues decreases to approximately 5% (Bray, 1980), and if exercise alone is used to achieve the weight loss there can actually be an increase in lean body mass (Zuti and Golding, 1976). Exercise will not, however, prevent the loss of lean tissue if the diet is a very low calorie diet (Krotkiewski, Toss, Bjorntorp and Holm, 1981).

The conservation of lean tissue, when caloric intake is adequate and exercise is employed in the weight control strategy, may well be due to increased fatty acid mobilization and utilization during and after exercie (Rodahl, Miller and Issekutz, 1964), which is mediated in part by the lypolytic effects of increased catecholamine and growth hormone secretion (Havel, 1971) and diminished concentration of serum insulin (Hunter and Sukkar, 1968). These and other exercise-induced metabolic alterations provide further justification for the role of exercise in the treatment of obesity. In fact, some metabolic changes occur with physical training even it there is only a moderate degree of fat loss. Many such metabolic changes are associated with a reduction in risk for specific health problems. For example, weight loss is known to reduce plasma insulin levels and improve glucose tolerance, thereby reducing the risk of type II diabetes. Consequently, Bjorntorp et al. (1970) report that when hyperplastic obese subjects were trained without losing fat, there was also a decrease in plasma insulin. The mechanisms for exercise-mediated reduction in serum insulin are unknown. However, Holm, Bjorntorp and Jagenburg (1978) have speculated that the acute effects of exercise on insulin secretion might eventually produce increased insulin sensitivity in muscle and other cells.

Regular physical activity is also associated with substantial decreases in serum triglycerides (Bjorntorp, 1976). More recently, Williams et al. (1983) have suggested that the metabolic consequences of exercise-induced weight change relative to plasma high density lipoproteins are different from the consequences of weight change in the sedentary state. According to their results, the weight change that was induced with increased physical activity was associated with increases in the HDL/C concentration that were predominantly due to increases in the reputedly anti-atherogenic HDL2 sub-component. Of even greater interest is the observation that these positive changes occurred in spite of only small weight losses ($X = 1.5$ kg).

Participation in regular exercise can promote an enhanced sense of well-being and increases the body's ability to handle physical and emotional stressors (Heinzelmann and Bagley, 1970). Exercise has also been shown to enhance self-esteem and other psychological attributes. These outcomes are significant for the treatment of obesity because the psychological and social hazards of obesity may be as serious as the medical hazards. There is a very strong bias against obese individuals. In fact, Brownell (1982) considers obesity to be a social disability. Obese people suffer from the stigma of their obesity and they are also blamed for their condition. Consequently, obese persons are characterized with labels such as lazy, weak, and self-destructive; with the implication being that if they had stronger character, they would not be obese. It is not surprising that many obese people detest their bodies and are preoccupied with weight (Stunkard, 1976).

Summary

Conceivably, participation in regular physical activity has the potential to ameliorate many psychological problems and help obese individuals develop more positive attitudes and behaviors. In addition, physical training seems to be able to favorably influence metabolism and thereby moderate certain health risk factors. Finally, because of its direct and indirect impact on caloric expenditure, exercise has the potential to help the obese individual lose fat weight and gain or at least spare lean tissues. In spite of this impressive theoretical basis for the utilization of exercise as a treatment strategy for obesity, the rate of long term compliance of obese individuals with regular exercise regimens is discouraging. In a follow-up investigation to their short term study on the effects of exercise on body composition, Mackeen et al. (1983) were disappointed to find that the majority of the middle-aged women in the study had regressed to their pre-exercising body weight and fatness when left on their own. Others have been equally discouraged with the long term compliance with physical training programs. This underscores the importance of integrating motivational strategies into any exercise program and emphasizes the relevance of preventing obesity, rather than treating obesity.

Since lifelong behavioral patterns are formed during childhood and children spend the majority of their waking hours in school-related activities, well conceived educational and motivational school-based programs which promote participation in regular physical activity seem to be the most feasible way of preventing obesity.

Summary

Insight into the influence of regular physical activity on body composition has long intrigued humankind. However, there have been a number of technical difficulties which have stymied our curiosity. Although a number of research investigations have been conducted to ascertain the influence of exercise on body composition, our body composition tools still pose major limitations. While addressing this issue, Tim Lohman (1983) said that, "We measure what we can, not what we should." He was referring to the limitations of the two component model of body weight. We should be evaluating the influence of physical activity on the individual lean tissues, rather than just the lean tissue mass. We also must be able to determine if exercise can alter the densities of specific tissues. Finally, there is a need to develop tools and procedures that are appropriate for evaluating the body composition of children and older adults whose bone densities and total body water are different from those of young adults.

References

Abraham, S. & Nordsieck, M. (1971). Relationship of excess weight in children and adults. *Public Health Report, 75,* 263-273.

American College of Sports Medicine. (1979). The recommended quantity and quality of exercise for developing and maintaining fitness in healthy adults. *Medicine and Science in Sport, 10,* 7-9.

Apfelbaum, M., Bostsarron, J., & Lacatis, D. (1971). Effect of caloric restriction and excessive caloric intake on energy expenditure. *American Journal of Clinical Nutrition, 24,* 1405-1409.

Avioli, L.V. (Ed.). (1983). *The Osteoporotic Syndrome: Detection, Prevention, and Treatment.* Orlando: Grune & Stratton, Inc.

Baecke, J.A.H., Van Staveren, W.A., & Burema, J. (1983). Food consumption, habitual physical activity, and body fatness in young Dutch adults. *American Journal of Clinical Nutrition, 37,* 278-286.

Behnke, A.R., & Wilmore, J.H. (1974). *Evaluation and Regulation of Body Build and Composition.* New Jersey: Prentice-Hall.

Bjorntorp, P. (1976). Exercise in the treatment of obesity. *Clinics in Endocriniology and Metabolism, 5,* 2-11.

Bjorntrop, P. (1978). Physical training in the treatment of obesity. *International Journal of Obesity, 3,* 261-279.

Bjorntrop, P. (1980). Physical training in the treatment of obesity. In G.A. Gray (Ed.), *Obesity: Comparative Methods of Weight Control* (pp. 51-58). Westport, CT: Technomic Publishing.

Bjorntorp, P., de Jounge, K., Sjostrom, L., & Sullivan, L. (1970). The effect of physical training on insulin production in obesity. *Metabolism, 19,* 631-640.

Borkan, G.A., Gerzof, S.G., Robbins, A.H., Hults, D.E., Silbert, C.K., & Silbert, S.E. (1982). Assessment of abdominal fat content by computed tomography. *American Journal of Clinical Nutrition, 36,* 172-177.

Bouchard, C., Savard, R., Despres, J.P., Tremblay, A., & Leblanc, C. (1982). Body fatness and lean body mass in unrelated and biological sibs. *Canadian Journal of Applied Sports Science, 7,* 244 (abstract).

Bray, G. (Ed.). (1980). *Obesity in America* (NIH Publication No. 80-359). Washington, DC: U.S. Government Printing Office.

Brewer, V., Meyer, B.M., Keele, M.S., Upton, S.J. & Hagan, R.D. (1983). Role of exercise in prevention of involutional bone loss. *Medicine and Science in Sport and Exercise, 15,* 445-449.

Brook, C.G.D., Huntley, R.M.C., & Slack, J. (1975). Influence of heredity and environment in determination of skinfold thickness in children. *British Medical Journal, 2,* 719-721.

Brownell, K.D. (1982). Obesity: Understanding and treating a serious, prevalent, and refractory disorder. *Journal of Consulting and Clinical Psychology, 50,* (6), 820-940.

Brownell, K.D., & Kaye, F.S. (1982). A school-based behavior modification, nutrition education, and physical activity program for obese children. *American Journal of Clinical Nutrition, 35,* 277-283.

Brozek, J. (1966). Body composition: models and estimation equations. *American Journal of Physical Anthropolgy, 24,* 239-250.

Brozek, J., Grande, F., Anderson, J.T., & Keyes, A. (1963). Densiotometric analysis of body composition: Revision of quantitative assumptions. *Annuals of New York Academy of Science, 110,* 113-140.

Brozek, J., & Keys, A. (1951). The evaluation of leanness-fatness in man: Norms and interrelationships. *British Journal of Nutrition, 5,* 194-206.

Coates, T.J., & Thoresen, C.. (1978). Treating obesity in children and adolescents: A review. *American Journal of Public Health, 68,* 143-151.

Davies, C.T.M., Barnes, C., & Godfrey, S. (1972). Body composition and maximal exercise performance in children. *Human Biology, 44,* 195-214.

Despres, J.P., Bouchard, C., Savard, R., Tremblay, A., Marcotte, M., & Theriault, G. (1984a). The effect of a 20-week endurance training program on adipose-tissue morphology and lipolysis in men and women. *Metabolism, 33,* 235-239.

Despres, J.P., Bouchard, C., Savard, R., Tremblay, A., Marcotte, M., & Theriault, G. (1984b). Level of physical fitness and adipocyte lipolysis in humans. *Journal of Applied Physiology, 56,* 1157-1161.

Despres, J.P., Bouchard, C., Savard, R. Prud'homme, D., Bukowiecki, L., & Theriault, G. (1983). Adaptive changes to training in adipose tissue lipolysis are genotype dependent. *International Journal of Obesity, 8,* 87-95.

Drinkwater, B.L., Nilson, K., Chesnut, C.H., Bremner, W.J., Shainholtz, S. and Southworth, M.B. (1984). Bone mineral content of amenorrheic and eumenorrheic athletes. *New England Journal of Medicine, 311,* 277-281.

Durnin, J.V., & Wormsley, J. (1974). Body fat assessed from total body density and its estimation from skinfold thickness: Measurements on 481 men and women aged 16 to 72 years. *British Journal of Nutrition, 32,* 77-79.

Epstein, L.H., Wing, R.R., Steranchak, L., Dickson, B., & Michelson, J. (1980). Comparison of family-based behavior modification and education for childhood obesity. *Journal of Pediatric Psychology, 5,* 25-36.

Evans, W.J., Bennett, A.S., Costill, D.L., & Fink, W.J. (1979). *Research Quarterly, 50,* 350-359.

Forbes, G.B (1975). Prevalence of obesity in childhood. In G.A. Bray (Ed.), *Obesity in Perspective,* DHEW Publication no. (NIH) 75-708. Washington, D.C.: US

Government Printing Office.

Forbes, G.B. (1978). Body composition in adolescence. In F. Falkner and J.M. Tanner (Eds.), *Human Growth Vol. 2: Postnatal Growth*. New York: Plenum Press.

Forbes, G.B., & Lewis, A.M. (1956). Total sodium, potassium and chloride in adult man. *Journal of Clinical Investigation, 35,* 596-600.

Forbes, G.L., Gallup, J., & Hursh, J.B. (1961). Estimation of total body fat from potassium 40 content. *Science, 113,* 101.

Franklin, B.A. (1984a). Exercise program compliance: Improvement strategies. In J. Storlie and H.. Jordan (Eds.), *Behavioral Management of Obesity* (pp. 105-136). New York: Spectrum Publications.

Franklin, B.A. (1984b). Myths and misconceptions in exercise for weight control. In J. Storlie and H.A. Jordan (Eds.), *Nutrition and Exercise in Obesity Management* (pp. 53-92). New York: Spectrum Publications.

Franklin, B., Buskirk, E., Hodgson, J., Gahagan, H., Kollias, J., & Mendez, J. (1979). Effects of physical conditioning on cardiorespiratory function, body composition and serum lipids in relatively normal-weight and obese middle aged women. *International Journal of Obesity, 3,* 97-109.

Franklin, B.A. & Rubenfire, M. (1980). Losing weight through exercise. *Journal of the American Medical Association, 244,*(4), 377-379.

Ginsberg-Fellner, F., & Carmel, H. (1974). The prevalence of obesity in nursery school children. Presented at the April 30, 1974 plenary session of the Ambulatory Pediatric Assocation.

Girandola, R.N. (1976). Body composition changes in women: Effects of high and low exercise intensity. *Archieves of Physical Medicine and Rehabilitation, 57,* 297-300.

Gwinup, G. Chelvam, R., & Steinberg, T. (1971). Thickness of subcutaneous fat and activity of underlying muscles. *Annals of International Medicine, 74,* 408-411.

Hammer, S.L. (1975). Obesity: Early identification and treatment. In P.J. Collip (Ed.), *Childhood Obesity*. Action, MA: Publishing Sciences Group, Inc.

Havel, R.J. (1971). Influence of intensity and duration of exercise on supply and use of fuels. In B. Pernow & B. Saltin (Eds.), *Muscle Metabolism during Exercise*. New York: Plenum Press.

Heinzelmann, F., & Bagely, W. (1970). Response to physical activity programs and their effects on health behavior. *Public Health Reports, 85* (10), 905-911.

Holm, G., Bjorntrop, P., & Jagersburg, R. (1978). Carbohydrate, lipid, and amino acid metabolism following physical exercise in man. *Journal of Applied Physiology, 45,* 128-132.

Hunter, W.M., & Sukkar, M.Y. (1968). Changes in plasma insulin levels during muscular exercise. *Journal of Physiology, 196,* 110-112.

Jackson, A.S., & Pollock, M.L. (1978). Generalized equations for predicting body density of men. *British Journal of Nutrition, 40,* 297-504.

Jackson, A.S., Pollock, M.L. & Ward, A. (1980). Generalized equations for predicting body density of women. *Medicine and Science in Sports and Exercise, 12,* 175-182.

James, W.P.T. & Trayhurn, P. (1981). Thermogenesis and obesity. *British Medical Journal, 37,* 43-48.

Johnson, M.L., Burke, M.S., & Mayer, J. (1956). Relative importance of inactivity and overeating in the energy balance of obese high school girls. *American Journal of Clinical Nutrition, 4,* 37-44.

Jung, R.T., Shetty, P.S., & James, W.P.T. (1979). Reduced thermogenesis in obesity. *Nature, 279,* 322-323.

Kannel, W.B. & Gordon, T. (1975). Some determinants of obesity and its impact as a cardiovascular risk factor. In A. Howard (Ed.), *Recent Advances in Obesity Research I*. London: Newman Publishing Ltd.

Katch, F.I., & McArdle, W.D. (1977). *Nutrition, Weight Control, and Exercise.* Boston: Houghton Mifflin.

Katch, F.I., Katch, V.L., & Behnke, A.R. (1980). The underweight female. *The Physician and Sportsmedicine, 8* (12), 55-60.

Katch, F.I., & Michael. E.D. (1971). Body composition of high school wrestlers according to age and wrestling weight category. *Medicine and Science in Sports, 3,* 190-194.

Kim, H.J., & Kalkhoff, R.K. (1975). Sex steroid influence on triglyceride metabolism. *Journal of Clinical Investigation, 56,* 888-896.

Krotkiewski, M., Aniansson, A., Grimby, G., Bjorntorp, P., & Sjostrom, L. (1979). The effect of unilateral isokinetic strength training on local adipose and muscle tissue morphology, thickness, and enzymes. *European Journal of Aplied Physiology, 42,* 271-281.

Krotkiewski, M., Toss, L., Bjorntorp, P., & Holm, G. (1982). The effect of a very-low-calorie diet with and without chronic exercise on thyroid and sex hormones, plasma proteins, oxygen uptake, insulin and c peptide concentrations in obese women. *International Journal of Obesity, 5,* 287-293.

Leighton, C.K., Shapiro, L.R., Crawford, P.B., & Huenemann, R.L. (1981). Body composition and physical activity in 8-year-old children. *American Journal of Clinical Nutrition, 34,* 2770-2775.

Lindberg, J.S., Fears, W.B., Hunt, M.M., Powell, M.R., Boll, D. and Wade, C.E. (1984). Exercise-induced amenorrhea and bone density. *Annals of Internal Medicine, 101* (5), 647-648.

Lohman, T.G. (1981). Skinfolds and body density and their relationship to body fatness: A review. *Human Biology, 53,* 181-225.

Lohman, T.G. (1983). Research progress in validation of laboratory methods of assessing body composition. *Medicine and Science in Sports and Exercise, 16,* 596-603.

Lucas, C.P. (1984). Medical indications for weight reduction. In J. Storlie and H.A. Jordan (Eds.), *Evaluation and Treatment of Obesity.* New York: Spectrum Publications.

Lukaski, H.C., & Johnson, P.E. (1985). A simple, inexpensive method of determining total body water using a tracer dose of D_2O and infrared absorbtion of biological fluids. *American Journal of Clinical Nutrition, 41,* 363-370.

MacKeen, P.C., Franklin, B.A., Nicholas, W.C., & Buskirk, E.R. (1983). Body composition, physical work capacity, and physical activity habits at 18-month follow-up of middle-aged women participants in an exercise intervention program. *International Journal of Obesity, 7,* 61-71.

Malina, R.L. (1980). The measurement of body composition. In F.E. Johnston, A.F. Roche and C. Susanne (Eds.), *Human Physical Growth and Maturation: Methodologies and Factors* (pp. 35-59). New York: Plenum Press.

Malina, R.M. (1983). Human growth, maturation, and regular physical activity. *Acta Medical Auxologia, 15,* 5-27.

Medical News. (1983). Those who 'eat and run' may lead healthier lives. *Journal of the American Medical Association, 250,* 2589-2590.

Moody, D.L., Wilmore, J.H., & Girandola, R.N. (1972). The effects of a jogging program on the body composition of normal and obese high school girls. *Medical and Science in Sports, 4,* 210-213.

Newsholme, E.A. (1980). A possible metabolic basis for the control of body weight. *New England Journal of Medicine, 302,* 400-405.

Osborne, R.H., & de George, F.V. (1959). Genetic Basis of Morphological Variation. Cambridge, MA: Harvard University Press.

Oscai, L.B. (1973). The role of exercise in weight control. In J.H. Whilmore (Ed.), *Exercise and Sport Sciences Reviews, Vol 1.* New York: Academic Press.

Oyster, N., Morton, M., & Linnell, S. (1984). Physical activity and osteoporosis in

post-menopausal women. *Medicine and Science in Sports and Exercise, 16,* 44-50.
Parizkova, J. (1977). *Body Fat and Physical Fitness.* The Hague: Martinus Nihoff.
Pollock, M.L., Cureton, T.K., & Greninger, L. (1969). Effects of frequency of training on working capacity, cardiovascular function, and body composition of adult men. *Medicine and Science in Sports, 1,* 70-74.
Presta, E., Wang, J., Harrison, G.G., Bjorntorp, P., Harker, W.H., & Van Itallie, T.B. (1983). Measurement of total body electrical conductivity: A new method for estimation of body composition. *Amercian Journal of Clinical Nutrition, 37,* 735-739.
Rodahl, K., Miller, H.I., & Issekutz, B. (1964). Plasma-free fatty acids in exercise. *Journal of Applied Physiology, 19,* 489-492.
Schade, M., Hellebrandt, F.A., Waterland, J.C., & Carns, M.L. (1962). Spot reducing in overweight college women. *Research Quarterly for Exercise and Sport, 33,* 461-471.
Segal, K.R. & Gutin, B. (1983). Thermic effects of food and exercise in lean and obese women. *Metabolism, 32*(6), 581-589.
Simko, V., Merrifield, H.H., & Stouffer, J.R. (1974). Mild exercise: Effect on body composition and metabolism. *New York State Journal of Medicine, 74,* 1563-1567.
Singer, R.N. (1973). Motor learning as a function of age and sex. In G.L. Rarick (Ed.), *Physical Activity: Human Growth and Development.* New York: Academic Press.
Sinning, W.E. (1974). Body composition assessment of college wrestlers. *Medicine and Science in Sports, 6,* 139-145.
Siri, W.E. (1956). Gross composition of the body. in J.H. Lawrence and C.A. Tobias (Eds.), *Advances in Biological and Medical Physics* (pp. 239-252). New York: Academic Press.
Sjostrom, L. (1980). Fat cells and body weight. In A.J. Stunkard (Ed.), *Obesity* (pp. 72-100). Philadelphia: W.B. Saunders Co.
Stukard, A.J. (1976). *The Pain of Obesity.* Palo Alto, CA: Bull Publishing Company.
Sutherland, W.H.F., Woodhouse, S.P., & Heyworth, M.R. (1981). Physical training and adipose tissue fatty acid composition in men. *Metabolism, 30,* 839-844.
Tanner, J.M. (1962). *Growth at Adolescence* (2nd ed.). Oxford: Blackwell.
Thompson, J.K., Jarvie, G., Lahey, B., & Cureton, K. (1982). Exercise and obesity: Etiology, physiology, and intervention. *Psychological Bulletin, 91* (1), 55-79.
Thorland, W.G., Johnson, G.O., Fagot, T.G., Tharp, G.D., & Hammer, R.W. (1981). Body composition and somatotype characteristics of Junior Olympic athletes. *Medicine and Science in Sports and Exercise, 13,* 332-338.
Upton, S.J., Hagan, R.D., Rosentswieg, J. & Gettman, L.R. (1983). Comparison of the physiological profiles of middle-aged women distance runners and sendentary women. *Research Quarterly for Exercise and Sport, 54,* 83-87.
Volz, P.A., & Ostrove, S.M. (1984). Evaluation of a portable ultra-sonoscope in assessing the body composition of college age women. *Medicine and Science in Sports and Exercise, 16,* 97-102.
Wade, G.N., & Gray, J.M. (1979). Gonadal effects on food intake and adiposity: A metabolic hypothesis. *Physiology of Behavior, 22,* 583-593.
Warwick, P.M., & Garrow, J.S. (1981). The effect of addition of exercise to a regime of dietary restriction on weight loss, nitrogen balance, resting metabolic rate and spontaneous physical activity in three obese women in a metabolic ward. *International Journal of Obesity, 5,* 25-32.
Webb, P. (1981). Energy expenditure and fat-free mass in men and women. *American Journal of Clinical Nutrition, 34,* 1816-1826.
White, G.M., & Young, R.J. (1978). Effect of a twelve week exercise program on cardiorespiratory and body composition variables in nonobese young and middle-aged females. *British Journal of Sports Medicine, 12,* 27-32.
Williams, P.T., Wood, P.D., Drauss, R.M., Haskell, W.L., Vranizan, K.M., Blair,

S.N., Terry, R., & Farquhar, J.W. (1983). Does weight loss cause the exercise-induced increase in plasma high density lipoproteins? *Atherosclerosis, 47,* 173-183.

Wilmore, J.H. (1982). *Athletic Training and Physical Fitness: Physiological Principles of the Conditioning Process* (2nd Ed.). Boston: Allyn and Bacon, Inc.

Wilmore, J.H. (1983a). Body composition in sport and exercise: directions for future research. *Medicine and Science in Sports and Exercise, 15,* 21-31.

Wilmore, J.H. (1983b). Appetite and body composition consequent to physical activity. *Research Quarterly for Exercise and Sport, 54,* 415-425.

Wilmore, J.H., & Haskell, W.L. (1972). Body composition and endurance capacity of professional football players. *Journal of Applied Physiology, 33,* 564-567.

Wilmore, J.H., & McNamara, J.J. (1974). Prevalence of coronary disease risk factors in boys, 8 to 12 years of age. *Journal of Pediatrics, 84,* 527-533.

Zuti, W.B. & Golding, L.A. (1976). Comparing diet and exercise as weight reduction tools. *Physician and Sports medicine, 4,* 49-53.

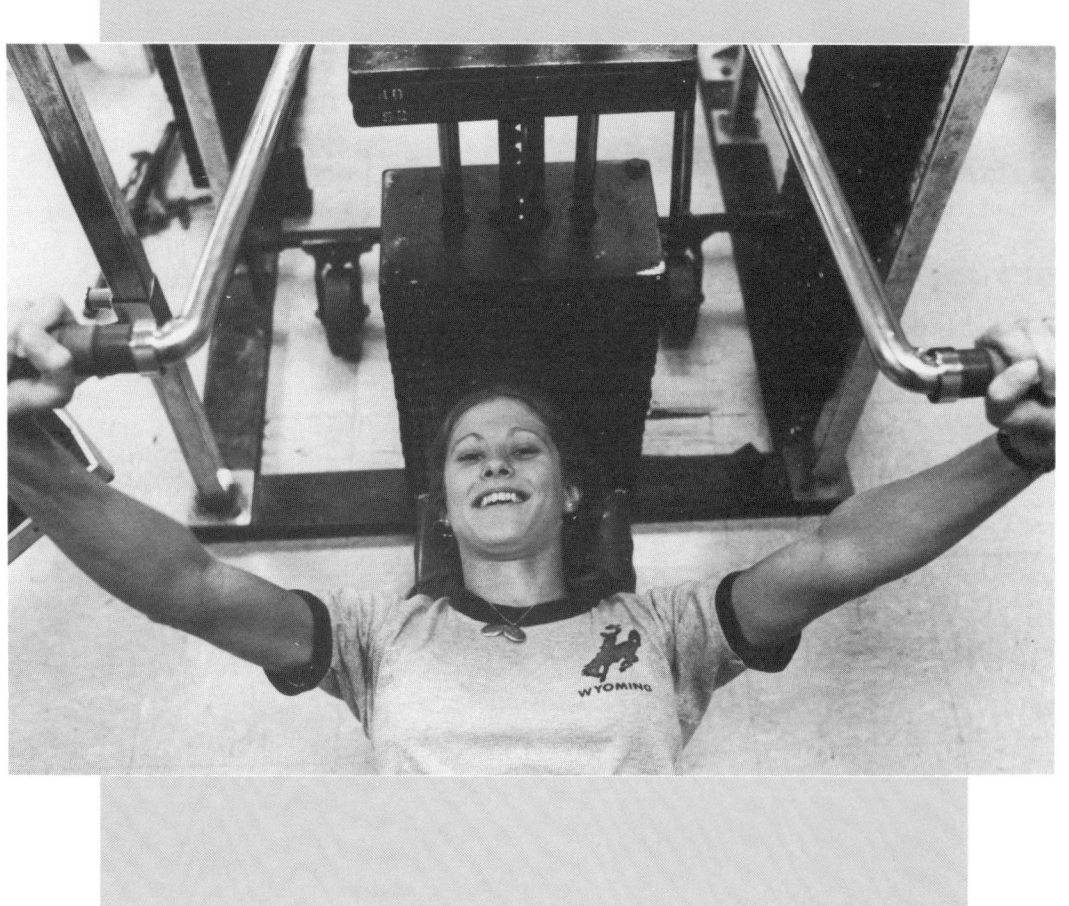

CHAPTER SEVEN

Neuromuscular Adaptations to High-resistance Exercise

Gary Kamen
Department of Physical Education
Indiana University
Bloomington, Indiana

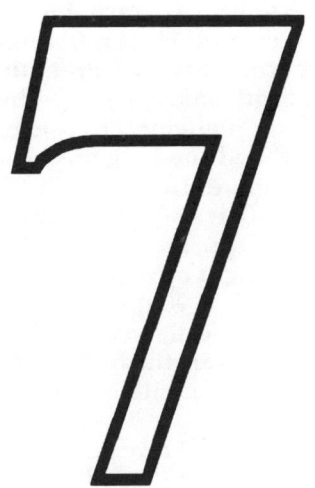

Ever since the story began to be told about Milo hoisting the bull high over his head, a search has continued for the perfect strength training regimen. The bulk of the strength-training research has been conducted in this century, although history records many prior attempts to increase strength through ergogenic aids such as lions' teeth and potions, as well as through regular physical exercise. This chapter will first review some of the current ideas concerning the effectiveness of various high-resistance exercise regimens in producing increases in muscular strength. In a later section, the effect of strengthening exercise on cellular components in muscles and nerves will be discussed, and finally, the last section will detail some of the neural adaptations which accompany regular high-resistance exercise. There are several earlier reviews on this topic to which the reader is referred for additional information (Atha, 1981; Clarke, 1973; McDonagh & Davies, 1984; Rasch, 1974).

Gross Adaptations in Muscle to High-resistance Exercise

Isometric Exercise

Before jogging was even considered a form of recreational activity, the first fitness wave to hit the U.S. involved Charles Atlas' system of isometric exercises. Here was a way a person could get some exercise, even while sitting on a train. While there were some earlier attempts at scientific investigation, two German investigators are generally credited with having documented the benefits of a program of isometric exercise. In 1953, Hettinger and Muller reported that the execution of just one 6-s isometric contraction at 2/3 maximal effort produced strength gains of five percent per week. At the time, it seemed incredulous to many people that so little time spent in strengthening exercise could produce such gains, and indeed, most investigations failed to substantiate the magnitude of strength gain demonstrated by Hettinger and Muller. Although there have been a few investigators who failed to find little if any effect resulting from isometric exercise (Bonde-Petersen, 1960; Mayberry, 1958), subsequent research focused on optimizing the training effect.

Contraction intensity. An early line of reasoning held that if 67% of maximal effort was sufficient to elicit a training effect, then perhaps 100% MVC would produce greater increases in strength. Rarick and Larsen (1958) found no differences in strength gains produced by either 67% or 80% MVC in prepubescent boys, although the higher intensity exercise resulted in greater strength retention. Cotten (1967) found similar gains using intensities of 50%, 75%, or 100% MVC, but found no training effect with the 25% MVC condition, confirming the suggestion made earlier that a 30% MVC level was the minimum intensity required from some strength increase (Hettinger & Muller, 1953). Davies and Young (1983) have also obtained strength increases following six weeks of isometric exercise at 30% MVC. Walters et al. (1960) presented somewhat contradictory data, suggesting that training isometrically with 100% MVC produced greater gains than training at 67% MVC; however, the bulk of the available evidence indicates that regular isometric exercise at an intensity greater than 30% MVC constitutes a sufficient training stimulus.

Contraction Duration. The effect of varying contraction duration was considered by Rohmert and Preising (1968) who found similar strength increases with a 1-s contraction to those reported earlier by Hettinger and Muller (1953) for 6-s contractions. Because many human muscle groups require longer than 1-s to reach maximum isometric tension (Atha, 1981; Kamen, 1983), the possibility exists that a 1-s contraction might be optimal for the elbow flexors (the muscle group used by Muller and Rohmert), while a 3-6 s isometric contraction might produce greater gains for other muscle groups.

Exercise Duration. The number of contractions performed during each training session seems to matter little. Meyers (1967) found no difference in the strength increases which resulted from using either 3 or 20 6-s isometric contractions per session. Similar results were obtained by Josenhans (1962).

Joint Angle Specificity. One of the criticisms leveled against isometric exercise as a training regimen concerns the observation that some degree of joint angle specificity seems to be present with isometric training. Training at one joint angle does seem to produce an increase in strength predominantly at that position (Gardner, 1963; Lindh, 1979). This criticism of isometric exercise may have been overstated, however, since others have reported general strength increases at all joint angles after isometric training (Belka, 1968; Darcus & Salter, 1955; Raitsin, 1976; Whitley, 1967). The study by Meyers (1967) helps to elucidate some of the reasons for these contrary findings. As indicated previously, Meyers trained one group using three 6-s contractions at 170° joint angle. Thus, while strength gains achieved through isometric exercise may be greatest at the muscle length at which contraction takes place, it seems that this aspect of isometric exercise specificity can be at least partially offset by a training program which considers both contraction number and contraction intensity. As well, a balanced isometric exercise program would include contractions at several joint angles.

Rehabilitation. Because it does not involve limb movement, there are several situations in which isometric exercise would seem to have some distinct advantages over isotonic training. For example, Rozier and Elder (1980) have shown that isometric exercise can be used in casted limbs to prevent disuse atrophy. Isometric exercise has also been used to effect strength gains in the contralateral unexercised musculature. This use of isometric exercise to produce a cross-transfer effect will be discussed later in the chapter.

Isotonic Exercise

While the preceding discussion indicates that isometric exercise can certainly be an effective high-resistance exercise protocol, recent studies have focused on the use of dynamic, isotonic exercise for increasing muscular strength. Credit for promoting research in isotonic exercise is generally given to Thomas DeLorme (1945) who described the principle of progressive resistance exercise (PRE) which remains an integral part of isotonic exercise programs.

DeLorme technique. DeLorme established the ten repetition maximum, the amount of weight which can be lifted ten times (10RM), as the basis for testing isotonic strength. Isotonic exercise programs were then planned using the 10RM load (DeLorme, 1945). His conclusion—that low-repetition, high-resistance exercise produces power, while high-repetition, low-resistance exercise produces endurance—forms the basis of current principles of exercise specificity. The standard exercise initially consisted of 10 sets using the 10RM load, with the weight increased as strength progressed (thus the term progressive resistance). DeLorme and Watkins (1948) later modified this schedule by reducing the number of sets to three, and increasing the load per set. Since DeLorme's initial investigations, other researchers have focused on optimizing the training schedule by altering such factors as contraction speed, exercise frequency, contraction intensity, and other aspects of the training schedule.

Oxford technique. In 1951, Zinovieff described the Oxford technique which involved a total of 100 contractions per training session. The first set used a load of 10RM. Ten repetitions were performed on each succeeding bout with a reduced load. The Oxford technique appears to result in significant strength gains similar to those achieved through DeLorme-type training (McMorris & Elkins, 1954).

During the 1960s, Berger sought to determine the optimal schedule for training with either isotonic or (in some experiments) isometric exercise. In a comparison of nine different exercise programs, he reported that the best schedule for isotonic exercise involved three bouts, with six repetitions per bout (Berger, 1962a). This was later confirmed in another study comparing isometric exercise with several different isotonic exercise programs (Berger, 1963). When one set of repetitions is performed, he recommended between three and nine repetitions (Berger, 1963).

Exercise load. The question of what exercise load should be used has produced conflicting results. Some researchers have suggested that maximal or near maximal loads are required for an optimal training effect (Berger & Hardage, 1967; Dons et al., 1979). However, other studies have produced substantial strength gains with submaximal loads. O'Shea (1966) found similar strength gains using either a 2RM, 5RM, or 10RM training load, and Withers (1970) found no differences among 3RM, 5RM or 7RM loads. Using a 12-week training program, Berger (1962b) produced the greatest strength gains using loads ranging from 4RM to 8RM, while Leighton et al. (1967) compared 10 different training programs and, in general, found that the higher loads seemed to produce the greatest strength gains. So it seems that maximal loads may not be necessary to produce strength gains, but some threshold load (approx. 2/3 of 1RM) is necessary to produce a strengthening effect, and the optimal load may differ among individuals of varying initial strength levels, lying somewhere between the threshold load and a 1RM load. Roman (1974) surveyed Bulgarian weight lifters and found the predominant use of loads ranging from 55% to 90% of maximum, with somewhat heavier loads used during the competitive periods. Loads greater than 90% of maximum were only lifted 8-15 times per month.

Exercise frequency. One aspect of the training schedule which has been confounded with load intensity is exercise frequency. Berger (1965) sought to determine the effect of load intensity on strength gain using loads of 66%, 80%, 90% and 100% of 1RM. Training frequency ranged between one and three times per week. Only the group training at the 66% of 1RM load, three times per week failed to gain strength. Berger concluded that the combination of near-maximal load and a weekly 1RM test were necessary for strength gain, but the effect of exercise frequency was unclear. Capen (1956) suggested that the optimal schedule involved three training sessions per week, three sets of exercise per session, five repetitions per set with a 5RM load. More recently, Gillam (1981) obtained greater gains using a five day/week program than exercise schedules of one, two, three or four days per week, although similar results were obtained with the three days/week and the five days/week program.

Constant resistance versus variable resistance exercise. Using conventional free weights, the torque measured at the joint changes as the joint angle changes due to the mechanics of the human lever system. Several pieces of commercial exercise equipment have been constructed which either maintain a constant resistance throughout the movement range or else vary the resistance applied at different muscle lengths due to the mechanics of the human lever system. Perhaps the first effort to design such a device was made by Noland and Kuckhoff (1954) who described its use in training the muscles of the upper leg. Using a specifically-constructed variable resistance device, Raitsin and Sarsaniya (1975) found the greatest gains at the shorter muscle length. Conventional weight training was more effective in producing strength increases throughout the range of movement. Stone et al. (1979) and Pipes (1978) also obtained strength gains using either constant or variable resistance training. However, the bulk of current evidence indicates that strength gains achieved using either variable resistance or constant resistance equipment are similar to those achieved with conventional free weights.

Isokinetics. Some exercise equipment has been designed to allow the muscle group to contract throughout the range of motion at a constant, pre-set velocity. The apparatus "accommodates" to the maximal force which the individual is capable of exerting at any muscle length, and thus the term "accommodating resistance exercise" has been proposed to describe this type of training (Thistle et al., 1967). The term "isokinetics" has been more widely used, although as Atha (1981) points out, isokinetics is hardly an appropriate term.

One of the first articles to report the effects of strength training using isokinetic equipment was published by Moffroid et al. (1969). Their results indicated that four weeks of isokinetic exercise involving contractions of the quadriceps and hamstrings muscles produced gains in isometric strength in both muscle groups. A later report (Moffroid & Whipple, 1970) showed that training at a low velocity caused strength gains which were not observed in subjects training at high velocity. Other researchers have verified that training at low velocities produces the greatest gains in isometric strength and torque at low velocities, while training at high velocities results in greater torque production at higher speeds of movement but lesser gains in isometric strength and torque at low velocities (Caiozzo et al., 1981; Coyle et al., 1981; Kanehisa & Mihashita, 1983; Lesmes et al., 1978). Thus, isokinetic exercise can be an effective means of increasing muscular strength, particularly in the velocity range at which performance occurs. Grimby (1982) stated the following advantages to isokinetic training: a) it allows maximal resistance through the whole range of motion; b) training at specific velocities is possible with resultant velocity-specific effects; c) agonist and antagonist muscles can be trained in series; and d) it offers less risk for overload, making isokinetic exercise especially useful as a therapeutic exercise modality.

Eccentric exercise. It has been repeatedly demonstrated that the force exerted in a lengthening or eccentric muscle contraction is greater than that which can be exerted in a shortening or concentric contraction (Asmussen et al., 1965; Doss & Karpovich, 1965) at a lower energy cost (Seliger et al., 1968). Strength researchers, reasoning that load intensity is a key component in high-resistance exercise training, have compared the strength gains produced by concentric exercise with those obtained using eccentric exercise. Bonde-Petersen (1960) found no effect of 10 eccentric contractions per day when subjects trained for 20-36 days. But he also reported no strength gain from isometric or concentric exercise. Singh and Karpovich (1967) showed that training with eccentric contractions could produce significant strength gains. Several other studies have indicated that strength gains from eccentric training are similar to those obtained using either concentric or isometric exercise (Johnson, 1972; Laycoe & Marteniuk, 1971; Mannheimer, 1969; Seliger et al., 1968).

Although Johnson (1972) indicated that subjects liked eccentric exercise and found it easier to perform than the shortening contractions, many subjects reported severe muscle soreness following the early stages of eccentric training (Friden, 1984a; Talag, 1973) which might cause an individual to cease pursuing a weight training program. Komi and Buskirk (1972) obtained significantly larger gains using eccentric exercise than concentric exercise. They indicated that greater muscle soreness was present in the eccentric-trained group than the isometric-trained group, but the soreness subsided considerably after a week and did not reappear. Hakkinen et al. (1981) reported greater strength increases using combined eccentric and concentric exercise than concentric exercise alone. Some recent experiments have indicated that there are some beneficial ultrastructural changes occurring following eccentric exercise which might enhance muscle contractility and reduce the risk for muscle injury (Friden, 1984b). The present evidence indicates that eccentric training produces increases in isometric and isotonic strength, with strength gains similar to those observed using other high-resistance exercise methods.

Plyometrics. Rapid stretch of a muscle allows the muscle to store elastic energy for release during a subsequent concentric contraction (cf. Cavagna, 1977). Plyometric exercises involve rapid lenthening contractions immediately followed by a concentric contraction. Such exercises are also called "depth jumping" and may involve jumping on and off low boxes (Wilt, 1975). Dobrovolski (1972) has shown strength increases with plyometric exercise; however, most other researchers have been concerned with the effect of plyometrics on such motor performance tests as the vertical jump (cf. Atha, 1981). Blattner and Noble (1979) found that plyometric exercises were effective in producing gains in vertical jumping, but no more effective than a program of isokinetic training.

Changes in the Training Regimen. Some investigators have considered whether strength gains might be achieved more rapidly by altering the exercise program periodically. DeLateur et al. (1968) trained two groups using high resistance/low repetition exercise and two groups using a low resistance/high repetition schedule. After 15 sessions, one of the high resistance groups shifted to low resistance exercise, and one of the low resistance groups shifted to high resistance exercise. After four additional exercise sessions the two cross-over groups displayed similar increments in muscular strength and endurance. In a subsequent investigation, DeLateur et al. (1972a) trained two groups using isometric exercise, and two with isotonic exercise. After 28 training sessions, two groups shifted to the alternate exercise type for an additional four training sessions. Strength assessments, conducted using an isotonic test, revealed that the group trained only with isotonic exercise had higher final strength levels than the other three groups. The authors concluded that ". . . the best training for a given type of task is that task itself. . . . "

Periodization. Stone et al. (1981) advocated a program designed by Eastern European weight lifting coaches called "periodization." They reasoned that since hypertrophied muscle possesses greater strength potential than non-hypertrophied muscle, the early phase of a strength training program should involve low resistance (perhaps three sets of 8-20RM). Following muscle hypertrophy, they suggest that a higher-resistance program (perhaps three to five sets of 2-6RM) would be more appropriate. A study designed to test this schedule did provide somewhat greater gains in squatting strength in a group using the "periodization" schedule, than in the group which used only three sets of 6RM exercise.

Comparisons Among High-resistance Exercise Techniques

Both Atha (1981) and Clarke (1973) reviewed the studies comparing isotonic with isometric exercise and found no evidence favoring one over the other. Of 49 studies considered by Atha (1981) prior to 1969, 11 favored isometrics, 12 favored isotonics, 19 favored neither technique, 2 favored a hybrid combination of exercise, and 5 required ". . . more complex interpretations. . . . " Since 1970, Atha found 2 studies which favored isometrics, 3 favoring isotonics, and 4 neither program.

There have been few comparisons of isokinetic exercise with other exercise programs, but most of these training regimens have yielded no clear advantage for isokinetics. DeLateur et al. (1972b) had subjects train using either isotonic or isokinetic exercise for 18 sessions, and then switch to the opposite exercise type. Both groups manifested similar strength gains. Stevens (1980) reported somewhat greater gains with isotonic exercise than with either isokinetic or combined isotonic-isokinetic exercise; however, no statistical analyses were provided. Using athletes or former athletes who had sustained knee injuries an average of 14 months prior to the experiment, Grimby et al. (1980) implemented an isokinetic exercise program with one group of subjects, an isotonic training schedule with another group. After six weeks, he noted markedly greater torques in the isokintic group than the isotonic group at angular velocities ranging from 0 deg/s to 120 deg/s.

Specificity of training. Any comparison among exercise programs must consider specificity of training and specificity of exercise effects. Several studies serve to exemplify the principle of specificity. Berger (1962c) trained one group using isotonic exercise, another using isometric exercise, and tested strength gains using both isotonic and isometric strength tests. The isotonic-trained group performed better when an isotonic test was used, while the isometric-trained group performed better under isometric test conditions. In his original reports, DeLorme (1945) indicated that high resistance/low repetition exercise produced the greatest gains in muscular strength, while a schedule involving low resistance/high repetition exercise resulted in the greatest increases in muscular endurance. Anderson & Kearney (1982) re-tested this idea recently, and found the greatest strength gains in the subjects who exercised using high-resistance/low-repetition training, although gains in muscular endurance were similar for both groups. Hickson (1980) trained one group using weight training exercises, while a second group trained for endurance using a bicycle ergometer and continuous running. A third group trained using both exercise programs. His findings showed that simultaneously training for both strength and endurance results in less strength gain than if only high-resistance exercise were performed. However, the ability to develop aerobic endurance was not affected.

Previous discussion of isokinetic exercise indicated that isometric strength and low velocity power gains were most evident when training was performed at low velocities, but training at high velocities had the greatest positive effect on performance at high velocity. In comparing subjects who train using either constant resistance or variable resistance procedures, Pipes (1978) found that the group training with constant resistance equipment scored better when tested using constant resistance equipment, while the group training with variable resistance equipment produced greater gains when tested under variable resistance procedures.

In summary, individuals will show the greatest stength gains when the strength assessment is made using the same kind of exercise and the same kind of equipment as that used during training. An effort to increase muscular strength should incorporate high-resistance exercise which is performed at the same speed and in the same general pattern as is required during normal motor performance.

Cellular Adaptations to High-resistance Exercise

Energy Utilization

One assumption of the specificity of exercise principle is that high-resistance exercise should enhance the ability to utilize immediate and short-term energy sources. Such an enhancement would be reflected by an increase in the biological activity of the enzyme systems needed for glycolysis and glycogenolysis, in the enzymes needed for muscle contraction, and in the resting levels of energy substrate required for immediate exercise demands. However, examination of training influences on resting energy levels and the capability to utilize immediate energy sources yields mixed results.

Energy substrate. Short-duration exercise lasting less than 10 seconds requires the breakdown of immediate muscle energy sources, including adenosine triphosphate (ATP) and creatine phosphase (CP) (Edington & Edgerton, 1976). One would logically expect high-resistance training to produce increased concentrations of these energy sources. Several studies using isometric, isokinetic, isotonic, sprinting, or eccentric bicycle training have produced no changes in either ATP or CP levels (Bonde-Petersen et al., 1973; Grimby et al., 1973; Grimby et al., 1980; Thorstensson et al., 1975). One possible explanation is that the duration of these experiments were too short to effect an adaptation. Indeed,

MacDougall et al. (1977) showed that five months of isotonic training could increase ATP (18%), CP (22%), muscle creatine (39%), and muscle glycogen (66%).

Utilization of immediate energy sources. As a result of training, one would expect the levels of enzymes required for immediate muscle contraction to increase. Some studies using swimming exercise have failed to demonstrate changes in myosin ATPase activity (Hearn & Gollnick, 1961; Rawlinson & Gould, 1959). However, other researchers have reported large increases (up to 44%) in myosin ATPase activity in rat muscle following swimming exercise (Wilkerson & Evonuk, 1971). Using a running exercise task, Bagby et al. (1972) were unable to demonstrate any change in myofibrillar myosin ATPase concentrations in the gastrocnemius muscle of either sprint-trained or endurance-trained rats. But Thorstensson et al. (1975) found that Mg^{++}-stimulated ATPase increased in four sprint-trained human beings following an eight-week exercise schedule.

Training rats using an isometric exercise regimen, Exner et al. (1973) found increased activity in creatine kinase in rectus femoris but no change in the soleus muscle, indicating that enzymatic adaptations could be fiber type-specific. Houston et al. (1983) reported that 10 weeks of isotonic exercise produced no change in creatine kinase or myofibrillar ATPase activities in the human quadriceps. Hakkinen et al. (1981) reported no change in creatine kinase in the quadriceps of subjects who trained for 16 weeks using a combination of eccentric and concentric exercise. It thus appears that experiments aimed at determining the response of immediate energy systems to training have produced somewhat equivocal results.

Adaptations in the glycolytic pathway. The question of whether improvements in glycolytic enzyme activities occur with high-resistance exercise is also somewhat controversial. The experiment by Houston et al. (1983) (discussed above) produced no significant increases in hexokinase or phosphofructokinase activities. Grimby et al. (1980) trained 30 patients who had recovered from knee surgery an average of 14 months. The patients trained for three weeks using either isokinetic or isotonic exercise. Neither group exhibited any change in myokinase or ATPase activity. The 16-week program utilized by Hakkinen et al. (1981) also produced no change in myokinase activity. But other investigations have shown improvements in phosphofructokinase (Costill et al., 1979; Fournier et al., 1982; Gillespie et al., 1982), citrate synthetase (Exner et al., 1973; Staudte et al., 1973), myokinase (Thorstensson et al., 1975), and hexokinase (Staudte et al., 1973) following high-resistance exercise training. Using isokinetic exercise, Costill et al. (1979) found increased phosphorylase activity in subjects who trained for seven weeks using ten 30-sec bouts each day. Six-second bouts produced no significant increase in phosphorylase.

Specificity of changes in enzyme activities. Adaptations in energy pathways have not always followed expected exercise specificity rules. Hickson et al. (1975) trained rats to run on a treadmill using either a sprint speed (99 m/min) or a slower speed for a more prolonged period of time to promote endurance. Enhancements in mitchondrial enzyme activities (indicated by a 42-45% increase in fumarase) were observed in both sprint- and endurance-trained groups. The authors concluded that ". . . similar enzyme adaptations occur over time with both types of training. . . ." Kowalski et al. (1969) also found that either running or weight lifting exercise can produce increases in oxidative enzymes (succinic dehydrogenase and cytochrome oxidase) in rat muscle. Roy et al. (1977) trained rats to perform a simple weight lifting task and found increases in the activity of several aerobic enzymes. Komi et al. (1978) showed that increases in both anaerobic and aerobic enzyme concentrations occurred following 12 weeks of weight training in four human subjects.

It seems that adaptations to high-resistance exercise may not be accurately reflected by alterations in enzyme activities. One important factor may be the duration of training necessary to produce a training effect. It may be plausible that adaptations in energy pathways might occur at varying rates. Considering the problems inherent in examining human muscle biopsy samples (Gollnick, 1982) and the small sample size often used in such experiments, further study seems warranted.

Muscle Hypertrophy

A logical assumption is that a muscle with larger diameter muscle fibers and/or a greater number of muscle fibers can produce greater muscular force. Thus, one important question is: what is the mechanism producing gross muscle hypertrophy?

Compensatory hypertrophy. In an effort to better study hypertrophy resulting from overload, an animal model was developed which was designed to produce rapid muscle hypertrophy. The typical experiment involves removing one or more muscles in a synergistic muscle group and observing the adaptations which occur in the remaining overloaded muscle(s). For example, only three days after sectioning the rat gastrocnemius tendon, increases in dry weight of the soleus muscle on the order of 25-30% have been observed (Mackova & Hnik, 1971).

There are several problems, however, which arise in generalizing the results from the compensatory hypertrophy model to potential benefits of high-resistance exercise. Decreases in tetanic tension, increases in twitch contraction time (Lesh et al., 1968), and decreases in ATPase activity (Gutmann et al., 1971) occur in muscles which have been overloaded following ablation of synergists. These changes, which would indicate a decrease in anaerobic potential, present a curious paradox, since hypertrophy is normally indicative of greater muscle power. Compensatory hypertrophy also occurs in denervated muscle (Schiaffino & Hanzlikova, 1970) but does not occur if the antagonist muscles are denervated (Mackova & Hnik, 1971). These observations coupled with the finding that stretch increases the rate of protein synthesis in muscle (Buresova et al., 1969) suggest that the hypertrophy produced from tenotomy or synergist removal can be attributed largely to the passive mechanical tension from antagonists.

Exercise-induced hypertrophy. One of the first demonstrations of exercise-induced hypertrophy was conducted by Morpurgo (1897) who indicated that the adaptation observed in dog sartorius muscle was due principally to an increase in the cross-sectional area of the overloaded muscle fibers. Subsequent investigations have generally confirmed the increase in muscle fiber cross-sectional area, usually in both fast-twitch (FT) and slow-twitch (ST) muscle fibers. For example, Hakkinen et al. (1981) found that 16 weeks of concentric and eccentric exercise produced an increase in FT fiber area with a somewhat smaller enhancement of ST fiber area.

However, there have been exceptions to the finding that high-resistance exercise produces muscle fiber hypertrophy. Grimby et al. (1980) trained subjects for six weeks using either isotonic or isokinetic exercise and found no significant change in muscle fiber areas. Thorstensson et al. (1976a) also noted no change in fiber areas after eight weeks of isotonic exercise, although 1 RM for the squat improved 67%. Fournier et al. (1982) found that three months of sprint training in adolescent males produced no significant alteration in muscle fiber area. One possible explanation for the latter finding is that sprint training may not present a sufficiently intense stimulus to induce muscle fiber hypertrophy. Alternatively, some quantitative differences may exist between adolescents and adults in the response of muscle to high-resistance exercise.

Some reports have indicated that FT fibers increase area faster and to a greater extent than ST fibers. Hamsters subjected to weight lifting exercise show greater hypertrophy in biceps and extensor digitorum longus muscles than in the red soleus (Goldspink & Howells, 1974). In a recent study involving human subjects, Houston et al. (1983) showed that 10 weeks of isotonic training with the knee extensors of one leg resulted in significant increases in FTa (21%) and FTb (18%) fiber areas, with no change in ST fiber area. Using isokinetic contractions, Krotkiewski et al. (1979) also found an increase in the area of FTb fibers, but no significant change in other fiber areas. The sprint training used by Thorstensson et al. (1975) produced hypertrophy in both FT and ST fibers.

Hyperplasia. It has been suggested that gross increases in muscle size can occur by means other than muscle fiber hypertrophy. The idea that high-resistance exercise can effect increases in muscle fiber number (or hyperplasia) is replete with controversy. Investigators have pointed to the existence of branching muscle fibers as evidence indicating the existence of longitudinal muscle fiber splitting. Workers in other laboratories have also presented data showing that muscle fibers are capable of splitting (Hall-Craggs, 1972; Hall-Craggs & Lawrence, 1970; Ho et al., 1977; Schiaffino et al., 1979; Van Linge, 1962).

A major impetus for the development of the compensatory hypertrophy model was the observation that many of the early training studies using an animal model failed to produce muscle hypertrophy or improvements in performance. In 1976, Gonyea and Ericson described an exercise regimen which produced gross muscle hypertrophy in amounts ranging from 7 to 34%. Using operant conditioning principles, cats were trained to move a weighted bar with their forelimb to obtain food. Subsequent studies in which cats were trained up to 34 weeks indicated that high-resistance training resulted in a 20.5% increase in the number of muscle fibers in the flexor carpi radialis, while low-resistance training resulted in no increase in fiber number (Gonyea et al., 1977; Gonyea, 1980).

Hypertrophy or hyperplasia? In solving the hypertrophy versus hyperplasia dilemma, an important methodological consideration concerns the technique used to count the number of muscle fibers. Most authors have used muscle cross-sections to obtain muscle fiber counts. However, Gollnick et al. (1981, 1983) have suggested that cross-sectional counts can lead to misleading results for several reasons. Following surgical removal of the gastrocnemius, rats were exercised on a treadmill for six to eight weeks. The combined muscle ablation/exercise treatment resulted in an enlargement of the soleus and plantaris muscles (25-45% compared to contralateral controls). Digesting the whole muscles with nitric acid allowed a direct count of the number of muscle fibers, and they found no change in the number of fibers compared to contralateral controls. Gollnick and his associates have concluded that muscle fiber hypertrophy and not hyperplasia is the mechanism by which gross increases in muscle size occur. Obviously, the hypertrophy versus hyperplasia question remains to be resolved.

Muscle Fiber Type Composition

Another area of controversy involves the extent to which muscle fibers can be transformed from one type to another. Muscle fiber transformations have been observed in animals following functional overloading (Lang et al., 1978; Muntener, 1982; Watt et al., 1984), longterm electrical stimulation (Salmons & Sreter, 1976) or exercise (Watt et al., 1982). Efforts to produce muscle fiber transformations in human beings following isokinetic (Costill et al., 1979; Seaborne & Taylor, 1981), isotonic (Dons et al., 1979; Hakkinen et al., 1981), or sprint training (Fournier et al., 1982; Thorstensson et al., 1975) have generally failed. In studies with monozygous and dizygous twins, Komi et al. (1977) have found high hereditability estimates for muscle fiber type composition, indicating that the relative percentage of fast and slow twitch fibers is largely genetically determined.

However, there have been some exceptions to the observation that fiber type composition in human beings is unalterable. An increase in the number of intermediate fibers and a decrease in FT fibers has been observed following training in long-distance skiers (Schantz et al., 1982; Schantz & Henriksson, 1983). Jansson et al. (1978) also reported an increase in type IIc (intermediate) fibers and a decrease in type I fibers following anaerobic-type interval training. Howald (1982) has criticized the earlier studies conducted in human beings suggesting that they may have been too short in duration to effect changes in muscle fiber type composition. It may well be that muscle fiber type composition is ultimately determined by a variety of both genetic and environmental factors.

Motoneuron Characteristics

There is also evidence of metabolic changes in the motoneuron as a result of chronic physical activity. Wedeles (1949) overloaded the medial gastrocnemius muscle in rabbits by denervating the lateral gastrocnemius, plantaris and soleus muscles and found an increase in both the total number of nerve fibers and total fiber area. He suggested that some of the unmyelinated fibers might have acquired myelination as a result of the treatment. Edds (1950) also found that synergist denervation resulted in larger nerve fibers and a greater number of myelinated nerves innervating the soleus. Similar to the compensatory hypertrophy studies discussed above, an exercise treatment seems to produce different changes in peripheral motor nerves. Treadmill exercise produced no change in nerve fiber diameter in guinea pigs (Andersson & Edstrom, 1957). Tomanek and Tipton (1967) reported smaller nerve fiber diameters and fewer nerve fibers in rat medial gastrocnemius nerve eight weeks after removal of the tendon than in control animals. Animals given a treadmill exercise program for eight weeks showed no changes in mean nerve fiber diameter or in the nerve fiber number.

Exercise also produces some metabolic changes in motoneurons. Gilliam et al. (1977) trained rats on a treadmill for 12 weeks using either endurance- or sprint-type training. Both training schedules resulted in smaller motoneuron cell bodies than in the sedentary control animals. Gerchman et al. (1975) reported greater concentrations of glucose-6-phosphaste dehydrogenase in ventral motoneuron cell bodies following 52 days of swimming exercise. These observations do not present clear interpretations, but they do show that motoneurons are indeed susceptible to adaptive plasticity following chronic exercise.

Neural Adaptations to High-resistance Exercise

Motor Learning and Muscular Strength

It is well known that high-resistance exercise can produce significant increases in limb girth, particularly in males (Hosler, 1977; O'Shea, 1966; Pipes, 1978). However, a common misconception is that muscle hypertrophy occurs with the same time course as muscular strength gains. In fact, some investigators have failed to observe any significant increases in muscle girth with exercise. For example, Ward & Fisk (1964) reported significant increases in strength of the elbow flexors and knee extensors following isometric and isotonic exercise with no change in circumference of either the upper arm or the thigh. Herbison et al. (1981) trained rats to carry a weight (up to 150 g) on their backs up a 50° incline over a six-week period and found no significant hypertrophy in the plantaris. Prolonged running or swimming exercise can actually decrease muscle size in rats (Gordon et al., 1967).

An important observation is that increases in muscle girth are usually more apparent during the later stages of strength training programs. Although Hakkinen et al. (1981) reported increases in thigh girth following eccentric and concentric training, most of the gross muscle and individual muscle fiber hypertrophy occurred during the second half of the 16-week experiment. The finding that morphological and enzymatic adaptations occur predominantly only after much of the initial increase in muscular strength would seem to indicate the existence of other factors accounting for the sizable gains in muscular strength during the initial phase of a strength training program.

Electromyographic Changes and Strength Training

Several investigators have alluded to the importance of the nervous system in strength training programs (Coyle et al., 1981; Hislop, 1963; Rasch & Morehouse, 1957; Ward & Fisk, 1964), but few studies have examined the neural changes which accompany strength gains. Studies of electromyographic changes accompanying strength gains provide some insight into the neural adaptations which occur during training.

Using the forearm flexors, Moritani and DeVries (1979) trained 15 subjects with progressive resistance exercise. During the initial training period there was no change in the EMG/force ratio. Instead, increases in muscular strength were accompanied by increases in total EMG activity, suggesting the existence of a neural mechanism operative during this period through which early strength gains were achieved by concomitant increases in EMG amplitude. After several weeks, further strength gains were achieved as the EMG/force ratio decreased. This decline in the EMG/force ratio was presented as evidence that muscle hypertrophy becomes a more important factor during the later stages of strength training.

Although Komi and Buskirk (1972) reported no significant increase in EMG amplitude following either concentric or eccentric exercise, most other studies have reported that strength training results in greater EMG amplitude during maximum effort (Hakkinen & Komi, 1983a; Moritani & DeVries, 1979) and less EMG activity at submaximal force levels (Komi et al., 1978; Thorstensson et al., 1976b). It would seem then, that the neuromuscular system is capable of adapting to the higher-resistance exercise stimulus by producing muscular force in a more economical and more efficient manner.

Other electromyographic evidence. Chronic high-resistance exercise also seems to alter the manner in which motor units are activated during activities requiring high levels of muscular force. Stepanov and Burlakov (1961) were among the first to suggest that strength training results in a synchronization of motor units. Gross EMG patterns were studied in cross-country skiers and weight lifters during dumbbell exercise resulting in fatigue. While the EMG pattern from the cross-country skiers appeared as a normal, random pattern of motor unit firing, the EMG activity from the muscles of the weight lifters appeared to be organized into distinct groups or bursts of motor units. This pattern of synchronized firing or simultaneous activation of motor units was assumed to be an adaptation designed to produce high levels of muscular force under conditions requiring little endurance. Milner-Brown et al. (1975) also reported a greater level of synchronization in weight lifters than non-athletes. Moreover, training a small finger muscle for 6 weeks produced a greater degree of synchronized motor unit firing.

Some researchers have also reported changes in motor unit firing frequency with training. Under standardized conditions, faster motor unit firing rates have been reported in sprinters than in untrained subjects (Saplinskas et al., 1979; Saplinskas & Yaschaninas, 1982). Cerquiglini et al. (1973) found an increase in frequencies greater than 120 Hz and less than 30 Hz in weight lifters and suggested that the lower frequencies might reflect an increase in the maximal firing frequency of active motor units. These observations support the idea that the pattern of motor unit activation can be altered as a result of long-term exercise.

Cross Transfer

Initially, it may seem difficult to believe that exercising a limb on one side of the body can result in strength increases in the contralateral limb. But many studies have verified that this phenomenon, termed "cross transfer" or "cross education", does indeed occur. Scripture et al. (1894) are generally credited with having made the initial discovery, demonstrating that exercise in the right arm could result in strength increases in the untrained left arm. It was later suggested that exercising the uninjured limb might be a useful treatment for the rehabilitation of injured and perhaps immobilized muscle groups (Klein, 1955; Klein & Williams, 1954).

Muscular strength. While there have been a few studies which failed to find any cross transfer effect (Gardner, 1963; Kruse & Mathews, 1958) most investigators have reported increases in the strength of the contralateral limb following either isometric or isotonic training (Carlson, 1973; Raitsin, 1976; Shaver, 1975; Walters et al., 1960). Lawrence et al. (1962) reported somewhat greater gains in the untrained quadriceps following isotonic than isometric exercise, but Coleman (1969) indicated that 12 weeks of either isometric or isotonic training using the forearm flexors produced significant strength gains in the untrained contralateral limb, with little difference between the two exercise conditions.

Muscular endurance. Mathews et al. (1956) trained subjects for four weeks using isotonic exercise and found strength gains in both the trained and untrained limbs but endurance gains only in the exercised limb. Shaver (1970) also found no contralateral increase in muscular endurance, but Slater-Hammel (1950) was able to obtain increases in muscular endurance of the untrained forearm flexors after only three weeks of isotonic exercise. It does appear then, that the cross transfer effect can extend to muscular endurance as well.

Mechanism for the cross transfer effect. Early researchers discussed the possibility that cross transfer resulted from a "diffusion of motor impulses" to the contralateral limb (Wissler & Richardson, 1900). Training using isokinetic exercise results in no change in fat-free weight, muscle fiber type distribution, or in the activity of several muscle enzymes (Mg-stimulated ATPase, myokinase, or lactate dehydrogenase) in the contralateral musculature (Krotkiewski et al., 1979). In the experiment conducted by Moritani and DeVries (1979) discussed above, the time course of muscle hypertrophy and EMG amplitude were also monitored in the contralateral, untrained muscle group. Although the training resulted in no increase in limb girth, the maximum EMG amplitude increased with approximately the same time course as the increase in strength of the contralateral arm. These results indicate that the strength gain in the untrained limb seems to be mediated by a neural mechanism affecting the efficiency through which motor units can be activated, rather than by some characteristic change in muscle.

Segmental and Long Loop Reflexes

Several efforts have been made to determine what adaptations occur in short-latency reflexes using the electrically-elicited Hoffman (H) reflex as well as the tendon tap (t) reflex. Francis and Tipton (1969) trained subjects using isotonic exercise for six weeks and observed a statistically significant five to six percent decrease in patellar reflex time. More recently, Hakkinen and Komi (1983b), using combined eccentric and concentric training, found no change in patellar reflex latency (interval between tendon tap stimulus and EMG onset) or electromechanical delay (interval between EMG onset and force initiation). However, there was a significant decrease in the EMG/force ratio which the authors attributed to a change in the sensitivity of muscle spindles.

Using the H reflex as an indication of motoneuron excitability, Ginet et al. (1975) reported a higher maximum H reflex amplitude in athletes than non-athletes. Expressed as a function of the maximum electrically-evoked EMG response (the M wave), the H/M ratio was also greater in the athletes. However, Rochcongar et al. (1979) found no difference in the H/M ratio between athletes and non-athletes.

Stimulation of a peripheral nerve often evokes a series of electrical events which appear to be potentiated by voluntary effort (Upton et al., 1971). The first electrical peak following the muscle (or M) response has a latency of approximately 25-30 msec and is termed the V1 wave. Upton and Radford (1975) defined an exitability coefficient (Z) based on the amplitude of the V1 wave at rest as well as during voluntary effort and found higher Z values for a group of sprinters than for a control group using the thenar, hypothenar and extensor digitorum brevis muscles. Milner-Brown et al. (1975) also reported that the late reflex responses in weight lifters were of greater amplitude than those observed in control subjects.

Sale et al. (1983a) found no differences in reflex potentiation between weight lifters and controls for either the V1 wave or the longer latency V2 response using the thenar and triceps surae muscles. However, an additional experiment in which subjects were trained using isometric or isotonic exercise for 9-21 weeks resulted in a potentiated V1 response for 13 out of 17 subjects, and a greater V2 wave in 8 out of 9 subjects, although for neither of the variables was the effect statistically significant (Sale et al., 1983b).

These results suggest that some enhancement of motoneuron excitability may be possible with high-resistance exercise. Milner-Brown et al. (1975) suggested that the site of enhancement may be the direct corticomotoneuronal synapses, resulting in additional motor unit synchronization. While this is certainly one possible adaptation site, the conditions under which these changes in motoneuron excitability occur, as well as the nature of the underlying changes in the nervous system, remain unclear.

Chronic Electrical Stimulation and Muscular Strength

Although few would argue that regular exercise involving muscular overload is an effective stimulus for enhancing muscular strength, efforts have continually been made to discover the ergogenic substance or phenomenon which will eliminate the slogan of weight coaches: "no pain, no gain." While electrical stimulation has been used since the 1700s for therapeutic purposes (cf. Hambrecht & Reswick, 1977), only recently have attempts been made to increase muscular strength using chronic electrical stimulation.

Much of the current interest in the use of electrical stimulation as a muscle strengthening modality can be attributed to the Russian investigator, Y.M. Kots, who has reported success in inducing strength increments of up to 40% over an eight week period (Kots, 1977). However, although Raitsin (1976) obtained slightly greater strength increases with electrical stimulation than with isometric exercise, other experimenters have indicated that stimulation produces strength gains similar to those produced through regular high-resistance training (Currier et al., 1979; Currier & Mann, 1983; Eriksson et al., 1981; Laughman et al., 1983). Electical stimulation does appear to produce muscle fiber hypertrophy (Munsat et al., 1976), as well as increases in capillary density (Sumida, 1984), and oxidative enzyme activity (Eriksson & Haggmark, 1979; Sumida, 1984).

The stimulation protocols used thus far seem to result in gains in isometric strength with lesser gains in dynamic strength (Currier & Mann, 1983; Eriksson et al., 1981; Romero et al., 1982). Although earlier reports failed to produce muscular strength gains from electrical stimulation (Massey et al., 1965), it now seems clear that properly applied electrical stimulation methods can be an effective strengthening stimulus. Because these strength increases appear to be similar (and in many cases inferior) to those achieved through appropriate high-resistance exercise methods, the most promising application of the stimulation treatment may lie in the rehabilitation of immobilized limbs to prevent disuse atrophy (cf. Houston, 1983).

Summary

1. Muscular strength can be increased by a regular program of *isometric exercise* performed at least three times per week using a load of at least 30% of maximal strength. Isometric contractions should be made at several different positions for each muscle group exercised, and should be held for at least six seconds.

2. A more popular method of implementing a high-resistance exercise program involves *isotonic exercise*, using either free weights or specialized weight machines. Isotonic exercise perfomed at least three times per week using loads ranging from 3RM (repetitions maximum) to 8RM generally results in significant gains in strength in 6 to 10 weeks.

3. *Isokinetic exercise* involves a muscle contraction performed at a constant pre-set velocity, using a machine which continually accommodates to the maximal force the individual is capable of exerting. Strength gains achieved using isokinetic exercise are somewhat specific to the velocity at which training occurs.

4. *Eccentric Exercise,* in which the muscle is lengthened during the contraction, produces strength gains similar to those produced by other high-resistance exercise techniques. Muscle soreness is more likely to follow the early stages of eccentric exercise. *Plyometric exercises* such as depth jumping, utilize the eccentric mode of contraction and can be effective in improving scores in the vertical jump and similar motor performance tasks.

5. Increases in the available energy substrate needed for high-resistance exercise, and in the concentration of anaerobic enzymes needed for short-duration activities can be demonstrated following chronic high-resistance training, provided the training is of sufficient duration.

6. Muscle fibers adapt to the chronic overload stimulus by increasing in diameter *(hypertrophy)* which increases overall muscular force capability. Some researchers contend that muscle fiber splitting occurs to produce a greater number of muscle fibers *(hyperplasia),* and this idea needs to be more fully explored.

7. Much of the improvement in muscular strength which occurs during the initial phase of a training program can be attributed to beneficial changes in motor unit firing patterns which result in more economical and more efficient motor performance. Alterations in muscle morphology and muscle metabolism seem to be more important during the later stages of high-resistance training.

8. Exercising one limb produces gains in muscular strength and endurance in the contralateral limb, a phenomenon known as *cross transfer*. The cross transfer effect seems to be mediated by a neural mechanism, and can be used as a rehabilitation treatment to reduce muscle atrophy which normally occurs in immobilized muscle groups.

9. Some improvements in muscular strength can occur through *chronic electrical stimulation*. Resultant strength gains are usually specific to very low velocity movements and similar to those achieved through regular physical exercise. Chronic electrical stimulation seems to be a suitable technique for the rehabilitation of injured and immobilized muscle.

References

Andersen, T., & Kearney, J.T. (1982). Effects of three resistance training programs on muscular strength and absolute and relative endurance. *Research Quarterly for Exercise and Sport, 53,* 1-7.

Andersson, Y., & Edstrom, J.E. (1957). Motor hyperactivity resulting in diameter decrease of peripheral nerves. *Acta Physiologica Scandinavica, 39,* 240-245.

Asmussen, E., Hansen, O., & Lammert, O. (1965). The relation between isometric and dynamic muscle strength. *Communications from the Testing and Observation Institute of National Association for Infantile Paralysis, 20*, 3-11.

Atha, J. (1981). Strengthening muscle. In D.I. Miller (Ed.), *Exercise and Sport Science Reviews* (pp. 1-73). Philadelphia: The Franklin Institute Press.

Bagby, G.J., Sembrowich, W.L., & Gollnick, P.D. (1972). Myosin ATPase and fiber composition from trained and untrained rat skeletal muscle. *American Journal of Physiology, 223*, 1415-1417.

Belka, D.E. (1968). Comparison of dynamic, static, and combination training on dominant wrist flexor muscles. *Research Quarterly, 39*, 244-250.

Berger, R. (1962a). Effect of varied weight training programs on strength. *Research Quarterly, 33*, 168-181.

Berger, R.A. (1962b). Optimum repetitions for the development of strength. *Research Quarterly, 33*, 334-338.

Berger, R.A. (1962c). Comparison of static and dynamic strength increases. *Research Quarterly, 33*, 329-333.

Berger, R.A. (1963). Comparison between static training and various dynamic training programs. *Research Quarterly, 34*, 131-135.

Berger, R.A. (1965). Comparison of the effect of various weight training loads on strength. *Research Quarterly, 36*, 141-146.

Berger, R.A., & Hardage, B. (1967). Effect of maximum loads for each of ten repetitions on strength development. *Research Quarterly, 38*, 715-718.

Blattner, S.E., & Noble, L. (1979). Relative effects of isokinetic and plyometric training on vertical jumping performance. *Research Quarterly, 50*, 583-588.

Bonde-Petersen, F. (1960) Muscle training by static, concentric and eccentric contractions. *Acta Physiologica Scandinavica, 48*, 406-416.

Buresova, M., Gutmann, E., & Klicpera, M. (1969). Effect of tension upon rate of incorporation of amino acids into proteins of cross-striated muscle. *Experientia, 25*, 144-145.

Caiozzo, V.J., Perrine, J.J., & Edgerton, V.R. (1981). Training-induced alterations of the in vivo force-velocity relationship of human muscle. *Journal of Applied Physiology, 51*, 750-754.

Capen, E.K. (1956). Study of four programs of heavy resistance exercises for development of muscular strength. *Research Quarterly, 27*, 132-142.

Carlson, B.R. (1973). Cross transfer during serial isometric trials. *American Corrective Therapy Journal, 27*, 36-39.

Cavagna, G.M. (1977). Storage and utilization of elastic energy in skeletal muscle. In R.S. Hutton (Ed.), *Exercise and Sport Sciences Reviews* (pp. 89-129). Santa Barbara: Journal Publishing Affiliates.

Cerquiglini, S., Figura, F., Marchetti, M., & Salleo, A. (1973). Evaluation of athletic fitness in weight-lifters through biomechanical, bioelectrical and bioacoustical data. In S. Cerquiglini, A. Venerando, & J. Wartenweiler (Eds.), *Medicine and Sport: Biomechanics III* (pp. 189-195). Basel: Karger.

Clarke, D.H. (1973). Adaptations in strength and muscular endurance resulting from exercise. In J.H. Wilmore (Ed.), *Exercise and Sport Sciences Reviews* (pp. 73-102). New York: Academic.

Coleman, A.E. (1969). Effect of unilateral isometric and isotonic contractions on the strength of the contralateral limb. *Research Quarterly, 40*, 490-995.

Costill, D., Coyle, E.F., Fink, W.F., Lesmes, G.R., & Witzmann, F.A. (1979). Adaptations in skeletal muscle following strength training. *Journal of Applied Physiology, 46*, 96-99.

Cotten, D. (1967). Relationship of the duration of sustained voluntary isometric contraction to changes in endurance and strength. *Research Quarterly, 38*, 366-374.

Coyle, E.F., Feiring, D.C., Rotkis, T.C., Cote, R.W., III, Roby, F.B., Lee, W., &

Wilmore, J.H. (1981). Specificity of power improvements through slow and fast isokinetic training. *Journal of Applied Physiology, 51,* 1437-1442.

Currier, D.P., Lehman, J., & Lightfoot, P. (1979). Electrical stimulation in exercise of the quadriceps femoris muscle. *Physical Therapy, 59,* 1508-1512.

Currier, D.P., & Mann, R. (1983). Muscular strength development by electrical stimulation in healthy individuals. *Physical Therapy, 63,* 915-921.

Darcus, H.D., & Salter, N. (1955). The effect of repeated muscle exertion on muscle strength. *Journal of Physiology, 12,* 325-336.

Davies, C.T.M., & Young, K. (1983). Effect of training at 30 and 100% maximal isometric force (MVC) on the contractile properties of the triceps surae in man. *Journal of Physiology, 336,* 22P-23P.

DeLateur, B., Lehmann, J., & Fordyce, W.E. (1968). A test of the DeLorme axiom. *Archives of Physical Medicine and Rehabilitation, 49,* 245-248.

DeLateur, B., Lehmann, J., Stonebridge, J., & Warren, C.G. (1972a). Isotonic versus isometric exercise: A double-shift transfer-of-training study. *Archives of Physical Medicine, 53,* 212-216

DeLateur, B., Lehmann, J.F., Warren, C.G., Stonebridge, J., Funita, G., Cokelet, K., & Egbert, S. (1972b). Comparison of effectiveness of isokinetic and isotonic exercise in quadriceps strengthening. *Archives of Physical Medicine and Rehabilitation, 53,* 60-64.

DeLorme, T.L. (1945). Restoration of muscle power by heavy-resistance exercises. *Journal of Bone & Joint Surgery, 27,* 645-667.

DeLorme, T.L., & Watkins, A.L. (1948). Techniques of progressive resistance exercise. *Archives of Physical Medicine, 29,* 263-273.

Dobrovolski, I. (1972). News in Strength Development. *Yessis Review of Soviet Physical Education and Sports, 7,* 71-75.

Dons, B., Bollerup, K., Bonde-Petersen, F., & Hancke, S. (1979). The effect of weight-lifting exercise related to muscle fiber composition and cross-sectional area in humans. *European Journal of Applied Physiology, 40,* 95-106.

Doss, W.S., & Karpovich, P.V. (1965). A comparison of concentric, eccentric and isometric strength of elbow flexors. *Journal of Applied Physiology, 20,* 351-353.

Edds, M.V.(1950). Hypertrophy of nerve fibers to functionally overloaded muscles. *Journal of Comparative Neurology, 93,* 259-275.

Edington, D.W., & Edgerton, V.R. (1976). *The biology of physical activity.* Boston: Houghton Mifflin.

Eriksson, E., & Haggmark, T. (1979). Comparison of isometric muscle training and electrical stimulation suplementing isometric muscle training in the recovery after major knee ligament surgery. *American Journal of Sports Medicine, 7,* 169-171.

Eriksson, E., Haggmark, T., Kiessling, K.H., & Karlsson, J. (1981). Effects of electrical stimulation on human skeletal muscle. *International Journal of Sports Medicine, 2,* 18-22.

Exner, G.U., Staudte, H.W., & Pette, D. (1973). Isometric training of rats: Effects upon fast and slow muscle and modification by an anabolic hormone (nandrolone decanoate). *Pflugers Archiv, 345,* 15-22.

Fournier, M., Ricci, J., Taylor, A.W., Ferguson, R.J., Montpetit, R.R., & Chaitman, B.R. (1982). Skeletal muscle adaptation in adolescent boys: Sprint and endurance training and detraining. *Medicine and Science in Sports and Exercise, 14,* 453-456.

Francis, P.R., & Tipton, C.M. (1969). Influence of a weight training program on quadriceps reflex time. *Medicine and Science in Sports, 1,* 91-94.

Friden, J. (1984a). Muscle soreness after exercise: implications of morphological changes. *International Journal of Sports Medicine, 5,* 57-66.

Friden, J. (1984b). Changes in human skeletal muscle induced by long-term eccentric exercise. *Cell and Tissue Research, 236,* 365-372.

Gardner, G.W. (1963). Specificity of strength changes of the exercised and nonexercised limb following isometric training. *Research Quarterly, 34,* 98-101.

Gerchman, L.R., Edgerton, V.R., & Carrow, R.E. (1975). Effects of physical training on the histochemistry and morphology of vental motor neurons. *Experimental Neurology, 49,* 790-801.

Gillam, G.M. (1981). Effects of frequency of weight training on muscle strength enhancement. *Journal of Sports Medicine and Physical Fitness, 21,* 432-436.

Gillespie, A.C., Fox, E.L., & Merola, A.J. (1982). Enzyme adaptations in rat skeletal muscle after two intensities of treadmill training. *Medicine and Science in Sports and Exercise, 14,* 461-466.

Gilliam, T.B., Roy, R.R., Taylor, J.F., Heusner, W.W., & Van Huss, W.D. (1977). Ventral motor neuron alterations in rat spinal cord after chronic exercise. *Experientia, 33,* 665-667.

Ginet, J., Guiheneuc, P., Prevot, M., & Vecchierini-Blineau, F. (1975). Etude comparative due recrutement de la response reflexe monosynaptique du soleaire (reflexe h) chez des sujets non entraines et chez des sportifs. *Medecine du Sport, 49,* 55-64.

Goldspink, G., & Howells, K.F. (1974). Work-induced hypertrophy in exercised normal muscles of different ages and reversibility of hypertrophy after cessation of exercise. *Journal of Physiology, 239,* 179-193.

Gollnick, P.D. (1982). Relationship of strength and endurance with skeletal muscle structure and metabolic potential. *International Journal of Sports Medicine, 3,* 26-32.

Gollnick, P.D., Parsons, D., Riedy, M., Moore, R.L., & Timson, B. F. (1983). An evaluation of mechanisms modulating muscle size in response to varying perturbations. In K.T. Borer, D.W. Edington, & T.P. White (Eds.), *Frontiers of Exercise Biology* (pp. 27-50). Champaign, IL: Human Kinetics.

Gollnick, P.D., Timson, B.F., Moore, R.L., & Riedy, M. (1981). Muscular enlargement and number of fibers in skeletal muscle of rats. *Journal of Applied Physiology, 50,* 936-943.

Gonyea, W.J. (1980). Role of exercise in inducing increases in skeletal muscle fiber number. *Journal of Applied Physiology, 48,* 421-426.

Gonyea, W.J., & Ericson, G.C. (1976). An experimental model for the study of exercise-induced skeletal muscle hypertrophy. *Journal of Applied Physiology, 40,* 630-633.

Gonyea, W.J., Ericson, G.C., & Bonde-Petersen, F. (1977). Skeletal muscle fiber splitting induced by weight-lifting exercise in cats. *Acta Physiologica Scandinavica, 99,* 105-109.

Gordon, E.E., Kowalski, K., & Fritts, M. (1967). Protein changes in quadriceps muscle of rat with repetitive exercise. *Archives of Physcial Medicine and Rehabilitation, 48,* 296-303.

Grimby, G. (1982). Isokinetic training. *International Journal of Sports Medicine, 3,* 61-64.

Grimby, G., Bjorntorp, P., Fahlen, M., Hoskins, T.A., Gook, O., Oxhoj, H., & Saltin, B. (1973). Metabolic effects of isometric training. *Scandinavian Journal of Clinical Laboratory Investigation, 31,* 301-305.

Grimby, G., Gustafsson, E., Peterson, L., & Renstrom, P. (1980). Quadriceps function and training after knee ligament surgery. *Medicine and Science in Sports and Exercise, 12,* 70-75.

Gutmann, E., & Hajek, I. (1971). Differential reaction of muscle to excessive use in compensatory hypertrophy and increased physical activity. *Physiologia Bohemoslovaca, 20,* 205-212.

Hakkinen, K., & Komi, P.V. (1983a). Electromyographic changes during strength training and detraining. *Medicine and Science in Sports and Exercise, 15,* 455-460.

Hakkinen, K., & Komi, P.V. (1983b). Changes in neuromuscular performance in voluntary and reflex contraction during strength training in man. *International Journal of Sports Medicine, 4*, 282-288.

Hakkinen, K., Komi, P.V., & Tesch, P.A. (1981). Effect of combined concentric and eccentric strength training and detraining on force-time, muscle fiber and metabolic characteristics of leg extensor muscles. *Scandinavian Journal of Sports Science, 3*, 50-58.

Hall-Craggs, E.C.B. (1972). The significance of longitudinal fibre division in skeletal muscle. *Journal of the Neurological Sciences, 15*, 27-33.

Hall-Craggs, E.C.B., & Lawrence, C.A. (1970). Longitudinal fibre division in skeletal muscle. A light and electron-microscopic study. *Zeitschrift fur Zellforschung, 109*, 481-494.

Hambrecht, T.T., & Reswick, J.B. (Eds.). (1977). *Functional Electrical Stimulation*. New York: Dekker.

Hearn, G.R., & Gollnick, P.D. (1961). Effects of exercise on the adenosine triphosphatase activity in skeletal and heart muscle of rats. *International Zeitschrift fur Angewandte Physiologie, 19*, 23-26.

Herbison, G.J., Jaweed, M.M., & Ditunno, J.F. (1981). Response of type I fibers to weight lifting in rat plantaris. *Archives of Physical Medicine and Rehabilitation, 62*, 342-344.

Hettinger, T., & Muller, E.A. (1953). Muskelleistung and Muskeltraining. *Internationale Zeitschrift fur Angewandte Physiologie einschleisslich Arbeitsphysiologie, 15*, 111-126.

Hickson, R.C. (1980). Interference of strength development by simultaneously training for strength and endurance. *European Journal of Applied Physiology, 45*, 255-263.

Hickson, R.C., Heusner, W.W., & Van Huss, W.D. (1975). Skeletal muscle enzyme alterations after sprint and endurance training. *Journal of Applied Physiology, 40*, 868-872.

Hislop, H.J. (1963). Quantitative changes in human muscular strength during isometric exercise. *Journal of the American Physical Therapy Association, 43*, 21-38.

Ho, K., Roy, R., Taylor, J., Heusner, W., Van Huss, W., & Carrow, R. (1977). Muscle fiber splitting with weight-lifting exercise. *Medicine and Science in Sports, 9*, 65.

Hosler, W.W. (1977). Electromyographic and girth considerations relative to strength training. *Perceptual and Motor Skills, 44*, 293-294.

Houston, M.E. (1983). Effects of electrical stimulation on skeletal muscle of injured and healthy athletes. *Canadian Journal of Applied Sport Sciences, 8*, 49-51.

Houston, M.E., Froese, E.A., Valeriote, S.P., Green, H.J., & Ranney, D.A. (1983). Muscle performance, morphology and metabolic capacity during strength training and detraining: a one leg model. *European Journal of Applied Physiology, 51*, 25-35.

Howald, H. (1982). Training-induced morphological and functional changes in skeletal muscle. *International Journal of Sports Medicine, 3*, 1-12.

Jansson, E., Sjodin, B., & Tesch, P. (1978). Changes in muscle fibre type distribution in man after physical training. *Acta Physiologica Scandinavica, 104*, 235-237.

Johnson, B.L. (1972). Eccentric vs. concentric muscle training for strength development. *Medicine and Science in Sports, 4*, 111-115.

Josenhans, W.K. (1962). An evaluation of some methods of improving muscle strength. *Revue Canadiennes Biologie, 21*, 315-323.

Kamen, G. (1983). The acquisition of maximal isometric plantar flexor strength: a force-time curve analysis. *Journal of Motor Behavior, 15*, 63-73.

Kanehisa, H., & Mihashita, M. (1983). Effect of isometric and isokinetic muscle training on static strength and dynamic power. *European Journal of Applied Physiology, 50*, 365-371.

Klein, K.K. (1955). A study of cross transfer of muscular strength and endurance resulting from progressive resistive exercise following injury. *Journal of the Association for Physical & Mental Rehabilitation, 9,* 159-161.

Klein, K.K., & Williams, H.E. (1954). Research: A study of cross transfer of muscular strength gains during reconditioning of knee injuries. *Journal of the Association for Physical & Mental Rehabilitation, 8,* 52-53.

Komi, P.V., & Buskirk, E.R. (1972). Effect of eccentric and concentric muscle conditioning on tension and electrical activity of human muscle. *Ergonomics, 15,* 417-434.

Komi, P.V., Viitasalo, J.T., Havu, M., Thorstensson, A., Sjodbin, B., & Karlsson, J. (1977). Skeletal muscle fibers and muscle enzyme activities in monozygous and dizygous twins of both sexes. *Acta Physiologica Scandinavica, 100,* 385-392.

Komi, P.V., Viitasalo, J.T., Rauramaa, R., & Vihko, V. (1978). Effect of isometric strength training on mechanical, electrical, and metabolic aspects of muscle function. *European Journal of Applied Physiology, 40,* 45-55.

Kots, Y.M. (1977). Unpublished lecture and laboratory notes, distributed by Numed, Inc., Joliet, IL.

Kowalski, K., Gordon, E.E., Martinez, A., & Adamek, J. (1969). Changes in enzyme activities of various muscle fiber types in rat induced by different exercises. *The Journal of Histochemistry and Cytochemistry, 17,* 601-607.

Krotkiewski, M., Aniansson, A., Grimby, G., Bjorntorp, P., & Sjostrom, L. (1979). The effect of unilateral isokinetic strength training on local adipose and muscle tissue morphology, thickness, and enzymes. *European Journal of Applied Physiology, 42,* 271-281.

Kruse, R.D., Mathews, D.K. (1958). Bilateral effects of unilateral exercise: Experimental study based on 120 subjects. *Archives of Physical Medicine and Rehabilitation, 39,* 371-376.

Lang, F., Govind, C.K., & Costello, W.J. (1978). Experimental transformation of muscle fiber properties in lobster. *Science, 201,* 1037-1039.

Laughman, R.K., Youdas, J.W., Garrett, T.R., & Chao, E.Y.S. (1983). Strength changes in the normal quadriceps femoris muscle as a result of electrical stimulation. *Physical Therapy,* 494-499.

Lawrence, M.S., Meyer, H.R., & Matthews, N.L. (1962). Comparative increase in muscle strength in the quadriceps femoris by isometric and isotonic exercise and effects on the contralateral muscle. *Journal of the American Physical Therapy Association, 42,* 15-20.

Laycoe, R.R., & Marteniuk, R.G. (1971). Learning and tension as factors in static strength gains produced by static and eccentric training. *Research Quarterly, 42,* 299-306.

Leighton, J.R., Holmes, D., Benson, J., Wooten, B., & Schmerer, R. (1967). A study on the effectiveness of ten different methods of progressive resistance exercise on the development of strength, flexibility, girth and body weight. *Journal of American Physical and Mental Rehabilitation, 21,* 78-81.

Lesh, M., Parmley, W.W., Hamosh M., Kaufmann, S., & Sonnenblick, E.J. (1968). Effects of acute hypertrophy on the contractile properties of skeletal muscle. *American Journal of Physiology, 214,* 685.

Lesmes, G.R., Costill, D.L., Coyle, E.F., & Fink, W.J. (1978). Muscle strength and power changes during maximal isokinetic training. *Medicine and Science in Sports, 10,* 266-269.

Lindh, M. (1979). Increase of muscle strength from isometric quadriceps exercises at different knee angles. *Scandinavian Journal of Rehabilitation Medicine, 11,* 33-36.

MacDougall, J.D., Ward, G.R., Sale, D.G., & Sutton, J.R. (1977). Biochemical adaptation of human skeletal muscle to heavy resistance training and immobilization. *Journal of Applied Physiology, 43,* 700-703.

Mackova, E., & Hnik, P. (1971). Compensatory muscle hypertrophy in the rat induced by tenotomy of synergistic muscles. *Experientia, 27,* 1039-1040.

Mannheimer, J.S. (1969). A comparison of strength gain between concentric and eccentric contractions. *Physical Therapy, 49,* 1201-1207.

Massey, B.H., Nelson, R.C., & Sharkey, B.C. (1965). Effects of high frequency electrical stimulation on the size and strength of skeletal muscle. *Journal of Sports Medicine & Physical Fitness, 5,* 136-144.

Mathews, D.K., Shay, C.T., Godin, F., & Hodgdon, R. (1956). Gross transfer effects of training on strength and endurance. *Research Quarterly, 27,* 206-212.

Mayberry, R.P. (1958). Isometric exercise and the cross-transfer of training effect as it related to strength. *Proceedings of the 62nd National College Physical Education Association for Men.* (pp. 155-158).

McDonagh, M.J.N., & Davies, C.T.M. (1984). Adaptive response of mammalian skeletal muscle to exercise with high loads. *European Journal of Applied Physiology, 52,* 139-155.

McMorris, R.O., & Elkins, E.C. (1954). A study of production and evaluation of muscular hypertrophy. *Archives of Physical Medicine and Rehabilitation, 35,* 420-426.

Meyers, C.R. (1967). Effects of two isometric routines on strength, size and endurance in exercised and nonexercised arms. *Research Quarterly, 38,* 430-440.

Milner-Brown, H.S., Stein, R.B., & Lee, R.G. (1975). Synchronization of human motor units: Possible roles of exercise and supraspinal reflexes. *Electroencephalography and Clinical Neurophysiology, 38,* 245-254.

Moffroid, M.T., & Whipple, R.H. (1970). Specificity of speed of exercise. *Physical Therapy, 50,* 1692-1700.

Moffroid, M.T., & Whipple, R.H., Hofkosh, J., Lowman, E., & Thistle, H. (1969). A study of isokinetic exercise. *Journal of the American Physical Therapy Association, 49,* 735-747.

Moritani, T., & DeVries, H.A. (1979). Neural factors versus hypertrophy in the time course of muscle strength gain. *American Journal of Physcial Medicine, 58,* 115-130.

Morpurgo, B. (1897). Uber Activitates-hypertrophie der willkurlichen muskeln. *Virchow's Archiv fur Pathologische anatomie und Physiologie, 150,* 522-554.

Munsat, T.L., McNeal, D., & Waters, R. (1976). Effects of nerve stimulation on human muscle. *Archives of Neurology, 33,* 608-617.

Muntener, M. (1982). A rapid and reversible muscle fiber transformation in the rat. *Experimental Neurology, 77,* 668-678.

Noland, R.P., & Kuckhoff, A. (1954). An adapted progressive resistance exercise device. *The Physical Therapy Review, 34,* 3233-338.

O'Shea, P. (1966). Effect of selected weight training programs on the development of strength and muscle hypertrophy. *Research Quarterly, 37,* 95-102.

Pipes, T.V. (1978). Variable resistance versus constant resistance strength training in adult males. *European Journal of Applied Physiology, 39,* 27-35.

Raitsin, L.M. (1976). The effectiveness of isometric and electro-stimulated training on muscle strength at different joint angles. *Yessis Review of Physical Education & Sports, 11,* 33-35.

Raitsin, L.M., & Saraniya, S.K. (1975). The influence of body position on effectiveness of strength training. *Theory and Practice of Physical Culture, 7,* 65-66.

Rarick, G.L., & Larsen, G.L. (1958). Observations on frequency and intensity of isometric muscular effort in developing static muscular strength in postpubescent males. *Research Quarterly, 29,* 333-341.

Rasch, P.J. (1974). The present status of negative (eccentric) exercise: A review. *American Corrective Therapy Journal, 28,* 77-94.

Rasch, P.J., & Morehouse, L.E. (1957). Effect of static and dynamic exercises on muscular strength and hypertrophy. *Journal of Applied Physiology, 11,* 29-34.

Rawlinson, W.A., & Gould, M.K. (1959). Biochemical adaptations as a response to exercise: Adenosine triphosphatase and creatine phosphokinase activity in muscles of exercised rats. *Biochemical Journal, 73,* 44-48.

Reitsma, W. (1970). Some structural changes in skeletal muscles of the rat after intensive training. *Acta Morphologica Neerlando-Scandinavica, 7,* 229-246.

Rochcongar, P., Dassonville, J., & LeBars, R. (1979). Modifications du Reflexe de Hoffmann en Fonktion de l'Entrainement chez le Sportif. *European Journal of Applied Physiology, 40,* 165-170.

Rohmert, W., & Preising, M. (1968). Rechts-Links vergleich bei isometrischem Armuskeltraining mit verschiedenem Trainingeriez. *Sportarzt und Sportmedizin, 19,* 43-55.

Roman, R.A. (1974). The training of Bulgarian weight lifters. *Yessis Review of Sports, 9,* 109-111.

Romero, J.A., Sanford, T.L., Schroeder, R.V., & Fahey, T.D. (1982). The effects of electrical stimulation of normal quadriceps on strength and girth. *Medicine and Science in Sports and Exercise, 14,* 194-197.

Roy, R., Ho, K., Taylor, J., Heusner, W., & Van Huss, W. (1977). Alterations in a histochemical profile induced by weight-lifting exercise. *Medicine and Science in Sports, 9,* 65.

Rozier, C.K., & Elder, J.D. (1980). Cross-training effects of isokinetic exercise on skeletal muscle. *International Journal of Rehabilitation Research, 3,* 71-73.

Sale, D.G., Upton, A.R.M., McComas, A.J., & MacDougall, J.D. (1983a). Neuromuscular function in weight-trainers. *Experimental Neurology, 82,* 521-531.

Sale, D.G., MacDougall, J.D., Upton, A.R.M., & McComas, A.J. (1983b). Effect of strength training upon motoneuron excitability in man. *Medicine and Science in Sports and Exercise, 15,* 57-62.

Salmons, S., & Sreter, F.A. (1976). Significance of impulse activity in the transformation of skeletal muscle type. *Nature, 263,* 30-34.

Saplinskas, J.S., Chobotas, M.A., & Yashchaninas, I.I. (1979). Discharge patterns of motor units during increasingly strong contraction of the rectus femoris muscle depending on level of training and athletic specialization. *Human Physiology, 5,* 639-642.

Saplinskas, J.S., & Yaschaninas, J.J. (1982). Activity of single motor units during prolonged muscle activity at various levels of contraction performed by nontrained persons and by highly specialized athletes. *Electromyography and Clinical Neurophysiology, 22,* 365-375.

Schantz, P., Billeter, R., Henriksson, J., & Jansson, E. (1982). Training-induced increase in myofibrillar ATPase intermediate fibers in human skeletal muscle. *Muscle & Nerve, 5,* 628-636.

Schantz, P., & Henriksson, J. (1983). Increases in myofibrillar ATPase intermediate human skeletal muscle fibers in response to endurance training. *Muscle & Nerve, 6,* 553-556.

Schiaffino, S., & Hanzlikova, V. (1970). On the mechanism of compensatory hypertrophy in skeletal muscles. *Experientia, 26,* 152-153.

Schiaffino, S., Pierobon Bormioli, S., & Aloisi, M. (1979). Fiber branching and formation of new fibers during compensatory muscle hypertrophy. In A. Mauro (Ed.), *Muscle Regeneration* (pp. 177-188). New York: Raven.

Scripture, E.W., Smith, T.L., & Brown, E.M. (1894). On the education of muscular control and power. *Studies Yale Psychological Laboratory, 2,* 114-119.

Seaborne, D., & Taylor, A.W. (1981). The effects of isokinetic exercise on vastus lateralis fibre morphology and biochemistry. *Journal of Sports Medicine and Physical Fitness, 21,* 365-370.

Seliger, V., Dolejs, L., Karas, V., & Pachlopnikova, I. (1968). Adaptation of trained athletes' energy expenditure to repeated concentric and eccentric muscle contractions. *Internationale Zeitschrift fur angewandte Physiologie einschleisslich Ar-

beitsphysiologie, 26, 227-234.

Shaver, L.G. (1970). Effects of training on relative muscular endurance in ipsilateral and contralateral arms. *Medicine and Science in Sports, 2,* 165-171.

Shaver, L.G. (1975). Cross transfer effects of conditioning and deconditioning on muscular strength. *Ergonomics, 18,* 9-16.

Singh, M., & Karpovich, P.V. (1967). Effect of eccentric training of agonists on antagonistic muscles. *Journal of Applied Physiology, 23,* 742-745.

Slater-Hammel, A.T. (1950). Bilateral effects of muscle activity. *Research Quarterly, 21,* 203-209.

Staudte, H.W., Exner, G.U., & Pette, D. (1973). Effects of short-term, high intensity (sprint) training on some contractile characteristics of fast and slow muscle of the rat. *Pflugers Archiv, 344,* 159-168.

Stepanov, A.S., & Burlakov, M.L. (1961). Electrophysiological investigation of fatigue in muscular activity. *Sechenov Physiological Journal of the USSR, 47,* 43-47.

Stevens, R. (1980). Isokinetic vs isotonic training in the development of lower body strength and power. *Scholastic Coach, 4* (6), 74-76.

Stone, M.H., Johnson, R.L., & Carter, D.R. (1979). A short term comparison of two different methods of resistance training on leg strength and power. *Athletic Training, 14,* 158-160.

Stone, M.H., O'Bryant, H., & Garhammer, J. (1981). A hypothetical model for strength training. *Journal of Sports Medicine and Physical Fitness, 21,* 342-351.

Sumida, Y. (1984). Effect of electrical stimulation on healthy skeletal muscles. *Hiroshima Journal of Medical Sciences, 33,* 35-46.

Talag, T.S. (1973). Residual muscular soreness as influenced by concentric, eccentric, and static contractions. *Research Quarterly, 44,* 458-469.

Thistle, H.G., Hislop, H.J., Moffroid, M., & Lowman, E.W. (1967). Isokinetic contractions: a new concept of resistive exercise. *Archives of Physical Medicine and Rehabilitation, 48,* 279-282.

Thorstensson, A., Hulten, B., von Dobeln, W., & Karlsson, J. (1976a). Effect of strength training on enzyme activities and fibre characteristics in human skeletal muscle. *Acta Physiologica Scandinavica, 96,* 392-398.

Thorstensson, A., Karlsson, J., Viitasalo, J.H.T., Luhtanen, P., & Komi, P.V. (1976b). Effect of strength training on EMG of human skeletal muscle. *Acta Physiologica Scandinavica, 98,* 232-236.

Thorstensson, A., Sjodin, B., & Karlsson, J. (1975). Enzyme activities and muscle strength after "sprint training" in man. *Acta Physiologica Scandinavica, 94,* 313-318.

Tomanek, R.J., & Tipton, C.M. (1967). Influence of exercise and tenectomy on the morphology of a muscle nerve. *Anatomical Record, 159,* 105-114.

Upton, A.R.M., Mccomas, A.J., & Sica, R.E.P. (1971). Potentiation of late responses evoked in muscles during effort. *Journal of Neurology, Neurosurgery & Psychiatry, 34,* 699-711.

Upton, A.R.M., & Radford, P.F. (1975). Motoneurone excitability in elite sprinters. In P.V. Komi (Ed.), *Biomechanics V-A* (pp. 82-87). Baltimore: University Park.

Van Linge, B. (1962). The response of muscle to strenuous exercise. *Journal of Bone and Joint Surgery, 44B,* 711-721.

Walters, E., Steward, C.L., & Leclaire, J.F. (1960). Effect of short bouts of isometric and isotonic contractions on muscular strength and endurance. *American Journal of Physical Medicine, 39,* 131-141.

Ward, J., & Fisk, G.H. (1964). The difference in response of the quadriceps and the biceps brachii muscles to isometric and isotonic exercise. *Archives of Physical Medicine and Rehabilitation, 45,* 614-620.

Watt, P.W., Goldspink, G., & Ward, P.S. (1984). Changes in fiber type composition in growing muscle as a result of dynamic exercise and static overload. *Muscle &*

Nerve, 7, 50-53.

Watt, P.W., Kelly, F.J., Goldspink, D.F., & Goldspink, G. (1982). Exercise-induced morphological and biochemical changes in skeletal muscles of the rat. *Journal of Applied Physiology, 53,* 1144-1151.

Wedeles, C.H.A. (1949). The effect of increasing the functional load of a muscle on the composition of its motor nerve. *Journal of Anatomy, 83,* 57.

Whitley, J.D. (1967). The influence of static and dynamic training on angular strength performance. *Ergonomics, 10,* 305-310.

Wilkerson, J.E., & Evonuk, E. (1971). Changes in cardiac and skeletal muscle myosin ATPase activities after exercise. *Journal of Applied Physiology, 30,* 328-330.

Wilt, F. (1975). Plyometrics: What it is—how it works. *Athletic Journal, 55*(76), 76, 89-90.

Wissler, C., & Richardson, W.W. (1900). Diffusion of the motor impulse. *Psychological Reviews, 7,* 29-38.

Withers, R.T. (1970). Effect of varied weight-training loads on the strength of university freshmen. *Research Quarterly, 41,* 110-114.

Zinovieff, .N. (1951). Heavy resistance exercise: The Oxford technique. *British Journal of Physical Medicine, 14,* 129-132.

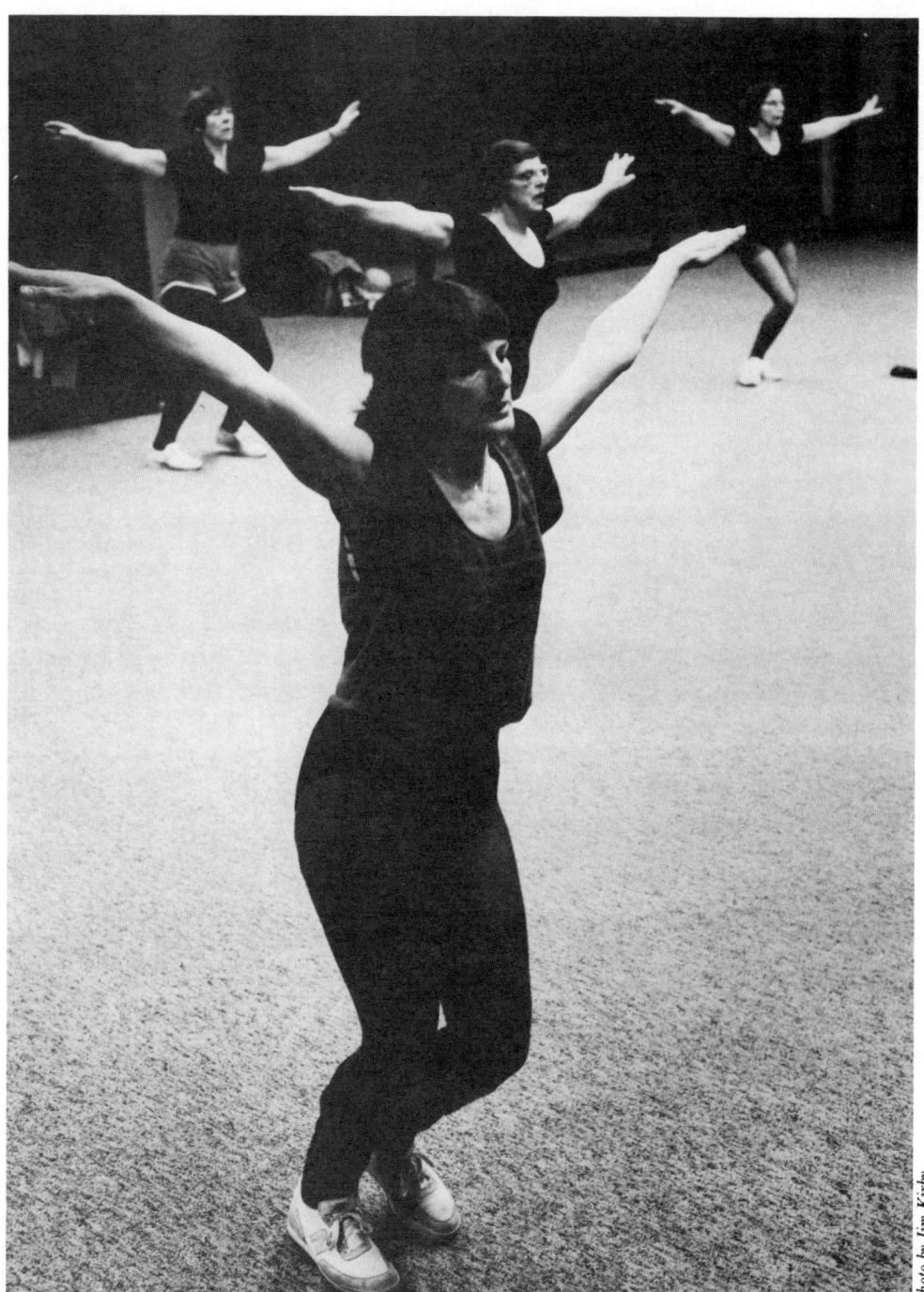

photo by Jim Kirby

CHAPTER EIGHT

Menstruation, Pregnancy, and Menopause

Christine L. Wells
Department of Health and Physical Education
Arizona State University
Tempe, Arizona

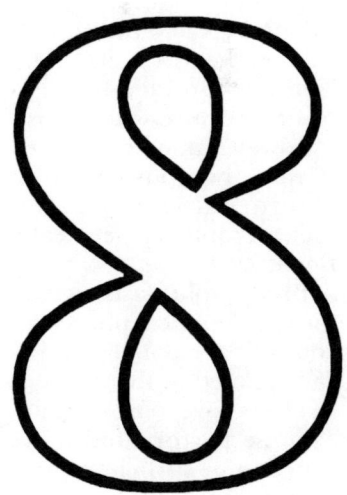

There are numerous myths regarding the interrelationships of exercise and menstrual function. Considerable misinformation exists about the effects of exercise on menstrual function, as well as the effects of menstrual function on exercise performance. For years the International Olympic Committee believed that sports training and competition were detrimental to proper reproductive function in women. This was the reason given for denying women the opportunity to participate in long-distance running in the Olympic Games. It was not until the American College of Sports Medicine published an opinion statement ("The Participation of", 1979) that virtually eliminated the medical objections to long-distance running by women that the 3000 meter and marathon races were added to the 1984 Olympic roster of events. This matter remains a major stumbling block to the active participation of girls and women in strenous physical activity. Despite much interest in the topic, however, there has not been a systematic review of the scientific literature regarding exercise and menstrual function until recently (Wells, 1985).

This chapter will review what is known about the female reproductive system and physical activity. The first part of the chapter will deal with the menstrual cycle and exercise; the middle part with pregnancy and exercise; and the last part with the nonmenstruating menopausal woman. For a comprehensive review of the basic anatomy and physiology of human menstrual function, see Wells (1985, Chapter 4).

The Menstrual Cycle and Physical Activity

Variations in physiological baseline due to the menstrual cycle. A large number of physical, biochemical, and systemic parameters have been reported to vary systematically with the three phases of the menstrual cycle. Unfortuately, not all investigators have agreed as to the direction of change or to the degree of change. Table 1, abstracted from an extensive review by Southam and Gonzaga (1965), describes some of the these changes.

The most consistent variation in physiological baseline is the alteration in basal body temperature. Following ovulation, basal body temperature rises, remains slightly elevated throughout the luteal phase, and falls at menstrual flow. In some women, heart rate is higher during the time that body temperature is elevated. There is considerable disagreement in the literature about variation in arterial blood pressure with menstrual function.

Lower values for hematocrit, hemoglobin, and red blood cell number are frequently reported during menstrual flow. However, these changes are more likely to reflect shifts in fluid volume than changes in red cell production. Nevertheless, capillary permeability and fragility are known to change with hormonal fluctuation.

Breast volume is significantly increased (by about 100 ml) in many women during the luteal phase. This is probably caused by a combination of hormonally controlled vascular and lymphatic changes, as well as structural changes specifically related to the influence of progesterone.

The above observations give rise to two important questions in regard to exercise performance: Are the reported variations in baseline with menstrual function of sufficient physiological significance to cause differences in exercise performance with menstrual phase? Or is there such individual variation that this question can only be answered for each woman independently of the next? The remainder of this part of the chapter is directed toward answering these questions.

The effects of the menstrual cycle on physical performance. Observations dealing with this question published prior to 1970 are equivocal. If one study reported a higher heart rate or blood pressure with a specific exercise task, another reported a contrary result with a similar task or subject group. More sophisticated investiga-

Table 1.
Changes in Physiological Baseline During the Menstrual Cycle

ITEM	CHARACTER OF CHANGE
Temperature	Decrease at time of ovulation then sharp rise to a plateau
Blood Pressure	Arterial pressure lower at midcycle
Respiration	Increased ventilation of lung with decreased arterial CO_2 tension in luteal phase
Weight	Some women gain in premenstrual period
Red Blood Cells	Decreased survival time in luteal phase
White Blood Cells	Decrease during menses and proliferative phase
Carbohydrate metabolism	Glucose tolerance less during menses; fasting blood glucose higher during menses
Lactic Acid	Increase at time of ovulation
Cholesterol	Total serum cholesterol rises following menses
Calcium	Lower in premenstrual phase, higher in ovulatory phase
Endocrine	Midcycle peak of total urinary gonadotropins
Thyroid	Premenstrual rise in basal metabolic rate and a fall during menses
Breast	Premenstrual hyperemia and increased size
GI Tract	Increased gastric motility during menses; defecation more frequent 1st and 2nd day of menses; gastric acids increased first half of cycle and fall second half of cycle
Physical Activity	Pedometer measured activity greater during post menstrual phase
Behavior and Emotion	Decreased mental efficiency in premenstrual phase, insomnia more frequent during menses; misdemeanors increase among school girls during menses; suicides and attempted suicides more frequent in premenstrual and menstrual phases; more crime committed same periods
Premenstrual Tension	Premenstrual complaints of breast pain and tenderness, abdominal discomfort, back pains, headache, and depression
Systemic Diseases	More susceptible to infectious diseases and to accidents in immediate premenstrual period; diabetic coma more frequent and insulin requirement increased during menses; allergic conditions worse during menses and premenstrual periods; urinary incontinence worse during luteal phase; more epileptic seizures during premenstrual and menstrual phases

Adapted from Southam, A.L. and F.P. Gonzaga. (1965). Systemic changes during the menstrual cycle. *American Journal of Obstetrics and Gynecology, 91,* 142-165.

tions (more variables, more elaborate equipment, sometimes more extensive experimental control) occurred after 1970, and only those studies will be reviewed here. Doolittle and Engebretsen (1972) studied variations in performance in the 12-minute run-walk, the 600-yard run-walk, the 1.5 mile run-walk, and maximal oxygen uptake in untrained university women. Differences in performance were not related to menstrual phase. Similarly, Stephenson, Kolka, and Wilkerson

(1982) studied variations in response to a series of exercise bouts to exhaustion on days 2, 8, 14, 20, and 26 of the menstrual cycle. They reported no differences relative to menstrual cycle day at any exercise intensity for oxygen uptake, carbon dioxide production, oxygen pulse, total respiratory volume, tidal volume, respiratory rate, or respiratory exchange ratio. In addition, there were no differences in exercise time to exhaustion. Slight elevations in core temperature (T_{re}) occurred during the luteal phase (days 14 and 20) at rest, *and* at submaximal and maximal exercise loads.

Investigations utilizing more highly trained and athletic subject groups have yielded similar metabolic results. Allsen, Parsons, and Bryce (1977) and Martin (1976) studied maximal oxygen uptake in college athletes, and concurred that there were no cyclic variations attributable to menstrual phase.

Schoene, Robertson, Pierson, and Peterson (1981) investigated the influence of progesterone on ventilation during exercise. Progesterone had previously been implicated as an agent causing hyperventilation in pregnancy and during the luteal phase of the menstrual cycle. It was conceivable, then, that the endogenous surge of progesterone during the luteal phase could stimulate the ventilatory drive during exercise. Because this could lead to premature respiratory fatigue, such a response could be deleterious to maximal performance. Schoene et al. (1981) studied this problem in three groups of women: six outstanding athletes with normal menstrual function; six sedentary controls with normal menstrual function; and a group of outstanding athletes who were amenorrheic.

Resting and exercise ventilation values were *elevated* in the luteal phase in the menstruating subjects. Both hypoxic (breathing air low in CO_2) and hypercapnic (breathing air high in CO_2) ventilatory responses were increased in the luteal phase, but the athletic subjects had a more blunted response than the sendentary subjects. These results were not duplicated in the amenorrheic subjects, who, of course, did not display cyclic variations in progesterone. Neither the menstruating athletes nor the amenorrheic athletes, however, displayed cyclic differences in oxygen uptake, carbon dioxide production, maximum exercise time, or onset of anaerobic threshold. The authors concluded that although ventilatory responses were elevated in menstruating women during the luteal phase, the increase in ventilation did not adversely affect the exercise performance of trained athletes.

Elevated basal body temperature during the luteal phase is thought to be the effect of progesterone on the hypothalmic "set-point". However, no menstrual phase differences were found for rectal temperature, mean skin temperature, mean body temperature, body heat content, sweating rate, evaporative heat loss, oxygen uptake, ventilation volume, or oxygen pulse in untrained and unacclimatized women walking in a hot-dry environment (48 C/118 F) (Wells & Horvath, 1973, 1974). In addition, there were no differences in plasma proteins, lactic acid, or serum sodium or potassium values with menstrual phase. These results were recently duplicated at lower work loads in three environments (28 C, 35 C, and 48 C) by Horvath and Drinkwater (1982). These investigators concluded that hormonal fluctuations in estradiol and progesterone during the menstrual cycle did *not* influence response to exercise in the heat.

Survey studies of athletes at World Championships and the Olympic Games have revealed that elite athletes do not believe menstrual function seriously affects their performance. This is borne out by the fact that women have achieved personal records, national records, Olympic records, and world records at every phase of the menstrual cycle. Of course, this doesn't mean that *all* women can perform at maximal capacity at any time during the menstrual cycle. There are as many individual responses to menstrual function as there are to exercise. Besides, athletic achievement is influenced by numerous physiological, psychological, and environmental variables that probably have more effect on performance than does menstrual phase.

The effects of exercise on the onset of menstrual function. A strenuous lifestyle such as that characteristic of a young athlete (8 to 14 years of age) is associated with a later age at menarche, the first menstrual flow. Puberty, the transitional period between childhood and adulthood, is marked by many physiological changes associated with reproductive development. Although the endocrinology of puberty is not thoroughly understood, the most prevalent theory is that the hypothalamus controls the onset of puberty. It is thought that the immature hypothalamus is extremely sensitive to the small amounts of steroid hormones (estrogens in the case of the female) produced by the gonads and acts to inhibit—in the manner of a negative feedback system—the development of the ovary and other reproductive organs. This occurs by inhibiting the release of luteinizing hormone releasing factor (LH-RF). The result is that follicle stimulating hormone (FSH) and luteinizing hormone (LH) are not produced by the anterior pituitary, and luteinizing hormone (LH) are not produced by the anterior pituitary, and the gonads remain small and undeveloped. Eventually, however, the hypothalamus becomes less sensitive to estrogen, and the system switches to a positive feedback mechanism. At that time, estrogen stimulates the release of LH-RF, and FSH and LH are produced by the pituitary. Shortly thereafter, the sexual organs mature and the secondary sex characteristics of advanced pubertal development become obvious. The subsequent increase in ovarian estrogen and progesterone production stimulate the growth and secretory functions of the endometrial lining of the uterus. Menarche, the first menstrual flow, occurs to slough off this lining. Average age at menarche in the United States ranges from 12.2 to 12.9 years of age.

Table 2. Factors Associated With Menarche	Table 3. Factors Associated With a Later Age at Menarche in Athletes
skeletal maturity (age)	age at entry into sport
breast and pubic hair development	low body fat
body weight	competitive skill level
body composition—body fat	diet
age at peak height velocity	
nutritional status	
family size	
socio-economic background	
altitude	
disease states	

Malina (1983) and Marker (1981) have reviewed the literature on menarche in the young athlete and concur that there is an apparent association between a later age at menarche in the young athlete and advanced competitive level. This is particularly evident in gymnasts, ballerinas, figure skaters, divers, and runners (Figure 1). Associated factors are listed in Table 3. Swimmers, who often visually appear more advanced in physical development at comparable chronological age, are often reported to have a *younger* age at menarche than other young athletes.

Two basic theories have been proposed to explain the later menarcheal age of highly competitive athletes. The "critical body fat" theory (Frisch & McArthur, 1974) holds that "a minimum level of stored, easily mobilized energy is necessary for ovulation and menstrual cycles in the human female" (p. 949). According to this theory, once the body attains a relative body fat level of 17%, menstrual function will begin. Advocates of this theory propose that the young girl athlete attains this prescribed body fat level at a slower rate than her age-matched sedentary counterpart. There has been considerable controversy regarding this theory, however, and few scientists currently subscribe to this explanation (Scott & Johnston, 1982; Malina, 1978; Trussell, 1978). Most now believe that relative body

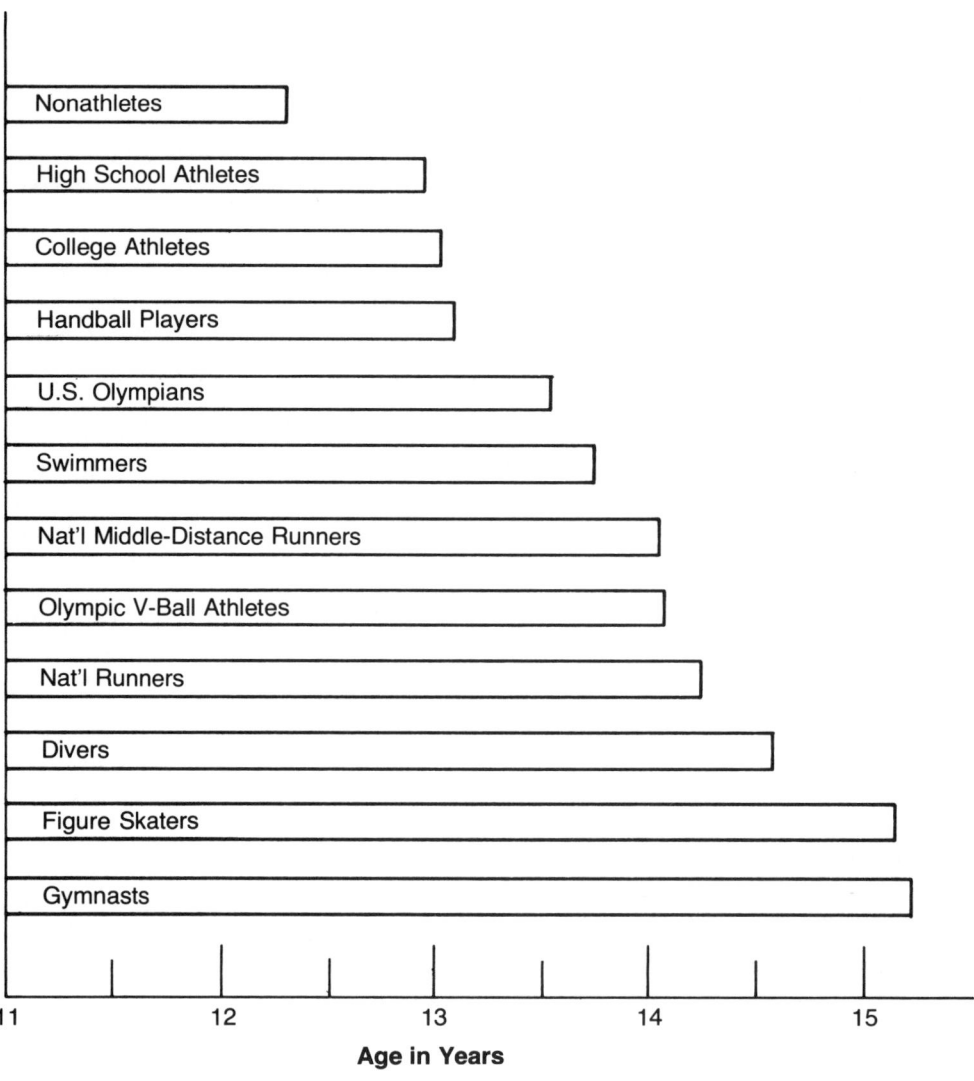

Fig. 1. Age at menarche. Data from Feicht et al., 1978; Malina et al., 1978; Waket & Sweeney, 1979; Märker, 1981.

fat is an associated factor, but *not* a causal variable in the delayed menarche observed in young athletes.

Advocates of the second theory (Malina, Spirduso, Tate, & Baylor, 1978; Malina, 1983) do not subscribe to the concept that there is a delay in menarche due to athletic training. Instead, they provide an explanation for why a more advanced age at menarche is seen in athletes. They point out that the biological characteristics associated with late maturity in females are generally those more suitable for athletic performance. The late maturer, for example, has longer legs, narrower hips, less weight per unit height, and less relative body fat than the early maturer—all factors recognized as advantageous to athletic performance (with the possible exception of swimming, see below). The young girl genetically programmed to be a later maturer is also more likely to be an athlete. And thus we observe that highly successful young female athletes have a later age at menarche. It is further suggested by the advocates of this concept, that the early maturing girls are "socialized away from sports competition through a myriad of social and status related motives" (Malina et al., 1978, p. 221).

This second theory, a genetically based explanation for the later age at menarche seen in athletic girls, also seems to explain the major exception to this observation—that exceptional girl swimmers more commonly have a mean age at menarche which approximates the average for nonathletes (Astrand et al., 1963; Malina, 1983). Early maturation appears to provide the young girl with a physique more suitable for swimming (more subcutaneous fat, more rounded contours) than does a later maturation.

The effects of exercise on menstrual disorders. This discussion will be limited to the most commonly cited menstrual disorders:
- dysmenorrhea—painful menstruation
- oligomenorrhea—irregular or infrequent menstruation
- secondary amenorrhea—absence or cessation of menses following menarche.

A survey of university freshmen revealed that the most physically active had the fewest menstrual complaints (Gendel, 1976), but some investigators have noted that girls who begin intensive training *before* menarche have an increased incidence of menstrual disorders (Erdelyi, 1976). Some contend that physical training does not affect menstruation (Zaharieva, 1972), others say that stressful sport activity *may cause* menstrual dysfunction (Erdelyi, 1976). While most believe that sports participation has a generally favorable effect on dysmenorrhea, Erdelyi (1976) states that certain sports may *cause* dysmenorrhea. His surveys indicate that among athletes, the incidence of dysmenorrhea is highest among swimmers. Approximately one-third of the young Swedish swimmers extensively studied by Astrand et al. in 1963 stated that strenuous swimming during menstruation caused pain in their lower abdomen. This sort of information should be obtained from young currently competing athletes. Training programs have changed considerably in the last 10 to 20 years, and so have attitudes toward training during menstruation. Updated information on dysmenorrhea in young athletes is needed to reevaluate this question.

The fact that highly trained women athletes often have oligomenorrhea or amenorrhea has received considerable attention in the last several years. Amenorrhea seems to be most common in athletes of slight build such as runners, ballerinas, and gymnasts, but participants in swimming, cycling, and crew also tend to have a higher incidence than the nonathletic norm. Estimates of incidence range from 4 to 52% depending partly on the stringency of the definitions used to classify these disorders and the type of population sampled (Erdelyi, 1976; Feicht, Johnson, Martin, Sparkes, & Wagner, 1978; Dale, Gerlach, & Wilhite, 1979; Baker, Mathur, Kirk, & Williamson, 1981; Lutter & Cushman, 1982). In contrast, oligo-amenorrhea occurs in about two to three percent of the nonathletic, nonpregnant, and nonlactating population.

A number of factors have been associated (correlation analysis) with the incidence of exercise related oligo-amenorrhea. Some have reported that menstrual irregularity or cessation is more likely to be seen in younger athletes (Speroff & Redwine, 1980; Baker et al., 1981; Lutter & Cushman, 1982), in those with a low body weight or a low percentage of body fat (Dale, Gerlach, & Wilhite, 1979; Baker et al., 1981, Lutter & Cushman, 1982), and in those who train intensively (greater mileage run) (Speroff & Redwine, 1980; Feicht et al., 1978; Feicht, Martin, & Wagner, 1980; Lutter & Cushman, 1982; Drinkwater, 1984; Dale, Gerlach, & Wilhite, 1979; Dale, Gerlach, Martin & Alexander, 1979). However, not all agree. Some have reported that athletes who lost a significant amount of body weight were more likely to experience menstrual disruption (Dale, Gerlach, Martin & Alexander, 1979; Speroff & Redwine, 1980). Others have failed to show a relationship between weight or body composition and amenorrhea in athletes (Feicht et al., 1978; Baker et al., 1981; Wakat, Sweeney, & Rogol, 1982). In two studies of ballerinas, menstrual function returned during vacations and periods of enforced rest due to injury without a gain in body weight or fat (Warren, 1980;

Abraham, Beaumont, Fraser, & Llewelyn-Jones, 1982). Other associated factors may be previous menstrual irregularity (Lutter & Cushman, 1982), nulliparity (Dale, Gerlach, & Wilhite, 1979; Baker et al., 1981), and an older age at menarche (Baker et al., 1981; Lutter & Cushman, 1982). It is obvious that not all investigators agree on the relationships of these variables with menstrual function.

While it is desirable to know about the variety of factors that are related to menstrual disruption such as those determined from the descriptive studies cited above, it is essential to study the direct effects of exercise on the hormonal cycles that make up the menstrual cycle. Not many investigators have been brave enough to attempt this enormous task. This type of study, however, is a more direct attempt to determine *casual* factors to explain exercise related oligo-amenorrhea.

Acute and chronic responses of the reproductive hormones to exercise. Acute androgen response to exercise has been studied in both men and women, with similar results. Androgenic hormones (testosterone and derivatives) rise significantly following strenuous exercise, but remain well within the normal limits for adult women (Sutton et al., 1973; Shangold et al., 1981). The acute influence of exercise on ovarian hormones seems to differ in trained and untrained subjects. In untrained women, both estradiol (E_2) and progesterone (P) levels increased following exercise (Jurkowski, Jones, Walker, Younglai, & Sutton, 1978; Bonen, Ling, MacIntyre, Neil, McGrail, & Belcastro, 1979; Hall, Younglai, Walker, Jones & Sutton, 1975). Usually, the absolute changes were large during the luteal phase. In the trained subjects, however, no significant elevations in E_2 or P were found. The acute effects of exercise on the plasma levels of ovarian hormones were apparently extinguished by training (Bonen et al., 1979). Chronically lower testosterone (T), estrogen, and progesterone levels have been reported in women runners (Dale, Gerlach, & Wilhite, 1979). Chronically lower levels of progesterone were reported in teenaged athletes (Bonen, Belcastro, Ling, & Simpson, 1981) and mature women runners (Shangold, Freeman, Thysen, & Gatz, 1979) with shortened luteal phases.

It is not known whether the acute elevations in T, E_2, and P were due to increased ovarian function, increased adrenal function, or to decreased clearance (removal) of these hormones from the plasma by the liver. However, blood flow to the liver is considerably reduced during heavy exercise in response to the sympathetic stimulation of norepinephrine (NorE). Because the concentration of most substances in the blood is a result of production, secretion, *and* removal, it is likely that reduced hepatic blood flow significantly contributes to these hormonal elevations following exercise. With training, there is a significant reduction in NorE in response to exercise, and a less significant decline in hepatic blood flow with exercise. This may be the explanation for the different response seen in the trained subjects of Bonen et al. (1979).

Whether exercise induced increments in T, E_2, or P are related to the incidence of menstrual cycle irregularities in athletes is not known. However, some athletes train strenuously three to five hours per day—sometimes in more than one training session. It is conceivable that these hormones remain elevated sufficiently long to exert an inhibitory effect on the gonadotrophic hormones, and consequently cause an alteration in menstrual function.

An acute rise in follicle stimulating hormone (FSH) was observed following exercise in the folicular phase (Jurkowski et al., 1978), but other investigators reported no changes in either FSH or luteinizing hormone (LH) during any menstrual phase (Bonen et al., 1979; Sutton, Coleman, Casey, & Lazarus, 1973). Under less controlled conditions, FSH levels were unchanged, but LH values were decreased following a marathon (Hale, Kosasa, Krieger, & Pepper, 1983). It is interesting that Shangold et al. (1979) found no difference in chronic FSH levels in normally menstruating runners compared to those with a short luteal phase. Dale, Gerlach, and Wilhite (1979), however, reported that anovulating runners, joggers, and control subjects displayed noncyclic hormonal patterns. It is obvious that confusion remains regarding the effects of exercise on the concentration of these important hormones.

A number of hypotheses have been proposed to explain exercise related oligo-amenorrhea. A brief explanation follows for those theories that have generated the most interest and study.

Proposed explanations for exercise related oligo-amenorrhea. The most commonly discussed and controversial concept of exercise related amenorrhea is called the "critical fat theory." This is an extension of the hypothesis that menarche is related to the attainment of a particular level of body fat (see menarche disussion above). Advocates of this theory propose that 17% body fat is needed for the onset of menstruation and 22% body fat is needed to restore or to maintain the menstrual cycle (Frisch & McArthur, 1974; Frisch, 1977, Frisch, Wyshak & Vincent, 1980). The logical application of this theory is that regular and strenuous training results in excessive leanness and a low percentage of body fat. The low amounts of body fat result in less aromatization (conversion) of testosterone to estrogen, preventing the LH surge required for ovulation. The result, say proponents of this theory, is chronically elevated T, low E, low FSH, low LH, and—amenorrhea.

The theory has considerable "face validity" because the incidence of amenorrhea is very high in the leanest of athletes (distance runners, ballerinas, gymnasts) and those with anorexia nervosa. In addition, the factor of weight (fat) loss has been associated with amenorrhea in a number of survey studies (see above). The theory, however, has been severely criticized, and is no longer seriously considered by most scientists. The data upon which the theory was based were obtained using a questionable technique for estimating body fat (Trussell, 1978; Reeves, 1979; Scott & Johnston, 1982; Loucks, Horvath, & Freedson, 1984). In addition, a number of studies have failed to show a relationship between body composition and oligo-amenorrhea in athletes (Baker et al., 1981; Feicht et al., 1978; Wakat et al., 1982; Lutter & Cushman, 1982; Loucks et al., 1984).

Hormonal theories of exercise-related oligo-amenorrhea are not particularly well developed, and remain experimentally untested. One concept suggests that the elevated ovarian hormones following exercise act to inhibit follicular development by activating the negative feedback mechanism between the ovary and the hypothalamic-pituitary axis, resulting in an inhibition of FSH and LH. Another theory is that exercise directly alters hypothalamic neurotransmitter activity. This would cause failure of ovulation because FSH would not stimulate the follicle to mature and secrete sufficient E_2 to complete the cyle. Obviously, if exercise affects the pituitary gland, the timing of the LH surge necessary for ovulation would be disrupted.

The classic example of the amenorrheic woman is the lactating woman. During lactation, elevated prolactin levels inhibit ovulation by prolonging the life of the corpus luteum, and therefore, cause amenorrhea. Prolactin has been shown to be markedly elevated following exercise by some (Hale et al., 1983; Shangold, Gatz, & Thysen, 1981; Brisson, Volle, DeCarufel, Desharnais, & Tanaka, 1980), but not by a group who studied swimmers (Bonen et al., 1981). It is postulated that exercise that jars the breast results in the stimulation of prolactin production and secretion.

Psychological stress has also been implicated as a possible cause of athletic-related amenorrhea. It is well known that stress factors such as changing jobs, marital conflicts, financial worries, imprisonment, heroin addition, and alcoholism are associated with amenorrhea (Wentz, 1977). However, only two studies have examined psychological stress in amenorrheic and eumenorrheic athletes. Neither study demonstrated significant differences between these two groups of subjects (Gray & Dale, 1983; Schwartz, Cumming, Riordan, Selye, Yen & Rebar, 1981).

Risks associated with exercise-related amenorrhea. It appears that exercise-related amenorrhea is a benign and reversible condition in most athletes. If amenorrhea is caused solely by exercise, menses usually reappears when serious training ceases or exercise intensity is decreased. However, Shangold (1982) states that amenorrheic athletes should not casually assume their amenorrhea is caused by exercise. There are many causes of amenorrhea—including ovarian cysts, endometrial tumors, and brain tumors. Every amenorrheic athlete, according to Shangold, should be thoroughly examined by a qualified physician if the amenorrhea has existed for more than a year.

In many cases, amenorrheic women are hypoestrogenic. If this is the case, several reports suggest that there may be enhanced risk of accelerated loss of bone mineral content (Cann, Martin, Genant, & Jaffee, 1984; Drinkwater, Nilson, Chesnut, Bremner, Shainholtz, & Southworth, 1984). Convincing evidence is available that low dose estrogen replacement therapy (ERT) is preventive of bone mineral loss in menopausal women. Every amenorrheic athlete should consult her physician about this matter, and consider ERT if she is shown to be hypoestrogenic.

Throughout a normal lifetime, a woman spends a great deal of time in the nonmenstruating state. She doesn't begin menstruating until sometime around the age of 12 years. For each child born thereafter, the woman is amenorrheic for about a year (possibly more if she breast feeds her baby). At about age 50, menopause occurs and a woman's reproductive period ends. A woman who has two children, and who lives to the age of 75 years will spend about 40 years of her life in the nonmenstruating state. The remainder of this chapter will focus on the physiological changes that occur in a woman during pregnancy, and at menopause. There is insufficient space for a totally comprehensive review of either topic, so emphasis will be placed on those changes that are most relevant to the performance of exercise.

Pregnancy and Exercise

Maternal responses to pregnancy and exercise. There are many structural and physiological changes that occur with pregnancy—many of which have a profound effect on exercise performance (see Wells, 1985 for a more extensive review). The most obvious, of course, is that the abdomin gradually becomes larger and heavier, causing a shift in the center of gravity. Postural changes occur to compensate for this. The most commonly seen change in posture is a combination of an increased lumbar curve, locked or hyperextended knees, and slight backward lean. This change in posture often results in backache. Exercises that strengthen the back and abdominal muscles usually relieve this condition.

As a result of these postural changes, sport movements gradually become more ponderous and awkward as pregnancy progresses and body weight increases. Athletes usually find that their skills are affected in the third trimester—rarely before, although they may have slowed down some before that. Running movements gradually become more lumbering or rolling in nature, but this is well tolerated by most women. Women who were regular runners prior to their pregnancy usually find it best to decrease their mileage and their speed by the end of the 6th month.

The ligamentous support of the sacroiliac joints and the pubis symphysis normally soften during the late stages of pregnancy under the influence of relaxin. This occurs to allow childbirth to take place. Sometimes, however, these joints separate slightly, causing considerable discomfort and pain with movement. When this happens, weight bearing exercise is contraindicated.

Changes in the cardiovascular system occur early in pregnancy to meet demands of the enlarging uterus and placenta for more blood and oxygen. The woman must now oxygenate the blood of a developing fetus as well as her own, and consequently, the heart works harder. Cardiac output ($\dot{Q}$) increases early in the first trimester, reaching levels approximately 20% above normal. In the second and third trimester, the increase in $\dot{Q}$ is more gradual. The increased $\dot{Q}$ is mediated by both an increase in heart rate (approximately 20%) and an increase in stroke volume (SV). Some investigators have reported an increase in SV by as much as 10 to 12%, but there is not agreement on this. In the last trimester, the heart is pushed upward and to the left by the elevation of the diaphragm.

There is a generalized vascular dilation and an increased venous distensibility as pregnancy progresses. This sometimes gives rise to the development of edema in the lower extremities, and an increased incidence of varicosities in the lower extremities, vulva and anus. However, there is relatively little change in blood pressure throughout pregnancy. Initially there is usually a slight decrease, followed by a rise before delivery.

There are marked changes in blood volume (BV) with pregnancy. In the first half of gestation, this increase is largely the result of a considerable increase in plasma volume (PV), and therefore, decreased values for hemoglobin and hematocrit are seen. Later, the red cell mass increases more rapidly than the PV, and some recovery is seen in these variables. Generally, however, the increase in PV exceeds the increase in red blood cell mass. If a woman has a low body iron store prior to pregnancy, as some athletes do, she may be at increased risk for the development of iron deficiency anemia at this time.

As the diaphragm rises with the enlargement of the uterus, the thoracic cavity compensates by increasing its dimensions so that more air can be inspired with each breath. This increase in tidal volume, in association with a constant respiratory rate, yields an increase in respiratory minute volume ($\dot{V}_E$) of about 40%. This is the usual *hyperventilation of pregnancy,* which causes a decreased concentration of carbon dioxide in the alveoli, and subsequently, in the blood. This leads to a *compensated respiratory alkalosis* and an elevation of blood pH (from 7.35 prior to pregnancy, to about 7.42 at term) (Quilligan & Kaiser, 1977; Alaily & Carrol, 1978). Similar (but not so large) changes are also seen during the luteal phase of the menstrual cycle, and are thought to be mediated by progesterone (see above).

Exercise is tolerated very well during pregnancy, but there is a loss of considerable cardiovascular-respiratory reserve. During the early months of pregnancy, cardiac output, oxygen uptake, and respiratory ventilation are markedly increased with exercise, even at relatively low levels of exertion. However, since the maximal values attainable for many variables decline as pregnancy progresses, the pregnant woman is at a considerable disadvantage in regard to high level athletic performance. Ueland, Novy, Peterson, & Metcalfe (1969) have shown that at moderate work (200 kpm·min^{-1} on a bicycle ergometer), the rise in SV and $\dot{Q}$ became progressively smaller with advancing pregnancy. They concluded that a progressive decrease in cardiac reserve as pregnancy advanced attributed to peripheral pooling of blood and obstruction of venous return. Guzman and Caplan (1970) noted that the heart had to work harder to meet the demands of exercise as pregnancy progressed, and that maximal cardiac output was reached at a lower level of work than when not pregnant.

There are some differences in response to exercise in the weight-bearing position and the nonweight-bearing position. Knuttgen and Emerson (1974) studied responses to grade walking (treadmill) and cycling (bicycle ergometer) during pregnancy, and again, postpartum. Oxygen uptake increased with pregnancy during walking, but not during cycling. The 13% $\dot{V}O_2$ increase with walking corresponded with a 15% increase in body weight. The investigators concluded that activities that do not involve lifting the body should not be expected to cause significant increases in energy cost during pregnancy. Another group of investigators, however, found an increase in $\dot{V}O_2$ and $\dot{Q}$ with comparable bicycle exercise in late pregnancy (Pernoll, Metcalfe, Schlenkar, Welch, & Matsumoto, 1975). They attributed this to the increased cost of hyperventilation and cardiac output as pregnancy progressed.

A pregnant woman often experiences considerable fatigue during pregnancy and finds that she wants to spend an increasing portion of her time sleeping. This may be related to her increased levels of progesterone, which in high doses can cause somnolence. Morning sickness (nausea and/or vomiting) may occur in the first trimester and is thought to be central in origin. In contrast, the second trimester is often associated with feelings of euphoria and well-being, while the third trimester is often associated with depression and chronic fatigue. Certainly these feelings and emotions are not universal. Many women go through pregnancy with few of these reactions. These responses are mentioned here primarily to point out that some women have increased difficulty maintaining an active lifestyle as pregnancy progresses. Often switching one's normal exercise time from morning to afternoon or early evening helps the woman continue her exercise program. Other problems that influence one's usual exercise habits include increased digestive difficulties due to lessened tone in the smooth muscle tissues of the gastrointestinal tract. Heartburn is common, as is constipation and flatulence. As the uterus enlarges, there is increased pressure on the bladder. This leads to frequent complaints of increased urination. With exercise, a pregnant woman may experience urinary incontinence. Wearing pads or panti-shields may contribute to a woman's level of security and confidence about this annoying, but harmless occurrence. There are major breast changes in pregnancy. There is a massive increase in ductal tissue and increased fat deposition. Tingling and soreness are not uncommon, and so good bra support is essential for comfort while exercising.

Physical fitness and pregnancy. Women who are physically fit prior to pregnancy are able to exercise at much higher work loads than women who are not physically fit. The most likely reason for this is that physical fitness increases one's cardiovascular-respiratory reserve and contributes to an expanded plasma volume. Although physical fitness was not found to be related to infant birth weight, length, head circumference, length of gestation, or complications of pregnancy, women with higher levels of fitness had significantly shorter periods of labor in pregnancies following their first child (Pomerance, Gluck, & Lynch, 1974).

Generally, it is best to begin an exercise program prior to pregnancy rather than while pregnant. However, two studies dealt with training during pregnancy in women unaccustomed to regular exercise prior to pregnancy (Curet & Collings, 1981; Erkkola, 1976). Both studies concluded that it was advantageous for pregnant women to exercise during pregnancy in an effort to offset the decrease in functional fitness while pregnant. No harm came to either the mother or the fetus in either investigation. Another study followed the progress of a woman beginning with her first pregnancy and concluding with the birth of her second child. Her running mileage, oxygen uptake, and weight gain were monitored to show the effects of training throughout pregnancy and lactation. The subject remained healthy throughout the investigation, and all aspects of pregnancy, delivery, and lactation were normal (Dressendorfer, 1978). Hutchinson, Cureton, and Sparling (1981) studied the metabolic and circulatory responses of a woman who had regularly engaged in running for eight years prior to pregnancy. $\dot{V}_E$, $\dot{V}O_2$, heart rate, and respiratory exchange ratio during steady state exercise increased substantially as pregnancy progressed. The increase in $\dot{V}O_2$ was proportional to weight gain, but the other changes were not. The investigators concluded that running became more stressful as pregnancy progressed, and recommended that pregnant women reduce their running speed to maintain a constant level of physiological strain throughout pregnancy.

Long-term effects of exercise on pregnancy and childbearing. Concern about the long-term effects of strenuous athletic training on pregnancy and childbearing has no basis in fact. Myths about ruptured and sagging organs from jumping or falling, or infertility have given way to evidence that women athletes are more likely to have normal pregnancies than sedentary women (Erdelyi, 1962; Zaharieva, 1965, 1972; Jokl, 1956; Eriksson, Engstrom, Karlberg, Lundin, Saltin, & Thoren, 1978). There are no recent assessments of the long-term effects of strenuous physical training on menstrual function, fertility, and childbearing even though training methods are considerably more strenuous now than when these reports were first published.

Fetal responses to maternal exercise. Of major concern in regard to exercise during pregnancy, of course, is the well-being of the baby. Few studies have dealt with this question because of the difficult nature of the research. Most data must be collected by noninvasive means so as not to endanger either the mother or the fetus. Technology limits us to observing only a few variables.

Normal fetal heart rates (FHR) range from 120 to 160 bpm. Dressendorfer and Goodlin (1980) studied FHR in third trimester women pedalling a bicycle ergometer. The women exercised at 150, 300, 450 and 600 kpm·min^{-1}. Maternal heart rates rose to 146 bpm and oxygen uptake to 1.85 l·min^{-1}. FHR at peak exercise averaged 149 bpm. This indicated that FHR increased approximately 1 beat for every 10 beat increase in the mother. Curet and Collings (1981) also measured FHR response to maternal cycling. Following 20 minutes of exercise. FHR was 148 bpm. These studies indicate that aerobic exercise that raises maternal heart rates to approximately 80% of maximum does not produce abnormal fetal heart rate responses.

Fetal breathing movements were observed to increase markedly during maternal exercise that did not elicit changes in FHR (Marsal, Lofgren, & Gennser, 1979). The investigators postulated that increased fetal breathing movements may be induced by acid-base alterations in placental blood, increased catecholamines, or stimuli from maternal muscle tone. The breathing movements were not related to changes in maternal pH, PCO_2, or PO_2. It was suggested that fetal breathing movements may be more sensitive to modifications in homeostatis than fetal heart rates, and thereby offer a higher resolution power than offered by the study of FHR.

Perhaps the most interesting question involved in the study of exercise during pregnancy is—what happens to uterine blood flow? Most of the information regarding this question, unfortunately, comes from the study of animal preparations. A good animal model for human pregnancy is the pregnant ewe. One report cited a significant increase in fetal pH and a decrease in PCO_2 reflecting respiratory alkalosis from maternal hyperventilation. A decrease in fetal PO_2 was also noted. The investigators spectulated that this was due to a decrease in uterine blood flow secondary to redistribution of regional blood flow due to exercise. Nevertheless, they concluded that the fetus tolerated maternal exercise quite well (Emmanouilides, Hobel, Yashiro, & Klyman, 1972).

Several investigations directly measured uterine blood flow in the exercising pregnant ewe. One group reported that uterine blood flow was not impaired, and in fact, *increased* 10% above resting values during tradmill exercise to exhaustion (Orr, Ungerer, Will, Wernicke, & Curet, 1972). A more detailed study from the same laboratory later revealed that total uterine blood flow in the ewe was not changed following exercise, but that blood distribution was altered in favor of the placenta (Curet, Orr, Rankin, & Ungerer, 1976). (Functionally speaking, there are two circulatory patterns in the pregnant uterus—one that serves the maternal side, and one that serves the fetal side.) Curet et al. (1976) suggested that this redistribution of blood might represent a compensatory mechanism for the fetus.

Another investigation disagreed with the two cited above. Four ewes were exercised 15 minutes twice daily during the last three to four months of gestation.

During treadmill exercise, fetal aortic PO_2 fell 19% and uterine blood flow decreased 59%. Fetal birth weights were significantly lower than in control animals. The investigators concluded that sustained moderate to heavy exercise may result in significant fetal hypoxia and cause intrauterine growth retardation (Longo, Hewitt, Lorijn, & Gilbert, 1978). Although a decrease in uterine blood flow (28%) was confirmed in another laboratory (Clapp, 1979), a compensatory increase (56%) in arteriovenous O_2 difference across the uterine circulation suggested that the fetus could tolerate exhaustive maternal exercise because it could extract more oxygen despite reduced uterine perfusion.

It is obvious that additional study of uterine blood flow during exercise is needed, and in particular, the study of exercising human subjects. Perhaps some of the recently developed clinical and investigative techniques will soon be available for exercise studies.

Suggested advice to pregnant women. There is no evidence that regular exercise during a normal pregnancy is contraindicated for either the mother or the fetus. Both are physiologically well equipped to tolerate the relatively minor reductions in cardiac reserve or uterine blood flow experienced with exercise. One question that remains unanswered is that of the effect of elevated maternal temperature, due to exercise, on the fetus. It is known that maternal fever can be a teratogen (an agent that may cause a malformation or functional abnormality) during the embryonic period (3rd to 8th week). This is often the period before a woman knows she is pregnant. For the safety of the developing fetus, it is probably wise to avoid an excessive body temperature gain due to exercise throughout pregnancy.

Physicians and exercise leaders probably should instruct their patients and clients to "listen to your body." If discomfort is experienced while exercising during pregnancy, then exercise intensity should be lowered. Perhaps exercise duration should be shortened as well. Problem signs include vaginal bleeding, high blood pressure, pain, rupture of membranes, or absence of fetal movements. If any of these warning signs appear, the pregnant women should consult her physician immediately.

The gradual gain of some 20 pounds is likely to cause additional muscular and ligamentous strain, especially if exercise activities involve bouncing or jarring movements. It is obvious that the pregnant woman should pay special attention to foot support and breast support during this time.

Pregnant women should avoid dehydration. Since the thirst mechanism is not sensitive enough to prevent dehydration in the heat or during exercise, the pregnant woman should be carefully instructed to drink fluids (especially water and fruit juices) before, during, and following exercise periods. Most women will notice an increase in thirst during pregnancy and lactation. Women who exercise during these periods should anticipate this indication of the need for additional body fluid.

Menopause and Exercise

The menopause represents the end of a woman's reproductive life span. It signals a series of physiological events that are often dreaded or feared, and consequently, may bring on a profound life crisis. Unfortunately, some women are victims of cultural attitudes that associate the menopause with being old, unwanted, having wrinkles and gray hair, and being useless. These women tend to view fertility as femininity. Other women view this period of life as a release from the burdens of the childbearing years. Whatever a woman's attitude toward menopause, there are profound physiological events and responses that occur during this phase of life that have significant interactions with the mental and emotional meanings of life.

More specifically, menopause refers to the final menstrual period, and occurs during the climacteric, a period of gradual change from the reproductive stage of life to the nonreproductive stage, a process that takes several years to fully accomplish. The climacteric is thus associated with "the change in life," and although it occurs in men as well as women, little attention has been paid to the male climacteric.

Menstruation stops when ovarian hormonal secretion diminishes to the extent that it fails to inhibit the pituitary gonadotropins, FSH and LH. Consequently, FSH and LH levels rise significantly, and the usual hypothalamic-pituitary-ovarian feedback system is altered sufficiently that normal menstruation terminates. This usually occurs between the ages of 45 and 55 years (Sloane, 1980).

Physiological changes occurring with menopause. Low tonic estrogen output, coupled with an elevation of serum gonadotropins, FSH, and LH, cause many changes in the reproductive system. Initially this period, called the perimenopause, is marked by considerable menstrual irregularity. Ovarian tissue continues, however, to secrete small amounts of androstenedione and testosterone so that there is a relative androgen excess in the postmenopausal woman's blood (Chang & Judd, 1981). Some of the resulting changes in the reproductive system include thinning of the vaginal lining, lessening of the strength and elasticity of the pelvic muscles and ligaments, and shrinkage of the genital organs including glandular breast tissue.

Changes occur in other systems as well. A classic symptom of the climacteric is the hot flash, or vasomotor flush. The hot flash is a sudden sensation of warmth that usually starts in the face and progresses to the neck and chest. It is followed by a reddening of the skin, and a drenching sweat. The episode is over in a few minutes. Hot flashes occur simultaneously with the pulsatile release of LH from the pituitary, and are thought to be the result of a disturbance in the vasomotor center located within the temperature regulation center in the hypothalamus. The vasomotor instability is attributed directly to estrogen deficiency (Bates, 1981). The similarity of menopause-associated hot flashes with the symptoms of catecholamine excess suggests a catecholaminergic basis for the hot flash. The hot flash, more frequently than any other symptom, often drives women to seek the therapeutic relief of replacement hormone therapy (RHT). The dramatic relief experienced with exogenous estrogen has led to RHT as the usual treatment of choice.

Medical statistics in this country have led to the common notion that estrogen "protects" the woman from coronary heart disease (CHD). However, the ratio of male to female deaths from CHD only favors the female in this country, an observation that throws doubt on the concept that estrogen has anything at all to do with the development of CHD. Study of mortality rates from heart disease indicates that the risk for women increases steadily with age, and that there is no abrupt upward trend at menopause (Jones & Wentz, 1977). Ryan (1976) suggests that the apparent decline with age of the sex advantage of women is due to a slower increment in the death rate of men in relation to a gradual increase in the death rate of women, and thus, there is no evidence that menopause places women at greater risk for the development of heart disease.

Postmenopausal women have higher plasma low-density lipoprotein cholesterol (LDL-chol) levels than men or premenopausal women, a factor associated with increased risk of atherosclerotic disease. Estrogen administration reduces elevated LDL-chol values in some women. Nevertheless, since results can be quite variable, there is no sound basis for the use of estrogen to control hyperlipidemia and the risk of CHD in postmenopausal women (Ryan, 1976). The upward trend in CHD with age in both men and women may be due to a multitude of factors—genetic endowment, hyperlipidemia, obesity, diabetes mellitus, hypertension, smoking, physical inactivity, and psychological stress. These factors make it difficult to study the influence of menopause on heart disease.

By inhibiting the effect of parathyroid hormone on the resorption of bone, estrogen also affects the well-being of the skeletal system. Peak bone mass is reached by both sexes at approximately age 35. After that age, both sexes gradually lose more bone mineral than is deposited. However, the rate of bone mineral loss at this time is greater in women, and is especially associated with menopause. As chronic estrogen levels decline with menopause, bone mineral losses accelerate. Postmenopausal osteroporosis is a common metabolic bone disease seen in elderly women. It is a reduction in bone mass per unit volume sufficient to cause spontaneous fracture. Osteoporosis leads to the characteristic posture of the humpbacked elderly woman. Estrogen therapy at menopause *slows* the rate of bone mineral loss, but it does not entirely prevent it.

Physiological changes occurring with menopause lead to an increased susceptibilty to vaginitis, bladder infections, uterine prolapse, osteroporosis, loss of elasticity of the skin (increased wrinkling), and elevated plasma LDL-cholesterol levels. Women often experience more fatigue following the menopause, become less physically active, and consequently, gain body fat.

Responses to exercise during the menopausal years. It is difficult to directly address the question of physiological response to exercise during the climacteric. While there are numerous studies documenting the gradual decline in the male's physical working capacity with age, there are relatively few studies of this nature on women. Furthermore, the very few studies on "master's women" dealt mostly with women under 40 or over 60. Only one study identified pre- or postmenopausal women (menstruating and nonmenstruating). For the most part, the studies indicate that women experience the same gradual reduction in the ability to tolerate heavy exercise as men, and that there is no sudden decrease in physiological reserve with menopause.

Wessel, Small, Van Huss, Anderson, and Cederquist (1968) reported a consistent trend for $\dot{V}O_2$, oxygen pulse, and $\dot{V}_E$ to be higher with increasing age for a low intensity treadmill walk. Using the same data, Wessel and Van Huss (1969) noted that these variables were positively related to age (r = .37 to .40), and negatively related to habitual physical activity level (r = −.52 to −.73). Their sample also showed a significant increase in body weight with age, and a lack of physical activity. Profant, Early, Nilson, Kusumi, Hofer, and Bruce (1972) tested the aerobic capacity of active and sedentary women in their fifth and sixth decades. $\dot{V}O_2$ max decreased significantly in the sedentary women, averaging 0.2 ml per kilogram of body weight per year. The active women outperformed the sedentary women, as might be expected. The active 40 to 49-year-old women had exercise duration and $\dot{V}O_2$ max values higher than those who were sedentary and in the 30 to 39 year age range; and the active 50 to 59-year-old women had values similar to those who were in the sedentary 40 to 49 year age range, demonstrating the "protective effect of approximately one decade of age in active women as noted before in men" (Profant et al., 1972, p. 500). Drinkwater, Horvath, and Wells (1975) studied a more physically fit group. In this study, each age group was divided into two activity classifications based on mean values for Canadian and Scandinavian women. The active subjects had $\dot{V}O_2$ max values 10 ml·kg^{-1} body weight higher than the moderately active subjects of Profant et al. (1972). The more active women also had lower body weight values than the sedentary subjects. The 40 to 49-year-old women had a lower $\dot{V}O_2$ max than the three younger groups, and the 50 to 59-year-old women were lower than all the other groups. But when aerobic power was expressed in absolute terms (L·min^{-1}), there was no significant relationship with age in the above average fitness women. In the women of below average fitness, there was a linear decline in $\dot{V}O_2$ with age. In general, the authors of this study found that there was a plateau for many variables during the years from 20 to 49, with a sharp decrement from age 50 on.

They further noted that 9 of the 12 women in the 50 to 59 year age group were past the menopause. Four of these women were above average in fitness, and five were below.

Plowman, Drinkwater, and Horvath (1979) added a longitudinal dimension to the study of the effect of age on aerobic power in women by studying some of Drinkwater's original sample six years later. All age groups showed a decrease in aerobic power expressed in L·min^{-1} and relative to body weight, but not relative to lean body mass. Since body fat had increased while body weight remained constant, this suggested that the loss of aerobic power was "related to a decrease in utilization of oxygen due to loss of muscle tissue" (p. 519).

A ten-week training program of three to four days per week of exercise intensity approximating 75 to 85% HR max resulted in improved cardiorespiratory fitness in sedentary middle-aged (28 to 50-year-old) women and men (Getchell & Moore, 1975). This indicates that sedentary middle-aged women (some of whom were in the climacteric years) can benefit from a systematic exercise program.

Vaccaro, Morris, and Clarke (1981) studied the physiological characteristics of outstanding masters distance runners, including some who were 45 to 49 years of age. These women were certainly perimenopausal, and some may have experienced menopause since the mean age for menopause is 50 years. Nevertheless, the aerobic capacities of these masters runners were comparable to values achieved by college basketball players (Vaccaro, Clarke, & Wrenn, 1979), and candidates for the U.S. Olympic speed skating team (Maksud, Hamilton, Coutts, & Wiley, 1971). The studies cited above seem to confirm Kilbom's suggestion (1971) that there are no sex differences in the ability to profit from physical training—at any age.

"Menopausal symptoms" and exercise. Although there is a dearth of documented evidence, some believe that women who exercise regularly experience fewer "menopausal symptoms" than sedentary women. Although the basis for this observation has not yet been established, there are several possible explanations. For example, regular exercise lowers plasma catacholamine levels. This is one reason why exercise is effective in reducing some forms of anxiety and depression. If the hot flash is mediated by a sudden release of catecholamines, perhaps exercise dampens the catecholamine release associated with the hot flash. If the hot flash is mediated by estrogen deficiency, possibly exercise reduces incidence of this symptom by increasing the concentration of E following exercise (Jurkowski et al., 1978; Bonen et al., 1979; Hall et al., 1975), thereby lessening the degree of menopausal estrogen deficiency. If the hot flash is caused by a pulsatile elevation in LH, then maybe exercise alleviates this symptom by reducing chronic LH concentrations. Dale, Gerlach, and Wilhite (1979) reported lower LH level in regular exercisers.

A recent study suggested that physical conditioning may delay the onset of menopause and change the climacteric symptomatology via mechanisms that increase serum estradiol concentrations (Wallace, Lovell, Talano, Webb, & Hodgson, 1982). Two groups of women classified as pre- or postmenopausal engaged in a six-week conditioning program set at 70% of maximum capacity. In both groups, E_2 increased significantly. Following the conditioning program the postmenopausal women had estrone:estradiol profiles characteristic of premenopause. Six weeks is a rather short training program, however, and the results of this study should be replicated before we extol exercise as the preventer of menopausal symptoms.

On the other hand, there is growing evidence that exercise, especially weight supported exercise that causes intermittent compression and deformation, *promotes* bone mineralization and hypertrophy (Chamay & Tschantz, 1972; Goodship, Lanyon, & McFie, 1979). As a result, exercise (as well as dietary calcium supplementation and estrogen replacement therapy) is commonly prescribed for the reduction of bone mineral loss in postmenopausal women, especially in those diagnosed as osteoporotic. Several studies have shown that regular exercise promotes an increase in bone mineral content (Smith, 1973; Smith, Reddan, & Smith, 1981) and positive calcium balance (Aloia, Cohn, Ostuni, Cane, & Ellis, 1978) in postmenopausal women. Although physical activity is only one of many factors in the development of osteoporosis in postmenopausal women, it is clear that bone loss in the aged female can be retarded and maintained at a higher level when sufficient physical activity is present (Smith, Reddan, & Smith, 1981; Smith, 1982).

Other "menopausal symptoms" include stress incontinence (the involuntary loss of a small amount of urine upon straining) and prolapse of the uterus, rectum, or bladder (the dropping and subsequent protrusion of these organs through their pelvic openings). These symptoms are related to the stretching or weakening of muscular and ligamentous support in the pelvic area due to multiple pregnancies or tearing of pelvic tissues at childbirth, coupled with the estrogen deficiency characteristic of menopause. Occasionally stress incontinence occurs following exercise if the already weakened tissues are subjected to the repeated pounding and jarring of bouncing activities (aerobic dance, jogging, etc.). Neither stress incontinence nor prolapse are *caused* by exercise, but exercise may aggravate both conditions. In the case of prolapse, strenuous weight bearing exercise is usually contraindicated. Stress incontinence is merely an annoying and possibly embarrassing incident. Sometimes stress incontinence can be treated with carefully performed pelvic exercises. Estrogen replacement usually controls it. Prolapse, on the other hand, can only be corrected by surgical repair. Often the required surgery is very minor and can be performed on an out-patient basis. Following the repair of a prolapse, strenuous weight bearing exercise can again be performed comfortably and safely. Menopausal women should not allow either symptom to limit their phsyical activity.

Exercise and the menopausal woman. Whether or not exercise actually alleviates menopausal symptoms is not known. Perhaps, the woman who regularly exercises is more tolerant of mild physical discomforts, and simply complains less. The years from 45 to 55, however, are often characterized by a gradual decline in physical activity level and a concomitant gain in body fat. If for no other reason, this is a good motive to continue or to begin a regular exercise program. Increasing body fat levels are not only unsightly, but are potentially detrimental to health. The menopausal years are often the same years in which adult onset diabetes, obesity, hyperlipidemia, and hypertension first appear.

Certainly the menopause or the climacteric period of one's life does *not* contraindicate regular stenuous exercise. On the contrary, all research findings indicate that exercise at this time of one's life is highly beneficial. The old adage is true: "exercise not only adds years to life, it adds life to years." Probably the most compelling evidence is that regular strenuous exercise retards the loss of bone mineral mass, and consequently, is protective of one's skeleton.

Summary

There are numerous baseline variations reported during the menstrual cycle. Whether or not these variations influence performance can only be examined on an individual basis.

Scientific investigations have not revealed differences in performance with menstrual cycle phase.

Menarche occurs at a later age in young girls who train strenuously. There are several correlated factors, but none of these are considered to have a cause-effect relationship. Possibly, late maturation in girls favors excellence in athletic performance.

Highly trained women athletes more frequently experience oligomenorrhea or amenorrhea than nonathletic, nonpregnant, and nonlactating women. A number of associated factors have been identified, but none are considered causal in nature.

The elevations in gonadal hormones seen with acute exercise may be due to changes in hepatic clearance rather than increased hormonal production or secretion.

The popular notion that low body fat levels, or a loss of body fat, is the *cause* of exercise related amenorrhea has been seriously questioned. Arguments against the "critical fat theory" are well established in the literature.

Exercise-associated amenorrhea appears to be a benign and reversible condition in most athletes, but every amenorrheic athlete should be thoroughly examined by a physician familiar with this phenomenon to rule out other causes.

There are many structural and physiological changes that occur with pregnancy. The enlarging abdomin causes a shift in the center of gravity and an increased lumbar curve. Skilled athletic movements gradually become more difficult, and gait often becomes more lumbering and rolling in nature.

Changes in the cardiovascular system occur to meet the demands of the uterus, placenta, and fetus for more blood and oxygen delivery. There are changes in $\dot{Q}$, HR, SV, venous distensibility, BV, and PV, which, in general, decrease the mother's cardiovascular reserve.

During pregnancy, $\dot{Q}$, $\dot{V}O_2$, and $\dot{V}_E$ are increased above their usual levels even at relatively low levels of exertion. Nevertheless, the fit and healthy pregnant woman can tolerate exercise quite well.

Women who are physically fit prior to pregnancy are able to exercise at higher levels than women who are not physically fit. Maternal physical fitness, however, does not appear to affect the baby.

Regular exercise during pregnancy is desirable to offset the decrease in functional fitness while pregnant. Studies indicate that exercise intensity is gradually lowered as pregnancy progresses. No harm occurs to either the mother or the baby as a result of strenuous and regular maternal exercise throughout a normal pregnancy.

Normal fetal heart rates range from 120 to 160 bpm. Aerobic exercise that raises maternal heart rates to approximately 80% of maximum does not produce abnormal fetal heart rate responses.

Pregnant women should be advised to reduce exercise intensity if unusual discomfort is experienced. Problem signs include vaginal bleeding, high blood pressure, pain, rupture of membranes, or absence of fetal movements. Dehydration and high body temperatures should be carefully avoided.

The final menstrual period—the menopause—signals a series of physiological events that are often dreaded or feared unnecessarily. The climacteric is a period of gradual change from the reproductive stage of life, and marks the diminution of ovarian hormone secretion.

The menopausal phase of life is marked by low tonic estrogen output coupled with elevations of FSH and LH. A relative androgen excess develops because ovarian tissue continues to secrete small amounts of androgenic substances.

Menopausal symptoms include thinning of the vaginal lining, loss of strength and elasticity of pelvic muscles and ligaments, shrinkage of the genital organs, reduced breast size, and hot flashes (vasomotor instability). Additional symptoms may include increased anxiety, sleep disturbance, increased bone mineral loss, stress incontinence, and prolapse of various pelvic organs. Replacement hormone therapy (low dose estrogen) often significantly reduces these signs and symptoms.

As chronic estogen levels decline, bone mineral losses accelerate. Postmenopausal osteoporosis is a common metabolic bone disease seen in elderly women. Reduction in bone mass per unit volume is often sufficient to cause spontaneous fractures that lead to the characteristic humpbacked posture of the elderly woman. Estrogen therapy, coupled with weightbearing exercise, and increased dietary calcium are usually prescribed to reduce bone mineral loss.

A review of the literature regarding the decline in physical working capacity with increasing age in women reveals that a gradually decreasing activity level and the subsequent gain in body fat and loss of lean body mass are probably more important factors than is increasing age, per se.

Descriptive studies of women "masters" athletes indicate that there are no sex differences in the ability to profit from physical training at any age.

The menopause or the climacteric years of one's life do *not* contraindicate regular stenuous exercise. All research findings indicate that exercise is highly beneficial to one's well-being at all phases of life and menstrual function.

References

Abraham, S.F., Beaumont, P.J.V., Fraser, I.S., & Llewellyn-Jones, D. (1982). Body weight, exercise, and menstrual status among ballet dancers in training. *British Journal of Obstetrics and Gynecology, 89,* 507-510.

Alaily, A.B., & Carrol, K.B. (1978). Pulmonary ventilation in pregnancy. *British Journal of Obstetrics and Gynecology, 85,* 518-524.

Allsen, P.E., Parsons, P. & Bryce, G.R. (1977). Effect of the menstrual cycle on maximum oxygen uptake. *The Physician and Sportsmedicine, 5*(7), 53-55.

Aloia, J.F., Cohn, S.H., Ostuni, J.A., Cane, R., & Ellis, K. (1978). Prevention of involutional bone loss by exercise. *Annals of Internal Medicine, 89,* 356-358.

Astrand, P.O., Engstrom, L., Eriksson, B.O., Karlberg, P., Nylander, I. Saltin, B., & Thoren, C. (1963). Girl swimmers, with special reference to respiratory and circulatory adaptation and gynaecological and psychiatric aspects. *Acta Paediatrica Scandinavica* (Supplementum 147).

Baker, E.B., Mathur, R.S., Kirk, R.F., & Williamson, H.O. (1981). Female runners and secondary amenorrhea: Correlation with age, pariety, mileage and plasma hormonal and sex hormone binding globulin concentration. *Fertility and Sterility, 36,* 183-187.

Bates, G.W. (1981). On the nature of the hot flash. *Clinical Obstetrics and Gynecology, 24,* 231-241.

Bonen, A., Belcastro, A.N., Ling, W.Y., & Simpson, A.A. (1981). Profiles of selected hormones during menstrual cycles of teenaged athletes. *Journal of Applied Physiology: Respiratory, Environmental, and Exercise Physiology, 50,* 545-551.

Bonen, A., Ling, W.Y., MacIntyre, K.P., Neil, R., McGrail, J.C., & Belcastro, A.N. (1979). Effects of exercise on the serum concentrations of FSH, LH, progesterone, and estradiol. *European Journal of Applied Physiology, 41,* 15-23.

Brisson, G.R., Dulac, S., Peronnet, F., & Ledoux, M. (1982). The onset of menarche: A late event in pubertal progression to be affected by physical training. *Canadian Journal of Applied Sport Sciences, 7,* 61-67.

Brisson, G.R., Volle, M.A., DeCarufel, D., Desharnais, M., & Tanaka, M. (1980). Exercise-induced dissociation of the blood prolactin response in young women according to their sports habits. *Hormones and Metabolic Research, 12,* 201-205.

Cann, C.E., Martin, M.C., Genant, H.K., & Jaffee, R.B. (1984). Decreased spinal mineral content in amenorrheic women. *Journal of the American Medical Association, 251,* 626-629.

Chamay, A., & Tschantz, P. (1972). Mechanical influence in bone modeling: Experimental research on Wolff's Law. *Journal of Bomechanics, 5,* 173-180.

Chang, R.J., & Judd, H.L. (1981). The ovary after menopause. *Clinical Obstetrics and Gynecology, 24,* 181-191.

Clapp, J. (1979). Acute exercise in the pregnant ewe. *Scientific Abstracts of the Society for Gynecological Investigation, 26.*

Curet, L.B., & Collings, C. (1981, April). *Acute and chronic effects of exercise on maternal, fetal and newborn well-being.* Paper presented at the American College of Obstetricians and Gynecologists, Las Vegas, NV.

Curet, L.B., Orr, J.A., Rankin, J.H.G., & Ungerer, T. (1976). Effect of exercise on cardiac output and distribution of uterine blood flow in pregnant ewes. *Journal of Applied Physiology, 40,* 725-728.

Dale, E., Gerlach, D.H., & Wilhite, A.L. (1979). Menstrual dysfunction in distance runners. *Obstetrics and Gynecology, 54,* 47-53.

Dale, E., Gerlach, D.H., Martin, D.E., & Alexander, D.R. (1979). Physical fitness profiles and reproductive physiology of the female distance runner. *The Physician and Sportsmedicine, 7*(1), 83-95.

Doolittle, T.L., & Engebretsen, J. (1972). Performance variations during the menstrual cycle. *Journal of Sports Medicine and Physical Fitness, 12,* 54-58.

Dressendorfer, R.H. (1978). Physical training during pregnancy and lactation. *The Physician and Sportsmedicine, 6*(2), 74-80.

Dressendorfer, R.H., & Goodlin, R.C. (1980). Fetal heart rate response to maternal exercise testing. *The Physician and Sportsmedicine, 8*(11), 91-95.

Drinkwater, B.L. (1984). Athletic amenorrhea: A review. *American Academy of Physical Education Papers, Exercise and Health, 17,* 120-131.

Drinkwater, B.L., Horvath, S.M., & Wells, C.L. (1975). Aerobic power of females, ages 10-68. *Journal of Gerontology, 30,* 385-394.

Drinkwater, B.L., Nilson, K., Chesnut, C.H., Bremner, W.J., Shainholtz, S., & Southworth, M.B. (1984). Bone mineral content of amenorrheic and eumenorrheic athletes. *The New England Journal of Medicine, 311*(5), 277-281.

Emmanouilides, G.C., Hobel, C.J., Yashiro, K., & Klyman, G. (1972). Fetal responses to maternal exercise in the sheep. *American Journal of Obstetrics and Gynecology, 112,* 130-137.

Erdelyi, G.J. (1976). Effects of exercise on the menstrual cycle. *The Physician and Sportsmedicine, 4*(3), 79-81.

Erdelyi, G.J. (1962). Gynecological survey of female athletes. *Journal of Sports Medicine and Physical Fitness, 2,* 174-179.

Eriksson, B.O., Engstrom, I., Karlberg, P., Lundin, A., Saltin, B., & Thoren, C. (1978). Long-term effects of previous swim training in girls: a 10-year follow-up on the "girl swimmers." *Acta Paediatrica Scandinavica, 67,* 285-292.

Erkkola, R. (1976). The influence of physical training during pregnancy on physical work capactiy and circulatory parameters. *Scandinavian Journal of Clinical and Laboratory Investigation, 36,* 747-754.

Feicht, C.B., Johnson, T.S., Martin, B.J., Sparks, K.E., & Wagner, Jr., W.W. (1978). Secondary amenorrhea in athletes (letter). *Lancet, 2*(8100), 1145-1146.

Feicht, C.B., Martin, B.J., & Wagner, Jr., W.W. (1980). Is athletic amenorrhea specific to runners. *Federation Proceedings, 39*(3), Part 1, 371. (Abstract 536).

Frisch, R.E. (1977). Fatness and the onset and maintenance of menstrual cycles. *Research in Reproduction, 6*(1), 1.

Frisch, R.E., & McArthur, J.W. (1974). Menstrual cycles: Fatness as a determinant of minimum weight for height necessary for their maintenance or onset. *Science, 185,* 494-951.

Frisch, R.E., Wyshak, G., & Vincent, L. (1980). Delayed menarche and amenorrhea in ballet dancers. *New England Journal of Medicine, 303,* 17-19.

Gendel, E.S. (1976). Psychological factors and menstrual extraction. *The Physician and Sportsmedicine, 4*(3), 72-75.

Getchell, L.H., & Moore, J.C. (1975). Physical training: Comparative responses of middle-aged adults. *Archives of Physical and Medical Rehabilitation, 56,* 250-254.

Goodship, A.E., Lanyon, L.E., & McFie, H. (1979). Functional adaptation of bone to increased stress. *Journal of Bone and Joint Surgery, 61-A,* 539-546.

Gray, D.P., & Dale, E. (1983). Variables associated with secondary amenorrhea in women runners. *Journal of Sports Sciences, 1,* 55-67.

Guzman, C.A., & Caplan, R. (1970). Cardiorespiratory response to exercise during pregnancy. *Amercian Journal of Obstetrics and Gynecology, 108,* 600-605.

Hale, R.W., Kosasa, T., Krieger, J., & Pepper, S. (1983). A marathon: The immediate effect on female runners' luteinizing hormone, follicle-stimulating hormone, prolactin, testosterone, and cortisol levels. *American Journal of Obstetrics and Gynecology, 146,* 550-554.

Hall, J.E., Younglai, E.V., Walker, C., Jones, N.L., & Sutton, J.R. (1975). Ovarian hormonal responses to exercise. *Medicine and Science in Sports, 7,* 65. (Abstract).

Horvath, S.M., & Drinkwater, B.L. (1982). Thermoregulation and the menstrual cycle. *Aviation, Space and Environmental Medicine, 53,* 790-794.

Hutchinson, P.L., Cureton, K.J., & Sparling, P.B. (1981). Metabolic and circulatory responses to running during pregnancy. *The Physician and Sportsmedicine, 9*(8), 55-61.

Jokl, E. (1956). Some clincial data on women's athletics. *Journal of the Association for Physical and Mental Rehabilitation, 10*(2), 48-49.

Jones, G.S., & Wentz, A.W. (1977). Adolescence, menstruation, and the climacteric. In D.N. Danforth (Ed.), *Obstetrics and Gynecology* (pp. 178-186). New York: Harper and Row.

Jurkowski, J.E., Jones, N.L., Walker, W.C., Younglai, E.V., & Sutton, J.R. (1978). Ovarian hormonal responses to exercise. *Journal of Applied Physiology: Respiration, Environmental and Exercise Physiology, 44,* 109-114.

Kilbom, A. (1971). Physical training in women. *Scandinavian Journal of Clinical and Laboratory Investigation, 28* (Suppl. 119), 1-34.

Knuttgen, H.G., & Emerson, Jr., K. (1974). Physiological response to pregnancy at rest and during exercise. *Journal of Applied Physiology, 36,* 549-553.

Longo, L., Hewitt, C.W., Lorijn, R.H.W., & Gilber, R.D. (1978). To what extent does maternal exercise affect fetal oxygenation and uterine blood flow? *Federation Proceedings, 37,* 905. (Abstract 3641).

Loucks, A.B., Horvath, S.M., & Freedson, P.S. (1984). Menstrual status and validation of body fat prediction in athletes. *Human biology, 56,* 383-392.

Lutter, J.M., & Cushman, S. (1982). Menstrual patterns in female runners. *The Physician and Sportsmedicine, 10*(9), 60-72.

Malina, R.M. (1978). Adolescent growth and maturation: Selected aspects of current research. *Yearbook of Physical Anthropology, 21,* 63-94.

Malina, R.M. (1983). Menarche in athletes: A synthesis and hypothesis. *Annals of Human Biology, 10,* 1-24.

Malina, R.M., Spirduso, W.W., Tate, C. & Baylor, A.M. (1978). Age at menarche and selected menstrual characteristics in athletes at different competitive levels and in different sports. *Medicine and Science in Sports, 10,* 218-222.

Maksud, M.G., Hamilton, L.H., Coutts, K.D., & Wiley, R.L. (1971). Pulmonary function measurements of Olympic speed skaters for the U.S. *Medicine and Science in Sports, 3,* 66-71.

Marker, K. (1981). Influence of athletic training on the maturity process of girls. *Medicine and Science in Sports, 3,* 117-126.

Marsal, K., Lofgren, O., & Gennser, G. (1979). Fetal breathing movements and maternal exercise. *Acta Obstetrics and Gynecology Scandinavica, 58,* 197-201.

Martin, F.L. (1976). Effects of the menstrual cycle on metabolic and cardiorespiratory responses. Unpublished dissertation, Ohio State University, Columbus, Ohio.

Orr, J., Ungerer, T., Will, J., Wernicke, K., & Curet, L.B. (1972). Effect of exercise stress on carotid, uterine, and iliac blood flow in pregnant and nonpregnant ewes. *American Journal of Obstetrics and Gynecology, 114,* 213-217.

Pernoll, M.L., Metcalfe, J., Schlenkar, T.L., Welch, J.E., & Matsumoto, J.A. (1975). Oxygen consumption at rest and during exercise in pregnancy. *Respiratory Physiology, 25,* 285-293.

Plowman, S.A., Drinkwater, B.L., & Horvath, S.M. (1979). Age and aerobic power in women: A longitudinal study. *Journal of Gerontoloy, 34*, 512-520.

Pomerance, J.J., Gluck, L., & Lynch, V.A. (1974). Physical fitness in pregnancy: Its effect on pregnancy outcome. *American Journal of Obstetrics and Gynecology, 119*, 867-876.

Profant, G.R., Early, R.G., Nilson, K.L., Kusumi, F., Hofer, V., & Bruce, R.A. (1972). Responses to maximal exercise in healthy middle-aged women. *Journal of Applied Physiology, 33*, 595-599.

Quilligan, E.J., & Kaiser, I.H. (1977). Maternal physiology. In D.N. Danforth, (Ed.), *Obstetrics and Gynecology,* 4th Ed. New York: Harper and Row, Publisher.

Reeves, J. (1979). Estimating fatness. *Science, 204,* 881.

Ryan, K.J. (1976). Estrogens and atherosclerosis. *Clinical Obstetrics and Gynecology, 19,* 805-815.

Schoene, R.B., Robertson, H.T., Pierson, D.J., & Peterson, A.P. (1981). Respiratory drives and exercise in menstrual cycles of athletic and nonathletic women. *Journal of Applied Physiology: Respiration, Environmental, and Exercise Physiology, 50,* 1300-1305.

Schwartz, B., Cumming, D., Riordan, E., Selye, M., Yen, S., & Rebar, R. (1981). Exercise-associated amenorrhea: A distinct entity? *American Journal of Obstetrics and Gynecology, 141,* 662-670.

Scott, E.C., & Johnston, F.E. (1982). Critical fat, menarche, and the maintenance of menstrual cycles: A critical review. *Journal of Adolescent Health Care, 2,* 249-260.

Shangold, M. (1982). Menstrual irregularity in athletes: Basic principles, evaluation, and treatment. *Canadian Journal of Applied Sport Sciences, 7,* 68-73.

Shangold, M., Freeman, R., Thysen, B., & Gatz, M. (1979). The relationship between long-distance running, plasma progesterone, and luteal phase length. *Fertility and Sterility, 31,* 130-133.

Shangold, M.M., Gatz, M.L., & Thysen, B. (1981). Acute effects of exercise on plasma concentrations of prolactin and testosterone in recreational women runners. *Fertility and Sterility, 35,* 699-702.

Sloane, E. *Biology of Women.* New York: John Wiley and Sons, 1980.

Smith, E.L. (1982). Exercise for prevention of osteoporosis: A review. *The Physician and Sportsmedicine, 10*(3), 72-83.

Smith, E.L. (1974). The effects of physical activity on bone in the aged. In R.B. Mazess, (Ed.), *International Conference on Bone Mineral Measurement.* (DHEW Publication No. (NIH) 75-683). Bethesda, MD: Public Health Service.

Smith, E.L., Reddan, W., & Smith, P.E. (1981). Physical activity and calcium modalities for bone mineral increase in aged women. *Medicine and Science in Sports, 13,* 60-64.

Southam, A.L., & Gonzaga, F.P. (1965). Systemic changes during the menstrual cycle. *American Journal of Obstetrics and Gynecology, 91,* 142-165.

Speroff, L., & Redwine, D.B. (1980). Exercise and menstrual function. *The Physician and Sportsmedicine, 8*(5), 42-52.

Stephenson, L.A., Kolka, M.A., & Wilkerson, J.E. (1982). Metabolic and thermoregulatory responses to exercise during the human menstrual cycle. *Medicine and Science in Sports and Exercise, 14,* 270-275.

Sutton, J.R., Coleman, M.J., & Casey, J.H. (1974). The adrenal cortical contribution to serum Androgens in physical exercise. *Medicine and Science in Sports, 6,* 72, (Abstract).

Sutton, J.R., Coleman, M.J., Casey, J., & Lazarus, L. (1973). Androgen responses during physical exercise. *British Medical Journal, 1,*520-522.

The Participation of the Female Athlete in Long-Distance Running. (1979). An opinion statement of The American College of Sports Medicine. *Medicine and Science in Sports, 11*(4), ix-xi.

Trussell, J. (1978). Menarche and fatness: Reexamination of the critical body composition hypothesis. *Science, 200,* 1506-1509.

Ueland, K., Novy, M.J., Peterson, E.N., & Metcalfe, J. (1969). Maternal cardiovascular dynamics. IV. The influence of gestational age on the maternal cardiovascular response to posture and exercise. *American Journal of Obstetrics and Gynecology, 104,* 856-864.

Vaccaro, P., Clarke, D.H., & Wrenn, J.P. (1979). Physiological profiles of elite women basketball players. *Journal of Sports Medicine and Physical Fitness, 19,* 45-54.

Vaccaro, P., Morris, A.F., & Clarke, D.H. (1981). Physiological characteristics of masters female distance runners. *The Physician and Sportsmedicine, 9*(7), 105-108.

Wakat, D.K., Sweeney, K.A., & Rogol, A.D. (1982). Reproductive system function in women cross-country runners. *Medicine and Science in Sports and Exercise, 14,* 263-269.

Wallace, J., Lovell, S., Talano, C., Webb, M.L., & Hodgson, J.L. (1982). Changes in menstrual function, climacteric syndrome, and serum concentrations of sex hormones in pre- and post-menopausal women following a moderate intensity conditioning program. *Medicine and Science in Sports and Exercise, 14,* 154. (Abstract).

Warren, M.P. (1980). The effects of exercise on pubertal progression and reproductive function in girls. *Journal of Clinical Endocrinology and Metabolism, 51,* 1150-1157.

Wells, C.L. (1985). *Women, Sport, and Performance: A Physiological Perspective.* Champaign, IL, Human Kinetics Publishers.

Wells, C.L., & Horvath, S.M. (1973). Heat stress responses related to the menstrual cycle. *Journal of Applied Physiology, 35,* 1-5.

Wells, C.L., & Horvath, S.M. (1974). Responses to exercise in a hot environment as related to the menstrual cycle. *Journal of Applied Physiology, 36,* 299-302.

Wentz, A.C. (1977). Psychogenic amenorrhea and anorexia nervosa. In R. Givens (Ed.), *Endocrine Causes of Menstrual Disorders,* Chicago: Year Book Medical Publishers.

Wessel, J.A., Small, A., Van Huss, W.D., Anderson, D.J., & Cederquist, D. (1968). Age and physiological responses to exercise in women 20-69 years of age. *Journal of Gerontology, 23,* 269-278.

Wessel, J.A., & Van Huss, W.D. (1969). The influence of physical activity and age on exercise adaptation of women, 20-69 years. *Journal of Sports Medicine and Physical Fitness, 9,* 173-180.

Zaharieva, E. (1972). Olympic participation by women: Effects on pregnancy and childbirth. *Journal of the American Medical Association, 221,* 992-995.

Zaharieva, E. (1965). Survey of Sportswomen at the Tokyo Olympics. *Journal of Sports Medicine and Physical Fitness, 5,* 215-219.

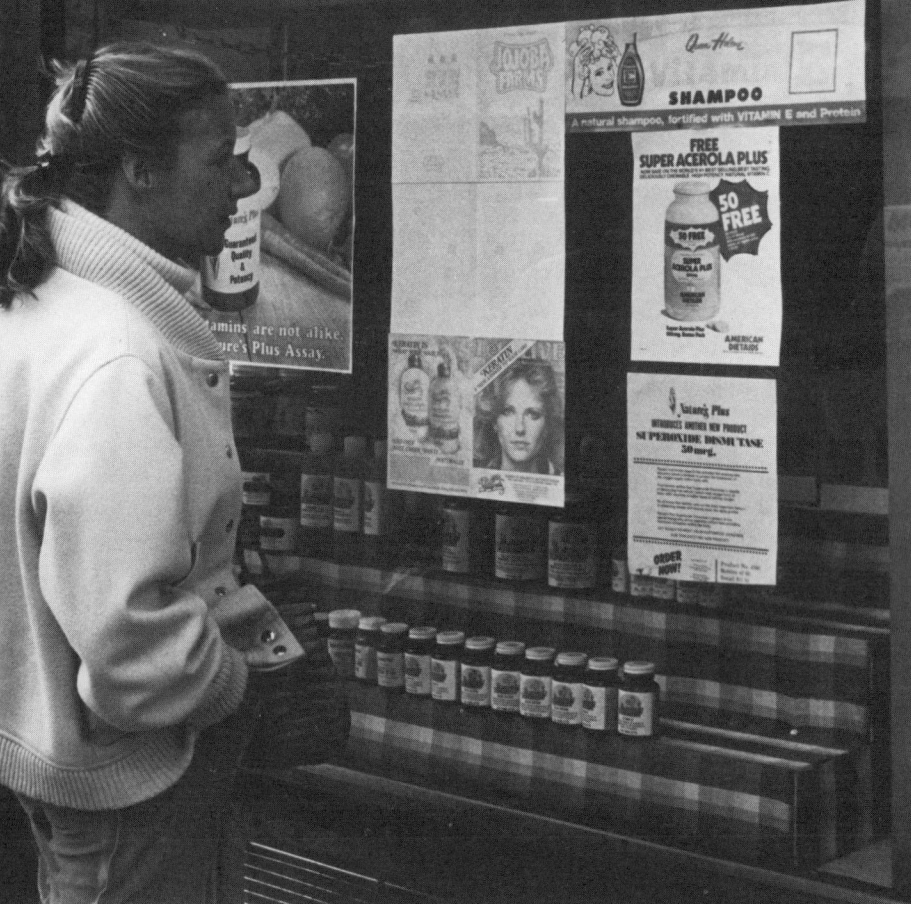

CHAPTER NINE

Nutrition and Ergogenic Aids

Emily M. Haymes
Department of Movement Science
and Physical Education
Florida State University
Tallahassee, Florida

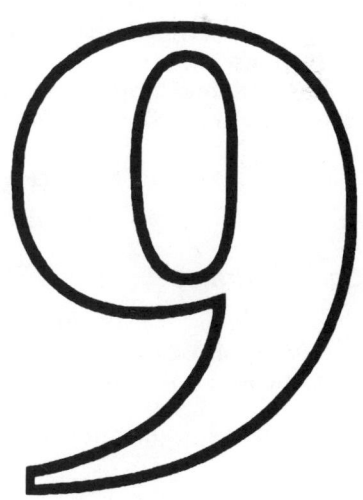

There are few areas related to sports and physical activity which have attracted more interest from coaches and athletes, including the weekend athlete, than the area of nutrition and ergogenic aids. The search for a magic formula which will improve performance beyond that achieved by daily training sessions probably began in the 19th century and continues even today. What began as a search for the main fuel for exercise in the 1860's and culminated in the carbohydrate loading studies of the 1960's has since broadened to include the use of drugs and blood doping to improve performance. Many "authorities" in the area have dismissed the research related to nutrition and performance by stating that the best diet for an athlete is one which is well balanced. This statement implies that the diet should contain all of the nutrients in sufficient quantity to meet the Recommended Dietary Allowance. Unfortunately, dietary surveys conducted during the late 1960's (Ten State Nutrition Survey, 1968-1970) and early 1970's (HANES, 1979) suggest that the average person in the United States is likely to be deficient in one or more of the nutrients.

Because adolescence is a time of rapid growth, the need for many nutrients will be greater than at any other time during the life span, with the exception of pregnancy and lactation for the female. Most nutritional surveys indicate that dietary deficiencies are more common among adolescents than in any other age group (Guthrie, 1979). Poor eating habits of teenagers are largely responsible for the inadequate nutrient intake. In general, males have fewer deficiencies than females because they consume more calories. It has been assumed that the teenage athlete might be even less prone to have a deficient diet than the average teenager because many activities require a large caloric expenditure. However, a recent survey of high school athletes suggests that the average athlete, male or female, is not eating a balanced diet (Douglas & Douglas, 1984). Although the theory that a well balanced diet is best for athletes may be correct, reality suggests that a majority of adolescents do not consume a balanced diet.

The first section of this chapter will examine the role that nutrients play in energy production and the various physiological systems that are stressed by physical activity. Evidence that nutritional deficiencies and supplements influence performance of physical activities will also be examined. The second section will examine the effects of some of the most commonly used drugs on the physiological responses of humans at rest and during activity. Use of physiological ergogenic aids (e.g. blood doping, oxygen administration) to alter performance will be examined in the final section of this chapter.

The Role of Nutrition in Health and Physical Activity

Carbohydrates

The primary role of carbohydrates (sugars and starches) in the diet is to supply energy for muscle contraction and metabolic reactions in most cells. Nerve tissue, in particular, relies almost exclusively on carbohydrates as its source of energy for metabolism. Under normal resting conditions, 50% of the energy used by the body will be supplied by the carbohydrate stores. During light physical activity the cells will continue to use a 50:50 mixture of fats and carbohydrates for energy. As the intensity of the activity increases, more of the energy will be derived from carbohydrates and less from fats because less oxygen is needed in the combustion of carbohydrate than fat (Figure 1). At the highest exercise intensities, carbohydrates are used almost exclusively as the fuel for energy.

Carbohydrates are stored in the liver and muscles as glycogen. Energy needs of the remaining cells are supplied by glucose which is derived from the carbohydrates in the diet or released from the liver glycogen stores. A small amount of

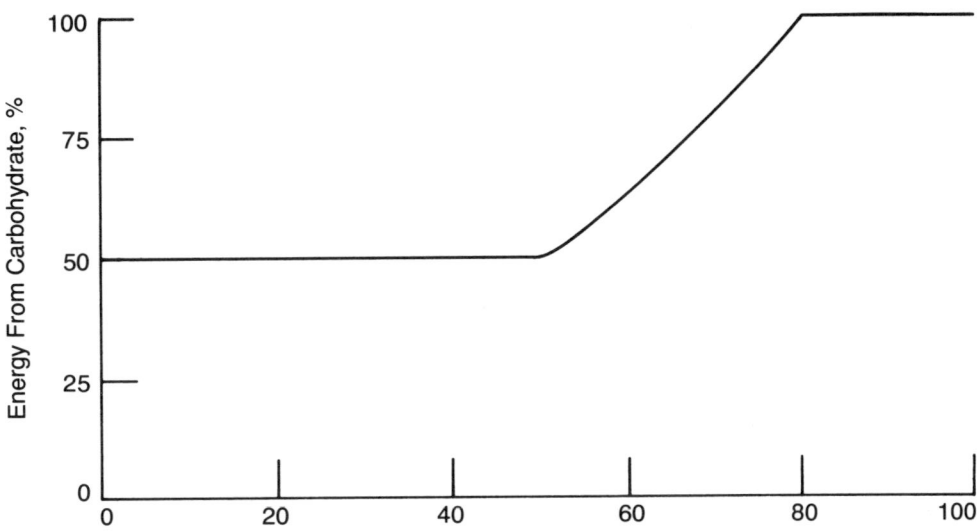

Fig. 1. Relationship between exercise intensity and energy derived from carbohydrate. (Adapted from the *Textbook of Work Physiology, 3rd ed.* by P.O. Astrand & K. Rodahl (1986). New York: McGraw-Hill).

glucose released from the liver is derived from other sources (e.g. lactic acid, amino acids) through gluconeogenesis. After a normal mixed diet, skeletal muscles will contain 300 g of glycogen and liver glycogen storage will range between 55 and 90 g (Saltin, 1978).

The actual source of energy used by the muscle for contraction is the high energy phosphate compound adenosine triphosphate (ATP).

$$ATP \rightarrow ADP + P + energy$$

When ATP is split into ADP and an inorganic phosphate (P), the energy stored in the chemical bond is released and part of it is used in the mechanical work of contraction. However, there is only a small quantity of ATP stored in any cell; enough for approximately two seconds work. ATP must be resynthesized by splitting other high energy compounds located in the muscle. Creatine phosphate (CP) is another high energy phosphate compound stored in muscle fibers. The energy stored in its chemical bond is used to resynthesize ATP from ADP.

$$CP + ADP \rightarrow ATP + C$$

Approximately four times as much creatine phosphate will be stored in muscle cells as ATP.

Glycogen and glucose can also supply energy for the resynthesis of ATP when they are broken into smaller molecules (Figure 2). If little oxygen is available to the muscle fiber, pyruvic acid will be converted to lactic acid with a net synthesis of two molecules of ATP. Pyruvic acid can only be converted to acetyle Co A and enter the Kreb's cycle when oxygen is present. Oxygen is needed at the final step of the Electron Transport System (ETS) to accept hydrogen ions (H^+) and electrons for the formation of water. In the transfer of electrons through the ETS, energy is released which is used to resynthesize ATP. The complete breakdown of glucose to carbon dioxide and water will yield a net synthesis of 38 ATP.

$$C_6H_{12}O_6 + 6\ O_2 \rightarrow 6\ CO_2 + 6\ H_2O + 38\ ATP$$

More energy is supplied when glucose is metabolized aerobically (with oxygen) than anaerobically (without oxygen).

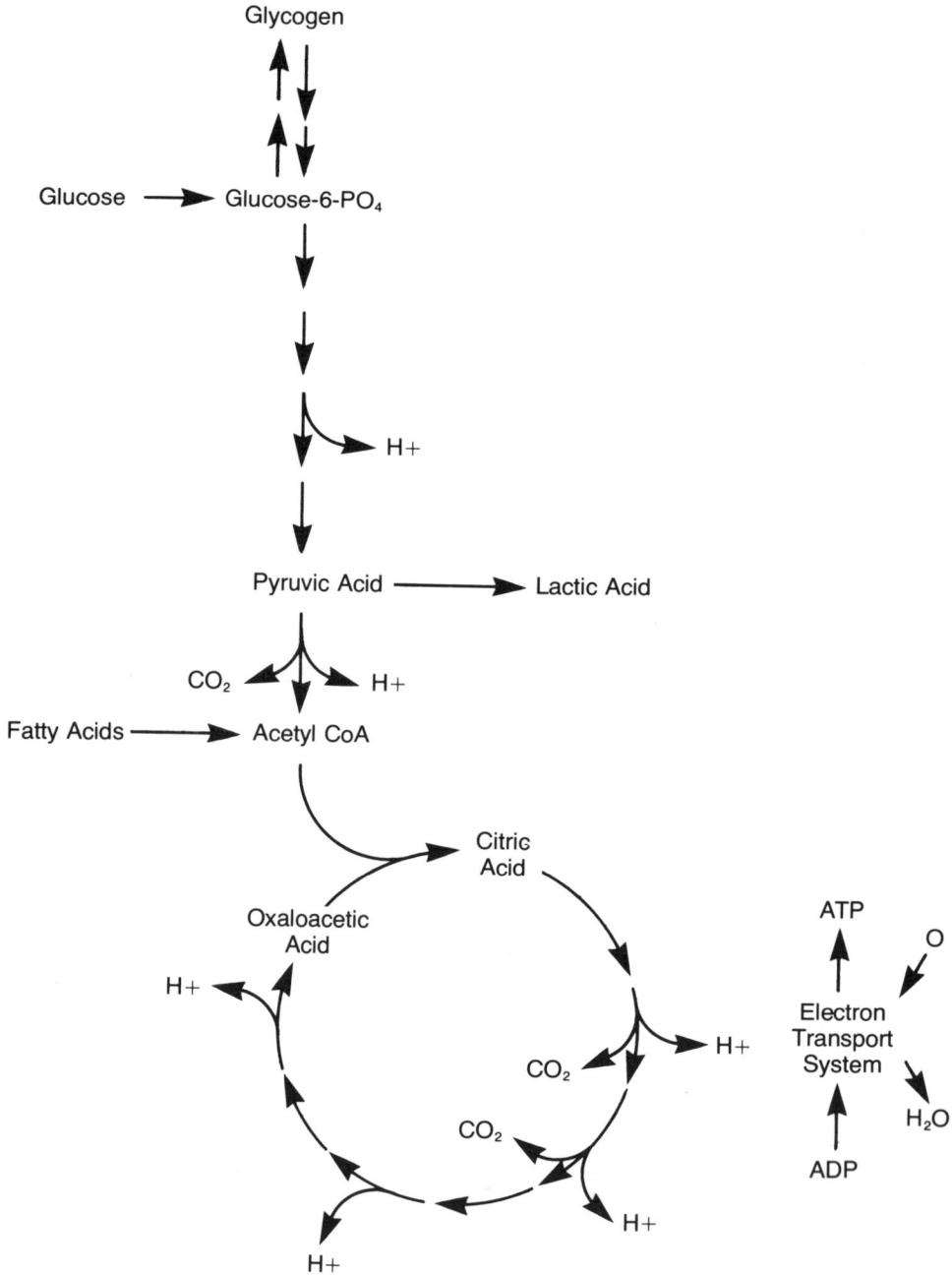

Fig. 2. The breakdown of carbohydrates through glycolysis and the Kreb's cycle of energy production.

Skeletal muscle glycogen stores are used for energy during physical activity. Glycogen stores in the vastus lateralis muscle of adult males were found to be nearly depleted after 90 minutes of exercise when the intensity was approximately 77% of the maximal oxygen uptake (Hermansen, Hultman, & Saltin, 1967). At lower exercise intensities the rate of glycogen depletion will occur more slowly. Children and adolescents have less glycogen stored in skeletal muscle than adults (Eriksson, 1980; Eriksson, Gollnick, & Saltin, 1973). The capacity to produce energy through anaerobic glycolysis is also limited in children because the amount of phosphofructokinase (PFK) in children's muscles is less than 50% that of adult males (Eriksson et al., 1973). Liver glycogen stores are also depleted during prolonged heavy exercise. When the liver glycogen stores are depleted, glucose will be produced for other sources, namely, lactic acid, certain amino acids, and glycerol.

Carbohydrate loading. Muscle glycogen stores can be increased by manipulating the diet. Early studies reported muscle glycogen stores were doubled by first depleting the stores by exercising to exhaustion, followed by three days on a high fat and protein diet (80% of the calories) and then three days on a high carbohydrate (80-90%) diet (Bergstrom, Hermansen, Hultman, & Saltin, 1967). The main drawback to this technique is the three days of low carbohydrate intake. Exercise is difficult when the glycogen stores are depleted. Liver glycogen stores will also be depleted using this technique, which may lead to low blood glucose levels. Recent evidence suggests that neither exercise to exhaustion nor three days of a high fat and protein diet are necessary for the muscle glycogen stores to increase (Sherman, Costill, Fink, & Miller, 1981). Subjects could increase the amount of glycogen stored in the muscle by tapering their training while consuming a mixed diet (50% carbohydrate) for three days and then increasing the cabohydrate intake to 70% for three days. This dietary manipulation would be preferred to the high fat and protein diet.

An increase in glycogen content does not necessarily mean that a person can run a race faster. Most studies indicate that races which are 20 miles or less will not be affected by increasing the muscle glycogen stores (Sherman et al., 1981). Speed in the latter stages of longer races (more than 20 miles) is increased by carbohydrate loading (Karlsson & Saltin, 1971). When the glycogen stores are depleted, a runner is forced to slow his/her pace so that fat can be burned for energy. By prolonging the time the glycogen can be used, a faster pace can be maintained for a greater distance. Endurance is also improved by carbohydrate loading. Subjects were able to double the length of time they could exercise following three days of a high carbohydrate diet compared to a mixed diet (Christiensen & Hansen, 1939). There is little evidence that carbohydrate loading improves performance in activites which are relatively short in duration such as sprinting, gymnastic events, or wrestling. However, if the glycogen stores are completely depleted, performance is likely to be reduced.

Glucose feeding before and during exercise. Use of a glucose soluton or solid sugar feeding prior to exercise has an adverse effect on the performer if it is eaten or drunk 15 minutes to two hours before participation. Glucose will be absorbed rapidly into the blood stream and the blood glucose level will rise stimulating an insulin response. When exercise begins, glucose will be removed by the cells at a faster rate than normal because of the combined effects of insulin and exercise. Blood glucose has been reported to fall below normal levels during the first 20 minutes of exercise in such instances (Costill, Coyle, Dalsky, Evans, Fink, & Hooper, 1977). The muscles will use carbohydrate as the preferred source of fuel when glucose is given prior to exercise. Because glucose is the main source of energy used by the nervous system, low blood glucose (hypoglycemia) can impair psychomotor performance, reduce endurance, and increase the feeling of fatigue (Brooke, 1978; Foster et al., 1979).

Glucose feedings which are delayed until after exercise begins do not stimulate an insulin response and will help maintain the blood glucose level during prolonged activity if taken at frequent intervals. However, glucose feeding during exercise will stimulate the use of glucose by the muscles (Ahlborg & Felig, 1977). An ideal solution would be one which contains no more than 25 g glucose per liter and is kept cold (Costill & Saltin, 1974). If the glucose solution is too concentrated, gastric emptying will be slowed. The amount of solution taken should not exceed

250 ml (1 cup) every 15 minutes, because larger quantities will remain in the stomach.

Glycogen replacement following activity. Many participants in strenuous activities are not aware of the need to replace glycogen stores following the activity. Several studies have shown that muscle glycogen stores are reduced after several days of running or skiing (Costill, Bowers, Branam, & Sparks, 1972; Nygaard, Andersen, Nilsson, Ericksson, Kjessel, & Saltin, 1978). Low levels of muscle glycogen during activity could impair training and increase the risk of injury. Apparently a mixed diet containing 40 to 50% carbohydrate is not adequate to replace glycogen losses. Recent work suggests that a diet containing 70% carbohydrate will replace the glycogen stores in 24 hours (Costill, Sherman, Fink, Maresh, Witten, & Miller, 1981). A greater amount of glycogen is stored over a 48 hour period if complex carbohydrates were consumed rather than simple sugars. In other words, starches found in cereals, pasta, and vegetables may be a better source of replacement carbohydrate than the sugars found in candy and soft drinks.

Lipids

Fats belong to the family of organic compounds known as lipids. The fats stored in the adipose tissue and most of the fat found in food are in the form of triglycerides. Triglycerides are composed of three fatty acids and a glycerol. Other lipids found in food and the body are phospholipids (e.g. lecithin) and sterols (e.g. cholesterol).

Slightly more than 50% of our energy is derived from fats when we are at rest. In order for fat to be used as an energy source, the triglycerides must first be mobilized from storage in the adipose tissue and released into the blood as free fatty acids (FFA) and glycerol. Cells which need a source of energy will then remove the FFA from the blood and break down the FFA to CO_2 and H_2O. During the metabolism of FFA a large amount of O_2 will be needed. The amount of ATP produced varies with the length of the FFA, but a typical FFA such as palmitic acid will yield 130 ATP. Per gram, fat is a better source of energy than carbohydrate. However, because more O_2 is needed to use fat, a person will be about 11% more efficient when using carbohydrate.

During light to moderate exercise (50% $\dot{V}O_2max$) nearly half of the energy produced will come from fats. At higher exercise intensities less energy will be derived from fats and more from carbohydrate (Figure 3). Trained endurance athletes are better able than untrained persons to use fats for energy as the exercise intensity increases. Increased FFA uptake by muscles begins almost immediately during light to moderate exercise. Blood FFA levels will drop initially, then rise as FFA are mobilized from storage sites. Increased FFA mobilization during exercise is thought to be due to norepinephrine released by the sympathetic nervous system (Havel, 1974). Mobilization of FFA can be enhanced by caffeine (Costill, Dalsky, & Fink, 1978) and inhibited by lactic acid (Miller, Issekutz, Paul, & Rodahl, 1964), insulin, and nicotinic acid (Carson, Havel, Ekelund, & Holmgren, 1963).

Dietary fat and blood lipids. Diets containing large quantities of fat with a high proportion of saturated fatty acids are associated with elevated serum cholesterol levels and an increased risk of coronary heart disease (CHD) (Kannelk, Doyle, & Ostfield, 1980). Total serum cholesterol can be subdivided into three fractions: very low density lipoprotein (VLDL) cholesterol; low density lipoprotein (LDL) cholesterol; and high density lipoprotein (HDL) cholesterol. LDL is thought to be the carrier of cholesterol which results in deposition of cholesterol on the walls of blood vessels and the formation of atherosclerotic plaques. HDL is believed to remove cholesterol to the liver for excretion. VLDL is the carrier for endogenous triglycerides. Elevated LDL and VLDL cholesterol levels are associated with an

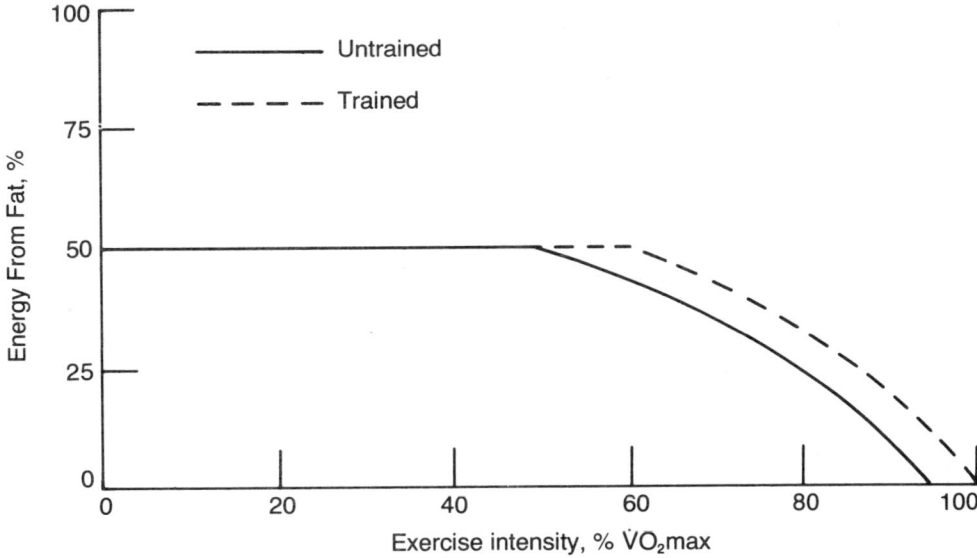

Fig. 3. Relationship between exercise intensity and energy derived from fats.

increased risk of CHD while elevated HDL cholesterol levels are associated with a low risk of CHD (Castelli et al., 1977).

Fats with a higher proportion of saturated fatty acids are found in meats, dairy products, and eggs. Most fats found in vegetables and grains contain a high proportion of polyunsaturated fatty acids. Vegetarians have lower levels of serum triglycerides, VLDL and LDL cholesterol than persons who eat meats and animal products (Sacks, Castelli, Donner, & Kass, 1975). Diets which lower VLDL and LDL cholesterol should reduce the incidence of CHD. Much emphasis has been placed on reducing the fat content of the American diet to no more than 30% of the total calories, the saturated fat content to 10% of the calories, and the cholesterol intake to 300 mg per day (Kannel et al., 1980). This would suggest that a diet high in carbohydrate (55 to 60% of the calories) would be beneficial in reducing serum lipid levels. However, recent evidence suggests that a diet high in polyunsaturated fatty acids may be more beneficial in lowering total serum cholesterol and triglyeride than either high carbohydrate or high saturated fat diets (Lukaski, Bolonchuk, Klevay, Mahalko, Milne, & Sandstead, 1984).

There is evidence that atherosclerosis and CHD may begin during childhood. Deposits of fat appear in the arteries of children and atherosclerotic plaque is frequently observed in the coronary arteries of young men in their 20's. Surveys of American adolescents have found that up to 20% had serum cholesterol levels exceeding 200 mg/dl (Glueck, Fallat, & Tsang, 1974). It has been suggested that dietary modification might be more beneficial in reducing serum cholesterol and triglyceride levels, and utimately CHD, if begun during childhood. Lower serum cholesterol levels have been observed when adolescent males consumed a diet which contained more polyunsaturated fat and less saturated fat and cholesterol (McGandy, Hall, Ford, & Stare, 1972). Reducing body weight to ideal weight has proved very effective in lowering serum triglyceride levels of children with hypertriglyceridema (Glueck, Fallat, & Tsang, 1975).

Ketogenic diets and physical activity. Among the most popular diets for losing weight are the low carbohydrate-ketogenic diets. Since little carbohydrate is consumed, muscle and liver glycogen stores are soon depleted. Approximately 3 g of water is stored with each g of glycogen. When the glycogen stores are used, the water is excreted. This is part of the reason why weight is lost rapidly on a low carbohydrate diet. As blood glucose levels decline, fat becomes the major source of energy. Excess fat metabolism leads to the formation of ketone bodies in liver which can be used by most cells, including the nervous system, for energy. Ketone bodies are also believed to depress the appetite and further reduce caloric intake.

Short term use (3 to 14 days) of low carbohydrate diets have a detrimental effect on endurance performance (Bergstrom et al., 1967; Pruett, 1970; Galbo, Holst, & Christiensen, 1979). Recent work has suggested that long term (28 days) adaptation to a ketogenic diet results in no loss of endurance (Phinney, Bistrain, Evans, Gervino, & Blackburn, 1983). However, the exercise intensity was slightly lower (64% $\dot{V}O_2$max vs. 70-75% $\dot{V}O_2$max) in the long term study than in the earlier studies. No improvement in endurance exercise at 85% $\dot{V}O_2$max was seen following 21 days of a low carbohydrate diet (Cooney, 1983). Athletes performing in activities requiring primarily glycogen as the source of energy are most likely to be affected by a low carbohydrate diet.

Protein

The need for protein during growth and development is reflected in the Recommended Dietary Allowance (RDA) for protein (Table 1). Protein is needed for the growth and repair of all cells and tissues including muscle cells. Lack of adequate protein results in smaller than normal muscle cells (Milner, 1976). In addition, protein is needed for the formation of hemoglobin, plasma proteins and antibodies, enzymes, and some hormones. Children suffering from protein-calorie malnutrition have been found to be smaller in stature, have lower aerobic capacities, and have higher heart rates at a given workload than children who were well nourished (Spurr, Barc-Nietro, & Maksud, 1978). Nutritional surveys conducted in the United States during the late 1960's and early 1970's suggest that most children and adolescents consume adequated protein in their diets. Low protein intakes were most often (10% or less) found in the diets of adolescent girls.

Protein as an energy source. The role of protein in supplying energy during exercise has long been disputed. Many exercise physiologists concluded that protein was not used for energy during exercise because the amount of urea excreted in the urine did not increase. However, recent studies suggest that significant amounts of urea are excreted in sweat during exercise (Dohm, Williams, Kasperek, & Van Rij, 1982; Lemon & Mullin, 1980). When protein is broken down and the individual amino acids are catabolized, the nitrogen containing amine group is converted to urea for excretion. The remainder of the original amino acid can be used for energy purposes or converted to glucose in the liver. It appears that the branched-chain amino acids (Leucine, Isoleucine, and Valine)

Table 1
Recommended dietary allowances for protein

	Age yrs	Protein g	g/kg
Children	4-6	30	1.5
	7-10	34	1.2
Males	11-14	45	1.0
	15-18	56	0.9
	19-22	56	0.8
Females	11-14	46	1.0
	15-18	46	0.9
	19-22	44	0.8

Source: Food and Nutrition Board, National Academy of Sciences-National Research Council Daily Dietary Allowance, Revised 1979.

are used directly by the muscle for energy, with the amine groups transferred to pyruvic acid to form alanine (a process known as transamination). Alanine leaves the muscle cell and is transported in the blood to the liver where it is converted to glucose. The amount of the energy supplied by protein could reach 10% of the total energy expenditure during prolonged exercise, once the glycogen stores are depleted (Lemon & Mullin, 1980).

There are several possible sources of the protein used during exercise. Amino acid levels in the blood are decreased following prolonged exercise, suggesting increased catabolism of the amino acid pool (Decombaz, Reinhardt, Anatharaman, Von Glutz, & Poortmans, 1979; Refsum, Gjessing, & Stromme, 1979). There is also evidence of increased liver protein destruction during exercise (Dohm, Puente, Smith, & Edge, 1978). Muscle protein catabolism appears to increase during recovery from strenuous exercise and last for 24 to 48 hours (Dohm et al., 1982). Increased catabolism is accompanied by an elevated rate of muscle protein synthesis during the recovery period (Dohm, Kasperek, Tapscott, Barakat, & Beecher, 1980). The rate of protein catabolism appears to be greatest during the first week of a training program and declines as training progresses (Gontzea, Sutzescu, & Dumitrache, 1975).

Protein intake and physical activity. Do athletes need more protein during training than the RDA of 0.8 g/kg for adults? Studies of young men undertaking a weight training program suggest that 0.5 g/kg is inadequate for building muscle mass and 0.8 g/kg is marginal (Marable, Hickson, Korslund, Herbert, Desjardins, & Thye, 1979; Torun, Scrimshaw, & Young, 1977). For the vast majority of adults undertaking physical activity programs a protein intake of 1.0 g/kg should be sufficient (Gontzea et al., 1975; Torun et al., 1977). If a man weighing 70 kg consumes 3000 kcal/day and 12% of the calories are from protein, then his protein intake will be 90 g or 1.3 g/kg. Similarly, a woman weighing 55 kg who consumes 2000 kcal per day of which 12% is protein will take in 60 g protein or 1.1 g/kg. However, if the caloric intake is restricted (e.g., 1500 kcal), a higher percentage of the intake must be protein in order to keep the person in positive nitrogen balance (Iyengar & Narasinga Rao, 1979).

Studies with highly trained weight lifters suggest that during periods of intense training a protein intake of 2.0 g/kg is needed to maintain positive nitrogen balance (Celejowa & Homa, 1970; Laritcheva, Yalovaya, Shubin, & Smirnov, 1978). Assuming a caloric intake of 4000 kcal/day, an 80 kg weight lifter who consumed 120 g protein (12% of 4000 kcal) would have a protein intake of 1.5 g/kg. In this example, a slightly higher percentage (16%) of the caloric intake should be from protein.

Children and adolescents have a greater requirement for protein than adults in order to support growth. The average 13-year-old girl or boy weighing 44 kg who consumes 12% of the calories as protein will take in 72 g on a 2400 kcal/day diet or 1.6 g/kg, which is substantially above the RDA of 1.0 g/kg. When physical activity increases, the caloric intake will also increase. If the protein intake is maintained at 12% of the total caloric intake, it should meet the needs of most children and adolescents during training.

Iron

Iron has several functions in the body. Almost ⅔ of the iron is found in the red blood cells as part of the hemoglobin molecule. It is also found in muscle cells in myoglobin and the cytochromes. The rest of the iron is stored as ferritin and hemosiderin in the bone marrow and liver. Men have approximately 1000 mg of iron in storage while women's iron stores are only 400 mg. The amount of iron needed to balance iron loss is 1.0 mg/day in adult males and children ages 4 to 10 years and 1.8 mg/day in male and female adolescents (ages 11-18 years) and adult females. Iron is needed for the formation of hemoglobin and the expansion of blood volume during the adolescent growth spurt. Females will lose approximately 0.5 mg iron/day through the menses once menarche is reached. Because only 10% of the dietary iron is normally absorbed, the RDA for children and adult males is 10 mg iron/day and for adolescents and adult females it is 18 mg iron/day (Table 2).

Table 2
Recommended dietary allowances for iron and calcium

	Age yrs	Iron mg	Calcium mg
Children	1-3	15	800
	4-6	10	800
	7-10	10	800
Males	11-14	18	1200
	15-18	18	1200
	19-22	10	800
Females	11-14	18	1200
	15-18	18	1200
	19-22	18	800

Source: Food and Nutrition Board, National Academy of Sciences-National Research Council Recommended Daily Dietary Allowances, Revised 1979.

Low dietary iron is the most common nutritional deficiency in the United States. According to the Ten State Nutrition Survey (1968-1970) more than 60% of adolescent females and 40% of adolescent males consume 12 mg iron or less per day. The average iron intake is 6 mg/1000 kcal. Over a long period of time, low iron intake will lead to a depletion of the iron stores. Assuming an iron loss of 1.5 mg/day, if a girl reaches menarche at age 12 and her iron intake is 12 mg/day, she should deplete her iron stores in four years. Low or absent iron stores can be detected by bone marrow biopsy or by low serum ferritin levels (12 ng/ml). Once the iron stores are depleted, hemoglobin formation will be depressed and the hemoglobin concentration in the blood will decrease. Anemia is defined as a hemoglobin level below 12 g/dl for women, children and adolescents and below 13 g/dl for adult men. Approximately 10% of the adolescent females and children and 14% of the adult females were found to be anemic in one population survey (Cook, Finch, & Smith, 1976). Less than 5% of the adult males and 2% of the adolescent males were anemic. Low serum ferritin levels were found in 24.5% of the adolescent females, 21% of the adult females, 18% of the children, 12% of the adolescent males, and less than 2% of the adult males.

Physical activity and iron status. Recent evidence suggests that many distance runners, male and female, have depleted iron stores (Clement & Asmundson, 1982; Hunding, Jordal, & Paulev, 1981; Plowman & McSwegin, 1981). The proportion of adolescent female cross-country runners found to have low serum ferritin levels (45%) was nearly twice that expected in the normal population (Nickerson & Tripp, 1983). Female athletes in other sports also appear to have lower than normal serum ferritin levels (Parr, Bachman, & Moss, 1984). Male distance runners have been found to have little or no iron stored in their bone marrow (Ehn, Carlmark, & Hoglund, 1980; Wishnitzer, Vorst, & Berrebi, 1983). Since male athletes have little difficulty meeting the RDA for iron of 10 mg, depleted iron stores suggest that iron is being lost at a faster rate in runners than in normal males. Ehn and associates (1980) calculated the rate of iron loss in male distance runners at 2 mg/day.

There are several reasons why iron may be lost at a faster rate during training. The amount of iron lost in the sweat has been estimated at 0.4 mg/liter of sweat (Veller, 1968). An athlete who loses 3 liters of sweat each day would also lose 1.2 mg of iron. Another possible source of iron loss is through the mechanical destruction of red blood cells, especially during running. Increased red blood cell fragility has been observed during the early phases of training and evidence of red blood cell destruction is frequently observed in distance runners (Dufaux, Hoederath, Streitberger, Hollmann, & Assmann, 1981; Hunding et al., 1981; Puhl, Runyan, & Kruse, 1981). Although most of the iron released during hemolysis should be recycled, small quantities may be lost through the urine. Recent evidence also suggests distance runners may lose some blood through the gastrointenstinal tract during running.

Iron deficiency and physical activity. Because iron is needed for hemoglobin formation and hemoglobin carries oxygen in the blood, low iron levels should reduce the maximal amount of oxygen transported to the tissues. Anemia is known to reduce maximal oxygen intake and physical work capacity (Gardner, Edgerton, Senewiratne, Barnard, & Ohira, 1977; Sproule, Mitchell, Miller, 1960). Blood lactate levels are elevated following strenuous work in anemic persons (Edgerton, Ohira, Hettiarachchi, Senewiratne, Gardner, & Barnard, 1981). At submaximal exercise intensities anemic persons can maintain oxygen transport by increasing heart rate and cardiac output (Davies, Chukweumeka, & Van Haaren, 1973).

Evidence from animal studies suggests that iron deficiency without anemia also has a detrimental effect on exercise performance. After iron deficient animals have had their hemoglobin levels restored to normal by transfusion, higher blood lactate levels are observed following exercise than in animals with normal iron status (Finch, Gollnick, Hlastala, Miller, Dillmann, & Mackler, 1979). Muscle fatigue occurs more rapidly in iron deficient animals than in controls (McLane, Fell, McKay, Winder, Brown, & Holloszy, 1981). Reduced levels of cytochrome c and cytochrome oxidase and a decreased respiratory capacity of skeletal muscle were observed in the iron deficient animals, suggesting that iron depletion affects tissue iron levels as well as bone marrow (McLane et al., 1981).

Iron supplements and physical activity. There is little question that iron therapy is beneficial in treating iron deficiency anemia. Not only are hemoglobin and iron levels elevated, but exercise performance is improved (Edgerton et al., 1981; Ohira, Edgerton, Gardner, Gunawardena, Senewiratne, & Ikawa, 1981; Ohira, Edgerton, Gardner, Senewiratne, Barnard, & Simpson, 1979). Recent evidence also suggests that iron therapy is beneficial in improving exercise tolerance of non-anemic iron deficient subjects. Lower heart rates and blood lactate levels were observed in iron deficient subjects following a few days of iron theapy (Ohira et al., 1981; Schoene, Escourrou, Robertson, Nilson, Parsons, & Smith, 1983). Muscle endurance increases and muscle lactate levels decline following a few days of iron supplementation in iron deficient rats (McLane et al., 1981). The improvement in endurance was accompanies by an increase in oxygen uptake by the muscles and increased levels of cytochrome c and cytochrome oxidase.

Because iron deficiency is fairly common among women athletes, there has been much interest in the routine use of iron supplements by athletes. Some studies of iron supplements failed to demonstrate any beneficial effects with athletes (Cooter & Mowbray, 1978; Haymes, Puhl, & Temples, 1983; Pate, Maguire, & Van Wyk, 1979). These studies used iron supplements containing 18-50 mg per day. Studies which used large supplements (60-270 mg iron) have been more successful in increasing iron and hemoglobin levels in iron deficient athletes (Hunding et al., 1981; Nickerson & Tripp, 1983; Plowman & McSwegin, 1981; Schoene et al., 1983). The problem with using supplements larger than 18 mg for long periods is that the excess iron will be stored and can become toxic. Large iron supplements should only be used after a person has been diagnosed as iron deficient. Because iron deficiency is so common among females of all ages, routine screening for low hemoglobin and ferritin levels should be a part of the annual physical exam for all female athletes. Routine use of an iron supplement containing 18 mg by female athletes may be beneficial in preventing iron deficiency from developing during training.

Calcium

Calcium is the most abundant mineral found in the body. Most of the body's calcium (99%) is stored in bones as calcium salts. Deposition of calcium salts in organic bone matrix during growth causes the bone to become hard or ossify. The remaining 1% of the calcium is free calcium and extremely important physiologically as it is needed for nerve conduction, muscle contraction, and blood clotting. Blood calcium levels are maintained within a narrow range, at the expense of calcium stores in bones. If blood calcium levels drop because of low calcium levels in the diet, calcium will be removed from the bones to maintain blood calcium levels.

The RDA for calcium is greatest during adolescence because of the rapid growth and ossification of bones during this period (Table 2). Approximately 25% of U.S. preschool children have calcium intakes which are inadequate (Guthrie, 1979). Supplementing the diet with foods rich in calcium increases bone growth in young children who have inadequate calcium in the diet (Rajalakshmi, Sail, Shah, & Ambady, 1973). Low calcium intake (less than 500 mg/day) has also been found in the diets of 25% of adolescent females and approximately 50% of women over 35 (Schuette & Linkswiler, 1984).

Calcium and bone mineral loss. Loss of calcium from bone begins after age 40 in both men and women, however, the rate of bone mineral loss is more than twice as great for women (8% per decade) as men (3% per decade) (Garn, Rohmann, & Wagner, 1967). Women begin to lose bone rapidly at the onset of menopause, due to the lack of estrogen. Loss of bone mineral content can ultimately lead to osteoporosis, a disorder in which the bones become brittle, and an increased risk of fractures. Osteoporosis is more common and occurs earlier in women, often soon after menopause. Fractures of the vertebrae are seen most commonly in women after menopause, while hip fractures occur later in life for both men and women (Warren, 1985). In addition to lack of estrogen, lack of physical activity and low calcium intake have been implicated in the development of osteoporosis.

The relationship of calcium intake to the development of osteoporosis is somewhat controversial. Little relationship between calcium intake and bone cortical thickness has been reported for men and women ages 25 to 85 (Garn et al., 1967). On the other hand, persons who traditionally have low calcium intakes have less bone cortical width and a greater frequency of fractures than persons who have higher calcium intakes (Matkovic, Kostial, Simonovic, Buzina, Brodarec, & Nordin, 1979). The RDA for calcium may be too low for women over age 35. It has been estimated that women prior to menopause and postmenopausal women receiving estrogen need approximately 1000 mg calcium daily, while untreated postmenopausal women need 1500 mg/day to maintain calcium balance (Heaney, Recker, & Saville, 1978). Once menopause occurs, estrogen therapy prevents the loss of bone mineral content, and calcium supplements slow the rate of bone loss (Recker, Saville, & Heaney, 1977). Both physical activity and a combination calcium and vitamin D supplement have been found to prevent bone loss in elderly persons (Smith, Reddan, & Smith, 1981).

Sodium, Potassium, and Chlorine

Three other minerals found in relatively large quantities in the body are sodium, potassium, and chlorine. All three ionize in solutions such as the body fluids and are frequently referred to as electrolytes. Sodium (Na$^+$) and chlorine (Cl$^-$) are found primarily in extracellular fluids outside the cell. Potassium (K$^+$) is found primarily in intracellular fluid inside the cell. One of the major functions of the electrolytes is to maintain water balance between the inside and outside of the cells. Other functions of these electrolytes include nerve impulse conduction and assisting in the maintenance of an acid/base balance. Under normal circumstances electrolyte concentrations are maintained within a narrow range by the renin-angiotensin-aldosterone system. If sodium levels decrease, sodium is conserved by the kidneys, and if it rises above normal levels, the excess sodium is excreted in the urine. Excess fluid loss through sweating, diuresis, vomiting, or diarrhea can substantially reduce the amount of one or more of the electrolytes.

There is no RDA for sodium, potassium, or cholrine, Instead, the Food and Nutrition Board suggests that adults should limit their sodium intake to 1.1-3.3 g per day and their salt (NaCl) intake to 3 to 8 g/day. Suggested sodium intake for children and adolescents is less than that of adults and increases with age and body growth. Average NaCl intake of adults in the U.S. ranges from 10 to 14.5 g/day (Fregly, 1984). Because most of the sodium in the diet is in the form of NaCl, the average sodium intake would be 3.9 to 5.7 g/day. In general, males consume more sodium than females because they have a higher caloric intake. There is some concern that high sodium intakes lead to the development of hypertension. Increased sodium retention leads to fluid retention and an expanded blood volume, which results in an increased blood pressure. Some studies comparing different populations report a positive relationship between sodium intake and hypertension while other studies have found no significant relationship (Fregly, 1984).

Sweating and electrolyte depletion. Sweat is a more dilute solution than plasma. The concentration of sodium and chlorine in sweat is only one-third of their concentration in plasma, while the concentration of potassium is approximately the same in plasma and sweat. However, since most of the potsssium is inside the cell, the potassium content of the plasma is quite low. An average liter of sweat contains 1150 mg Na, 1420 mg Cl, and 195 mg K (Veller, 1968). If a person exercising vigorously in a warm climate loses 3 liters of sweat (6.6 lbs), the sodium and chloride losses of 3450 mg and 4260 mg respectively will still be less than the normal daily NaCl intake of 10 to 14 g. When sweat loss is 4 liters (8.8 lbs), electolyte losses result in a 5% deficit in the body's sodium, a 7% chloride deficit and a 1% potassium deficit (Fink, 1982). Prolonged exercise in the heat leading to sweat losses exceeding 4 liters would produce a greater depletion of the body's electrolyte content. Repeated daily exposure to exercise in the heat could lead to substantial losses of sodium and chloride from the body. As a result, the person may experience heat cramps or salt depletion heat exhaustion while exercising in the heat.

The total amount of potassium lost through sweating is much smaller than for sodium and chloride. There is some evidence that potassium depletion can occur with repeated daily exercise in hot environments (Knochel, 1977). However, potassium depletion is more likely to occur after excessive fluid loss through vomiting and diarrhea or when diuretics are used. Potassium depletion may increase a person's susceptibility to heat stroke during exercise (Knochel, 1977).

Electrolyte replacement. How much salt does a person who exercises in a hot environment need? Men who do heavy work in the heat every day need approximately 15 g NaCl (Taylor, Henschel, Mickelson, & Keys, 1944). Because this amount is only slightly greater than the normal dietary intake, very little extra salt is needed. Increasing the salt intake to 30 g results in excretion of the excess sodium. If a person loses more than 4 liters of sweat per day, a slight increase in NaCl should be added to the diet. This can best be accomplished by adding a few more shakes from the salt shaker to food or by choosing a few foods which are high in sodium (e.g. pretzels, potato chips, ham). Salt tablets are not advisable because they often irritate the digestive tract. In order for a salt tablet to pass from the stomach to the small intestine, it must first be diluted to the proper osmolarity. Unless a sufficient quantity of water is ingested with the salt tablet, one pint of water per salt tablet, the salt tablet will remain in the stomach until sufficient body fluids are drawn into the stomach to dilute it.

Since the average potassium intake is 2 to 5 g/day, there appears to be little need for an increase in potassium intake during exercise in hot environments. Excess potassium in the diet is excreted if sodium intake is adequate (Costill, Cote, & Fink, 1982).

Glucose-electrolyte drinks for replenishing body fluids during exercise have been widely advertised as beneficial. These drinks contain a small amount of sugar (glucose, sucrose, or fructose), sodium, chloride, potassium, and sometimes magnesium in addition to water. The amount of sugar and electrolytes affects the osmolarity of the solution. Some glucose-electrolyte drinks contain too much sugar for rapid emptying and should be diluted for faster entry into the small intestine. Cold drinks will empty more rapidly from the stomach than warm ones (Costeill & Saltin, 1974). While the small amount of glucose may be beneficial during endurance events, there is little evidence that glucose-electrolyte drinks are superior to water in maintaining core temperature during exercise (Costill, Kammer & Fisher, 1970).

Water

Water is the single most important and abundant compound found in the body, comprising between 50 and 60% of the total body weight. Approximately ⅔ of the water is found inside cells, while the remaining ⅓ is extracellular. Included in the extracellular water is the plasma volume, 2.5 to 3 liters, and the interstitial fluid surrounding the cells, another 12 liters. During physical activty plasma is needed to transport nutrients to the cell and waste products from the cell. In addition, heat which is produced in the muscles during metabolism must be removed and transferred to other parts of the body. Because water is an excellent conductor of heat and has a high specific heat (i.e. can absorb a large quantity of heat without changing temperature), most of the heat is removed from the muscles by plasma. When heat is removed by fluid movement, the process is known as convection. In a cold environment, heat transported by the plasma is used to maintain tissue temperature in less active regions of the body. In warm environments, most of the heat will be transferred to the skin through superficial blood vesels. If the ambient air temperature is below skin temperature, heat will be transferred to the surrounding enviornment through convention, radiation and evaporation.

Evaporation is the process of changing water from a liquid to a gaseous state. In order for evaporation to occur, heat must be added. Evaporation of one liter of water requires 580 kilocalories (kcal). Sweat is formed from the interstitial fluid and is composed mostly of water, with a small quantity of elecrolytes and other substances. The amount of sweat produced during exercise primarily depends upon the intensity of the exercise bout, the ambient temperature, and the relative humidity. In general, the greater the intensity of the exercise or the higher the ambient temperature, the higher the sweat rate. More sweat will be produced in dry climates than humid climates because the presence of moisture on the skin suppresses sweating. Because sweat is more dilute than interstitial fluid, as sweating continues the interstitial fluid becomes more concentrated and draws water from both the plasma and intracellular water. A reduction of plasma volume reduces the total amount of blood available for circulation to the tissues. This usually results in a decrease in stroke volume, the amount of blood pumped per beat. In order to maintain cardiac output and blood flow to the tissues under these conditions, the heart rate must increase.

Hypohydration and heat illness. During prolonged exercise such as running a marathon, athletes may lose six liters of sweat or more (Costill et la., 1970). In the typical marathon runner, a weight loss of this magnitude could represent 10% of the total body weight. Failure of athletes to replace water losses in excess of 3% of body weight leads to elevated rectal temperatures (Wyndham & Strydom, 1969). The increase in rectal temperature is directly proportional to the percent body weight lost. Dehydration is one of the primary causes of heat illness among athletes. Heat stroke and heat exhaustion cases occur during distance races in warm weather and occasionally even on relatively cool days (Hanson & Zimmerman, 1979; Hughson, Green, Houston, Thomsom, MacLean, & Sutton, 1980; England, Fraser, Hightower, Tirinnanzi, Greenberg, Powell, Slovis, & Varsha, 1982).

Unfortunately, many persons do not voluntarily replace fluid loss during exercise (Bar-Or, Dotan, Inbar, Rotshtein, & Zonder, 1980; Wyndham & Strydom, 1969). Thirst is often satisfied before body fluid replacement is completed. In children, the rate of increase in rectal temperature is greater per percent body weight loss than for adults (Bar-Or et al., 1980). Most children will not voluntarily replace the amount of fluid lost through sweating. Children are less tolerant of exercise in hot environments than adults even though fluid replacement is forced (Drinkwater, Kupprat, Denton, Crist, & Horvath, 1977; Haymes, Buskirk, Hodgson, Lundegren, & Nicholas, 1974; Haymes, McCormick, & Buskirk, 1975). The inability of children to maintain thermal equilibrium in hot environments is most likely due to the child's large ratio of surface area to body mass. More heat will be gained from the environment by the child, in proportion to the mass which must absorb it, than in the adult. In order to achieve thermal equilibrium the child will have to supply more blood to the skin and produce a greater amount of sweat per unit of surface area than the adult. Blood flow to the skin is higher in children than adults, but this results in a lower stroke volume and cardiac output for the child (Drinkwater et al., 1977). Prepubertal children appear unable to produce as much sweat as adults in hot environments (Bar-Or, 1980; Haymes et al., 1975).

Fluid replacement and physical activity. Drinking small quantities (100 to 200 ml) of fluids at intervals of 5 to 20 minutes during exercise results in lower rectal temperatures than exercise without fluid replacement (Costill et al., 1970; Gisolfi & Copping, 1974). Although fluid loss is likely to exceed this rate of fluid replacement during heavy exercise, the rate of gastric emptying limits the amount of fluid intake. Larger quantities of fluid intake are likely to stay in the stomach and may produce sensations of gastric distress. The osmolarity and temperature of the fluid determine the rate at which fluids empty from the stomach. Water and solutions containing sugar and/or electroltyes with an osmolarity of 200 mOsmol/liter or less will empty most rapidly from the stomach (Costill & Saltin, 1974). Cold fluids (5°C) empty at a faster rate than warm fluids.

Hyperhydration during the 30 minute period before exercise is also beneficial. If fluids are consumed in large quantities more than 30 minutes prior to activity, the kidneys begin excreting the excess water load in the urine. For best results, hyperhydration should be combined with fluid intake during activity (Gisolfi & Copping, 1974).

Dehydration and weight loss. In sports such as wrestling and boxing, where weight classifications are used, athletes frequently lose large amounts of weight prior to weigh-in before the event. Much of this weight loss is accomplished by dehydration. The athlete may sit in a sauna or exercise in a rubber suit to sweat off excess pounds, restrict fluid intake as well as caloric intake for several days, or use a diuretic. Such procedures result in a reduction of plasma volume and increased heart rate during exercise (Costill & Sparks, 1973), a reduction in physical work capacity (Herbert & Ribisl, 1972), and decreased muscular strength (Houston, Marrin, Green, & Thomson, 1981).

During the one to five hours between weigh-in and competition, the athlete attempts to rehydrate. Plasma volume is not always restored over the period of rehydration, although heart rate during exercise returns to normal after more than 60% of the body weight loss is replaced (Costell & Sparks, 1973). Muscular strength and physical work capacity are still likely to be below normal following rehydration (Houston et al., 1981; Herbert & Ribisl, 1972). The American College of Sports Medicine has taken a position stand discouraging fluid deprivation and dehydration in wrestling (American College of Sports Medicine, 1976).

Vitamins

Nutrients classified as vitamins are divided into two groups—those which are water soluble and those which are fat soluble. Water soluble vitamins include all of the vitamins in the B complex family and vitamin C, while the fat soluble vitamins include vitamins A, D, E and K. The B complex vitamins serve as coenzymes for metabolic reactions and are involved mostly in either the breakdown of other nutrients for energy purposes or the formation of substances such as hemoglobin. Vitamin C is involved in the formation of collagen, a tough protein which gives strength to connective tissues including tendons, ligaments, and bone. Vitamin A is necessary for the formation of rhodopsin, needed for night vision. Vitamin D plays a major role in the absorption of calcium from the diet. One of the major functions of vitamin E in human beings is to serve as an antioxidant, preventing the oxidation of the unsaturated fatty acids in the cell membrane. The major function of vitamin K is the formation of prothrombin, a plasma protein involved in blood coagulation.

Table 3
Recommended dietary allowances for selected vitamins

Vitamin	Children		Males			Females		
	4-6	7-10	11-14	15-18	19-22	11-14	15-18	19-22
Thiamin, mg	0.9	1.2	1.4	1.4	1.5	1.1	1.1	1.1
Riboflavin, mg	1.0	1.4	1.6	1.6	1.7	1.3	1.3	1.3
Niacin, mg	11	16	18	18	19	15	14	14
B_6, mg	1.3	1.6	1.8	2.0	2.2	1.8	2.0	2.0
B_{12}, ug	2.5	3.0	3.0	3.0	3.0	3.0	3.0	3.0
C, mg	45	45	50	60	60	50	60	60
A, ug R.E.	500	700	1000	1000	1000	800	800	800
D, ug	10	10	10	10	7.5	10	10	7.5
E, mg αT.E.	6	7	8	10	10	8	8	8

Source: Food and Nutrition Board, National Academy of Sciences-National Research Council Recommended Daily Dietary allowances, Revised 1979.

The RDA's for most of the vitamins for children and adolescents are listed in Table 3. As the child grows, the need for most vitamins increases. The need for three of the B complex vitamins—thiamin, riboflavin, and niacin—is directly related to the amount of energy expenditure. All three of these vitamins are involved in the breakdown of carbohydrates, fats and proteins for energy. Thiamin becomes the coenzyme TPP involved in the removal of CO_2 from pyruvic acid, alpha ketoglutarate, and the branched chain amino acids. Niacin becomes NAD and riboflavin is converted to FAD, both coenzymes in the electron transport system. When energy expenditure increases, such as training for a competitive sports team, the need for these three vitamins also increases.

Vitamin B_6 is also involved in energy formation. Most of the vitamin B_6 in mammals is found in muscle in the enzyme glycogen phosphorylase (Henderson, 1984). Glycogen phosphorylase is necessary for the breakdown of glycogen for energy. Another B complex vitamin, pantothenic acid, is converted to coenzyme A which is necessary for aerobic catabolism of carbohydrates, as well as the breakdown of fatty acids. There is no RDA for pantothenic acid, but the suggested daily intake is 4 to 7 mg. The average intake for children is 4 to 5 mg (Olson, 1984). Folacin and vitamin B_{12} are both involved in the formation of hemoglobin.

Vitamin deficiencies and physical activity. The potential detrimental effects of a deficiency in one or more of the B complex vitamins were investigated in several studies during the early 1940's. Diets deficient in thiamin and probably low in other B complex vitamins such as niacin, riboflavin, and B_6 were assoicated with decreased endurance, in some studies (Archdeacon & Mulin, 1944; Barborka, Foltz, & Ivy, 1943; Berryman, Henderson, Wheeler, Cogswell, & Sinella, 1947; Johnson, Darling, Forbes, Brouha, Egana, & Graybiel, 1942) but not in others (Keys, Henschel, Mickelsen, & Brozek, 1943; Keys, Henschel, Taylor, Mickelsen, & Brozek, 1944). In the studies which demonstrated a detrimental effect, supplementing the diet with brewers' yeast which is a good source of thiamin, riboflavin, pantothenic acid, niacin, and B_6 or with one or more of the individual B vitamins restored performance.

Little information is available on diets deficient in other vitamins. Restricting vitamin C intake to less than 40 mg for up to one week has little effect on recovery heart rate or strength of men exposed to a hot climate (Henschel, Taylor, Brozek, Mickelsen, & Keys, 1944.).

Vitamin supplements and physical activity. There is some evidence that supplementing the diet of young men training in the heat with a multiple B vitamin will reduce fatigue (Early & Carlson, 1969). On the other hand, supplementing boys' diets with vitamin B_{12} has no effect on running performance (Montoye, Spata, Pickeny, & Barron, 1955) and vitamin B_6 supplements do not improve swimming performance (Lawrence, Smith, Bower, & Riehl, 1975). Use of megavitamin doses of niacin in its nicotinic acid form inhibits mobilization of free fatty acids and reduces fat utilization (Carlson, Havel, Ekelund, & Homgren, 1963). When the muscle glycogen stores are depleted, a large dose (1.2 g) of nicotinic acid reduces the amount of work that can be done (Pernow & Saltin, 1971).

Vitamin C supplements ranging from 2 mg/kg weight to 1000 mg/day have been reported to improve mechanical efficiency (Hoogerwerf & Hoitink, 1963; Spioch, Kobza, & Mazur, 1966) and reduce heart rate during exercise (Howald, Segesser, & Korner, 1975; Van Huss, 1966), but appear to have little effect on maximal oxygen uptake or performance in the 12 minute run (Gey, Cooper & Bottenberg, 1970; Keren & Epstein, 1980). In several of the studies which reported improved performance with vitamin C supplements, the improvement could also be due to a training effect.

There is little evidence that vitamin E supplements have a beneficial effect on performance or maximal oxygen uptake under normal environmental conditions (Lawrence et al., 1975; Shephard, Campbell, Pimm, Stuart, &Wright, 1974; Watt, Romet, McFarlane, McGuey, Allen, & Goode, 1974). However, there is some evidence that vitamin E supplements may improve aerobic performance at altitude (Shephard, 1980). Vitamin E may also have a protective effect against the oxidant effects of air pollutants, both at rest and during exercise (Dillard, Litov, Savin, Dumelin, & Tappel, 1978).

Vitamin supplements and toxicity. Because the fat soluble vitamins are stored by the body, there is some danger that megadoses of these vitamins may have toxic effects. Vitamin A can be quite toxic, especially in children, either in a single dose (30,000 ug and above) or over a period of several months in daily doses of 10,000 ug or more (McLaren, 1984). An acute toxic response is associated with elevated intracranial pressure, headache, and vomiting. Symptoms of chronic toxicity are anorexia, dry itchy skin, liver and spleen enlargement, and bone cortex thickening in the short and long bones. Vitamin D is toxic when the daily intake exceeds 1000 ug. Because vitamin D increases calcium absorption, too much vitamin D leads to calcium deposits in soft tissues. There is little evidence at present that megadoses of vitamin E are toxic; however, some persons experience nausea when taking large doses of this vitamin. The water soluble vitamins are not thought to be toxic in large doses. There are some reported side effects to megavitamin doses of vitamin C including hypoglycemia and excessive iron absorption (Sauberlich, 1984).

Effects of Pharmacological Ergogenic Aids

Pharmacological ergogenic aids are those drugs that are believed to improve performance in mental and physical activities. Included among these drugs are recreational drugs such as alcohol, cocaine, and marijuana, synthetic hormones known as anabolic steroids, drugs found in many medications such as decongestants and cold remedies, and caffeine which is found in several drinks and food consumed daily. Use of some of these drugs is illegal, as is the case with both cocaine and marijuana, while alcohol is legal only when a certain age is reached, 21 years in most states. Many of the drugs thought to have an erogenic effect, such as the amphetamines, can be obtained with a prescription, while others like caffeine and ephedrine are available as over-the-counter drugs.

Use of drugs by athletes to improve performance has been of concern to the International Olympic Committee (IOC) since 1962 when the first resolution against "doping" was passed (Ryan, 1984). In 1968 the IOC issued its first list of banned drugs and began drug testing at the Mexico City Olympics. Table 4 contains a partial list of drugs which are currently banned by the IOC.

Research on the effects of various drugs on performance in sporting events has been conducted since the beginning of the 20th century. Many of the early studies were poorly controlled and did not include a placebo. Placebos are necessary to control for any psychological effects a drug may have on the user. If a person thinks the substance is going to help, the improvement in performance may be due to psychological factors instead of any physiological changes. Some recent, well-controlled studies may appear to contradict each other. Factors which can

Table 4
Partial list of drugs banned by the International Olympic Committee

Psychomotor Stimulant Drugs	Over-the-Counter Drugs
Amphetamine	Pseudoephedrine HCl and Sulfate
Benzphetamine	Phenylpropanolamine HCl
Cocaine	Phenylephrine HCl
Dimethylamphetamine	Propylhexedrine
Methylamphetamine	Narcotic Analgesics
Norpseudoephedrine	Codeine
Central Nervous Stimulants	Heroin
Caffeine (greater than 15 ug/ml in urine)	Methadone HCl
Doxapram	Morphine Sulfate
Strychnine Nitrate	Naloxone HCl
Sympathomimetic Amines	Anabolic Steroids
Ephedrine Sulfate	Methandienone
Isoproternol	Methyltestosterone
Methylephedrine	Testosterone
Metaproterenol	

affect responses to drugs include the size of the drug dose used, the intensity and duration of the exercise bouts, the body weights of the subjects and their tolerance for the drug. For ethical reasons, studies conducted on human subjects restrict drug dosages to levels not thought to be toxic. Athletes, on the other hand, may consume drugs in much larger dosages.

Caffeine

The most widely used drug by children and adults is caffeine. Caffeine is a member of the methylxanthine family, which also includes theophylline and theobromine. Caffeine is found in many drinks including coffee, tea, hot chocolate, and cola. Table 5 lists the average amount of caffeine found in commonly used drinks, food, and drugs. Average caffeine consumption by adults in the United States is approximately 227 mg/day and caffeine consumption by children ages 6-17 years is estimated to be 101 mg/day (Graham, 1978). The amount of caffeine excreted in the urine of normal coffee drinkers rarely exceeds 7 ug/ml (Delbeke & Debackere, 1984). Most caffeine is metabolized to 1-methyl uric acid before excretion.

Table 5
Estimated caffeine content of beverages, food & drugs

Source	Caffeine Content
Coffee, brewed	90-120 mg/cup
Coffee, instant	66-74 mg/cup
Coffee, decaffinated	1-6 mg/cup
Tea, leaf	70 mg/cup
Tea, instant	30 mg/cup
Cocoa	6-24 mg/cup
Chocolate milk	48 mg/8 oz glass
Colas, Dr. Pepper, Mountain Dew	48 mg/12 oz can
Chocolate candy	20 mg/oz
Anacin, aspirin	32 mg/tablet
No Doz	100 mg/tablet

Source: Graham, 1978; MacCornack, 1977; Van Handel, 1983.

Caffeine is absorbed rapidly by the body, with peak blood levels occurring one hour after ingestion. Physiological responses to caffeine include stimulation of the central nervous system, stimulation of cardiac muscle, relaxation of smooth muscle, stimulation of gastric acid secretion, and diuresis. Although caffeine stimulates the heart, the heart rate may decrease with low doses of caffeine (50-200 mg) because the vagal centers in the medulla are also stimulated (MacCornack, 1977). Elevated heart rates are usually seen with large doses of caffeine (200-500 mg). Caffeine and theophylline will relax the smooth bronchial muscles of the lungs and are used as bronchodilators during bronchial asthma attacks.

The effects of caffeine on the central nervous system appear to be dose dependent. In small quantities (up to 200 mg) caffeine increases alertness, increases excitability, increases the attention span, reduces fatigue, decreases dowsiness, and improves simple reaction time (Stephenson, 1977, Wenzel & Rutledge, 1962). However, when the caffeine dose exeeds 200 mg, complex reaction time is slowed, hand steadiness decreases, and nervousness and irritability increase.

Effect on exercise. Caffeine doses (4-5 mg/kg) increase the amount of work that can be performed during exercise (Ivy, Costill, Fink, & Lower, 1979), and the length of time that prolonged exercise can be performed (Costill, Dalsky, & Fink, 1978). However, exercise bouts of short duration appear not to be affected by caffeine (Perkins & Williams, 1975; Powers, Byrd, Talley, & Callender, 1983). The increase in endurance in prolonged exercise bouts is thought to be due to a glycogen sparing effect of caffeine (Essig, Costill, & Van Handel, 1980). During prolonged exercise, FFA are mobilized and fat utilization is elevated (Costil et al., 1978; Ivy et al., 1979). The amount of muscle glycogen used during submaximal exercise is reduced and muscle triglyceride utilization is increased following caffeine ingestion (Essig et al., 1980). Perception of effort during prolonged exercise bouts also appears to be reduced by a caffeine dose of 330 mg (Costill et al., 1978).

Adverse effects of caffeine. Large doses of caffeine may produce a condition know as caffeinism. Symptoms of this disorder include anxiety, nervousness, irritability, insomnia, heart palpitations, arrhythmias, diuresis, and gastric distrubances (Stephenson, 1977). Even children who consume excessive amounts of caffeine may experience insomnia and tachycardia. Sleep disturbances including loss of sleep, increased frequency of awakening, and reduced amount of deep sleep have been observed in older adults when 300 mg of caffeine is consumed before bedtime (Stephenson, 1977). Non-coffee drinkers are more more likely to experience sleep disturbances following caffeine ingestion than coffee drinkers, suggesting that coffee drinkers are less sensitive to the effects of caffeine. Headaches can occur from excessive use of caffeine or from caffeine withdrawal.

There appears to be little evidence that "heavy" coffee consumption is related to an increased risk of coronary artery disease or precipitates myocardial infractions (MacCornack, 1977). Early epidemiological studies which suggested an association between caffeine intake and heart disease failed to control for the effects of cigarette smoking. Studies which controlled for the effects of cigarette smoking reported little relationship between coffee drinking and the incidence of coronary artery disease.

Toxic levels of caffeine produce symptoms of convulsions, nausea and vomiting. Caffeine can be fatal if doses exceed 10 g in adults and 5 g in children (Graham, 1978; Stephenson, 1977).

Alcohol

Next to caffeine, the most commonly used drug is alcohol. It is estimated that more than 50% of all students entering junior high school have already experimented with alcohol and 90% have used it by the time they reach their senior year in high school (Hamilton & Whitney, 1979). Alcohol is also the most widely abused drug in the United States. Problem drinking begins in the teenage years and it is estimated that there are 3.3 million teens (ages 14-17) with a drinking problem. Approximately 8-9% of college students will become problem drinkers or alcoholics during their lifetime.

Alcoholic beverages contain ethyl alcohol, a source of energy which yields 7 kcal/g. The alcohol content of beer, wine, and liquor is listed in Table 3. In addition to alcohol, beer and wine contain carbohydrate, a small quantity of protein, and trace amounts of some B vitamins and minerals. Because the amount of nutrients other than carbohydrate is quite small, alcoholic beverages are known as "empty calories". Alcohol is absorbed directly from the stomach and small intestine and is metabolized exclusively by the liver. The rate of oxidation is 75 mg alcohol/kg body weight/hour regardless of the amount of alcohol present in the blood (Gastineau, 1984).

Effects on psychomotor performance. Alcohol is a depressant of the central nervous system. However, one of the first areas of the brain to be affected is the reticular activating system. Since many of the inhibitory pathways arise from this area of the brain, the effect is one of reduced inhibitions and greater activity in other areas of the brain which is often thought to be stimulating (Williams, 1985). As blood alcohol levels rise, other areas of the brain become anesthetized, accompanied by a loss of reasoning ability, impaired vision, balance, and motor control.

Numerous studies have demonstrated that alcohol has a detrimental effect on psychomotor peformance. Reaction time is slowed and hand-eye coordination is reduced by even small amounts of alcohol (Carpenter, 1962). Alcohol is a factor in 50% of all fatal automobile accidents. Most states consider a person to be legally intoxicated when the blood alcohol level (BAL) exceeds 0.10. Although alcohol was one of the drugs originally banned by the IOC in 1968, it was removed from the banned list in 1972 and is not on the current list. It is banned, however, by the federation which governs the pentathalon (Williams, 1985). Alcohol has been used by participants in shooting events, including the pentathalon, to relax and reduce muscular tension during competition. There is little reason to believe that performance in sporting events requiring coordination, balance, or quick reactions would be helped by the ingestion of alcoholic beverages even though self confidence may be improved.

Effects on physical performance. Most studies of the effects of low (BAL .04-.05) and moderate (BAL = .10) doses of alcohol have reported no beneficial or detrimental effects on muscular strength and endurance (Williams, 1969), or on heart rate, blood pressure, oxygen uptake, perceived exertion, and blood lactate during progressively increasing exercise workloads (Bond, Franks, & Howley 1983; Williams, 1972). During prolonged exercise in a cold environment, ingestion of alcohol increases heat loss from the body by vasodilating skin blood vessels and reduces blood glucose levels (Graham, 1981; 1983; Haight & Keatinge, 1973). The reduction in blood glucose is due to a reduction in gluconeogenesis and release of glucose from the liver. Recently, the American College of Sports Medicine (1982) issued a position statement on the use of alcohol in sports recommending continued "efforts should be made to educate athletes, coaches, health and physical educators, physicians, trainers, the sports media, and the general public regarding the effects of acute alcohol ingeston upon human physical performance and on the potential acute and chronic problems of excessive alcohol consumption."

Effects of habitual use. Habitual use of alcohol is addictive and can lead to dependence—alcoholism. Chronic abuse of alcohol can lead to fatty liver and cirrhosis, cardiomyopathy, dementia and other neurologic conditions, pancreatitis, malnutrition, and anemia (Gastineau, 1984). Acute ingestion of a large dose of alcohol results in intoxication. In addition to increasing the risk of an automobile accident while driving, accidents on the job and in the home are increased following acute intoxication.

There have been some suggestions that chronic consumption of moderate amounts of alcohol may increase HDL cholesterol levels in men and therefore have a protective effect against coronary heart disease. A recent study reported that the consumption of 24 oz. of beer per day increased HDL cholesterol levels in sedentary men but not in men who normally ran or jogged (Hartung, Foreyt, Mitchell, Mitchell, Reeves, & Gotto, 1983). At the present time there is little evidence that alcohol actually decreases the risk of CHD.

Amphetamines

Amphetamines are sympathomimetic drugs which have similar actions in the body as the hormones epinephrine and norepinephrine. However, amphetamines are more potent stimulators of the central nervous system than the hormones. In low dosages they decrease fatigue, decrease appetite, increase confidence, elevate mood, and produce euphoria. With large doses a person may become apprehensive, aggressive, impulsive, or even psychotic. There are legitimate medical uses for amphetamines in the treatment of obesity, narcolepsy, and children with hyperkinesis (Council on Scientific Affairs, 1978). Prescriptions for drugs containing amphetamines are strictly controlled. The other source of "bennies," "dexies," and "speed" are street drug dealers. Prior to 1971 when the National Football League banned the use of the drug, it was estimated that the average amphetamine consumption for one NFL team was 60-70 mg/player/game (Mandell, Stewart, & Russo, 1981).

Effects on physical performance. Most studies indicate that amphetamines improve performance in endurance events (Chandler & Blair, 1980; Laties & Weiss, 1981). Since maximal oxygen uptake was not increased, but blood lactate levels were higher, the increased time to exhaustion was most likely due to amphetamines masking the symptoms of fatigue. Improvements in muscular strength and distance throws by weight throwers and shot putters have also been observed with amphetamine use (Chandler & Blair, 1980; Laties & Weiss, 1981; Lovingood, Blyth, Peacock, & Lindsay, 1967). Although amphetamines are known as "speed", it would appear that they have a greater effect on the initial acceleration than on the average velocity of running. Amphetamines have been banned by the IOC since 1968 and by the NFL since 1971. However, there is evidence that some professional football players are still using them (Marshall, 1979). Many colleges and universities have begun testing athletes periodically for the presence of drugs in the urine. While amphetamines do improve performance, their use without a prescription is illegal.

Adverse effects. Use of large doses of amphetamines over a prolonged time period produces a tolerance for the drug and the need for even larger doses. Large doses can result in high blood pressure, tachycardia, elevated body temperatures, sleep loss, anorexia, convulsions, mood changes and psychotic episodes (Council on Scientific Affairs, 1978). When used during physical activity in a hot environment, amphetamines can lead to hyperthermia and death. Because amphetamines mask symptoms of fatigue and pain, a person may become seriously injured and not even be aware of it. Withdrawal of the stimulant may result in depression, anxiety, or intense tiredness and sleepiness.

Anabolic Steroids

The functions of the male sex hormone, testosterone, are both androgenic and anabolic. These include development of the sex organs, growth of body and facial hair, enlargement of the larynx and lengthening the vocal cords, accerlerating the growth of bones and skeletal muscles, and increasing the number of red blood cells. Anabolic steroids are synthetic hormones which are primarily anabolic (stimulating protein formation), but do have an adrogenic effect on the sex organs. These drugs are beneficial in promoting weight gain in underweight persons, in the treatment of osteoporosis and arthritis, and stimulating tissue repair following surgery (Stone & Lipner, 1980). Because anabolic steroids stimulate muscle growth, they are popular among athletes who wish to gain body weight and strength.

Effects on muscle growth and strength. Numerous studies have been conducted on the effects of anabolic steroids on muscle growth and strength in both men and animals. At the present time there are no published studies on the effects of anabolic steroids on women. The results of studies with normal male animals suggest that anabolic steroids have no beneficial effect on increasing muscle size or strength (Stone & Lipner, 1980). Studies with human males (athletes, trained men, and untrained men) are almost evenly divided between those which demonstrated an increase in muscle strength and body weight and those which found no significant difference between subjects receiving anabolic steroids and those in the placebo group (Lamb, 1983). Double blind studies are difficult to perform with anabolic studies. Unfortunately, it is very easy for a subject to determine when they are receiving an anabolic steroid because of changes in urine color and odor, retention of body water, acne, and changes in mood.

It has been suggested that the improvment in strength observed in many athletes using anabolic steroids may be due to their effects on the central nervous system. Athletes are more aggressive, more tolerant of stress, and euphoric when using anabolic steroids, which may allow them to use greater intensity and more frequent training bouts (Stone & Lipner, 1980). Many athletes also use much larger doses of the anabolic steroids, often combining two or more steroids (known as "stacking") than used in the experimental studies (Burkett & Falduto, 1984; Strauss, Wright, Finerman, & Catlin, 1983). Most of the athletes reported obtaining drugs through the "black market" although some athletes received them from physicians.

Use of anabolic steroids is banned by the Internatonal Olympic Committee and many of the sports federations. Elaborate tests for the presence of anabolic steroids were introduced at the Pan American Games in 1983 in an attempt to prevent their use by athletes. Unfortunately, this is only likely to serve as a deterrent to the highest caliber athletes competing in international or national meets. The American College of Sports Medicine (1984) has recently adopted a position stand deploring "the use of anabolic-androgenic steroids by athletes" because such use "is contrary to the rules and ethical principles of athletic competition as set forth by many of the sports governing bodies." Ryan (1981) suggests that educating athletes, coaches, trainers, and physicians about the adverse side effects of anabolic steroids may be more effecitve in preventing their use than testing and disqualifications.

Adverse side effects. Most of the evidence of adverse side effects of anabolic steroid use comes from patients who received therapeutic doses of the drugs. Included among the side effects are pathological changes in the liver, a decrease in HDL cholesterol which may increase the risk of coronary heart disease, decreased spermatogenesis, depressed libido, decreased testosterone levels, acne, and hair loss from the scalp (Wright, 1981). Malignant tumors in the liver have been linked to the therapeutic use of anabolic steriods. Recently, a young body builder who had been taking anabolic steriods for four years became the first known case of an athlete dying of liver cancer (Overly, Dankoff, Wang, & Singh, 1984). Athletes also report increased aggressive behavior and irritability when using steroids (Strauss et al., 1983).

Use of anabolic steroids by growing children and adolescents results in early closure of the epiphyses and a reduction in bone length and height. Virilization, including increased activity of the sebacceous and sweat glands, voice deepening, facial hair, and clitoral enlargement has been reported among women receiving anabolic steroids (Wright, 1981). Most of these changes are not reversible when anabolic steroid use is discontinued.

Marijuana

Next to alcohol the most widely used recreational drug is marijuana (also know as grass or pot). Marijuana, which comes from the hemp plant, cannabis sativa, is either smoked or ingested in foods like brownies. The active ingredient which produces the high is tetrahydrocannabinol (THC). Based on surveys, it is estimated that 20% of U.S. college athletes use marijuana (Smith, 1983). Approximately 25% of the U.S. population has used the drug at some time and 10% of high school seniors use it daily (National Institute on Drug Abuse, 1983).

The physiological responses to marijuana include increases in heart rate and both systolic and diastolic blood pressures (Steadward & Singh, 1975). Physical work capacity measured following marijuana use was significantly reduced, probably due to the elevation in heart rate (Steadward & Singh, 1975). Psychological effects include euphoria and distortions of time and space. Performance of complex motor skill tasks, including driving, is impaired when under the influence of marijuana (National Institute on Drug Abuse, 1983).

Adverse effects. Physical addiction to marijuana does not occur; however, a person may become psychologically dependent upon the drug. With excessive use learning, thinking, concentration, and memory are adversely affected. Some individuals may become anxious or irritable while under the influence of marijuana. The by-products of marijuana are stored in body fat and remain in the body for several weeks after use. Chronic use increases the risk of lung cancer and other lung diseases and may impair heart function (National Institute on Drug Abuse, 1983). Although animal studies have suggested that marijuana has adverse effects on the reproductive and immune systems, studies on human beings are inadequate for conclusions to be made. More research is needed on the long-term effects of marijuana on human health.

Effects of Physiological Ergogenic Aids

Blood Doping

The amount of oxygen used by the body during physical activity is dependent upon the amount of oxygen transported to the tissues through the blood and the extraction of oxygen from the blood by the tissues. Oxygen transport is determined by the cardiac output and the oxygen content of the blood. Hemoglobin, a protein found within the red blood cell, carries most of the oxygen in the blood. Normal hemoglobin levels are 14 g/dl blood for women and 15.5 g/dl for men. In blood doping, the hemoglobin level is raised by the infusion of red blood cells which were removed several weeks earlier and stored or from a blood donor. Theoretically, by increasing the hemoglobin concentration, the amount of oxygen transported and used by the body is also increased.

Effects on endurance. Numerous studies have examined the effects of removing 450-1200 ml of blood, storage of the blood for three to twelve weeks, and reinfusion of the red blood cells for maximal oxygen uptake and endurance performance. Those studies which used 450-500 ml of blood or allowed only three weeks for new red blood cells to be formed by the bone marrow reported little or no improvement in maximal oxygen uptake and endurance (Glendhill, 1982). Three weeks is an insufficient time period for the red blood cells to be completely replaced. In North America red blood cells must be frozen if they are stored for more than three weeks. Most of the studies which allowed seven weeks or longer before reinfusion of the red blood cells reported significant improvements in maximal oxygen uptake and endurance time (Buick, Glendhiil, Froese, & Spriet, 1982; Williams, Wesseldine, Somma, & Schuster, 1981).

Hazards of blood doping. The safest method of blood doping is to use a person's own cells which have been stored for a period of time before reinfusion. Blood transfusion from another person involves some danger because of the possibility of transmitting hepatitis or other blood-borne infections of mismatching blood types (Glendhill, 1982). At the 1984 Olympics in Los Angeles, seven members of the U.S. Cycling Team received transfusions of whole blood from relatives or persons with the same blood type a few days before competition began. Two of the cyclists reportedly became sick shortly after receiving the transfusions. At the time of the 1984 Olympics, blood doping was not banned by the IOC. The International Olympic committee banned the practice of blood doping in the spring of 1985.

Oxygen

Another method of possibly increasing the amount of oxygen transported in the blood would be to increase oxygen content of the blood by raising the oxygen pressure in the gas being breathed. The pressure of an individual gas in a gas mixture is equal to the product of the percentage of gas in the mixture and the total gas pressure (barometric pressure):

$$PO_2 = \%O_2 \times BP$$

Air contains 21% O_2 and the barometric pressure at sea level is 760 torr or one atmosphere (1 ATA). This means that the air being inhaled has a PO_2 of 160 torr. You can increase the PO_2 by either breathing an air mixture with a higher percentage of O_2 or by raising the barometric pressure. For example, breathing 100% O_2 raises the PO_2 to 760 torr. Scuba divers breathing compressed air experience an increase in PO_2 during dives because the barometric pressure increases 1 ATA for every 33 feet in depth. Thus, a dive to a depth of 132 feet (5 ATA) with compressed air would be the equivalent of breathing pure O_2 at sea level.

As altitude increases above sea level, the percentage of O_2 in the air remains constant at 21%, but the barometric pressure decreases. This results in lower PO_2 at higher altitudes (Table 6). At sea level, 97% of the hemoglobin will be saturated with oxygen when the blood leaves the lungs. The amount of oxygen bound to hemoglobin is described by the oxygen disociation curve (an S shaped curve). With increases in altitude, oxygen saturation of hemoglobin decreases slowly at first and then more rapidly at the higher altitudes (Table 6). A mountain climber reaching the summit of Mount Everest breathing air would have hemoglobin less than 50% saturated with oxygen. In other words, oxygen transport would be reduced more than 50%.

Table 6
PO_2 and hemoglobin saturation with oxygen at different altitudes

Location	Altitude m.	Barometric Pressue torr	PO_2 torr	Hb Saturation with O_2 %
Sea level	0	760	159	97
Denver	1600	630	132	94
Leadville	3100	530	101	90
Pikes Peak	4300	440	82	82
Mount Everest	8850	250	42	48

Adapted from The Environment and Human Performance by E. M. Haymes & C. L. Wells (1986). Champaign: Human Kinetics.

Oxygen use during physical activity. Breathing gas mixtures with an elevated oxygen content during exercise has been shown to be beneficial in increasing the length of time that maximal exercise can be performed (Cunningham, 1966; Wilson & Welch, 1975; 1980). Because hemoglobin is already 97% saturated with oxygen, increasing the O_2 percentage in the gas results in only a slight increase in the oxygen transported by the blood. Nevertheless, reductions in oxygen debt and blood lactate levels, post exercise, were found when subjects breathed oxygen during exercise (Cunningham, 1966). Another explanation for the improvement in performance could be a reduction in the cost of breathing during maximal exercise when breathing oxygen (Wilson & Welch, 1980). Peripheral chemoreceptors located in the carotid arteries are stimulated by decreases in blood PO_2 and depressed by increasing the O_2 percentage in the gas mixture above 21%. When the chemoreceptors are depressed, ventilation decreases. During heavy exercise approximately 10% of the total energy cost will be used by the respiratory muscles for ventilation. Thus, a reduction in ventilation during exercise while breathing oxygen would reduce the energy cost of breathing.

The question is not wheather oxygen breathing is beneficial during exercise, but whether it is practical. In order to breathe oxygen during exercise the person must either remain stationary on a treadmill or cycle erogometer near a tank of gas or carry the gas tank along while moving as in scuba diving and mountain climbing. Only in the case of climbing at very high altitudes do the benefits of oxygen breathing outweigh the increased energy cost of carrying the tank. Until 1978 the only successful ascents to the summit of Mount Everest were achieved by climbers breathing oxygen.

Oxygen use during recovery from physical activity. How often have you observed a football player who has just left the playing field standing on the sideline breathing from a tank containing O_2? Breathing oxygen immediately following exercise does not speed up the recovery process. Studies have reported little reduction in heart rate or blood lactate with oxygen breathing during recovery (Hagerman, Bowers, Fox, & Ersing, 1968; Weltman, Stamford, Moffat, & Katch, 1977). There also appears to be no improvement in subsequent exercise performance following oxygen breathing (Weltman et al., 1977).

Passive Heating and Cooling

Application of both heat and cold is useful in the treatment of sports injuries. There have also been suggestions in the literature that heating and cooling muscles could improve performance. Passive heating modalities include hot packs or water baths, diathermy, radiant heating, and massage. Theoretically, heating would raise the temperature of the body, which would reduce viscosity of body fluids and decrease resistance to movement. There is little evidence that passive heating benefits isometric strength (Binkhorst, Hoofd, & Vissers, 1977; Falls, 1972). However, the rate at which force develops increases with passive heating (Binkhorst et al. 1977; Davies, Mecrow, & White, 1982). On the other hand, endurance appears to be reduced by passive heating (Falls, 1972). The application of heat results in vasodilation of skin blood vessels, which shunts blood from the muscles. This may result in an accumulation of metabolites in the muscle, which interferes in the contraction process. In order to maintain blood flow to both muscles and skin, cardiac output must either increase or blood flow must be shunted from other body organs.

Cooling can take the form of ice packs, cold water baths, cold showers, or air cooling. When the skin is cooled, skin blood vessels vasoconstrict, shunting more blood into the deep vessels, which increases venous return to the heart. This usually results in a lower heart rate during activity and is beneificial in a hot environment (Falls, 1972). Muscular endurance also appears to improve if the muscles cool slightly, but muscle temperatures below 27 C are associated with reduced endurance (Clarke, Hellon, & Lind, 1958). Dynamic strength at fast velocities and jumping and sprinting performance decrease as muscle temperature decreases (Bergh & Ekblom, 1979). Cooling a muscle decreases the rate of force development, which could be due to increased viscosity of the sarcoplasm and/or a slowing of the chemical reactions. Nerve conduction velocity is also reduced with cooling and can even be blocked at skin temperatures below 7 C (Vangaard, 1975). Decreases in muscular strength and endurance at low muscle temperatures could be due to the mobilization of fewer muscle fibers.

Warm-up

Physical warm-up refers to an increase in body temperature through physical activity. The type of warm-up takes one of two forms: direct, where the warm-up used is similar to the activity, and indirect, where the warm-up is dissimilar to the activity. Jogging prior to a 100-yd sprint would be an example of a direct warm-up while calisthenics before a high jump would be an example of an indirect warm-up. Both types of warm-up result in increased muscle temperature if activity is sustained for a few minutes. The physiological benefits of increased muscle temperature include a decrease in viscosity of the sarcoplasm, vasodilation of blood vessels in the muscle, and a shift in the oxygen dissociation curve to the right, which allows hemoglobin to release more O_2 to the muscle tissue.

Direct warm-up also provides practice of the skill to be used in the physical activity. This may aid the performer in achieving the optimal mental set (Franks, 1983). Another benefit of physical warm-up is an increase in arousal. However, activities requiring fine motor control require less arousal than high intensity gross motor skills (Franks, 1983).

Numerous studies support the theory that physical warm-up is beneficial to performance in many types of physical activity if the warm-up is of sufficient duration and intensity to actually increase muscle temperature. The major exception appears to be endurance activites. If the intensity of the warm-up is high, fatigue becomes a factor. In endurance activities, high intensity warm-up reduces performance (Bonner, 1974; Gutin, Wilkerson, Horvath, & Rochelle, 1981). Prolonged warm-up may also be detrimental in high intensity activities, such as the vertical jump (Richards, 1968). Fatigue in this case could be due to depletion of the creatine phosphate stores and/or an accumulation of metabolites in the muscle.

Improvement in performance following warm-up may also be psychological. Many persons believe that warm-up is beneficial, especially in preventing injuries. These individuals may not be willing to give an all-out effort when exercising in the no warm-up trials. To control for this effect, several studies have attempted to use subjects who were naive about the true purpose of the study (Bonner, 1974; Richards, 1968). In both studies, warm-up was beneficial if it was at low intensity (Bonner, 1974) or of short duration (Richards, 1968). Massey, Johnson, and Kramer (1961) hypnotized subjects prior to warm-up or no warm-up and found no significant differences in performance between the two conditions.

There is no direct research evidence that warm-up prevents injuries because investigators will not deliberately set-up situations where an indiviudal would likely be injured. However, there is evidence that low intensity warm-up is beneficial in preventing abnormal ECG's during more intense activities (Barnard, Gardner, Diaro, Macalpin, & Kattus, 1973). Because ischemia is the most likely cause of the abnormal ECG's, the primary benefit of low intensity warm-up appears to be the gradual increase in blood flow to the cardiac muscle.

Summary

Nutritionally inadequate diets are most common among adolescents.

Carbohydrate, stored as glycogen, is the main source of energy during heavy exercise.

Muscle glycogen stores limit the amount of heavy exercise that can be accomplished. Children have smaller glycogen stores than adults and produce less lactic acid. Glycogen storage can be increased by consuming a high (70%) carbohydrate diet for several days after first depleting the glycogen stores.

Glucose ingestion prior to exercise stimulates an insulin response and a reduction in blood glucose during exercise.

Fat is a major source of energy at low exercise intensities. Endurance training increases fat mobilizaton and utilization. Ingestion of diets high in saturated fat is associated with elevated serum cholesterol levels.

Protein needs are greater relative to body weight for children and adolescents than adults. Protein needs of athletes are covered by a balanced diet.

Inadequate iron intake is the most common nutritional deficiency in the U.S. and is especially common among females. Depletion of the iron stores leads to iron deficiency anemia and reduced oxygen transport to the tissues. Iron supplements increase iron stores in iron deficient persons.

Low calcium intakes are frequently observed among females. Bone mineral loss occurs in both men and women, but at a faster rate in women after age 40.

Adequate water intake during exercise is necessary for maintaining blood volume and body temperature. Electrolyte drinks should be dilute, osmolarity of 200 mOsm or less, for rapid emptying from the stomach. Dehydration is a primary cause of heat illness.

There is little evidence that vitamin supplements improve performance when the diet is adequate.

Drugs like caffeine, amphetamines, and anabolic steroids which may improve performance are banned by the International Olympic Committee and many sports federations.

Use of alcohol and marijunana can lead to addiction or a psychological dependency. Chronic heavy use can have an adverse effect on health.

Blood doping can increase oxygen transport if adequate time is allowed before reinfusion for red blood cells to regenerate. The IOC recently banned blood doping.

Active warm-up is beneficial in improving performance in some activities and may prevent injuries.

References

Ahlborg, G., & Felig, P. (1976). Influence of glucose ingestion on fuel-hormone response during prolonged exercise. *Journal of Applied Physiology, 41,* 683-688.

American College of Sports Medicine. (1982). Position statement of the use of alcohol in sports. *Medicine and Science in Sports and Exercise, 14* ix-xi.

American College of Sports Medicine. (1984). Position stand on the use of anabolic-androgenic steroids in sports. *Sports Medicine Bulletin, 19(3), 1.*

American College of Sports Medicine. (1976). Position stand on weight loss in wrestlers. *Medicine and Science in Sports and Exercise, 8*(2), xi-xiii.

Archdeacon, J., & Murlin, J. (1944). The effect of thiamin deletion and restoration on muscular efficiency and endurance. *Journal of Nutrition, 28,* 244-254.

Barborka, C.J., Foltz, E.E., & Ivy, A.C. (1943). Relationship between vitamin B complex intake and work output in trained subjects. *Journal of the American Medical Association, 122,* 717-720.

Barnard, R.J., Gardner, G.W., Diaro, V.V., MacAlpin, R.N., & Kattus, A.A. (1973). Cardiovascular responses to sudden strenuous exercise: Heart rate, blood pressure, and ECG. *Journal of Applied Physiology, 34,* 833-837.

Bar-Or, O. (1980). Climate and the exercising child: A review. *International Journal of Sports Medicine, 1,* 53-65.

Bar-Or, O., Dotan, R., Inbar, O., Rotshtein, A., & Zonder, H. (1980). Voluntary hypohydration in 10- to 12-year-old boys. *Journal of Applied Physiology: Respiratory, Environmental, Exercise Physiology, 48,* 104-108.

Bergh, U., & Ekblom, B. (1979). Influence of muscle temperature on maximal muscle strength and power output in human skeletal muscles. *Acta Physiologica Scandinavia, 107,* 33-37.

Bergstrom, J., Hermansen, L., Hultman, E., & Saltin, B. (1967). Diet, muscle glycogen and physical performance. *Acta Physiologica Scandinavia, 71,* 140-150.

Berryman, G.H., Henderson, C.R., Wheeler, N.C., Cogswell, R.C., & Spinella, J.R. (1947). Effects in young men consuming restricted quantities of B complex vitamins and proteins, and changes associated with supplementation. *American Journal of Physiology, 148,* 618-647.

Binkhorst, R.A., Hoofd, L., & Vissers, C.A. (1977). Temperature and force-velocity relationship of human muscles. *Journal of Applied Physiology, 42,* 471-475.

Bond, V., Franks, B.D., & Howley, E.T. (1983). Effects of small and moderate doses of alcohol on submaximal cardiorespiratory function, perceived exertion and endurance performance in abstainers and moderate drinkers. *Journal of Sports Medicine, 23,* 221-228.

Bonner, H.W. (1974). Preliminary exercise: a two factor theory. *Research Quarterly, 45,* 138-147.

Brooke, J.D. (1978). Carbohydrate nutrition and human performance. In J. Parizkova & V.A. Rogozkin (Eds.), *Nutrition, Physical Fitness, and Health.* Baltimore: University Park Press.

Buick, F.J., Glendhill, N., Froese, A.B., & Spreit, L.I. (1982). Red cell mass and aerobic performance at sea level. In J.R. Sutton, N.L. Jones, & C.S. Houston (Eds.), *Hypoxia: Man at Altitude.* New York: Thieme-Stratton, Inc.

Burkett, L.N., & Falduto, M.T. (1984). Steroid use by athletes in a metropolitan area. *Physician and Sportsmedicine, 12* (8), 69-74.

Carlson, L.A., Havel, R.J., Ekelund, L.G. & Holmgren, A. (1963). Effect of nicotinic acid on the turnover rate and oxidation of the free fatty acids of plasma in man during exercise. *Metabolism Clinical and Experimental, 12,* 837-845.

Carpenter, J. (1962). Effects of alcohol on some psychological processes. *Quarterly Journal of Studies of Alcohol, 23,* 274-314.

Castelli, W.P. et al. (1977). HDL cholesterol and other lipids in coronary heart disease: The cooperative lipoprotein phenotyping study. *Circulation, 55,* 767-772.

Celejowa, I. & Homa, M. (1970). Food intake, nitrogen and energy balance in Polish weight lifters, during a training camp. *Nutrition and Metabolism, 12,* 259-274.

Chandler, J.V. & Blair, S.N. (1980). The effect of amphetaimines on selected physiological components related to athletic success. *Medicine and Science in Sports and Exercise, 12,* 65-69.

Christensen, E.H. & Hansen, O. (1939). Respiratorischer quoteint and O_2-aufnahme. *Scandinavian Archives of Physiology, 81,* 180-189.

Clarke, R.S.J., Hellon, R.F., & Lind, A.R. (1958). The duration of sustained contractions of the human forearm at different muscle temperatures. *Journal of Physiology, 143.* 454-473.

Clement, D.B. & Asmundson, R.C. (1982). Nutritional intake and hematological parameters in endurance runners. *Physician and Sportsmedicine, 10* (3), 37-43.

Cook, J.D., Finch, C.A., & Smith, N.J. (1976). Evaluation of the iron status of a population. *Blood, 48,* 449-455.

Cooney, M.M. (1983). *The effects of a low carbohydrate-ketogenic diet in trained females.* Unpublished doctoral dissertation, Florida State University.

Cooter, G.R. & Mowbray, K.W. (1978). Effects of iron supplementation and activity on serum iron depletion and hemoglobin levels in female athletes. *Research Quarterly, 49,* 114-118.

Costill, D.L., Bowers, R., Branam, G., & Sparks, K. (1971). Muscle glycogen utilization during prolonged exercise on successive days. *Journal of Applied Physiology, 31,* 834-838.

Costill, D.L., Cote, R., & Fink, W.J. (1982). Dietary potassium and heavy exercise:

Effects on muscle water and electrolytes. *American Journal of Clinical Nutrition, 36,* 266-275.

Costill, D.L., Coyle, E.F., Dalsky, G., Evans, W., Fink, W.J., & Hooper, D. (1977). Effects of elevated plasma FFA and insulin in muscle glycogen usage during exercise. *Journal of Applied Physiology, 43,* 695-699.

Costill, D.L., Dalsky, G., & Fink, W.J. (1978). Effects of caffeine ingestion on metabolism and exercise performance. *Medicine and Science in Sports, 10,* 155-158.

Costill, D.L., Kammer, W.F., & Fisher, A. (1970). Fluid ingestion during distance running. *Archives of Environmental Health, 21,* 520-525.

Costill, D.L. & Saltin, B. (1974). Factors limiting gastric emptying during rest and exercise. *Journal of Applied Physiology, 37,* 679-683.

Costill, D.L., Sherman, W.M., Fink, W.J., Maresh, C., Witten, M. & Miller, J.M. (1981). The role of dietary carbohydrates in muscle glycogen resynthesis after strenuous running. *American Journal of Clinical Nutrition, 34,* 1831-1836.

Costill, D.L. & Sparks, K.E. (1973). Rapid fluid replacement following thermal dehydration. *Journal of Applied Physiology, 34,* 299-303.

Council on Scientific Affairs, (1978). Clinical aspects of amphetamine abuse. *Journal of the American Medical Association, 240,* 2317-2319.

Cunningham, D.A. (1966). Effects of breathing high concentrations of oxygen on treadmill performance. *Research Quarterly, 37,* 491-494.

Davies, C.T.M., Chukwenmeka, A.C., & Van Haaren, J.P.M. (1973). Iron deficiency anemia: its effect on maximal aerobic power and responses to exercise in African males aged 17-40 years. *Clinical Science, 44,* 555-562.

Davies, C.T.M., Mecrow, I.K., & White, M.J. (1982). Contractile properties of the human triceps surae with some observations on the effects of temperature and exercise. *European Journal of Applied Physiology, 49,* 255-269.

Decombaz, J., Reinhardt, P., Anantharaman, K., von Glutz, G., & Poortmans, J.R. (1979). Biochemical changes in a 100 kg run: Free amino acids, urea, and creatinine. *European Journal of Applied Physiology, 41,* 61-72.

Delbeke, F.T. & Debackere, M. (1984). Caffeine: use and abuse in sport. *International Journal of Sports Medicine, 5,* 179-182.

Dillard, C.J., Litov, R.E., Savin, W.M., Dumelin, E.E., & Tappel, A.L. (1978). Effects of exercise, vitamin E, and ozone on pulmonary function and lipid peroxidation. *Journal of Applied Physiology: Respiratory, Environmental, Exercise Physiology, 45,* 927-932.

Dohm, G.L., Puente, F.R., Smith, C.P., & Edge, A. (1978). Changes in tissue protein levels as a result of endurance exercise. *Life Sciences, 23,* 845-850.

Dohm, G.L., Kasperek, G.J., Tapscott, E.B., Barakat, H.A., & Beecher, G.R. (1980). Protein synthesis in liver and muscle during recovery from exhaustive exericse. *Federation Proceedings, 3,* 290.

Dohm, G.L., Williams, R.T., Kasperek, G.J., & van Rig, A.M. (1982). Increased excretion of urea and N-methylhistidine by rats and humans after a bout of exercise. *Journal of Applied Physiology: Respiratory, Environmental, Exercise Physiology, 52,* 27-33.

Douglas, P.D. & Douglas, J.C. (1984). Nutrition knowledge and food practices of high school athletes. *Journal of the American Dietetic Association, 84,* 1198-1202.

Drinkwater, B.L., Kupprat, I.C., Denton, J.E., Crist, J.L., & Horvath, S.M. (1977). Response of prepubertal girls and college women to work in the heat. *Journal of Applied Physiology: Respiratory, Environmental, Exercise Physiology, 43,* 1046-1053.

Dufaux, B., Hoederath, A., Streitberger, I., Hollmann W., & Assmann, G. (1981). Serum ferritin, transferrin, haptoglobin, and iron in middle- and long-distance runners, elite rowers, and professional racing cyclists. *International Journal of Sports Medicine, 2.* 43-46.

Early, R.G. & Carlson, B.R. (1969). Water-soluble vitamin therapy in the delay of fatigue from physical activity in hot climatic conditions. *International Zeitschrift fur Angewandte Physiologie, 27,* 43-50.

Edgerton, V.R., Ohira, Y., Hettiarachchi, J., Senewiratne, B., Gardner, G.W., & Barnard, R.J. (1981). Elevation of hemoglobin and work tolerance in iron-deficient subjects. *Journal of Nutrition Science and Vitaminology, 27,* 77-86.

Ehn, L., Carlmark, B., & Hoglund, S. (1980). Iron status in athletes involved in intense physical activity. *Medicine and Science in Sports and Exercise, 12,* 61-63.

England, A.C., Fraser, D.W., Hightower, A.W., Tirinnanzi, R., Greenberg, D.J., Powell, K.E., Slovis, C.M., & Varsha, R.A. (1982). Preventing severe heat injury in runners: Suggestions from the 1979 peachtree road race experience. *Annals of Internal Medicine, 97,* 196-201.

Eriksson, B.O.(1980). Muscle metabolism in children: A review. *Acta Paediatrica Scandinavia,* Supplement 283, 20-27.

Eriksson, B.O., Gollnick, P.D., & Saltin, B. (1973). Muscle metabolism and enzyme activities after training in boys 11-13 years old. *Acta Physiologica Scandinavia, 87,* 485-497.

Essig, D., Costill, D.L., & Van Handel, P.J. (1980). Effects of caffeine ingestion on utilization of muscle glycogen and lipid during leg erogometer cycling. *International Journal of Sports Medicine, 1,* 86-90.

Falls, H.B. (1972). Heat and cold applications. In W.P. Morgan (Ed.), *Ergogenic Aids and Muscular Performance.* New York: Academic Press.

Finch, C.A., Gollnick, P.D., Hlastala, M.P., Miller, L.R., Dillman, E., & Mackler, B. (1979). Lactic acidosis as a result of iron deficiency. *Journal of Clinical Investigation, 64,* 129-137.

Fink, W.J. (1982). Fluid intake for maximizing athletic performance. In W. Haskell, J. Scala, & J. Whittam (Eds.), *Nutrition and Athletic Performance.* Palo Alto: Bull Publishing.

Foster, C., Costill, D.L., & Fink, W.J. (1979). Effects of preexercise feedings on endurance performance. *Medicine and Science in Sports and Exercise, 11,* 1-5.

Franks, B.D. (1983). Physical warm-up. In M.H. Williams (Ed.), *Ergogenic Aids in Sport.* Champaign: Human Kinetics Publishers.

Fregly, M.J. (1984). Sodium and potassium. In *Present Knowledge in Nutrition* (5th ed.). Washington, DC: The Nutrition Foundation.

Galbo, H., Holst, J.J., & Christensen, N.J. (1979). The effect of different diets and insulin on the hormonal response to prolonged exercise. *Acta Physiologica Scandinavica, 107,* 19-32.

Gardner, G.W., Edgerton, V.R., Senewiratne, B., Barnard, R.J., & Ohira, Y. (1977). Physical work capacity and metabolic stress in subjects with iron deficiency anemia. *American Journal of Clinical Nutrition, 30,* 910-917.

Garn, S.M., Rohmann, C.G., & Wagner, B. (1967). Bone loss as a general phenomenon in man. *Federation Proceedings, 26,* 1729-1736.

Gastineau, C. (1984). Nutritional implications of alcohol. In *Present Knowledge in Nutrition* (5th ed.). Washington, DC: The Nutrition Foundation, Inc.

Gey, G.O., Cooper, K.H., & Bottenberg, R.A. (1970). Effect of ascorbic acid on endurance performance and athletic injury. *Journal of Applied Physiology, 211* 105.

Gisolfi, C.V. & Copping, J.R. (1974). Thermal effects of prolonged treadmill exercise in the heat. *Medicine and Science in Sports, 6,* 108-113.

Glendhill, N. (1982). Blood doping and related issues: A brief review. *Medicine and Science in Sports and Exercise, 14,* 183-189.

Glueck, C.J., Fallat, R.W., & Tsang, R. (1974). Hypercholesterolemia and hypertriglyceridemia in children. *American Journal of Diseases in Children, 128,* 569-576.

Glueck, C.J., Fallat, R.W., & Tsang, R. (1975). A pediatric approach to atherosclerosis prevention. In M. Winick, (Ed.), *Childhood Obesity*. New York: John Wiley & Sons.

Gontzea, I., Sutzescu, R., & Dumitrache, S. (1975). The influence of adaptation to physical effort on nitrogen balance in man. *Nutrition Reports International, 11*, 231-236.

Graham, D.M. (1978). Caffeine—its identity, dietary sources, intake and biological effects. *Nutrition Reviews, 36*, 97-102.

Graham, T.E. (1981). Thermal and glycemic responses during mild exercise in +5 to −15°C environments following alchohol ingestion. *Aviation, Space, and Environmental Medicine, 52*, 517-522.

Graham, T.E. (1983). Alcohol ingestion and sex differences on the thermal responses to mild exercise in a cold environment. *Human Biology, 55*, 463-476.

Guthrie, H.A. (1979). *Introductory Nutrition*. (4th ed.). St. Louis: C.V. Mosby.

Gutin, B., Wilkerson, J.E., Horvath, S.M., & Rochelle, R.D. (1981). Physiologic response to endurance work as a function of prior exercise. *International Journal of Sports Medicine, 2*, 87-91.

Hagerman, F.C., Bowers, R.W., Fox, E.L., & Ersing, W.W. (1968). The effects of breathing 100 percent oxygen during rest, heavy work and recovery. *Research Quarterly, 39*, 965-974.

Haight, J.S.J. & Keatinge, W.R. (1973). Failure of thermoregulation in the cold during hypoglycaemia induced by exercise and ethanol. *Journal of Physiology, 229*, 87-97.

Hamilton, E.M. & Whitney, E. (1979). *Nutrition: Concepts and Controversies*. St. Paul: West Publishing Co.

HANES I. (1979). *First health and nutrition examination survey 1971-1974*. DHEW Publication No. (PHS) 79-1221. Hyattsville, MD: National Center for Health Statistics.

Hanson, P.G. & Zimmerman, S.W. (1979). Exertional heatstroke in novice runners. *Journal of the American Medical Association, 242*, 154-157.

Hartung, G.H., Foreyt, J.P., Mitchell, R.E., Mitchell, J.G., Reeves, R.S., & Gotto, A.M. (1983). Effect of alcohol intake on high-density lipoprotein cholesterol levels in runners and inactive men. *Journal of the American Medical Association, 249*, 747-750.

Havel, R.J. (1974). The fuels for muscular exercise. In W.R. Johnson & E.R. Buskirk (Eds.), *Science and Medicine of Exercise nad Sport, 2nd ed.* New York: Harper & Row.

Haymes, E.M., Buskirk, E.R., Hodgson, J.L., Lundegren, H.M., & Nicholas, W.C. (1974). Heat tolerance of exercising lean and heavy prepubertal girls. *Journal of Applied Physiology, 36*, 556-571.

Haymes, E.M., McCormick, R.J., & Buskirk, E.R. (1975). Heat tolerance of exercising lean and obese prepubertal boys. *Journal of Applied Physiology, 39*, 457-461.

Haymes, E.M., Puhl, J.L., & Temples, T.E. (1983). Training for cross-country skiing and iron status. *Medicine and Science in Sports and Exercise, 15*, 133.

Heaney, R.P., Recker, R.R., & Saville, P.D. (1978). Menopausal changes in calcium balance performance. *Journal of Laboratory Clinical Medicine, 92*, 953-963.

Henderson. I.M. (1984). Vitamin B6. In *Present Knowledge in Nutrition, 5 ed.* Washington: The Nutrition Foundation.

Henschel, A., Taylor, H.L., Brozek, J., Mickelsen, O., & Keys, A. (1944). Vitamin C and ability to work in hot environments. *Amercian Journal of Tropical Medicine, 24*, 259-265.

Herbert, Wmoom. & Ribisl, P.M. (1972). Effects of dehydratiHerbert, W.G. & Ribisl, P.M. (1972). Effects of dehydration upon physical work capacity of wrestlers under competitive conditions. *Research Quarterly, 43*, 416-422.

Hermansen, L., Hultman, E., & Saltin, B. (1967). Muscle glycogen during prolonged severe exercise. *Acta Physiologica Scandinavica, 71*, 129-139.

Hoogerwerf, A. & Hoitink, A.W.J.H. (1963). The influence of vitamin C administration on the mechanical efficiency of the human organism. *Internationale Zeitschrift fur Angewandte Physiologie, 20*, 164-172.

Houston, M.E., Marrin, D.A., Green, H.J., & Thomson, J.A. (1981). The effect of rapid weight loss on physiological functions in wrestlers. *The Physician and Sportsmedicine, 9*(11), 73-78.

Howald, H., Segeser, G., & Korner, W.F. (1975). Ascorbic acid and athletic performance. *Annals of the New York Academy of Sciences, 258*, 458-463.

Hughson, R.L., Green, H.J., Houston, M.E., Thomson, J.A., MacLean, D.R., & Sutton, J.R. (1980). Heat injuries in Canadian mass participation runs. *Canadian Medical Association Journal, 122*, 1141-1144.

Hunding, A., Jordal, R., & Paulev, P.E. (1981). Runner's anemia and iron deficiency. *Acta Medica Scandinavia, 209*, 315-318.

Ivy, J.L., Costill, D.L., Fink, W.J., & Lower, R.W. (1979). Influence of caffeine and carbohydrate feedings on endurance performance. *Medicine and Science in Sports, 11*, 6-11.

Iyengar, A. & Narasinga Rao, B.S. (1979). Effect of varying energy and protein intake on nitrogen balance in adults engaged in heavy manual labour. *British Journal of Nutrition, 41*, 19-25.

Johnson, R.E., Darling, R.C., Forbes, W.H., Brouha, L., Egana, E., & Graybiel, A. (1942). The effects of a diet deficient in part of the vitamin B complex upon men doing manual labor. *Journal of Nutrition, 24*, 585-596.

Kannel, W.B., Doyle, J.T., & Ostfield, A.M. (1980). Risk factors and coronary disease. *Circulation, 62*, 449A-455A.

Karlsson, J. & Saltin, B. (1971). Diet, muscle glycogen, and endurance performance. *Journal of Applied Physiology, 31*, 203-206.

Keren, G. & Epstein, Y. (1980). The effect of high dosage vitamin C intake on aerobic and anaerobic capacity. *Journal of Sports Medicine, 20*, 145-148.

Keys, A., Henschel, A.F., Mickelsen, O., & Brozek, J.M. (1943). The performance of normal young men on controlled thiamine intakes. *Journal of Nutrition, 26*, 399-415.

Keys, A., Henschel, A.F., Taylor, H.L., Mickelsen, O., & Brozek, J. (1944). Absence of rapid deterioration in men doing hard physical work on a restricted intake of viatmins of the B complex. *Journal of Nutrition, 27*, 485-496.

Knochel, J.P. (1977). Potassium deficiency during training in the heat. *Annals of the New York Academy of Sciences, 301*, 175-182.

Lamb, D.R. (1983). Anabolic steroids. In M.H. Williams (Ed.), *Ergogenic Aids in Sport*. Champaign: Human Kinetics Publishers.

Laritcheva, K.A., Yalovaya, N.I., Shubin, V.I., & Smirnov, P.V. (1978). Study of energy expenditure and protein needs of top weight lifters. In J. Parizkova & V.A. Rogozkin (Eds.), *Nutrition, Physical Fitness, and Health*. Baltimore: University Park Press.

Laties, V.G. & Weiss, B. (1981). The amphetamine margin in sports. *Federation Proceedings, 40*, 2689-2692.

Lawrence, J.D., Smith, J.L., Bower, R.C., Riehl. W.P. (1975). The effect of α-tocopherol (vitamin E) and pyridoxine HC1 (vitamin B_6) on the swimming endurance of trained swimmers. *Journal of the American College Health Association, 23*, 219-222.

Lemon, P.W.R. & Mullin, J.P. (1980. Effect of initial muscle glycogen levels on protein catabolism during exercise. *Journal of Applied Physiology: Respiratory, Environmental, Exercise Physiology, 48*, 624-629.

Lovingood, B.W., Blyth, C.S., Peacock, W.H., & Lindsay, R.B. (1967). Effects of d-amphetamine sulfate, caffeine, and high temperature on human performance. *Research Quarterly, 38*, 64-71.

Lukaski, H.C., Bolonchuk, W.W., Klevay, L.M., Mahalko, J.R., Milne, D.B., & Sandstead, H.H. 1984. Influence of type and amount of dietary lipid on plasma lipid concentrations in endurance athletes. *Amercian Journal of Clinical Nutrition, 39*, 35-44.

MacCornack, F.A. (1977). The effects of coffee drinking on the cardiovascular system: Experimental and epidemiological research. *Preventive Medicine, 6*, 104-119.

Mandell, A.J., Stewart, K.D., & Russo, P.V. (1981). The Sunday syndrome: From kinetics to altered consciousness. *Federation Proceedings, 40*, 2693-2698.

Marable, N.L., Hickson, J.F., Korslund, M.K., Herbert, W.G., Desjardins, R.F., & Thye, F.W. (1979). Urinary nitrogen excretion as influenced by a muscle-building exercise program and protein intake variation. *Nutrition Reports International, 19*, 795-805.

Marshall, E. (1979). Drugging of football players curbed by central monitoring plan, NFL claims. *Science, 203*, 626-628.

Massey, B.H., Johnson, W.R., & Kramer, G.F. (1961). Effect of warm-up exercise upon muscular performance using hypnosis to control the psychological variable. *Research Quarterly, 32*, 63-71.

Matkovic, V., Kostial, K., Simonovic, I., Buzina, B., Brodarec, A., & Nordin, B.E.C. (1979). Bone status and fracture rates in two regions of Yugoslavia. *American Journal of Clinical Nutrition, 32*, 540-549.

McGandy, R.B., Hall, B., Ford, C., & Stare, F.J. (1972). Dietary regulation of blood cholesterol in adolescent males: A pilot study. *American Journal of Clinical Nutrition, 25*, 61-66.

McLane, J.A., Fell, R.D., McKay, R.H., Winder, W.W., Brown, E.B., & Holloszy, J.O. (1981). Physiological and biochemical effects of iron deficiency on rat skeletal muscle. *American Journal of Physiology, 241*, C47-C54.

McLaren, D.S. (1984). Vitamin A Deficiency and toxicity. In *Present Knowledge in Nutrition* (5th ed.). Washington, DC: The Nutrition Foundation, Inc.

Miller, H.L., Issekutz, B., Paul, P., & Rodahl, K. (1964). Effect of lactic acid on plasma free fatty acids in pancreatectomized dogs. *American Journal of Physiology, 207*, 1226-1230.

Milner, R.D.G. (197ilner, R.D.G. (1976). Protein-calorie malnutrition. In *Present Knowledge in Nutrition* (4th ed.). New York: The Nutrition Foundation, Inc.

Montoye, H.J., Spata, P.J., Pickney, V., & Barron, L. (1955). Effects of vitamin B_{12} supplementation on physical fitness and growth of young boys. *Journal of Applied Physiology, 7*, 589-592.

National Institute on Drug Abuse. (1983). Marijuana and health: 1982. In M.E. Kelleher, B.K. MacMurray, & T.M. Shapiro (Eds.), *Drugs and Society*, (pp. 199-207). Dubuque: Kendall/Hunt Publishing Company.

Nickerson, H.J. & Tripp, A.D. (1983). Iron deficiency in adolescent cross-country runners. *Physician and Sportsmedicine, 11*(6), 60-66

Nygaard, E., Andersen, P., Nilsson, P., Eriksson, E., Kjessel, T., & Saltin, B. (1978). Glycogen depletion pattern and lactate accumulation in leg muscles during recreational downhill skiing. *European Journal of Applied Physiology, 38*, 261-269.

Ohira, Y., Edgerton, V.R., Gardner, G.W., Gunawardena, K.A., Senewiratne, B., & Ikawa, S. (1981). Work capacity after iron treatment as a function of hemoglobin and iron deficiency. *Journal of Nutrition Science and Vitaminology, 27*, 87-96.

Ohira, Y., Edgerton, V.R., Gardner, G.W., Senewiratne, B., Barnard, R.J., & Simpson, D.R. (1979). Work capacity, heart rate and blood lactate responses to iron treatment. *British Journal of Hematology, 41*, 365-372.

Olson, R.E. (1984). Pantothenic acid. In *Present Knowledge in Nutrition, 5 ed.* Washington: The Nutrition Foundation.

Overly, W.L., Dankoff, J.A., Wang, B.K., & Singh, U.D. (1984). Androgens and hepatocellular carcinoma in an athlete. *Annals of Internal Medicine, 100,* 158-159.

Parr, R.B., Bachman, L.A., & Moss, R.A. (1984). Iron deficiency in female athletes. *Physician and Sportsmedicine, 12*(4), 81-86.

Pate, R.R., Maguire, M., & Van Wyk, J. (1979). Dietary iron supplementation in women athletes. *Physician and Sportsmedicine, 7* (9), 81-88.

Perkins, R. & Williams, M.H. (1975). Effect of caffeine upon maximal muscular endurance of females. *Medicine and Science in Sports, 7,* 221-224.

Pernow, B. & Saltin, B. (1971). Availability of substrates and capacity for prolonged heavy exercise in man. *Journal of Applied Physiology, 31,* 416-422.

Phinney, S.D., Ristrian, B.R., Evans, W.J., Gervino, E., & Blackburn, G.L. (1983). The human metabolic response to chronic ketosis without caloric restriction: Preservation of submaximal exercise capability with reduced carbohydrate oxidation. *Metabolism, 32,* 769-776.

Powers, S.K., Byrd, R.J., Tulley, R., & Calender, T. (1983). Effects of caffeine ingestion on metabolism and performance during graded exercise. *European Journal of Applied Physiology, 50,* 301-307.

Plowman, S.A. & McSwegin, P.C. (1981). The effects of iron supplementation on female cross country runners. *Journal of Sports Medicine, 21,* 407-416.

Pruett, E.D.R. (1970). Glucose and insulin during prolonged work stress in men living on different diets. *Journal of Applied Physiology, 28,* 199-208.

Puhl, J.L., Runyan, W.S., & Kruse, S.J. (1981). Erythrocyte changes during training in high school women cross-country runners. *Research Quarterly for Exercise and Sport, 52,* 484-494.

Rajalakshmi, R., Sail, S.S., Shah, D.G., & Ambady, S.K. (1973). The effects of supplements varying in carotene and calcium content on the physical, biochemical and skeletal status of preschool children. *British Journal of Nutrition, 30,* 77-86.

Recker, R.R., Saville, P.D., & Heaney, R.P. (1977). Effect of estrogens and calcium carbonate on bone loss in postmenopausal women. *Annals of Internal Medicine, 87,* 649-655.

Refsum, H.E., Gjessing, L.R., & Stromme, S.B. (1979). Changes in plasma amino acid distribution and urine amino acids excretion during prolonged heavy exercise. *Scandinavian Journal of Clinical Laboratory Investigation, 39,* 407-413.

Richards, D.K. (1968). A two-factor theory of the warm-up effect in jumping performance. *Research Quarterly, 39,* 668-673.

Ryan, A.J. (1981). Anabolic steroids are fool's gold, *Federation Proceedings, 40,* 2682-268.

Ryan, A.J. (1984). Drug problem building since 1952 Olympics. *Physician and Sportsmedicine, 12*(7), 119-124.

Sacks, F.M., Castelli, W.P., Donner, A., & Kass, E.H. 1975. Plasma lipids and lipoproteins in vegetarians and controls. *New England Journal of Medicine, 292,* 1148-1151.

Saltin, B. (1978). Fluid, elecrolyte, and energy losses and their replenishment in prolonged exercise. In J. Parizkova & V.A. Rogozkin (Eds.), *Nutrition, Physical Fitness, and Health.* Baltimore: University Park Press.

Sauberlich, H.E. (1984). Ascorbic acid. In *Present Knowledge in Nutrition, 5 ed.* Washington: The Nutrition Foundation.

Schonene, R.B., Escourrou, P., Robertson, H.T., Nilson, K.L., Parsons, J.R., & Smith, N.J. (1983). Iron repletion decreases maximal exercise lactate concentrations in female athletes with minimal iron-deficiency anemia. *Journal of Laboratory Clinical Medicine, 102,* 306-312.

Schutte, S.A. & Linkswiler, H.M. (1984). Calcium. In *Present Knowledge in Nutrition* (5th ed.). Washington, DC: The Nutrition Foundation.

Shepard, R.J. (1980). Vitamin E and physical performance. In G.A. Stull (Ed.),

Encyclopedia of Physical Education, Fitness and Sports: Training, Environment, Nutrition, and Fitness. Salt Lake City: Brighton.

Shephard, R.J., Campbell, R., Pimm, P., Stuart, D., & Wright, G. (1974). Vitamin E, exercise and the recovery from physical activity. *European Journal of Applied Physiology, 33,* 119-126.

Sherman, W.M., Costill, D.L., Fink, W.J., & Miller, J.M. (1981). The effect of exercise and diet manipulation on muscle glycogen and its subsequent utilization during performance. *International Journal of Sports Medicine, 2,* 114-118.

Smith, E.L., Reddan, W., & Smith, P.E., (1981). Physical activity and calcium modalities for bone mineral increase in aged women. *Medicine and Science in Sports and Exercise, 13,* 60-64.

Smith, G. (1983). Recreational drugs in sports. *Physician and Sportsmedicine, 11* (9), 75-82.

Spioch, F., Kobza, R., & Mazur, B. (1966). Influence of vitamin C upon certain functional changes and the coefficient of mechanical efficiency in humans during physical effort. *Acta Physiologica Polonica, 17,* 204-215.

Sproule, B.J., Mitchell, J.H., & Miller, W.F. (1960). Cardiopulmonary physiological responses to heavy exercise in patients with anemia. *Journal of Clinical Investigation, 39,* 378-388.

Spurr, G.B., Barc-Nieto, M., & Maksud, M.G. (1978). Childhood undernutrition: implications for adult work capacity and productivity. In L.H. Folinsbee, J.A. Wagner, J.F. Borgia, B.L. Drinkwater, J.A. Gliner, & J.F. Bedi (Eds.), *Environmental Stress: Individual Human Adaptations.* New York: Academic Press.

Steadward, R.D., & Singh, M. (1975). The effects of smoking marijuana on physical performance. *Medicine and Science in Sports, 7,* 309-311.

Stephenson, P.E. (1977). Physiologic and psychotropic effects of caffeine on man: a review. *Journal of the American Dietetic Association, 71,* 240-247.

Stone, M.H., & Lipner, H. (1980). The use of anabolic steroids in athletics. *Journal of Drug Issues, 10,* 351-359.

Strauss, R.H., Wright, J.E., Finerman, G.A.M., & Catlin, C.H. (1983). Side effects of anabolic steroids in weight-trained men. *Physician and Sportsmedicine, 11* (12), 87-98.

Taylor, H.L., Henschel, A., Mickelsen, O., & Keys, A. (1944). The effect of the sodium chloride intake on the work performance of man during exposure to dry heat and experimental heat exhaustion. *American Journal of Physiology, 140,* 439-451.

Ten-State Nutrition Survey 1968-1970. V-Dietary. (1972). DHEW Publication No. (HMS) 72-8133. Atlanta: Center for Disease Control.

Torun, B., Scrimshaw, N.S., & Young, V.R. (1977). Effect of isometric exercises on body potassium and dietary protein requirements of young men. *American Journal of Clinical Nutrition, 30,* 1983-1993.

Vangaard, L. (1975). Physiological reactions to wet-cold. *Aviation, Space, and Environmental Medicine, 46,* 33-36.

Van Handel, P. (1983). Caffeine. In M.H. Williams (Ed.), *Ergogenic Aids in Sport.* Champaign: Human Kinetics Publishers.

Van Huss, W.D. (1966). What made the Russians run ? *Nutrition Today, 1,* 20-23.

Vellar, O.D. (1968). Studies on sweat of nutrients. I. Iron content of whole body sweat and its association with the sweat constituents, serum iron levels, hematological indices, body surface area, and sweat rate. *Scandinavian Journal of Clinical Laboratory Investigation, 21,* 157-167.

Warren, R.A. (1985). Osteoporosis. *Contemporary Nutrition, 10,* 1-2.

Watt, T., Romet, T.T., McFarlane, I., McGuey, D., Allen, C., & Goode, R.C. (1974). Vitamin E and oxygen consumption. *Lancet, 2,* 354-355.

Weltman, A., Stamford, B.A., Moffat, R.J., & Katch, V.L. (1977). Exercise recovery, lactate removal, and subsequent high intensity exercise performance.

Research Quarterly, 48, 786-796.

Wenzel, D.G., & Rutledge, C.O. (1962). Effects of centrally-acting drugs on human motor and psychomotor performance. *Journal of Pharmaceutical Science, 51,* 631-644.

Williams, M.H. (1969). Effect of selected doses of alcohol on fatigue parameters of the forearm flexor muscles. *Research Quarterly, 40,* 832-840.

Williams, M.H. (1972). Effect of small and moderate doses of alcohol on exercise heart rate and oxygen consumption. *Research Quarterly, 43,* 94-104.

Williams, M.H. (1985). *Nutritional Aspects of Human Physical and Athletic Performance. 2nd ed.* Springfield: Charles C. Thomas.

Willams, M.H., Wesseldine, S., Somma, T., & Schuster, R. (1981). The effect of induced erythrocythemia upon 5-mile treadmill time. *Medicine and Science in Sports and Exercise, 13,* 169-175.

Wilson, G.D., & Welch, H.G. (1975). Effects of hyperoxic gas mixtures on exercise tolerance in man. *Medicine and Science in Sports, 7,* 48-52.

Wilson, G.D., & Welch, H.G. (1980). Effects of varying concentrations of N_2/O_2 and He/O_2 on exercise tolerance in man. *Medicine and Science in Sports and Exercise 12,* 380-384.

Wishnitzer, R., Vorst, E., & Berrebi, A. (1983). Bone marrow iron depression in competitive distance runners. *International Journal of Sports Medicine, 4,* 27-30.

Wright, J.E. (1981). Anabolic steriods and athletics. In R.S. Hutton & D.I. Miller (Eds.), *Exercise and Sport Sciences Reviews.* Philadelphia: Franklin Institute Press.

Wyndham, C.H. & Strydom, N.B. (1969). The danger of an inadequate water intake during marathon running. *South African Medical Journal, 43,* 893-896.

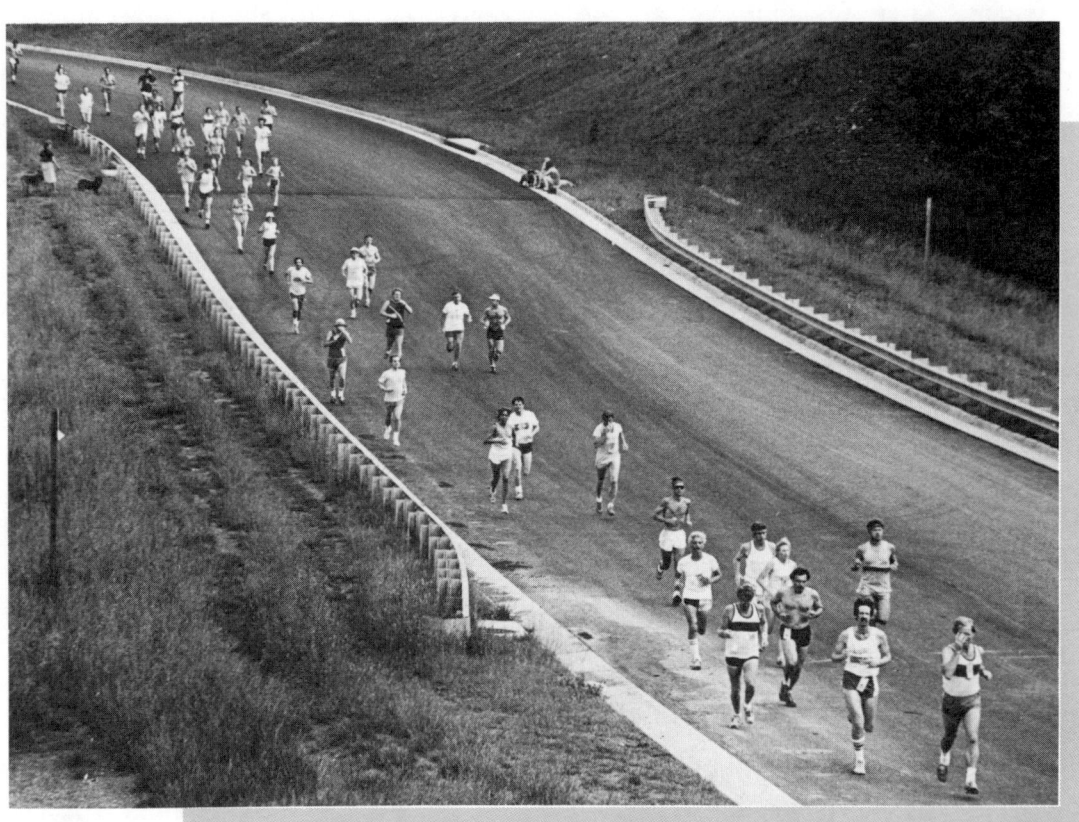

photo by Jim Kirby

CHAPTER TEN

Cardiorespiratory Adaptations to Chronic Endurance Exercise

Russell R. Pate and
J. Larry Durstine
Department of Physical Education
University of South Carolina
Columbia, South Carolina

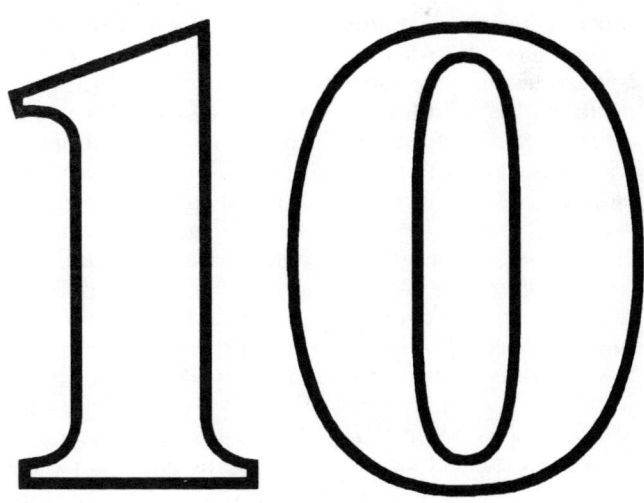

Exercise scientists have long been interested in the effects of endurance exercise on the cardiorespiratory system. In fact, elucidation of the cardiorespiratory adaptations to exercise has been a central theme in exercise physiology since its inception as a scientific discipline. The prolonged and intense interest of exercise scientists in this field is due to two key beliefs. First, it has long been known that performance level in endurance physical activities is related to certain elements of cardiorespiratory structure and function. Second, the Western cultures have long held to the belief that regular exercise carries important health benefits for the organs and tissues of the cardiorespiratory system. Accordingly, the research in this field has focused on explaining: (a) the effects of exercise training on those aspects of cardiorespiratory function that might be associated with endurance performance, and (b) the effects of chronic exercise on the health status of the cardiorespiratory system.

This chapter summarizes the scientifically documented effects of endurance exercise training on the structure, function and health status of the cardiorespiratory system. Specifically, the effects of exercise training on skeletal muscle tissue and on the major components of the cardiorespiratory system (i.e., heart, blood, blood vessels, lungs) will be discussed. Major sections of the chapter will focus on effects of training on cardiorespiratory functional capacity and on cardiovascular health. In addition, the unique adaptive responses of females, children, and the elderly will be noted. In beginning the discussion, a brief review of the principles of endurance exercise training will be provided.

Principles of Endurance Training

The Training Stimulus

It has long been recognized that physiological systems are capable of adapting to increased functional demands. Accordingly, "overload" is one of the most fundamental principles of exercise training. In the present context, overload might be defined as performance of exercise that is more demanding than that to which the individual is already accustomed. Systematic applications of overloading exercise causes physiological adaptations that result in increased functional capacities.

The term "cardiorespiratory endurance" refers to the ability to perform large-muscle, whole-body, moderate-to-high intensity activity for extended periods of time. Over the past three decades researchers have expended great effort in studying various approaches to training for improved cardiorespiratory endurance (CRE). The result of this effort is a general consensus regarding the nature of the training stimulus that can be expected to increase cardiorespiratory endurance (see Table 1). This stimulus most typically has been described in terms of four factors: mode, frequency, duration, and intensity of exercise.

Mode of exercise. As a general principle, activity that involves rhythmic, large-muscle exercise, if employed with adequate frequency, duration, and intensity, can be expected to increase cardiorespiratory endurance. This general principle has been derived primarily from studies of continuous, aerobic activities such as walking, jogging or running, cycling, and swimming (American College of Sports Medicine [ACSM], 1978). Much less research has been focused on relatively discontinuous activities such as team games and racket sports. Therefore, firm claims about the training effects of participation in these activities should await publication of relevant studies. Some evidence indicates that circuit weight training can increase CRE in some participants, although the training response is less marked than with activities such as running or cycling (Gettman, Ayres, Pollock, & Jackson, 1978; Wilmore et al., 1978).

Frequency. CRE is usually increased significantly with training regimens that involve three or more exercise sessions per week (Pollock, Cureton, & Greninger,

Table 1
Components of a training program for enhancement of cardiorespiratory endurance

Effective cardiorespiratory endurance training programs usually meet the following criteria:

Mode of Exercise:
  Rythmic activity involving large-muscle groups and movements of the whole body or large segments of the body (i.e., an "aerobic activity").

Frequency of Training:
  Three to seven training sessions per week.

Duration of the Training Session:
  Fifteen to sixty minutes of vigorous activity per session.

Intensity of Exercise:
  Metabolic rate is elevated to 50-80% of maximal aerobic power (usually corresponds to 60-90% of maximal heart rate)

1969). The rate of increase is somewhat greater with more frequent exercise sessions; however, risk of orthopedic injury is also elevated with higher frequency programs (Pollock et al., 1977). Training at frequencies less than three sessions per week can be expected to increase CRE in previously sedentary and low-fit persons. However, reductions in percentage of body fat tend not to occur with these lower frequency training programs (Pollock, 1978).

Duration. Relatively prolonged bouts of exercise are required to increase CRE. The minimal duration required to improve CRE in most beginning exercisers is in the range of 15-20 minutes (Milesis et al., 1976). Longer durations of activity are needed to maintain or improve CRE in previously active and/or younger, more athletic groups. Exercise durations approximating 30 minutes are most commonly recommended for the healthy adult participant whose aim is development and maintenance of an adequate functional capacity.

Intensity. It is well documented that increases in CRE occur only in response to exercise training sessions that require substantially elevated rates of energy expenditure. Considerable attention has been focused on identifying the minimal exercise intensity needed to simulate the desired adaptive response. It has been demonstrated that the required intensity is a function of the individual's fitness level (i.e., maximal aerobic power). The consensus is that the minimal intensity is in the range of 50-60% of individual maximal aerobic power ($\dot{V}O_2$max) (Karvonen, Kentala, & Mustala, 1957; ACSM, 1978). That is, the overall average rate of aerobic energy expenditure ($\dot{V}O_2$) during the exercise session should be equivalent to 50-60% $\dot{V}O_2$max. In most persons this exercise intensity elevates heart rate to 60-70% of its maximum.

Factors Modifying the Training Adaptation

The physiological adaptations to endurance training are determined largely by the magnitude of the training dose applied (i.e., combined effects of frequency, duration, and intensity of exercise). However, scientists and practitioners alike have frequently noted that different individuals may adapt differently to the same training program. This section addresses several of the factors, besides training dose, that affect the adaptation to training.

Initial fitness level. In general, previously sedentary and/or lower fit individuals tend to adapt more markedly to exercise training than do persons who are already active or more fit (Moody, Wilmore, Girandola, & Royce, 1972). Less fit persons manifest functional states that are further below their genetically determined upper limit and, therefore, tend to have a greater potential for improvement than do higher fit individuals. However, it also should be noted that lower fit persons typically have a lower tolerance for exercise training and consequently tend to experience greater stress than more fit persons when both are exposed to the same training program. This higher stress level may precipitate higher frequencies of injury and illness in lower fit or previously sedentary persons.

Specificity. An extensive body of research has demonstrated that the physiological response to endurance training is highly specific to the mode of exercise that is performed in the training process (Stromme, Ingjer, & Meen, 1977). For example, it has been shown that training with the arms (e.g., arm cranking, swimming) has little effect on the muscle metabolic and cardiorespiratory responses to exercise with the legs such as bicycling or running (McKenzie, Fox, & Cohen, 1978).

Developmental stage. Age and developmental status apparently affect the magnitude of the response to endurance training. While much more study of this issue is needed, available evidence suggests that pre-pubertal children and the elderly tend to manifest adaptations to endurance training that are smaller in absolute magnitude than those seen in young and middle-aged adults (deVries, 1970; Stewart & Gutin, 1976). A more detailed discussion of this topic will be presented later in this chapter.

Adaptations of Skeletal Muscle to Endurance Exercise Training

This chapter will focus primarily on the cardiorespiratory adaptations to endurance training. However, mounting evidence indicates that the cardiorespiratory adaptations to training are inextricably linked to the adaptations that occur in the skeletal muscle tissue. Indeed, many of the changes in "central" cardiorespiratory function that occur with training are apparently secondary to changes that occur in the "peripheral" muscle tissue. Consequently, we shall summarize here the skeletal muscle adaptations to endurance training (see Table 2).

Table 2
Skeletal muscle adaptations to endurance exercise training

Chronic participation in endurance training results in the following changes in skeletal muscle structure and functions:

    Increased number and size of mitochondria
    Increased activity of enzymes of Krebs cycle and electron transport system
    Increased intracellular storage of glycogen and triglycerides
    Increased capacity for fat utilization during submaximal exercise
    Increased capillary density

Skeletal muscle tissue adapts to endurance training principally by increasing its "oxidative capacity" (Holloszy, 1973). That is, the constituents of the muscle fiber that are involved in aerobic metabolism adapt in such a way as to increase the maximum rate at which oxygen can be utilized in provision of the chemical energy that is expended during muscle contraction. The result is an increase in the rate of power output that the muscle can sustain for a prolonged period. Several specific adaptations have been shown to contribute to this increase in skeletal muscle oxidative capacity.

Mitochondrial Enzyme Systems

The aerobic metabolic pathway consists of an extensive series of chemical reactions that result in the complete oxidation of cellular energy sources such as glucose and free fatty acids. Each of the many chemical reactions involved in aerobic metabolism is catalyzed by a specific enzyme. These enzymes control the rate of the chemical reactions which they catalyze. The total amount and activity of an enzyme present in a medium determines the maximum rate at which its chemical reaction can proceed. The enzymes of aerobic metabolism form two linked sub-systems: the Krebs cycle and the electron transport system. The enzymes which form these two sub-systems are located within the mitochondria, sub-cellular organelles which are present in large numbers in skeletal muscle fibers.

Extensive evidence indicates that the enzyme systems of aerobic metabolism adapt to the metabolic demands imposed by endurance exercise training (Holloszy & Booth, 1976). The number of mitochondria present in muscle (i.e., mitochondrial density) increases with endurance training (Gollnick & King, 1969) and some reports indicate that the size of the individual mitochondria also increase (Howard, 1975). Certain key enzymes in the aerobic pathway increase in activity with endurance training. For example, succinic dehydrogenase and cytochrome oxidase, enzymes in the Krebs cycle and electron transport system, respectively, typically manifest increased activity with training (Gollnick, Armstrong, Saubert, Piehl, & Saltin, 1972).

Storage of Energy Substrates

The principle energy substrates utilized in aerobic muscle metabolism are glycogen and triglycerides. Both of these substances are stored within the muscle fiber and therefore are immediately available to the metabolic apparatus of the muscle fiber at the onset of exercise. With endurance training the intracellular pools of glycogen and triglycerides stored within muscle fibers expand. Resting glycogen concentrations are roughly two to three times as great in trained subjects as in sedentary persons (Gollnick et al., 1973). The intramuscular free fatty acid concentration has been shown to increase by 50% with training (Hoppeler, Luthi, Claassen, Weibel, & Howard, 1973). This increased capacity for storage of energy substrates is of particular benefit during performance of prolonged exercise which can deplete muscle glycogen stores.

Energy Substrate Utilization Patterns

Several factors affect the relative contributions of carbohydrate (glycogen or glucose) and fat (triglycerides) to the muscle metabolic process during exercise. Among these are intensity of exercise, duration of exercise, and nutritional state of the individual. Endurance training causes adaptations in the fat metabolic pathway that result in greater utilization of fat as an energy substrate during submaximal exercise (Mole, Oscai, & Holloszy, 1971). The trained individual's greater fat utilization during submaximal exercise manifests as a lower respiratory exchange ratio (ratio of CO_2 production to O_2 consumption, $\dot{V}CO_2/\dot{V}O_2$). This adaptation is potentially beneficial due to its "glycogen-sparing" effect. Increased fat utilization proportionally decreases glycogen use and reduces the rate at which the muscle's finite glycogen pool is depleted. In addition, decreased glycogen use may facilitate an increase in the rate of energy expenditure at which anaerobic glycolysis and lactic acid production begin. More detail on the effects of training on this "anaerobic threshold" will be presented later in this chapter.

Capillarization

Skeletal muscle tissue is infiltrated by an extensive network of blood vessels. The individual muscle fibers are surrounded by capillaries, across the wall of which the oxygen and other nutrients needed for muscle metabolism move. The ratio of capillaries to muscle fibers has been shown to be about 50% greater in endurance trained persons than in untrained subjects (Hermansen & Wachtlova, 1971). Likewise, increased capillary density has been observed in response to controlled endurance training (Andersen, 1975). This adaptation is thought to facilitate rapid delivery of oxygen to the muscle fiber. An added benefit may be an enhanced rate of clearance of lactic acid from the muscle during high intensity exercise.

Adaptations of the Cardiorespiratory System to Endurance Training

Endurance training has a profound impact on cardiorespiratory function. It is well documented that both central (heart and pulmonary function) and peripheral (blood and vascular function) adaptations occur (Rowell, 1974; Clausen, 1977; Dowell, 1983). This section presents the training-induced adaptations that are observed in the structure and function of the heart, blood vessels, blood and pulmonary system. These adaptations are summarized in Table 3.

Table 3
Cardiorespiratory adaptations to endurance training

Chronic participation in endurance training induces the following changes in the structure and function of the cardiorespiratory system:

Heart
   Decreased heart rate during rest and submaximal exercise
   Increased stroke volume during rest, submaximal exercise and maximal exercise
   Increased maximal cardiac output

Vascular System
   Decreased blood pressure during submaximal exercise
   Decreased total peripheral resistance during exercise

Blood
   Increased total blood volume
   Increased red cell mass
   Increased total hemoglobin

Pulmonary System
   Decreased ventilation during submaximal exercise
   Increased ventilation at maximal exertion

Heart Structure and Function

Heart Rate. Resting heart rate is reduced by as much as 15 percent following 20 weeks of endurance training 30 minutes a day five days a week (Gettman et al., 1976). The mechanism for this decrease is not entirely understood, but it may be related to changes in autonomic nervous system activity. Endurance training may create a change in the balance between sympathetic and parasympathetic activity favoring a dominance of vagal, parasympathetic influences (Winder, Hagberg, Hickson, Ehsani, & McLane, 1978). Also, training may reduce the intrinsic activity of the sino-atrial node of the heart (Scheuer, Penparqkul, & Bhan, 1974).

After training, decreased heart rate is also observed during performance of standard, submaximal exercise (Saltin, 1969). As with the reduction in resting heart rate, the decrease in submaximal exercise heart rates may be related to increased parasympathetic activity. Training does cause a reduction in the circulating levels of epinephrine and norepinephrine during submaximal work loads, but the decrease in exercise heart rate is not associated with the reduction in these hormones (Winder et al., 1978).

Maximal heart rate is either unchanged (Gettman et al., 1976) or reduced slightly (Pollock, 1973; Saltin, 1969) by endurance training. Thus, maximal heart rate seems to be quite stable and can be used as a reliable marker for maximal levels of exertion (Pollock, 1973).

Stroke volume. Endurance training has been reported to cause increases in volume of blood ejected with each contraction of the heart at rest and during exercise (Saltin, 1969; Ekblom, 1969a). This increased stroke volume has been attributed to three mechanisms that may act independently or together. Increased stroke volume at rest may be secondary to the longer diastolic period associated with the reduced resting heart rate (Wolfe, Cunningham, Rechnitzer, & Nichol, 1979). A greater filling if the ventricles with blood would stretch the cardiac fibers and more properly align the actin and myosin filaments resulting in a greater contractile force and increased stroke volume (Frank-Starling mechanism). A second possible explanation for increased stroke volume is enlargement of the heart (Stein, Michielli, Diamond, Horwitz, & Krasnow, 1980; Zeldis, Morganroth, & Rubler, 1978). Greatest hypertrophy is found in the left ventricle (Kanakis & Hickson, 1980). The type of physical activity seems to be particularly important in determining the nature of the hypertrophy response of the heart. Morganroth, Maron, Henry, and Epstein (1975), using echocardiography, found that the hearts of athletes who were involved in dynamic endurance exercise (running or swimming) showed increased left ventricular end-diastolic volume and mass, but normal wall thickness. In contrast, athletes participating in high resistance exercises (wrestling and shot-putting) has increased left ventricular wall thickness and mass, but normal end-diastolic volume. An increase in the left ventricle end-diastolic volume could mean greater stroke volume.

A third possible mechanism for increased stroke volume is an increased contractile state of the heart. Greater stroke volume has been found without increased heart volume (Barnard, 1975; Barnard, Duncan, Baldwin, Grimditch, & Buckberg, 1980; Schaible & Scheuer, 1979; Tibbits, Barnard, Baldwin, Cugalj, & Roberts, 1981). Therefore, endurance training must have some effect on stroke volume that is independent of hypertrophy. Tibbits et al. (1981) suggest that training causes increased intracellular levels of calcium in cardiac muscle cells. This change could result in increased force of contraction.

Greater values for stroke volume at submaximal and maximal work loads following endurance training have been reported (Ekblom, Astrand, Saltin, Stenberg, & Wallstrom, 1968; Saltin et al., 1968; Rowell, 1974; Barnard, 1975). With one exception, the same mechanisms that account for the changes in resting stroke volume have been proposed to explain the changes during exercise. Maximal heart rate does not change following training and, therefore, a greater diastolic period during maximal exercise cannot occur.

Cardiac output. Resting cardiac output is not changed following endurance training (Clausen, 1977; Ekblom et al., 1968; Saltin et al., 1968). Cardiac output during standard submaximal exercise following training has typically been observed to be unchanged or slightly decreased (Clausen, Klausen, Rasmussen, & Trap-Jensen, 1973; Saltin et al., 1968; Kilbom & Astrand, 1971). However, cardiac output at maximal workloads following training is considerably increased by training (Ekblom et al., 1968; Gleser, 1973; Hartley et al., 1969; Clausen et al., 1973). Since maximal heart rate does not change, the increase in maximal cardiac output is due to increased maximal stroke volume.

Blood pressure. Active people tend to have lower systolic and diastolic blood pressures than inactive persons (Blair, Goodyear, Gibbons, & Cooper, 1984; Haskell 1984a; Cooper et al., 1976). However, controlled training studies have typically found minimal changes in blood pressure in initially normotensive subjects. Other studies have reported decreased systolic pressures in borderline hypertensive patients following endurance training (Choquette & Ferguson, 1973; Roman, Camuzzi, Villalon, & Klenner, 1981).

Some authors have reported that blood pressure during standard, submaximal exercise is decreased as a result of endurance training (Choquette & Ferguson, 1973; Kilbom, 1971; Haskell, 1984a). Other authors have reported no changes in submaximal exercise blood pressure (Clausen et al., 1973; Hartley et al., 1969; Kilbom & Astrand, 1971; Saltin et al., 1968). If there is a reduction in submaximal blood pressure, the mechanisms remain undetermined. Decreased blood pressure could be due to a decrease in sympathetic nervous activity during submaximal exercise, and there is some experimental evidence to support this hypothesis (Cousineau, Ferguson, deChamplain, Gautheir, & Bourassu, 1977). There is evidence that maximal blood pressure is not changed after endurance training (Ekblom et al., 1968; Gleser, 1973; Hartley et al., 1969; Pollock, 1973).

Total peripheral resistance. The term "total peripheral resistance" (TRP) refers to the impediment to blood flow through blood vessels. This variable, which is primarily dependent on the diameter of the arterioles, cannot be measured by any direct means. However, an estimate may be obtained by the following equation:

TRP = mean arterial pressure / cardiac output

Because resting blood pressure and cardiac output are not affected by endurance training, resting peripheral resistance is not changed. However, if we assume that blood pressure in response to standardized submaximal work loads following endurance training is reduced and that cardiac output has remained the same, then total peripheral resistance must be reduced. Likewise, total peripheral resistance during maximal exercise is reduced by endurance training (Clausen, 1977). This follows from the observations that maximal cardiac output is increased but maximal blood pressure is unchanged.

Blood

Blood, the fluid medium that circulates through the vascular system, consists primarily of plasma and red blood cells. Plasma is an aqueous solution that functions as the transport medium for numerous metabolites. Red blood cells carry hemoglobin, the red-pigminted protein that plays a central role in transportation of oxygen and carbon dioxide. Blood also functions to transport heat from warmer to cooler regions of the body and to transport regulatory substances such as hormones.

Endurance training results in increases in total blood volume, red cell mass and total amount of hemoglobin (Oscai, Williams, & Hertig, 1968). These adaptations probably enhance endurance performance by facilitating venous return of blood to the heart and thereby contribute to the increase in stroke volume of the heart that occurs with training. Also, increased blood volume may help maintain blood flow to the active skeletal muscle during exercise in heat stress, which tends to divert blood to the skin.

Although both plasma volume and red cell mass tend to increase with training, hemoglobin concentration (Hb) and hematocrit (Hct) do not. With moderate doses of training Hb and Hct change very little, indicating that plasma volume and red cell mass have changed, proportionally. However, with high levels of endurance training Hb and Hct tend to decrease (Pate, 1983). The physiological mechanism underlying this "sports anemia" is presently unclear but it may be related to an increase in plasma volume that is proportionally greater than the increase in total hemoglobin and/or disturbances in iron metabolism. Likewise, the functional significance of a moderate decrease in Hb concomitant with an expanded blood volume is uncertain.

Pulmonary system

The primary function of the pulmonary system (lungs and associated air passages) is to maintain normal partial pressures of oxygen and carbon dioxide in arterial blood. During exercise, which necessitates increased rates of oxygen utilization and carbon dioxide production, ventilation of the lung must increase at least in proportion to the increase in the rates of oxygen consumption and cardiac output. In the person with a normal, healthy pulmonary system the capacity for responses to the ventilatory demands of exercise is more than adequate. That is, maximal breathing capacity typically is greater than the maximal rate of ventilation observed during exhaustive endurance exercise.

The high ventilatory capacity observed in healthy persons suggests: (a) that pulmonary function normally is not a limiting factor in endurance performance, and (b) improvements in endurance performance may occur without marked adaptations in the structure or function of the pulmonary system. Experimental and descriptive studies support the validity of these concepts. Descriptive studies comparing trained and sedentary persons have reported marginally greater static lung volumes and resting pulmonary function scores in endurance trained in comparison to untrained subjects (Raven, 1977). However, experimental training studies have tended to observe that static lung volumes and resting pulmonary function change very little with chronic endurance activity (Bachman & Horvath, 1968). These observations indicate that endurance training does not cause marked adaptations in the structure of the pulmonary system.

In contrast, pulmonary *function* during exercise does change with training, although the observed changes are probably secondary to adaptations in the skeletal muscles and cardiovascular system. During standard submaximal exercise, ventilation decreases with training (Martin, Sparks, Zwillich, & Weil, 1979). This reduction is probably due, at least in part, to the decreased ventilatory drive associated with lower rates of lactic acid production (Sutton & Jones, 1979). At maximal exertion, ventilation is increased after endurance training (Ekblom, 1969a). This increase tends to be highly correlated with the increase in maximal aerobic power and probably indicates only that the trained person is capable of tapping a greater fraction of the maximal breathing capacity.

Impact of Endurance Training on Functional Capacity

The most readily observable adaptation to chronic participation in endurance exercise is an increase in the participant's cardiorespiratory endurance. This increased tolerance for prolonged, moderate-to-high intensity activity is manifested through numerous physiological adaptations observed during both submaximal and maximal exercise. This section summarizes the adaptations observed during these two types of activity.

Adaptations Observed During Maximal Exercise

For purposes of this discussion, "maximal exercise" is defined as physical activity that results in exhaustion at the conclusion of a graded exercise test. It is assumed that the exercise mode involves large-muscle, rhythmic activity and that the total duration of the exercise test is in the range of five to twenty minutes.

Endurance training is well documented to cause an increase in the individual's absolute rate of power output at maximal exercise (Ekblom, 1969a). For example, an individual who trains via endurance running would be expected to manifest an increase in the speed of running that could be tolerated prior to encountering exhaustion during a graded, treadmill running test. The magnitude of the increase in power output varies markedly among individuals and, of course, depends on the mode, frequency, duration, and intensity of the training dose.

The training-induced increase in power output at maximal exercise is closely associated with an increased maximal rate of aerobic energy expenditure (Ekblom, 1969a). The physiological marker for aerobic energy expenditure is oxygen consumption ($\dot{V}O_2$). The rate of oxygen consumption observed at maximal exercise, the maximal aerobic power ($\dot{V}O_2$ max), has long been taken as the "gold standard" for measurement of cardiorespiratory endurance. Maximal aerobic power is one of the most extensively studied variables in exercise physiology and a vast body of research has demonstrated that it tends to increase with endurance training (Pollock, 1973). Examination of the numerous controlled training studies that have observed the impact of endurance training on $\dot{V}O_2$ max lead to the conclusion that previously sedentary adults tend to manifest 10-15% increase in $\dot{V}O_2$ max with programs that last for 4 to 8 months (ACSM, 1978). Greater increases in maximal aerobic power may occur with very heavy training doses, with very prolonged programs and with persons who begin in a very deconditioned state (Saltin et al., 1968).

Increases in maximal aerobic power are due to adaptations in both the trained skeletal muscle tissue and the cardiorespiratory system. The major cardiovascular and muscle metabolic adaptations to training were discussed in proceeding sections of this chapter. This section considers these adaptations in the context of the contribution they make to the increases in maximal aerobic power and maximal power output that are observed with training.

As shown in Equation 1, oxygen consumption can be computed as the product of cardiac output ($\dot{Q}$) and arteriovenous oxygen difference (AVD). AVD is the difference between the oxygen contents of arterial and venous blood and is a reflection of the percentage of the arterial blood oxygen that is unloaded to the peripheral tissues. It is typically quantified as milliliters of oxygen unloaded per 100 milliters of blood circulated through the tissues.

$$\dot{V}O_2 \text{ (ML/MIN)} = \dot{Q} \text{ (ML/MIN)} \cdot AVD \text{ (ML/ML BLOOD)} \quad (1)$$

Accordingly, maximal oxygen consumption can be computed from maximal cardiac output and AVD at maximal exercise:

$$\dot{V}O_2 \text{ max (ML/MIN)} = \dot{Q} \text{ max (ML/MIN)} \cdot AVD \text{ max (ML/ML BLOOD)} \quad (2)$$

As discussed in a preceding section, maximal cardiac output increases with endurance training. This increase is due to an increased maximal stroke volume which, in turn, is secondary to increases in total blood volume and myocardial contractility. Also, maximal arteriovenous oxygen difference, expressed as milliliters of oxygen per 100 milliliters of blood, is somewhat increased by endurance training (Ekblom, et al., 1968). AVD is expressed relative to the volume of blood circulated, and this volume is increased by training (i.e., increased $\dot{Q}$ max). The ability of the skeletal muscles to increase their rate of extraction of oxygen from the blood, even with an increased rate of blood flow, is probably a reflection of the increased oxidative capacity of the muscle tissue.

Adaptations Observed During Submaximal Exercise

The term "submaximal exercise" will be defined here as physical activity that involves a specified, constant rate of power output and which requires a rate of aerobic energy expenditure that is less than the individual's maximal aerobic power ($\dot{V}O_2$ max). A large volume of research supports the conclusion that endurance training increases tolerance for submaximal exercise. This increased tolerance is manifested as either (a) an increased work time to exhaustion when exercising at a specified submaximal intensity, or (b) an increased submaximal rate of power output that can be tolerated for a specified period of time before exhaustion is encountered. The training induced increase in work time to exhaustion at a standard submaximal exercise intensity is secondary to increased maximal aerobic power and, in some cases, to a decreased oxygen cost of activity (i.e., increased efficiency). Tolerance for submaximal exercise is highly and negatively correlated with the percentage of the maximal aerobic power that is required during its performance (Costill, Thomason, & Roberts, 1973; Pate & Kriska, 1984). As shown in Equation 3, work time to exhaustion during submaximal exertion is directly related to maximal aerobic power and inversely related to the oxygen cost of the activity (i.e., inverse of the % $\dot{V}O_2$ max required by the activity).

$$\text{WORK TIME TO EXHAUSTION} \approx \left(\frac{\dot{V}O_2}{\dot{V}O_2 \text{ max}}\right)^{-1} \quad (3)$$

As discussed above, training increases $\dot{V}O_2$ max. Increased efficiency of exercise manifests as a decreased oxygen cost ($\dot{V}O_2$) of activity. In activities that involve relatively novel skills (e.g., swimming), in which mechanical efficiency can be improved substantially with practice, efficiency may improve markedly. In more familiar skills such as walking, running and cycling, training may not result in large improvements in efficiency.

In any case, increased tolerance for submaximal exercise does *not* result from an increased rate of oxygen utilization during performance of the activity. As noted above, $\dot{V}O_2$ during standard, submaximal exercise is either unchanged or decreases with endurance training (Ekblom et al., 1968). Nonetheless, a training induced increase in $\dot{V}O_2$ max contributes to improved tolerance for submaximal exercise by decreasing the percent $\dot{V}O_2$ max required by the activity. A partial explanation for this observation may lie in the phenomenon that has been labelled "anaerobic threshold."

Anaerobic threshold. Definition of the term "anaerobic threshold" is a controversial issue that has been discussed in detail elsewhere (Skinner & McLellan, 1980). In this chapter, anaerobic threshold is defined as the rate of power output at which the product of anaerobic glycolysis, lactic acid, begins to accumulate in the blood. Evidence indicates that endurance training increases anaerobic threshold (Davis, Frank, Whipp, & Wasserman, 1979). However, the physiological mechanism that underlies this adaptation has not been fully elucidated. Among the factors which may contribute to an increased anaerobic threshold are: (a) decreased use of glycogen as an energy substrate due to increased fat utilization, (b) increased rate of clearance of lactic acid from the blood and, (c) increased number of mitochondria and increased aerobic enzyme activity in skeletal muscle.

Impact of Endurance Exercise Training On Risk of Chronic Cardiovascular Disease

Diseases of the circulatory system were responsible for approximately one-half of the total mortality in the United States in the year 1982 (American Heart Association, 1985). Coronary heart disease (CHD) was the single most frequent cause of death due to cardiovascular disease. Atherosclerosis is the predominant underlying cause of cardiovascular disease, and is the form of ateriosclerosis that most frequently causes CHD. Although the precise pathophysiologic basis of these clinical manifestations is not understood, there are a number of factors that are associated with an increased risk for development of the disease. The primary risk factors are elevated blood cholesterol, hypertension, and cigarette smoking. Secondary risk factors include obesity, physical inactivity, psychological stress, and diabetes (American Heart Association, 1985).

Persons engaged in regular endurance training programs generally demonstrate fewer clinical manifestations of CHD than their sedentary counterparts. When cardiac events occur in active persons, they tend to be less severe and to appear at an older age (Costas, Garcia-Palmieri, Nazario, & Sorlie, 1978; Morris, Everitt, Pollard, Chave, & Semmence, 1980; Paffenbarger, Wing, & Hyde, 1978; Salonen, Puska, & Tuomilehto, 1982; Haskell, 1984a). Data from these studies demonstrate an inverse association between habitual physical activity level and risk of CHD. However, it should be noted that no adequately designed clinical trial has been completed which clearly demonstrates a cause and effect relationship between exercise and reduced CHD risk (Haskell, 1984a).

The issue that remains to be resolved is how exercise might provide a "cardioprotective effect." The resolution to this issue clearly is not simple and probably involves several complex, interacting explanations. One mechanism whereby endurance training could delay the development of atherosclerosis is by modifying the risk factors that are associated with CHD. Other mechanisms could involve physiological adaptations that improve oxygen supply to the myocardium and/or factors that decrease myocardial work and the need for increased oxygen supply to the myocardium during exercise (Haskell, 1984a). Following are discussions of the effects of endurance training of CHD risk factors and on myocardial oxygen supply and demand. These effects are summarized in Table 4.

Table 4
Mechanisms by which endurance exercise training may reduce risk for development of coronary heart disease

The following adaptations to endurance training may contribute to reduced coronary heart disease risk:

Increased plasma HDL cholesterol and HDL cholesterol/total cholesterol ratio
Decreased resting blood pressure in borderline hypertensive patients
Decreased percentage of body fat
Decreased myocardial oxygen demand during rest and submaximal exercise

Blood lipids. A succinct review of the hypothesized role of blood lipids in the atherosclerotic process has been provided by McMillan (1978). The "lipid hypothesis" is based on the following observations: (a) frequent occurrence of excessive amounts of cholesterol and lipid in atherosclerotic lesions, (b) the positive association between elevated serum lipids and atherogenesis in human beings and in animals, and (c) the association of dietary saturated fats and cholesterol with atherogenesis in human beings and experimental animals (McMillan, 1978). The accumulation of lipid in atherosclerotic plaque involves the introduction of excessive amounts of plasma lipoproteins through the endothelial barrier into the intimal layer of the arterial wall. Plasma lipoproteins are the transport vehicles for synthesized and dietary lipids. These are discrete water-soluable macromolecular complexes containing cholesterol, triglyceride, phospholipid, and protein. Classification of lipoproteins is based on their gravitational density by ultracentrifugation with four major classes identified: chylomicrons, very low density lipoprotein (VLDL), low density lipoproteins (LDL), and high density lipoproteins (HDL). Concentrations of VLDL and LDL cholesterol have been directly related to risk of CHD (Kannel, Castelli, & Gordon, 1979). HDL cholesterol has been inversely related to CHD risk (Miller & Miller, 1975; Kannel et al., 1979). In the formation of plaque, LDL are internalized by smooth muscle as well as connective tissue cells. Lipid components accumulate in the cells and with progressive cellular lipid accumulation, cellular necrosis may occur, causing lipid to be dispersed into the extracellular portions of the arterial wall. Thus, lipid may accumulate both intracellularly and extracellularly and may act as a local cause of injury (McMillan, 1978).

An extensive review of the effect of endurance training on plasma lipids and liproproteins has been provided by Haskell (1984b). In general, active persons do not demonstrate lower levels of total plasma cholesterol than do inactive persons (Adner & Castilli, 1980; Durstine, Smith, Dover, Fronsoe, Manno, Goodyear,

Lambert, & Pate, 1984; Lehtonen & Viikari, 1978). Likewise, measurements of blood lipids made before and following endurance training have produced no clear change in total cholesterol. Most studies using short term training periods (less than 12 weeks) have reported no changes in total plasma cholesterol (Huttunen et al., 1979; Williams, Logue, Lewis, Barton, Stead, Wallace & Pizzo, 1980) while some studies using longer training periods have produced decreases in total cholesterol (Kiens et al., 1980; Kilbom et al., 1969). However, plasma triglycerides are usually found to be lower in active than sedentary persons (Durstine et al., 1984; Martin, Haskell & Wood, 1977; Wood et al., 1976; Lehtonen & Viikari, 1978).

Also, mounting evidence indicates that plasma lipoproteins are affected by endurance training. VLDL is the primary carrier of triglyceride in the blood. Since triglyceride levels are lower following endurance training, it is not surprising that the VLDL fraction is also decreased with training (Nye, Carlson, Kirstein, & Rossner, 1981; Huttunen et al., 1979). Endurance training has only a small impact on LDL cholesterol concentration. In general, LDL cholesterol is reduced by about 10% in response to endurance training (Brownell, Bachorik, & Ayerle, 1982; Huttunen et al., 1979; Peltonen, Marniemi, Hietanen, Vuori, & Ehnholm, 1981). In contrast and perhaps most importantly, the cholesterol associated with HDL typically has been found to be higher in active than inactive persons. Relatively high levels of HDL cholesterol have been reported in runners (Adner & Castilli, 1980; Durstine et al., 1984), cross-country skiers (Enger, Herbjornsen, Krikssen, & Fretland, 1977), speed skaters (Farrell, Maksud, Pollock, Foster, & Anholm, 1982), and soccer players (Lehtonen & Viikari, 1980). The magnitude of the change induced by endurance training is about 10 percent (Nye et al., 1979).

These findings indicate that endurance training modifies the blood lipoproteins so as to reduce risk for developing CHD. Although total cholesterol remains about the same, the amount of cholesterol that is carried by the various lipoprotein fractions is beneficially altered by endurance training. This effect may be a key explanation for the lower CHD risk observed in physically active persons.

Hypertension. It is estimated that 20 to 30 million persons in the United States have high blood pressure (systolic and diastolic values that exceed 140/90 mmHg at rest) (Ward, 1980). Persons suffering from hypertension face an increased risk for several health problems including stroke, heart failure, renal failure, vascular lesions, and myocardial infarction (Folkow & Neil, 1971). The mechanism by which hypertension contributes to development of atherosclerotic plaque is not thoroughly understood. Hypertension may injure the intimal layer of the vessel and lead to migration of smooth muscle cells from the medial layer of the intima. It is known that proliferation of smooth muscle cells in the intima is a key step in the atherogenic process.

Epidemiological studies have observed that active persons tend to have lower levels of systolic and diastolic pressure (Cooper et al., 1976; Paffenbarger et al., 1978). Their results indicate that the heavier the individual for a given height, the greater the likelihood for becoming hypertensive. Furthermore, the more hours per week given to physical activity, the lower the incidence of hypertension. However, it is nonetheless clear that some highly fit individuals do develop hypertension (Blair et al., 1984).

Endurance exercise training has been recommended as therapy for hypertension (Tipton, 1984; Haskell, 1984a). Endurance training studies utilizing normotensive subjects have typically found no effect on resting blood pressure, or slight decreases in persons whose initial pressures are at the upper end of the normal range (greater than 125/85 mm Hg) (Tipton, 1984). In borderline hypertensives (pressures between 140/90 mmHg and 155/100 mmHg), there appears to be a reasonable chance that resting blood pressure will be decreased by an endurance training program (Tipton, 1984). However, endurance training studies utilizing fully hypertensive patients demonstrate that it is unlikely that blood pressure will be normalized without pharmacological therapy (Tipton, 1984).

Obesity. Obesity has been implicated as a risk factor in the development of cardiovascular disease (Kannel & Gordon, 1979; Bray, 1984). Although obesity is not considered a primary CHD risk factor, data collected in the Framingham Heart Study indicate that maintaining optimal body weight decreases CHD risk by 35 percent.

In recent years endurance exercise training has become accepted as an important component of obesity prevention and treatment regimens (Wilson, 1984). Physical activity is an important component of weight control programs because of its impact on the body's metabolic rate. Endurance training increases overall caloric expenditure, minimizes the amount of lean tissue loss, and may increase resting metabolic rate (Scheuer & Tipton, 1977; Apflebaum, Bostsarron, & Lacatis, 1971). An important reason for including exercise in weight loss programs is that caloric restriction diets can reduce resting metabolic rate (Wooley, Wooley, & Dyrenforth, 1979). This reduction may be offset by repeated bouts of exercise.

Improved Myocardial Oxygen Supply

It has been hypothesized that endurance exercise training may reduce risk of heart attack by improving the supply of oxygen to the myocardium. This could occur through increased development of collateral coronary blood vessels. Some support for this possibility has come from studies of animals (Eckstein, 1957; Stevenson, Feleki, Rechnitzer, & Beaton, 1964). However, studies on human beings, using coronary arteriography, have failed to provide comparable evidence (Ferguson, Petitclerc, Choquette, Chaniotis, Gauthier, Hout, Allard, Jankowski, & Campean, 1974). Likewise, studies of coronary blood flow in cardiac patients following endurance training do not support this notion (Ferguson, Cote, Gautheir, & Bourassa, 1978). Scheuer (1982) has reviewed this topic and concludes that there may, in fact, be an increased coronary collateral growth in response to endurance training in animals, but that the data in human beings is equivocal. Studies on human beings are limited in that the methods used to measure coronary blood flow may not be sufficiently sensitive. Also, appropriate training programs may not have been used. Nonetheless, it is very possible that training in human beings does not induce changes in coronary vasculature.

Reduced Myocardial Oxygen Demand

Direct measurement of myocardial oxygen consumption requires invasive and technically difficult procedures (Froelicher, 1983). However, myocardial oxygen consumption can be approximated from the "double product" (heart rate × systolic blood pressure) (Amsterdam et al., 1977). As noted previously, resting heart rate is reduced with endurance training and this probably indicates a lower oxygen demand by the myocardium. In addition, both heart rate and blood pressure typically are reduced during submaximal workloads following endurance training and this leads to reduced oxygen demand by the heart during submaximal exercise. Angina pectoris results from an imbalance between myocardial oxygen supply and demand and is usually associated with coronary atherosclerosis (Amsterdam et al., 1977). Endurance training increases the exercise intensity necessary to elicit angina (i.e., "anginal threshold") (Ehsani, Heath, Hagberg, Sobel, & Holloszy, 1981) and this is generally taken as an indication of decreased myocardial oxygen demand. This effect of training is not fully understood but it is probably related primarily to reduced heart rate at rest and during standard, submaximal exercise. As noted previously, this training-induced bradycardia may be due to cardiac hypertrophy, increased myocardial contractility and/or increased blood volume (Haskell, 1984a).

Endurance Training in the Elderly

Functional Changes and Aging

Aging of the cardiovascular system involves an increased deposition of connective tissue, with loss of the elastic properties of the walls of both the heart and arteries (Gerstenblith, Lakatta, & Weisfeldt, 1976). Associated with these changes are increases in total peripheral resistance and systolic and diastolic blood pressures. The result is a greater demand for work by the myocardium (Granath, Johnsson, & Strandell, 1964). This increased work load can result in an enlargment of the heart without a concommitant adaptation in the vascular bed (Roskamm, 1967).

Resting heart rate either decreases slightly or stays the same as aging proceeds (Landin, Linnemeier, Rothbaum, Chappelear, & Noble, 1985; Jose & Collison, 1970). However, resting cardiac output decreases steadily with advancing age (Brandfonbrener, Landowne, & Shock, 1955). The primary reason for this decrease in cardiac output is reduced stroke volume (Kennedy & Caird, 1981; Astrand, 1968). The mechanism of this age-related loss of stroke volume is not clear, but it may be related to a diminished contractile state of the heart, increased peripheral resistance, and/or loss of vessel elasticity (Kennedy & Caird, 1981).

With aging the cardiovascular system loses some of its ability to adjust to exercise. During submaximal exercise, the heart rate may be similar to that in younger adults, but stroke volume and cardiac output are reduced (Astrand, 1960; Niinimaa & Shepherd, 1978). Systolic and diastolic pressures are increased in response to exercise, but tend to be higher with older persons (Astrand, 1968; Granath et al., 1964). Total peripheral resistance is higher at the beginning of exercise in older adults, but the decrease in TPR observed with acute execise is similar as that seen in younger adults (Julius, Amery, Whitlock, & Conway, 1967). During maximal exercise heart rate, stroke volume, and cardiac output are lower in the older adult (Amery, Julius, Whitlock, & Conway, 1967; Astrand, 1968). Systolic and diastolic blood pressure during maximal exercise are similar in older adults when compared to young adults, but the rate of rise in systolic blood pressure during graded exercise is higher in the older persons (Julius et al., 1967).

Endurance Training and Aging

Several excellent reviews of the literature on aging and exercise have been published (Skinner, Tipton, & Vailus, 1982; Landin et al., 1985; Shepherd, 1981; Sidney, 1981). (For a comprehensive review of the interaction between aging and physical activity see Chapter 5 of this volume by W. Spirduso). Improvements in cardiovascular function can occur with endurance training in older persons (Sidney, 1981). However, the number of research studies focusing on this age group are not as numerous as for young groups, and the available data are at times conflicting and difficult to interpret. A common adaptation to training in young adults is a reduction in resting heart rate; however, this is not always the case in older persons. Resting heart rate may not be changed (Buccola & Stone, 1975; Emes, 1979) and only in some cases is there a slight increase in stroke volume (Skinner et al., 1982). As in young adults, no changes in resting systolic and diastolic blood pressures are seen in older persons who are normotensive (Skinner et al., 1982). While reduction in blood pressure is more likely in persons with elevated blood pressure, there remains much uncertainty about the effect of enduance training on blood pressure in elderly persons (Sidney, 1981).

Cardiac function in the older adult is improved during submaximal and maximal exercise following endurance training. Prolonged training has been shown to reduce heart rate (Niinimaa & Shepherd, 1978) and to increase stroke volume (Skinner, 1970) during performance of submaximal exercise. Systolic pressure has been reported to decrease or remain the same during submaximal exercise following endurance training (Sidney, 1981; Skinner et al., 1982). As would be expected from experience with younger persons, maximal heart rate in older persons does not change with training (Sidney, 1981). However, maximal stroke volume and cardiac output do increase with prolonged endurance training programs (Adams & deVries, 1973; deVries, 1970).

Endurance training brings about increases in maximal aerobic power in the elderly. $\dot{V}O_2$max has been directly measured in relatively few studies of training adaptations in older persons. However, available data indicate that the rate of change in $\dot{V}O_2$max and the relative increase in this variable (10-15%) are similar to the adaptations seen in younger persons. The aforementioned cardiovascular adaptations are probably key factors in the increased maximal aerobic power that results from training in the elderly. Also, increased oxidative capacity of skeletal muscle has been observed with training in older persons (Suominen, Heikkinen, & Parkatti, 1977).

Endurance Training in Females

Gender Differences in Cardiorespiratory Function

In general, lower levels of cardiorespiratory endurance are observed in females than in comparably trained males (Sparling & Cureton, 1983). This gender difference in CRE has been explained primarily on the basis of male-female differences in $\dot{V}O_2$ max. Available evidence indicates that gender differences in work efficiency and anaerobic threshold (expressed relative to $\dot{V}O_2$max) are not marked and, thus, probably do not explain much of the inter-gender variance in CRE (Pate & Kriska, 1984).

The gender difference in $\dot{V}O_2$ max (expressed relative to body weight) can be explained largely by inter-gender differences in body composition and in several basic cardiorespiratory variables (Wells & Plowman, 1983). In general, females manifest higher percentages of body fat than males and therefore must generate a greater rate of energy expenditure relative to the mass of active muscle tissue. Also, females tend to manifest lower blood hemoglobin concentrations and smaller hearts than males (Pate & Kriska, 1984). Thus, in general, peak rates of systemic oxygen tranportation are lower in females than males.

Adaptations to Endurance Training

Available evidence indicates that females and males adapt to endurance training in similar ways. Training studies using previously sedentary female subjects have reported significant increases in maximal aerobic power, maximal stroke volume and maximal cardiac output (Kilbom, 1971; Cunningham & Hill, 1975). As is the case in males, the effect of training on maximal arteriovenous oxygen difference in females is somewhat controversial. It has been suggested that AVD max may increase only with relatively long term training regimens (Wells, 1985). The magnitudes of the training adaptations in females apparently are comparable to those observed in males, as long as the changes are expressed as percentages of the initial values. Because females often manifest initially lower values for functional variables such as $\dot{V}O_2$ max, absolute changes with training may be less in females than males. Direct comparisons of training adaptations in females and males are rare and, therefore, final conclusions about the gender differences in the time course and magnitude of training adaptations must await additional research.

Endurance Training in Children

Cardiorespiratory Responses to Exercise in Children

Cardiorespiratory responses to acute endurance exercise in children are qualitatively similar to those observed in adults. However, the developmental process is accompanied by functionally important changes in the magnitudes of the responses to acute exercise. For example, in comparing the responses of adults and children to performance of a standard absolute exercise workload, children show lower cardiac output, higher arteriovenous oxygen difference, lower stroke volume and higher heart rate (Bar-Or, 1983). At maximal exercise children manifest higher heart rates, but lower stroke volumes and cardiac outputs (Eriksson & Koch, 1973a).

The metabolic responses of children to acute submaximal and maximal exercise have been studied extensively. During submaximal work performed against an external resistance (e.g., bicycle ergometer) children attained rates of oxygen consumption that were similar to those seen in adults (Shephard, Allen & Bar-Or, 1969). However, during exercise that involves movement of the whole body (e.g., walking or running at a specified speed) weight-relative $\dot{V}O_2$ is higher in children than adults (Astrand, 1952). Thus, in activities like running, children are considered to be less "efficient" than adults.

In response to maximal exertion, children demonstrated lower absolute rates of oxygen consumption than adults (BAR-Or, 1983). This lower $\dot{V}O_2$ max ($1 \cdot min^{-1}$) dictates that the child's absolute maximal rate of work output, as might be observed with bicycle ergometer exercise, is lower than that of the adult. However, weight-relative $\dot{V}O_2$ max is typically observed to be as high in children as in young adults (Pate & Blair, 1978). Mean values for maximal aerobic power ($\dot{V}O_2$ max, $ML \cdot KG^{-1} \cdot MIN^{-1}$) in the range of 45-55 have been frequently reported for young males. Somewhat lower values have been observed in young females (Bar-Or, 1983). Despite their relatively high weight-relative $\dot{V}O_2$ max, children do not perform as well as adults in tasks such as distance running. This performance decrement is probably explained by the child's lower running efficiency (i.e., higher oxygen cost of activity).

Adaptations to Endurance Training in Children

The effects of endurance training on maximal aerobic power in children have not been fully elucidated. Several studies have observed increases in $\dot{V}O_2$max with endurance training (Ekblom, 1969b; Eriksson, 1972) while others have reported no change in this variable (Daniels & Oldridge, 1971; Stweart & Gutin, 1976). Two factors seem to discriminate between these two groups of studies: (a) initial fitness level of the subjects, and (b) length and severity of the training program. Available evidence suggests that significant increases in maximal aerobic power can be expected only in children who are relatively unfit and/or those who are exposed to quite heavy and prolonged training regimens (Pate & Blair, 1978).

Training-induced increases in maximal aerobic power are accompanied by physiological adaptations that are similar to those seen in adults. Heart volume, stroke volume, maximal cardiac output, blood volume and total hemoglobin have been reported to increase with training in children, particularly those that are postpubertal (Eriksson & Koch, 1973b). In contrast to observations made with adults, arteriovenous oxygen difference has not been observed to change with training in children (Bar-Or, 1983). As is the case in adults, endurance training induces skeletal muscle adaptations in children. Oxidative enzyme activities and muscle glycogen stores increase (Eriksson, Gollnick, & Saltin, 1974).

Summary

Cardiorespiratory endurance usually can be improved in initially inactive participants with training programs that employ aerobic activity, three or more sessions per week, for at least 20 minutes per session, at an intensity corresponding to at least 50-60% of maximal aerobic power. Skeletal muscle tissue adapts to endurance training by increasing oxidative capacity through increased activity of the enzymes of aerobic metabolism, increased number of mitochondria, increased storage of glycogen and triglycerides, increased utilization of fat as an energy providing substrate and increased capillary density.

In response to endurance training, the stroke volume of the heart is increased. This increase is associated with decreased heart rate during rest and submaximal exercise and with increased maximal cardiac output.

Total blood volume, plasma volume, red cell mass and total hemoglobin increase with endurance training.

Endurance training results in increased power output at maximal exertion. This increase is due primarily to increased maximal aerobic power ($\dot{V}O_2$ max) which is, in turn, secondary to increases in maximal cardiac output and maximal arteriovenous oxygen difference.

Tolerance for sustained, submaximal exercise is improved with training. This improvement results from increases in anaerobic threshold and, in some cases, increased work efficiency.

Endurance training tends to reduce the risk for premature development of the atherosclerotic diseases such as coronary heart disease. This effect may be due to improved blood lipid profile, decreased blood pressure in persons with borderline hypertension, decreased percentage of body fat and a decreased myocardial oxygen demand.

Cardiorespiratory endurance tends to decrease with aging in adults. However, endurance training can improve functional capacity and associated cardiorespiratory variables in the elderly.

Due to their greater body fatness, lower blood hemoglobin concentration, and smaller heart, females, as a group, manifest lower cardiorespiratory endurance than males. Training causes a percentage increase in maximal aerobic power in females that is comparable to that seen in males.

Children have a lower tolerance for endurance exercise than young adults. This difference is due to the child's lower absolute maximal aerobic power ($1 \cdot min^{-1}$) and lower efficiency in activities like walking and running. Children are physiologically responsive to endurance training if the program is sufficiently demanding and prolonged.

References

Adams, G.M. & de Vries, H.A. (1973). Physiological effects of an exercise training regimen upon women aged 52-79. *Journal of Gerontology, 28,* 50-55.

Adner, M.M., & Castili, W.P. (1980). Elevated high-density lipo-protein levels in marathon runners. *The Journal of the American Medical Association. 242,* 534-536.

American College of Sports Medicine (1978). The recommended quantity and quality of exercise for developing and maintaining fitness in healthy adults. *Medicine and Science in sports, 10*(3), vii-x.

American Heart Association (1985). *Heartfacts.* Dallas, TX.

Amery, A., Julius, S., Whitlock, L.S., & Conway, J. (1967). Influence of hypertension on the hemodynamic response to exercise. *Circulation, 36,* 231-237.

Amsterdam, E.A., Price, J.E., Berman, D., Hughes, J.L., Riggs, K., DeMaria, A.N., Miller, R.R., & Mason, D.T. (1977). Exercise testing in the indirect assessment of myocardial oxygen consumption: Application for evaluation of mechansims and therapy of angina pectoris. In E.A. Amsterdam, J.H. Wilmore & A.N.

DeMaria (Eds.), *Exercise in cardiovascular health and disease* (pp. 218-233). New York: Yorke Medical Books.

Andersen, P. (1975). Capillary density in skeletal muscle of man. *Acta Physiologica Scandinavica, 95,* 203-205.

Apflebaum, M., Bostsarron, J., & Sactia, D. (1971). Effect of caloric restriction and excessive caloric intake on energy expenditure. *American Journal of Clinical Nutrition, 24,* 1405-1409.

Astrand, I. (1960). Aerobic work capacity in men and women with special preference to age. *Acta Physiologica Scandinavia, 49,* (Supp. 169), 1-92.

Astrand, P.O. (1952). *Experimental studies of physical working capacity in relation to sex and age.* Copenhagen: Munksgaard.

Astrand, P.O. (1968). Physical performance as a function of age. *Journal of the American Medical Association, 205,* 729-733.

Bachman, J., & Horvath, S. (1968). Pulmonary function changes which accompany athletic conditioning programs. *Research Quarterly, 39,* 235-239.

Barnard, R.J. (1975). Long-term effects of exercise on cardiac function. In J.H. Wilmore & J.F. Keogh (Eds.), *Exercise and Sport Sciences Reviews: Vol. 3* (pp. 113-133). New York: Academic Press.

Barnard, R.J., Duncan, H.W., Baldwin, K.M., Grimditch, G., & Buckberg, G.D. (1980). Effects of intensive exercise training on myocardial performance and coronary blood flow. *Journal of Applied Physiology, 49,* 444-449.

Bar-Or, O. (1983). *Pediatric sports medicine for the practitioner,* (pps. 1-65). New York: Springer-Verlag.

Blair, S.N., Goodyear, N.N., Gibbons, L.W., & Cooper, K.H. (1984). Physical fitness and incidence of hypertension in healthy normotensive men and women. *Journal of the American Medical Association, 252,* 487-490.

Brandfonbrener, M., Landowne, M., & Shock, N.W. (1955). Changes in cardiac output with age. *Circulation, 12,* 557-566.

Bray, G.A. (1984). The role of weight control in health promotion and disease prevention. In. J.D. Matarazzo, Sh.M. Weiss, J.A. Herd, N.E. Miller, & St. M.Weiss (Eds.), *Behavioral Health: Handbook of Health Enhancement and Disease Prevention* (pp. 632-656). New York: John Wiley and Sons.

Brownell, K.D., Bachorik, P.S., & Ayerle, R.S. (1982). Changes in plasma lipid and lipoprotein levels in men and women after a program of moderate exercise. *Circulation, 65,* 477-484.

Buccola, V.A., & Stone, W.J. (1975). Effects of jogging and cycling program on physiologicaly and psychological variables in aged men. *Research Quarterly, 46,* 134-139.

Choquette, G., & Ferguson, R.J. (1973). Blood pressure reduction in borderline hypertensives following physical training. *Canadian Medical Association Journal, 108,* 699-703.

Clausen, J.P. (1977). Effect of physical training on cardiovascular adjustments to exercise in man. *Physiological Reviews, 57,* 779-815.

Clausen, J.P., Klausen, K., Rasmussen, B., & Trap-Jensen, J. (1973). Central and peripheral circulatory changes after training of the arms or legs. *American Journal of Physiology, 225,* 675-682.

Cooper, K.A., Pollock, M.L., Martin, R.P., White, S.R., Linnerud, A.C., & Jackson, A. (1976). Physical fitness levels vs. selected coronary risk factors. A Cross Sectional Study. *Journal of the American Medical Association, 236,* 166-169.

Costas, R., Jr., Carcia-Palmieri, M.N., Nazario, E., & Sorlie, P.D. (1978). Relation of lipids, weight and physical activity to incidence of heart diesease: A Puerto Rico heart study. *American Journal of Cardiology, 42,* 653-658.

Costill, D., Thomason, H., & Roberts, E. (1973). Fractional utilization of the aerobic capacity during distance running. *Medicine and Science in Sports, 5,* 248-252.

Cousineau, D., Ferguson, R.J., de Champlain, J., Gauthier, P.C., & Bourassu M. (1977). Catecholamines in coronary sinus during exercise in an before and after training. *Journal of Applied Physiology, 43*, 801-806

Cunningham, D.A., & Hall, J.S. (1975). Effect of training on cardiovascular response to exercise in women. *Journal of Applied Physiology, 39*, 891-895.

Daniels, J. & Oldridge, N. (1971). Changes in oxygen consumption of young boys during growth and running training. *Medicine and Science in sports, 3*, 161-165.

Davis, J.A., Frank., M.H., Shipp, B.J., & Wasserman, K. (1979). Anaerobic threshold alterations caused by endurance training in middle-aged men. *Journal of Applied Physiology, 46*, 1039-1046.

deVries, H.A. (1970). Physiological effects of an exercise training regimen upon men aged 52-88. *Journal of Gerontology, 25*, 325-336.

Dowell, R.T. (1983). Cardiac adaptations to exercise. In R.J. Terjung (Ed.), *Exercise and Sport Science Reviews, Vol. II* (pp. 99-117). Franklin Institutute.

Durstine, J.L., Smith, P.E., Dover, E.V., Fronsoe, M.S., Manno, E.M., Goodyear, L.J., Lambert, M.I., & Pate, R.R. (1984). Women, exercise and changes in high-density lipoprotein subfractions (HDL_2 and HDL_3) and other plasma lipids. *Medicine and Science in Sports and Exercise, 16*, 202-203.

Eckstein, R.W. (1957). Effect of exercise on coronary artery narrowing and coronary collateral circulation. *Circulation Research, 5*, 230-235.

Ehsani, A., Heath, G., Hagberg, J., Sobel, B., & Holloszy, J. (1981). Effects of 12 months of intense exercise training on ischemic ST-segment depression in patients with coronary artery disease. *Circulation, 64*, 1116-1124.

Ekblom, B. (1969a). Effect of physical training on oxygen transport system in man. *Acta Physiologica Scandinavia* (suppl. 328), 1-45.

Ekblom, B. (1969b). Effect of physical training in adolescent boys. *Journal of Applied Physiology, 27*, 350-355.

Ekblom, B., Astrand, P., Saltin, B., Stenberg, J., & Wallstrom, B. (1968). Effect of training on circulatory response to exercise. *Journal of Applied Physiology, 24*, 518-528.

Emes, C.G. (1979). The effects of a regular program of light exercise on seniors. *Journal of Sports Medicine, 19*, 185-190.

Enger, S.C., Herbjornsen, K., Krikssen, J., & Fretland, A. (1977). High-density lipoprotein (HDL) and physical activity: The influence of physical exercise, age, and smoking on HDL-cholesterol and HDL-total cholesterol ratio. *Scandinavian Journal of Clinical and Laboratory Investigation, 37*, 251-255.

Eriksson, B.O. (1972). Physical training, oxygen supply and muscle metabolism in 11-13 year old boys. *Acta Physiologica Scandinavica Supplementation, 384.*

Eriksson, B.O., Gollnick, P.D., & Saltin, B. (1973). Muscle metabolism and enzyme activities after training in boys 11 to 13 years old. *Acta Physiologica Scandinavica, 87*, 485-487.

Eriksson, B.O. & Koch, G. (1973a). Cardiac output and intra-arterial blood pressure at rest and during submaximal and maximal exercise in 11 to 13 year old boys before and after physical training. In O. Bar-Or (Ed.), *Pediatric work physiology* (pps. 139-150). Natanya: Wingate Institute.

Eriksson, B.O. & Koch, G. (1973b). Effect of physical training on hemodynamic response during submaximal and maximal exercisein 11-13 year old bosy. *Acta Physiologica Scandinavica, 87*, 27-39.

Farrell, P.A., Maksud, M.G., Pollock, M.L., Foster, C., & Anholm, J. (1982) A comparison of plasma cholesterol, triglycerides and high density lipoprotein-cholesterol in speed skaters, weight lifters and non-athletes. *European Journal of Applied Physiology and Occupational Physiology, 48*, 77-82.

Ferguson, R.J., Cote, P., Gauthier, P., & Bourassa, M.G.)1978). Changes in exercise coronary sinus blood flow with training in patients with angina pectoris, *Circulation, 58*, 41-47.

Ferguson, R.J., Petitclerc, R., Choquette, G., Chaniotis, P., Gauthier, R., Huot, R., Allard, C., Jankowski, L., & Champeau, L. (1974). Effect of exercise capacity collateral circulation and progression of coronary disease. *American Journal of Cardiology, 34,* 769.

Falkow, B. & Neil, E. (1971). *Circulation* (pp. 1-19, 560-568). London: Oxford.

Froelicher, V.F. (1938). *Exercise testing and training.* Chicago: Yearbook Medical Publishers.

Gerstenblith, G., Lakatta, E.G., & Weisfeldt, M.L. (1976). Age changes in myocardial function and exercise response. *Progress in Cardiovascular Disease, 19,* 1-21.

Gettman, L.R., Ayres, J.J., Pollock, M.L., & Jackson, A. (1978). The effect of circuit weight training on strength, cardiorespiratory function and body composition of adult men. *Medicine and Science in Sports, 10,* 171-176.

Gettman, L.R., Pollock, M.L., Durstine, J.L., Ward, A., Ayres, J., & Linnerud, A.C. (1976). Physiological responses of men to 1, 3 and 5 day per week training programs. *Research Quarterly, 47,* 638-646.

Gleser, M.A. (1973). Effects of hypoxia and physical training on hemodynamic adujustments to one-legged exercise. *Journal of Applied Physiology, 34,* 655-659.

Gollnick, P., Armstrong, R., Saltin, B., Saubert, C., Sembrowich, W., & Shepherd, R. (1973). Effect of training on enzyme activity and fiber composition of human skeletal muscle. *Journal of Applied Physiology, 34,* 107-111.

Gollnick, P., Armstrong, R., Saubert, C., Piehl, K., & Saltin, B. (1972). Enzyme activity and fiber composition of untrained and trained men. *Journal of Applied Phsyiology, 33,* 312-319.

Gollnick, P. & King, D. (1969). Effects of exercise and training on mitochrondria of rat skeletal muscle. *American Journal of Physiology, 216,* 1502-1509.

Granath, A., Johnson, B. & Strandell, T. (1964). Circulation in healthy old men studied by right heart catheterization at rest and during exercise in supine and sitting position. *Acta Medica Scandinavica, 176,* 425-446.

Hartley, L.H., Grimby, G., Kilborn, A., Nilsson, N.J., Astrand, I., Bjure, J., Ekblom, B., & Saltin, B. (1969). Physical training in sedentary middle age and older men III. Cardiac output and gas exchange at submaximal and maximal exercise. *Scandinavian Journal of Clinical and Laboratory Investigation, 24,* 335-344.

Haskell, W.L. (1984a). Overview: Health benefits of exercise. In J.D. Matarazzo, Sh.M. Weiss, J.A. Herd, N.E. Miller, & St.M. Weiss (Eds.), *Behavioral Health: A Handbook of Health Enhancement and Disease Prevention* (pp. 409-423). New York: John Wiley and Sons.

Haskell, W.L. (1984b). The influence of exercise on the concentrations of triglyceride and cholesterol in human plasma. In R.J. Terjung (Ed.), *Exercise and Sport Sciences Reviews: Vol. 12* (pp. 205-244). Lexington, MA: D.C. Heath.

Hermansen, L. & Wachtlova, M. (1971). Capillary density of skeletal muscle in well-trained and untrained men. *Journal of Applied Physiology, 30,* 860-863.

Holloszy, J.O. (1973). Biochemical adaptations to exercise: aerobic metabolism, In: J.H. Wilmore (Eds.), *Exercise and Sport Sciences Reviews, Vol. 1* (pp. 46-71). New York: Academic Press.

Holloszy, J.O. & Booth, F.W. (1976). Biochemical adaptations to endurance exercise in muscle. *Annual Reviews of Physiology, 38,* 273-291.

Hoppeler, H., Luthi, P., Claassen, H., Weibel, E.R., & Howard, H. (1973). The ultrastructure of the normal human skeletal muscle: A norphometric analysis on untrained men, women and well-trained orientees. *Pflugers Archives, 344,* 217-232.

Howard, H. (1975). Ultrastructural adaptation of skeletal muscle to prolonged physical exercise. In H. Howard & J.R. Poortmans (Eds.), *Metabolic adaptation to Prolonged Physical Exercise* (pp. 372-383). Basel: Birkhauser Verlag.

Huttunen, J.K., Lansimies, E., Voutilainen, E. Ehnholm, C., Hietanen, E. Rentilla,

Siitonen, O., & Rauvamaa, R. (1979). Effect of moderate physical exercise on serum lipoproteins. *Circulation, 60,* 1220-1229.

Jose, A.D. & Collision, D.L. (1970). The normal range and determinants of the intrinsic heart rate in man. *Cardiovascular Research, 4,* 160-167.

Julius, S., Amery, A., Whitlock, A.S., & Conway, J. (1967). Influence of age on the hemodynamic response to exericse. *Circulation, 36,* 222-230.

Kanakis, C. & Hickson, R.C. (1980). Left ventricular responses to a program of lower limb strength training. *Chest, 78,* 618-621.

Kannell, W.B., Castelli, W.P. & Gordon, T. (1979). Cholesterol in the prediction of atherosclerotic disease. *Annals of Internal Medicine, 90,* 85-91.

Kannel, W.B. & Gordon, T. (1979). Physiological and medical concomitants of obesity: The Framingham Study. In G.A. Bray (Ed.), *Obesity in America* (DHEW Publication No. (NIH) 79-359). Washington, DC: US Government Printing Office.

Karvonen, M., Kentala, K., & Mustala, O. (1957). The effects of training heart rate: A longitudinal study. *Annals of Medicine and Experimental Biology Tenn., 35,* 307-315.

Kennedy, R.D. & Caird, F.I. (1981). Physiology of aging of the heart. In R.J. Noble & D.A. Rothbaum (Eds.), *Geriatric Cardiology* (pp. 1-8). Philadelphia: F.A. Davis.

Kiens, B., Jorgenson, I., Lewis, S., Jensen, G., Lithell, H., Vessby, B. Hoe, S., & Schnoher, P. (1980). Increased plasma HDL-cholesterol and apo A-1 in sedentary middle-aged men after physical conditioning. *Scandinavian Journal of Clincial and Laboratory Investigation, 10,* 203-209.

Kilbom, A. (1971). Physical training in women. *Scandinavian Journal of Clincial and Laboratory Investigation, 28* (Suppl. 119), 7-34.

Kilbom, A. & Astrand, I. (1971). Physical training with submaximal intensities in women II. Effect on cardiac output. *Scandinavian Journal of Clincial and Laboratory Investigation, 28,* 163-175.

Kilbom, A., Hartley, L.H., Stin, B., Hore, J.B., Grimby, G., & Astrand, I. (1969). Physical training in sedentary middle-aged older men. *Scandinavian Journal of Clinical and Laboratory Investigation, 24,* 315-322.

Landin, R.J., Linnemeier, T.J., Rothbaum, D.A., Chappelear, J., & Noble, R.J. (1985). Exercise testing and training of the elderly patient. In N.K. Wenger & A.N. Buest (Eds.), *Exercise and the heart* (2nd ed.) (pp. 201-218). Philadelphia: F.A. Davis.

Lehtonen, A. & Viikari, J. (1978). Serum triglycerides and cholesterol and serum high density lipoproten cholesterol in highly physically active men. *Acta Medica Scandinavia, 204,* 111-114.

Martin, B.J., Sparks, K.E., Zwillich, V.W., & Weil, J.V. (1979). Low exercise ventilation in endurance athletes. *Medicine and Science in Sports, 11,* 181-185.

Martin, R.P., Haskell, W.L., & Wood, P.D. (1977). Blood chemistry and lipid profiles of elite distance runners. In P. Milvy (Ed.) *Annals of New York Academy of Science Vol. 301.* The marathon: Physiological, medical, epidemiological and psychological studies. New York: New York Academy of Science.

McKenzie, D.C., Fox, E.L., & Cohen, K. (1978). Specificity of metaboic and circulatory responses to arm or leg interval training. *European Journal of Applied Physiology, 39,* 241-248.

McMillan, G.C. (1978). Atherogenesis: The process from normal to lesion. In A.B. Chandler, K. Euvenius, G.C. McMillan, C.B. Nelson, C.J. Schwartz & S. Wessler (Eds.), *The Thrombotic Process in Atherogenesis* (pp 3-10). New York: Plenum.

Milesis, C.A., Pollock, M.L., Bah, M.D., Ayres, J.J., Ward. A, & Linnerud, A.C. (1976). Effects of different durations of training on cardiorespiratory function. Body composition and serum lipids. *Research Quarterly, 47,* 716-725.

Miller, G.J. & Miller, N.E. (1975). Plasma high density lipoprotein concentration and development of ischemic heart disease. *Lancet, 1,* 16-19.

Mole, P., Oscai, L., & Holloszy, J. (1971). Adaptations of muscle to exercise. Increased in levels of palmityl CoA synthetase, carnitine palmitgltransferase and palmityl CoA dehydrogenases and in the capacity to oxidize fatty acid. *Journal of Clinical Investigation, 50,* 2323-2330.

Moody, D.L., Wilmore, J.H., Girandola, R.N., & Royce, J.P. (1972). The effects of a jogging program on the body composition of normal and obese high school girls. *Medicine and Science in Sports, 4,* 210-213.

Morganroth, J., Maron, B.J., Henry, W.L., & Epstein, S.E. (1975). Comparative left ventricular dimension in trained athletes. *Annals of Internal Medicine, 82,* 521-524.

Morris, J.N., Everitt, M.G., Pollard, R., Chave, S.P.W., & Semmence, A.M.W., (1980). Vigorous exercise in leisure-time: Protection against coronary artery disease. *Lancet, 2,* 1207-1210.

Niinimaa, V. & Shephard, R.J. (1978). Training and oxygen conductance in the elderly. I. The respiratory system. II. The cardiovascular system. *Journal of Gerontology, 33,* 354-367.

Nye, E.R., Carlson, K., Kirstein, P., & Rossner, S. (1981). Changes in high density lipoprotein subfractions and other lipoproteins induced by exercise. *Clinica Chimica Acta, 113,* 51-57.

Oscai, L.B., Williams, B.T., & Hertig, B.A. (1968). Effect of exercise on blood volume. *Journal of Applied Physiology, 24,* 622-624.

Paffenbarger, R.S., Jr., Wing, A.W., & Hyde, R.T. (1978). Physical activity as an index of heart attack risk in college alumni. *American Journal of Epidemiology, 108,* 161-175.

Pate, R.R. (1983). Sports anemia: A review of the current research literature. *The Physician and Sportsmedicine, 11(2),* 115-131.

Pate, R.R. & Blair, S.N. (1978). Exercise and the prevention of atherosclerosis: pediatric implications. In W.B. Strong (Ed.), *Atherosclerosis: Its Pediatric Aspects,* (pp. 287-300).

Pate, R.R. & Kriska, A. (1984). Physiological basis of the sex difference in cardiorespiratory endurance. *Sports Medicine, 1,* 87-98.

Peltonen, P., Marniemi, J., Hietanen, E., Vuori, I., & Ehnholm, C. (1981). Changes in serum lipids, lipoproteins and heparin releasable lipolytic enzymes during moderate physical training in men: A longitudinal study. *Metabolism Clinical and Experimental, 30,* 518-526.

Pollock, M.L. (1978). How much exercise is enough? *The Physician and Sportsmedicine, 6(6),* 50-64.

Pollock, M.L. (1973). The quantification of endurance training programs. In J.H. Wilmore (Ed.), *Exercise and Sport Sciences Reviews,* Vol. 1 (pp. 155-188). New York: Academic Press.

Pollock, M.L., Cureton, T.K., & Greninger, L. (1969). Effects of frequency of training on work capacity, cardiovascular function and body composition of adult men. *Medicine and Science in Sports, 1,* 70-74.

Pollock, M.L., Gettman, L.R., Milesis, C.A., Bah, M.D., Durstine, J.L., & Johnson, R.B. (1977). Effects of frequency and duration of training on attrition and incidence of injury. *Medicine and Science in Sports, 9,* 31-36.

Raven, P.B. (1977). Pulmonary function of elite distance runners. *Annals of the New York Academy of Sciences, 301,* 371-381.

Roman, O., Camuzzi, A.L., Villalon, E., & Klenner, C. (1981). Physical training program in arterial hypertension. A long term prospective follow-up. *Cardiology, 67,* 230-243.

Roskamm, H. (1967). Optimum patterns of exercise for healthy adults. In *Proceedings of the international symposium on physical and cardiovascular health. Canadian Medical Association Journal, 96,* 895-899.

Rowell, L.B. (1974). Human cardiovascular adjustments to exercise and stress.

Physiological Reviews, 54, 75-159.

Salonen, J.T., Puska, P., & Tuomilehto, J. (1982). Physical activity and risk of myocardial infarction, cerebral stroke and death. *American Journal of Epidemiology, 115,* 526-537.

Saltin, B. (1969). Physiological effects of physical conditioning. *Medicine and Science in Sports, 1,* 50-56.

Saltin, B., Blonquist, G., Mithcell, J.H., Johnson, R.L., Widenthal, K., & Chapman, C.B. (1968). Response to exercise after bedrest and after training. *Circulation, 38* (Supp. 7), 7.1-7.78.

Schaible, T.F. & Scheuer, J. (1979). Effects of physical training by running or swimming on ventricular performance of rats. *Journal of Applied Physiology, 40,* 854-860.

Scheuer, J. (1982). Effects of physical training on myocardial vascularity and perfusion. *Circulation, 66,* 491-495.

Scheuer, J., Penpargkul, S., & Bhan, A.K. (1974). Experimental observations on the effects of physical training upon intrinsic cardiac physiology and biochemistry [special issue]. *American Journal of Cardiology, 33,* 745-751.

Scheuer, J. & Tipton, C.M. (1977). Cardiovascular adaptations to physical training. *Annual Review of Physiology, 39,* 221-251.

Shephard, R.J. (1981). Cardiovascular limitations in the aged. In. E.L. Smith, & R.C. Serfass (Eds.), *Exercise and Aging: The Scientific Basis* (pp. 19-29). Hillside, NJ: Enslow.

Shephard, R.J., Allen, C. & Bar-Or, O. (1969). The working capacity of Toronto school children. *Canadian Medical Association Journal, 100,* 560-566.

Sidney, K.H. (1981). Cardiovascular benefits of physical activity in the exercising aged. In. E.L. Smith & R.C. Serfass (Eds.), *Exercise and Aging: The Scientific Basis* (pp. 131-147). Hillside, NJ: Enslow.

Skinner, J. (1970). The cardiovascular system with aging and exercise. In. D. Brunner & E. Jokl (Eds.), *Medicine and Sport: Vol. 4. Physical Activity and Aging* (pp. 100-108). Baltimore: University Park.

Skinner, J.S. & McLellan, T.H. (1980). The transition from aerobic to anaerobic metabolism. *Research Quarterly for Exercise and Sport, 51,* 234-248.

Skinner, J.S., Tipton, C.M. & Vailas, A.C. (1982). Exercise, physical training and the aging process. In A. Viidik (Ed.), *Lectures on Gerontolgy: Vol 1B* (pp. 407-439). London: Academic Press.

Sparling, P.B. & Cureton, K.J. (1983). Biological determinants of the sex difference in 12 min. run performance. *Medicine and Science in Sports and Exercise, 15,* 218-223.

Stein, R.A., Michielli, D., Diamond, J., Horwitz, B., & Krasnow, N.)1980). The cardiac response to exercise training: Echocardiographic analysis at rest and during exercise. *American Journal of Cardiology, 46,* 219-225.

Stevenson, J.A.S., Feleki, V., Rechnitzer, P., & Beaton, J.R. (1964). Effects of exercise on coronary tree size in the rat. *Circulation Research, 15,* 256-269.

Stewart, K.J. & Gutin, B. (1976). Effects of physical training on cardiorespiratory fitness in children. *Research Quarterly, 47,* 110-120.

Stromme, S.B., Ingjer, F., & Meen, H.D. (1977). Assessment of maximal aerobic power in specifically trained athletes. *Journal of Applied Physiology, 42,* 833-837.

Suominen, H., Heikkinen, E., & Parkatti, T. (1977). Effect of eight weeks' physical training on muscle and connective tissue of the m. vastus lateralis in 69-year-old men and women. *Journal of Gerontology, 32,* 33-37.

Sutton, J.R. & Jones, N.L. (1979). Control of pulmonary ventilation during exercise and mediators in the blood: CO_2 and hydrogen ion. *Medicine and Science in Sports, 11,* 198-203.

Tibbits, G.F., Barnard, R.J., Baldwin, K.M., Cugalj, N., & Roberts, N.K. (1981). Influence of exercise on excitation—contraction coupling in rat myocardium.

American Journal of Physiology, 240, H472-H480.

Tipton, C.M. (1984). Exercise training and hypertension. In. R.L. Terjung (Ed.), *Exercise and Sport Sciences Reviews: Vol. 12* (pp. 245-306). Lexington, MA: D.C. Heath.

Ward, G.W.(1980). An overview of the national high blood pressure educational program in the United States. In. Th. Phillips, & A. Distler (Eds.), *Hypertension Mechanisms and Management* (pp. 231-244). Berlin: Springer-Verlag.

Wells, C.L. (1985). *Women, Sport and Performance: A Physiological Perspective.* Champaign, IL: Human Kinetics Publishers.

Wells, C.L. & Plowman, S.A. (1983). Sexual differences in athletic performance: biological or behavioral? *The Physician and Sportsmedicine, 11(8),* 52-63.

Williams, R.S., Logue, E.E., Lewis, J.L., Barton, T., Stead, N.W., Wallace, A.G., & Pizzo, S. V. (1980). Physical conditioning augments the fibrinolytic response to venus occlusion in health adults. *New England Journal of Medicine, 302,* 987-991.

Wilmore, J.H., Parr, B., Girandola, R.N., Ward, P., Vodak, P.A., Barstow, T.J., Pipes, T.V., Romero, G. T., & Leslie, P. (1978). Physiological alterations consequent to circuit weight training. *Medicine and Science in Sports, 10,* 79-84.

Wilson, T.G. (1984). Weight control treatments. In J.D. Matarazzo, S.M. Weiss, J.A. Herd, N.E. Miller, & St.M. Weiss (Eds.), *Behavioral Health: A Handbook of Health Enhancement and Disease Prevention* (pp. 409-423). New York: John Wiley and Sons.

Winder, W.W., Hagberg, J.M., Hickson, R.C., Ehsani, A.A., & McLane, J.A. (1978). Time course of sympathoadrenal adaptation to endurance exercise training in man. *Journal of Applied Physiology, 45,* 370-374.

Wolfe, L., Cunningham, D.A., Rechnitzer, P.A., & Nichol, M. (1979). Effects of endurance training on left ventricular dimensions in healthy men. *Journal of Applied Physiology, 47,* 207-211.

Wood, P.D., Haskell, W., Klein, H., Lewis, S., Stern, M.P., & Farquhar, J.W. (1976). The distribution of plasma lipoproteins in middle-aged male runners. *Metabolism Clinical and Experimental, 25,* 1249-1257.

Wooley, S.C., Wooley, O.W., & Dyrenforth, S.R. (1979). Theoretical, practical and social issues in behavioral treatments of obesity. *Journal of Applied Behavioral Analysis, 12,* 3-25.

Zeldis, S.M., Morganroth, J., & Rubler, S. (1978). Cardiac hypertrophy in response to dynamic conditioning in female athletes. *Journal of Applied Physiology, 44,* 849-852.

Section III

SOCIAL AND PSYCHOLOGICAL PERSPECTIVES

- Mental Health
- Social Development
- Moral Development

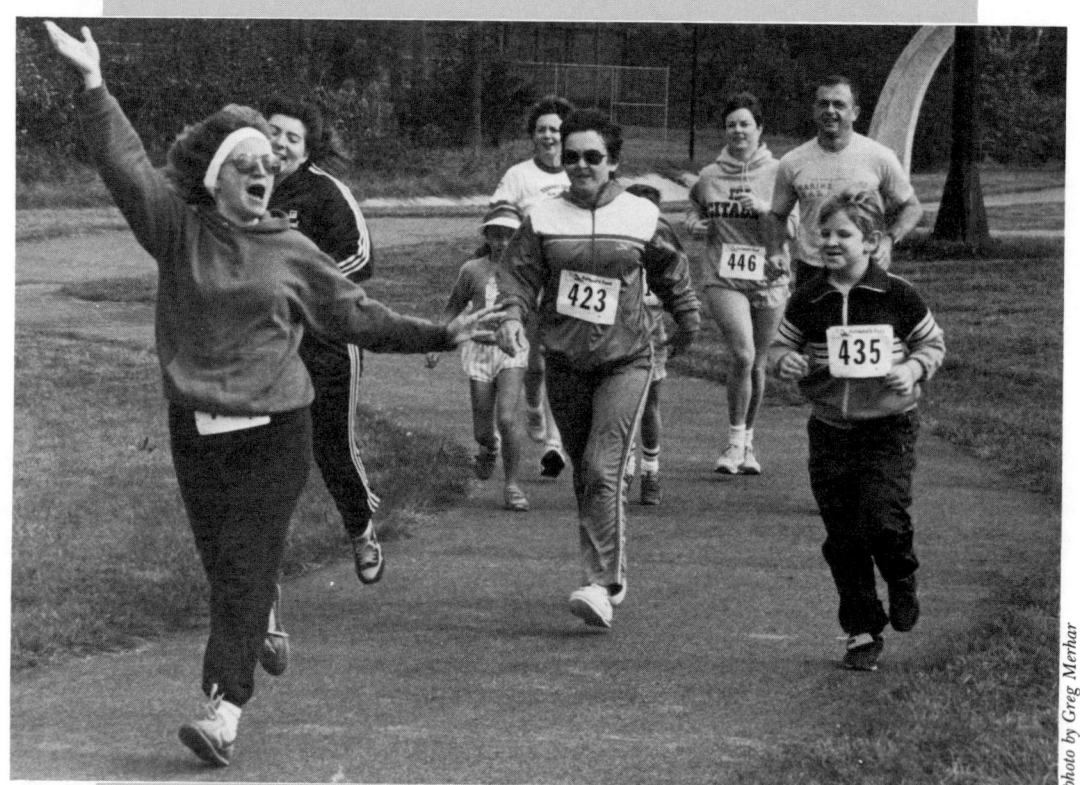

photo by Greg Merhar

CHAPTER ELEVEN

Mental Health

Rod K. Dishman
Department of Physical Education
The University of Georgia
Athens, Georgia

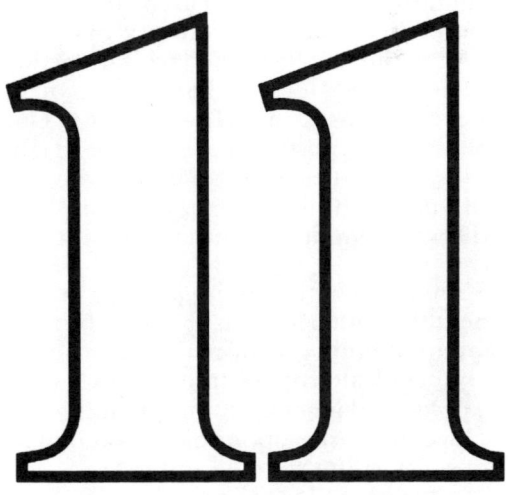

> *Avoid exercising either mind or body without the other, and thus preserve an equal and healthy balance between them.*
>
> **Plato, 427-347 B.C.**
> **Greek Philosopher**

> *The most beneficial of all types of exercise is physical gymnastics to the point that the soul becomes influenced and rejoices.*
>
> **Rabbi Moses Maimonides, 1135-1204**
> **Jewish Philosopher-Physician**

Mens Sana in Corpore Sano, a healthy mind in a healthy body, has been a common wisdom through most of recorded history; it is a philosophy long synonymous with physical activity. Hippocrates, hailed as the father of medicine, is known to have prescribed exercise for patients suffering from mental illness (Ryan, 1984). In recent times, though, advances in specific therapies by the fields of medicine and psychology promoted a more dualistic view of mental and physical health; the role of exercise diminished. Psychopathology refined diagnoses while psychopharmacology and neurobiology produced more effective drugs for prevalent disorders such as depression, anxiety, and schizophrenia. Professional services by clinical psychologists expanded with the development of behavior modification and psychotherapy. Only a small academic and professional interest in exercise for mental health was maintained, and this was largely seen only in physical education, therapeutic recreation, and psychosomatic medicine.

The situation has begun to change. Scientific studies of modern disease have reaffirmed many of the health philosophies of old: good nutrition, rest, and exercise (Matarazzo, Weiss, Herd, Miller, & Weiss, 1984). The result is a renaissance of physical activity as a mental health behavior. In the past seven years, scholarly reviews of research on the psychological effects of exercise have appeared in the literatures of psychiatry (Morgan, 1979), general psychology (Folkins & Sime, 1981), behavioral medicine (Morgan, 1982), sport psychology (Weinstein & Meyers, 1983), sports medicine (Morgan, 1985; Sonstroem, 1984), preventive medicine (Hughes, 1984; Goff & Dimsdale, 1985), health psychology (Sime, 1984), post-graduate medicine (Dishman, 1985), and public health (Taylor, Sallis, & Needles, 1985). These reviews confirm that physical activity is associated with mental health, but they also illustrate that much remains to be learned about who can benefit from what types of exercise under which circumstances—and why.

The goals of this chapter are to: (a) provide a rationale for viewing exercise as a mental health behavior; (b) describe the prevalence rates, symptomatologies, and apparent etiologies of major disorders for which exercise might be an effective adjunct or alternative intervention; (c) review and evaluate existing research on exercise and mental health; (d) outline proposed mechanisms or enabling circumstances that are responsible for mental health outcomes that accompany exercise; (e) contrast the benefits and risks of exercise with conventional treatments when possible; and (f) propose an agenda for future studies of exercise in mental health promotion and disease prevention that considers age, gender, and mental health status. The overall objective is to provide a representative view of what is scientifically known within a conceptual framework that can guide attempts to know more. Better theory can aid more effective professional services, public health promotion, and self-regulation by the individual.

A Rationale for Exercise

The renewed interest in physical activity by mental health professionals stems from several sources. First, academic curiosity among physical educators spawned the field of sport psychology. This curiosity helped maintain a slow but steady accumulation of scientific knowledge during the past 15 years. A recent history of sport psychology by Ryan (1981) attributes much of this mental health impetus to William P. Morgan of the University of Wisconsin.

Second, the popular trend toward self-help and away from dependence on health care professionals was paralleled in clinical psychology by the development of cognitive-behavior modification. The emphasis on *therapy* and an exclusive reliance on a service provider shifted to include *prevention* and self-regulation by the client to carry out, monitor, and reinforce adaptive plans. This added focus on coping skills and personal responsibility fostered health promotion; the past emphasis in behavior modification and psychotherapy had been illness reduction.

Third, it became empirically clear that lifestyle behaviors, moreso than human biology, the environment, or the health care system combined, account for years lived (from ages 1 to 65), and the quality of years lived. The Institute of Medicine of the National Academy of Sciences determined that much of the morbidity and mortality for modern day chronic disease and suffering is linked to behavior and stress (Hamburg, Elliot, & Parron, 1982). An understanding of how people appraise situations as stressful and how they cope with stress when it is experienced was recognized as a necessary aid to developing effective interventions for prevention and therapy. Exercise, and the settings where it takes place, has potential for changing the appraisal of stress and for coping when stress occurs. This potential prompted the National Institute of Mental Health to recently sponsor a workshop for leading researchers on exercise to examine its effectiveness for coping with mental stress (Morgan & Goldston, in press).

Fourth, the role of life style and mental stress in modern day health has fueled the growth of new fields such as behavioral medicine and health psychology. Their efforts to prevent illness and promote health include exercise as both an intervention and a research modality. In each instance, mental health is a key concern.

Fifth, despite successes, the prevalence of misdiagnosis, recidivism, and nonspecific or undesired effects for psychoanalysis, psychotherapy, and drugs has led psychiatry to reexplore adjunctive treatments like exercise for certain disorders. Also, because physical activity has been a strong predictor of other chronic diseases (Dishman, in press), the search for precursors of mental disorders by psychiatric epidemiology will likely include activity history in future studies.

The sixth and overriding reason for renewed interest in exercise for the prevention and treatment of mental disorders is the cost effectiveness of exercise, were it found to be therapeutically effective. The financial cost of mental illness in the United States has risen to 40 billion dollars annually during the past several years (Levine & Willmer, 1976; Schweiker, 1981) with direct annual costs of mental health services ranging from 14 to 20 billion dollars (Califano, 1978; Eisenberg & Parron, 1979; Hodgson & Kopstein, 1984; Levine & Willmer, 1976; Waldo & Gibson, 1982). This cost has been 8-15% of all national health costs and has amounted to 1 percent of the Gross National Product. Containment of medical costs remains a high priority for public health policy. Exercise could offer a low cost, seemingly low risk alternative or adjunct for reducing the fiscal cost of mental health problems.

The human costs of mental disorders and their total impact on healthful living are more difficult to gauge. Current rates are not available, but in 1975 mental disorders were the top cause of days spent in hospitals (260 million days or 30% of the total). They were the third leading cause of social security disability, the ninth reason for office visits to physicians, the ninth cause of activity restriction, and the tenth leading contributor to missed days of work (Eisenberg & Parron, 1979). It is believed that depression accounts for up to 60% of suicide, which in 1977 tied arteriosclerosis as the nation's 10th leading cause of death (Harris, 1981). Estimates suggest that as much as 50% of the complaints seen by primary care physicians have roots in anxiety and depression, and even among general surgery patients the primary or secondary diagnosis is often stress related (Kuyler & Dunner, 1976; Poe, Lowell, & Fox, 1966).

The stress emotions (e.g. anger, anxiety, depression) that characterize many mental disorders are also implicated in the etiology of several physical disorders that are prevalent health concerns. Cardiovascular diseases, which remain the leading cause (over 50%) of premature death in the United States, and their major risk factors (hypertension, cholesterolemia, obesity, and coronary-prone behavior) are linked to behavior in part through emotions and neuroendocrine stress. Convincing epidemiologic studies confirm that mental health influences physical health (Berkman & Syme, 1979; Vaillant, 1979). For these reasons, exercise could exert a positive physical health impact through mental means.

There is also a growing population of American elders who may benefit from low cost preventive medicine. An estimated 17 million Americans, aged 65 and over, live independently and are in moderately good health (Skinner & Vaughan, 1983). As Spirduso describes in chapter 5, the psychological and behavioral role of exercise in the health of the aged population is only beginning to be explored in a systematic way. However, the behaviors that influence mortality in the young and middle aged do not appear to be risk factors in the elderly (Branch & Jette, 1984). For this reason, the benefits of physical activity for older people may be equally important as a means for enhancing mental health and subjective well-being than for decreasing the known risk factors that impede physical health and longevity.

Prevalence of Mental Health Problems

It was estimated in 1979 that at some time in his or her life, one in four American adults suffers from moderate depression, anxiety, or symptoms of affective disorder (Califano, 1979). Within a year, 10% to 15% of the population were victims of mental disease (Califano, 1978). Anxiety and depression affected 10 to 15 million Americans annually (Harris, 1981). Among inpatient admissions to state and local mental hospitals, depressive illness ranked behind only schizophrenia and alcohol disorders as the most prevalent diagnosis (Meyer, 1977). These problems are often intertwined.

A recent population survey completed by the National Institute of Mental Health (Regier, Myers, Kramer, Robins, Blazer, Hough, Eaton, & Locke, 1984) confirmed a similar pattern. Detailed interview responses by about 10,000 representative Americans over 18 years of age were compared with criteria for mental disorders found in the Diagnostic and Statistical Manual of Mental Disorders (DSM-III) of the American Psychiatric Association. Results indicated that during a six-month span, 29 million adults, (20% of the adult population) experienced mental disturbance. Anxiety, including phobic, panic, and obsessive-compulsive disorders, were highest in incidence and affected 8.3% (13.1 million) of the adult population. Alcohol and substance abuse followed, affecting 6.4% (10 million), while depression ranked third, affecting 6% (9.4 million). Schizophrenia accounted for 1.5 million cases or 1% of the population over 18 (Myers, Weissman, Tischler, Holzer, Leaf, Orvaschel, Anthony, Boyd, Burke, Kramer, & Stoltzman, 1984). According to these rates, 29% to 38% of American adults can expect a mental problem of psychiatric significance at some point in their lifetimes (Robins, Helzer, Weissman, Orvaschel, Gruenberg, Burke, & Regier, 1984). During an episode, however, just one in five will seek professional services, and this will usually involve a primary care physician, not a psychiatrist or clinical psychologist (Shapiro, Skinner, Kessler, Vonkorff, German, Tischler, Leaf, Benham, Cottler, & Regier, 1984). These facts highlight a potential role for exercise as an effective and implementable coping behavior.

Prescribing Exercise

Of the 1,750 primary care physicians who responded to a recent survey by the professional magazine, *The Physician and Sportsmedicine* (November, 1983, p. 10), 85% said they prescribe exercise for depression, 60% for anxiety, and 43% for chemical dependence. Each of these disorders can be stress related and the figures are consistent with earlier surveys of internists (Byrd, 1963a) and psychiatrists (Byrd, 1963b) on the use of exercise in tension control. Among primary care physicians, walking is the most commonly prescribed form of exercise, followed by swimming, bicycling, strength training, and running.

There are, however, stark contrasts to this medical emphasis on exercise for alleviating mental stress. Among an estimated 1.16 billion visits to office-based physicians during 1980 and 1981 (National Center for Health Statistics, 1983), over 69 million (6%) involved one or more psychotropic drugs for prevention, diagnosis, or treatment: 60.4% were anxiolytics, sedatives, and hypnotics (mainly benzodiazepines and barbituates); 25.9% were antidepressants (mainly tricyclics, monoamine oxidase inhibitors and lithium carbonate); and 14.1% were antipsychotic and antimanic agents (e.g. phenothiazines). Two primary care providers, the general practitioner and the internist, accounted for 66% of antianxiety, 59% of antidepressant, and 45% of antipsychotic prescriptions.

These figures are noteworthy because psychotropic drugs can have unpleasant and dangerous side effects, often require prolonged use, and can produce withdrawal symptoms when treatment is reduced or stopped (Gilman, Goodman & Gilman, 1984). For some individuals, exercise might diminish or remove the need for medication and pose less apparent risk. Figures are not available regarding the incidence of prescriptions combining both exercise and psychopharmacologic agents, and the important issue of exercise and drug interactions has only recently been studied (Morgan & Goldston, in press). However, SNS beta-blocking drugs are commonly prescribed (to lower exertional heart rate) for cardiac patients involved in rehabilitative exercise, and their psychogenic side effects for some patients (e.g. depressed mood and decreased anxiety symptoms with cardiac non-selective blockers like propanolol) are clinically well known.

Exercise and Mental Disorders

Although there are many areas of living where physical activity might exert an influence on mental health, the NIMH workshop on exercise and mental stress (Morgan & Goldston, in press) identified anxiety, depression, mental stress tolerance, self-esteem, psychoses, eating disorders, sleep disorders, and alcohol and drug abuse as topics of immediate concern.

Anxiety

Most individuals worry or feel tension from time to time. Periodic anxiety is a normal stress emotion and when it is moderate in intensity and frequency, it is merely part of our response to the hassles of the day and to the aspirations and frustrations of pursuing goals and rewarding relationships with others. At times though, the anticipation of physical or emotional threats can become so strong or recurrent that they reach clinical magnitude. They can distract attention from work, family, and personal development, foster maladaptive behaviors, and lead to painful symptoms. When this occurs, it frequently becomes necessary to make a life change or seek professional help. Often, it is necessary to learn new ways to evaluate the causes and expected consequences of life events and develop new skills for coping with stress.

For some, anxiety can be classically conditioned to an event or object. This can even occur by observational learning in the absence of direct experience. This process is clearly revealed in *phobias*. Phobias are usually specific to single or narrow ranges of stimuli, and they often respond well to behavior modification therapies.

At times, exaggerated anxiety can be provoked with little warning or apparent cause; it does not seem linked to a phobic stimulus. This often describes an anxiety neurosis or *panic disorder*, in which attacks are typically characterized by an acute fear of impending doom, tremor, tachycardia, palpitations, hyperventilation, and paresthesias (tingling sensations). In some cases, when behavior modification or psychotherapy fail, drugs can help control the symptoms of phobic anxiety and panic.

Other individuals experience a lower grade anxiety to a wider range of events. This *generalized anxiety* is usually cognitively learned by personal or observed exposures to physical threats or negative evaluations and failures. When the response is chronic, it is referred to as *trait anxiety*. This indicates an individual experiences anxiety states often and in many circumstances. Trait anxiety can also be situationally restricted to a narrow range of behaviors or settings such as public speaking, test taking, job interviews, and writing chapters for books. Most cognitively learned anxieties have in common apprehension over a valued but uncertain outcome that will be gauged against a standard of achievement or will affect the social reinforcement received from another person. Often there is a transient feeling of lack of control and low confidence. *State anxiety* is the immediate response and can be manifested by ruminations about undesirable outcomes, self-critical thoughts and self-doubts, avoidance behavior, and somatic symptoms and signs such as elevated heart rate, sweating, muscle tension, visceral motility, and narrowed or broken concentration.

Although there appears to be a biological basis for some anxiety disorders, cognitively learned anxiety can respond to psychotherapy that attempts to block, restructure, or replace the irrational, incomplete, or poorly formed assumptions that people hold about the sources or potential consequences of events (Tuma & Maser, 1985). In recent years, a more preventive or self-regulatory approach to anxiety management, called cognitive-behavior modification, has attempted to teach coping skills that the individual can use to avoid situations that produce anxiety, to change thought patterns that create worry and self-criticism, and to substitute new behaviors that are incompatible with anxiety.

It can be difficult to determine what part of anxiety is conditioned and requires therapy by counterconditioning through behavioristic techniques. It is also difficult to generalize and maintain cognitive and behavioral therapy outcomes in daily living. Thus, drugs are often the frontline treatment for anxiety. Effective treatments, however, may require a blending of behavior modification, psychotherapy, and drug therapy (Tuma & Maser, 1985).

The importance of developing behavioral skills for coping with anxiety is reinforced by estimates that less than one in four of the 13 million sufferers of anxiety will seek professional treatment (Shapiro et al., 1984). Periodic exercise provides an effective option for controlling some forms of anxiety in some people. It can be comparable or preferred to other cognitive and somatic alternatives such as biofeedback, hypnotic suggestions, meditation, progressive relaxation, and distracting rest. Exercise apparently shares anxiety reducing components found in other therapies and coping behaviors. It may help manage anxiety by (a) regulating the sympathetic tone of the autonomic nervous system, (b) distracting

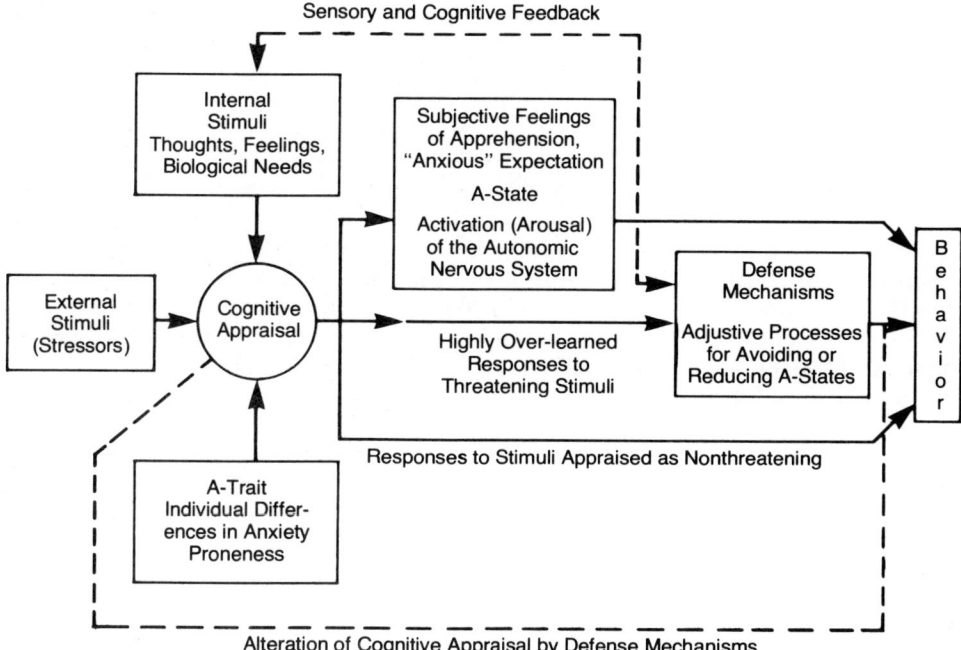

Fig. 1. A trait-state conception of anxiety. From Spielberger, C.D. (1966). Theory and research on anxiety. In *Anxiety and Behavior* (p. 17). New York: Academic Press.

anxiety ruminations, and (c) relabeling the cognitive appraisal of arousal symptoms.

Exercise and anxiety. Rhythmic endurance-type exercise of moderate and vigorous intensities using at least one half of the body's muscle mass is accompanied by reduced tension when tension is measured by neurophysiological recording devices. This is a pronounced effect for individuals who experience clinically elevated symptoms, but it also occurs in those who are asymptomatic. Walking, jogging, cycling, and bench stepping for 5 to 30 minutes at 30% (in middle aged and elderly men and women) to 60% (in young adults) of maximum heart rate are associated with acute reductions in skeletal muscle action-potential when it is measured by resting electromyograms in biceps brachii, Hoffman reflex, and achilles tendon reflex (deVries, 1982). These changes can persist for about one hour following cessation of the exercise. Twenty minutes of aerobic exercise at 40% or 75% of $\dot{V}O_2$ max has yielded a 13% and 22% reduction, respectively, in Hoffman reflex activity among men aged 20 to 45 years (Darabos & Bulbulian, 1986). In asymptomatic adults, transient increases in alpha brain wave activity measured by electroencephalograms can occur after submaximal and maximal stationary bicycle rides (Farmer, Olewine, & Comer, 1978), while brain waves become more synchronous across hemispheres during and following submaximal treadmill running (Daniels & Fernhall, 1984; Fernhall & Daniels, 1984) and stationary bicycling at 40-60% $\dot{V}O_2$ maximum (Weiss, Singh, & Yeudall, 1983).

Local tension reduction with exercise seems to be specific to skeletal muscle but it is not due to fatigue, because electromyograms become elevated, not depressed, in a fatiguing muscle. The effect is also not dependent on fusimotor feedback from sensory receptors in muscle (deVries, Simard, & Wiswell, 1982). For these reasons, reduced muscle tension with exercise seems to reflect a central (corticospinal) relaxation effect. However, generalization to other muscle groups where clinical symptoms of tension occur (e.g. frontalis) is not reliable for either trait anxious or non-anxious individuals. Exercise has been as effective as Meprobamate, a now obsolete sedative (deVries & Adams, 1972), and yields effects that are comparable to biofeedback but are no greater than distracting rest (deVries, Burke, & Hooper, 1977).

These studies indicate that a neurological relaxation response can accompany acute aerobic exercise. However, personality and life history influence the neurophysiological patterns people experience during stress. Because of this, exercise responses will also vary (Balog, 1983; deVries, Wiswell, Bulbulian, & Moritani, 1981; Dienstbier, Crabbe, & Johnson, 1981; Farmer, Olewine, & Comer, 1978; Lake, Suarez, Tocci, & Schneiderman, 1985; Sime, 1977).

Similar reductions occur for animals when tension is measured by behavior (Tharp & Carson, 1975; Weber & Lee, 1968) and for human beings when subjective anxiety is assessed. Endurance athletes such as distance runners, rowers, and wrestlers report lower state anxiety at rest than do others of the some age (Morgan, 1980). Because endurance athletes are not lower than average in trait anxiety (Eysenck, Nias & Cox, 1982), this finding probably reflects an exercise effect moreso than a characteristic brought to exercise. Also, endurance athletes typically report increased anxiety when they must interrupt their conditioning program (Thaxton, 1982; Robbins & Joseph, 1985). This implies their low anxiety is due to activity.

Self-selection may, however, influence the degree to which anxiety reductions will occur with exercise. In one study (Schwartz, Davidson, & Coleman 1978), habitual joggers reported fewer bodily symptoms (e.g. tension) but more cognitive symptoms (e.g. worry) of anxiety than did a group of meditators. Because exercisers and meditators each chose their activity, and a measure of trait anxiety was used, this study supports the view that exercise is a preferred coping behavior for certain types of people. Passive methods may be preferred by others. Also, exercise might facilitate reduction of somatic symptoms moreso than cognitive aspects of anxiety. In fact, one cross-sectional study of a large medical sample (Collingwood, Bernstein, & Hubbard, 1983) found that treadmill endurance during graded exercise testing was inversely related to somatic symptoms in certain patients, while others who were inactive and unfit complained of physical symptoms, but were not subjectively tense. However, none of these cross-sectional comparisons of static groups determine whether exercise leads to reduced anxiety or if low anxious people choose to be active. A recent prospective experiment (Long, 1984) comparing exercise training and cognitive-behavior modification found both were effective for anxiety, but neither had an advantage for cognitive or somatic symptoms.

Other prospective studies of group change, non-equivalent control group comparisons, and randomized experiments confirm, however, that exercise can reduce state anxiety. Both acute and chronic exercise of vigorous intensities consistently are associated with a reduction in state anxiety following graded and continuous treadmill exercise and exercise in natural settings (Morgan, 1979; Berger & Owen, 1983). These effects can last as long as four to six hours but are quite variable during this time (Morgan, 1982). Changes in trait anxiety following chronic exercise training are much less reliable. An equal number of studies show decreases and no change, while a few show increases (Dishman, 1985).

These studies do not, however, account for the mitigating impact of other personality traits and life stressors on exercise effects and do not contrast the pattern of chronic response to exercise against a chronic baseline life stress response. Exercise might not make people better, but it could keep them from getting worse.

Exercise effects may not be different from other effective interventions. Experimental study has shown, for example, that both chronic exercise and cognitive anxiety management training (AMT) can reduce state anxiety and systolic blood pressure among self-referred anxiety disorders, but only AMT reduced trait anxiety (Lobitz, Brammell, & Stoll, 1983). Exercise can be as effective as group counseling in reducing anxiety, but benefits seen after a few months may not persist (Stern, Gorman, & Kaslow, 1983). Thus, it appears that exercise is best viewed as one method for intermittent coping with daily events or thoughts that provide an anxiety response. Exercise is less likely to alter anxiety traits or presistent sources of stress.

Exercise appears as effective as other self-help approaches such as meditation (Bahrke & Morgan, 1978), group counseling (Stern et al., 1984), cognitive-behavioral methods (Driscoll, 1976; Lobitz, Brammell, & Stoll, 1983; Long, 1984), or distracting rest (Bahrke & Morgan, 1978). However, the effects of exercise on subjective anxiety are not reliable for mild exercise intensities, and it appears that an intensity exceeding 70% of $\dot{V}O_2$ max or age-adjusted HR_{max} for at least 20 minutes is needed to insure an acute reduction.

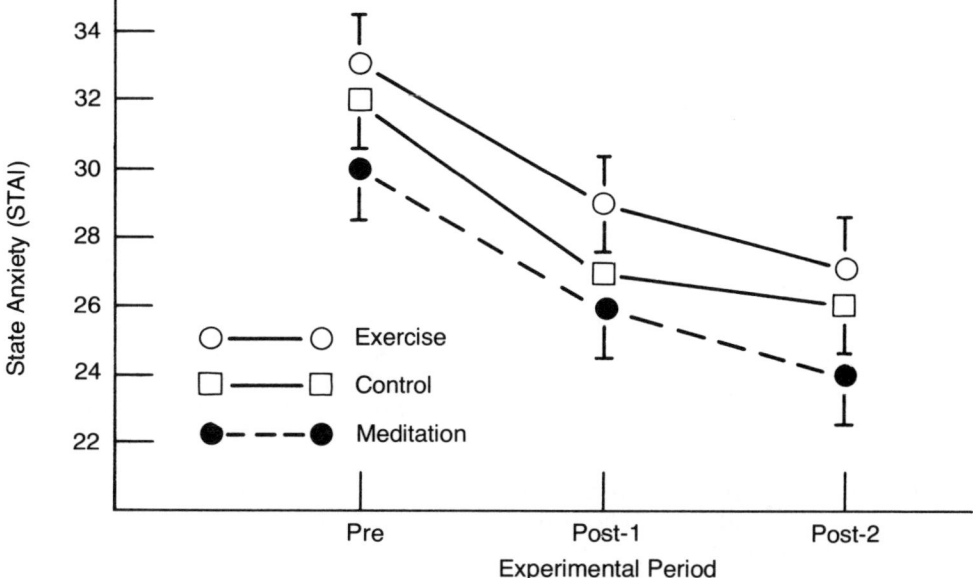

Fig. 2. State anxiety before and following exercise, meditation, and control treatments. From Bahrke, M.S. & Morgan, W.P. (1978). Anxiety reduction following exercise and meditation. *Cognitive Therapy and Research, 2,* 326.

A maximal aerobic effort can lead to a temporary increase in state anxiety, but this should not be a clinical concern because both trait anxious individuals (Morgan, 1979) and schizophrenic outpatients (Ross & Levin, 1981) experience normal anxiety during graded exercise testing. Despite reports that intravenous injections of sodium dl- lactate can induce panic attacks in anxiety neurotics (Gorman, Levy, Liebowitz, McGrath, Appleby, Dillon, Davies, & Klein, 1983; Margraf, Ehlers, & Roth, 1986), exercise intensities that elevate blood lactate four to five times above resting levels do not cause anxiety attacks or elevate state anxiety in either anxiety prone or normal individuals (Morgan, 1979). Moreover, case data (Driscoll, 1976; Muller & Armstrong, 1975; Orwin, 1973, 1974) show that chronic exercise can be an effective adjunct for treating phobias. These discrepancies probably reflect the unique metabolic and acid-base state induced by exercise, compared with buffered lactate injection, and the problems in distinguishing between generalized anxiety disorders, panic disorder, and phobias.

Although peripheral biochemical correlates of fitness and exercise responsivity are related to subjective anxiety (Peronnet, Blier, Brisson, Diamond, Ledoux, &

Volle, 1986), current evidence suggests that exercise reduces state anxiety when it, or the exercise setting, (1) distracts attention from anxiety-provoking thoughts, (2) competes with the perception of anxiety symptoms, (3) helps redefine the subjective meaning of arousal, or (4) alters physiological measures of autonomic nervous system arousal. These effects may not be reliable when anxiety is a symptom of primary affective disorder or when it is superimposed on a life-threatening illness.

Depression

It is normal to experience temporary mood swings. Most people get the blues or feel down from time to time. When depression is diagnosed as a primary psychiatric disorder, however, it is usually characterized by symptoms that endure for at least one month. These include dysphoric mood, anorexia, insomnia or hypersomnia, chronic fatigue, psychomotor retardation, apathy, diminished libido, lowered self-esteem, confusion, and cognitive impairment. Recurrent thoughts of suicide are common, and estimates indicate that 10% to 20% of depression leads to suicide. In some types of depression there is a chronic over stimulation of the sympathetic nervous system or an exaggerated autonomic response to physical or emotional challenge. Depressive symptoms can also be secondary to, or superimposed upon, pre-existing psychiatric illnesses not involving mood. They may also coincide with life-threatening or incapacitating medical/surgical illness (Akiskal & McKinney, 1975).

Depression can be *reactive* (precipitated by life events) or *endogenous* (precipitating events are unknown). Neurotic or moderate depression is typically reactive and unipolar (episodes involve mood downswings only), while melancholia and bipolar manic-depressive (alternating episodes of elation with mood downswings) psychoses usually are independent of precipitating life events.

Mild depression will often subside quickly without intervention. Likewise, some cases of moderate depression will experience spontaneous remission within six months of onset. Although psychotherapy is often effective with mild and moderate depression, it usually must be augmented with antidepressive medication. For severe depression, drugs are nearly always indicated. For unipolar disorders, tricyclic and tetracyclic antidepressants are preferred, but monoamine oxidase (MAO) inhibitors can be used with some success, as can lithium for recurrent unipolar episodes. Lithium is the drug of choice for manic-depressive disorders. Neither psychotherapy nor drug therapy can be expected to work with psychotic depressions. These respond best to electroconvulsive therapy (ECT).

There are undesirable complications in the course of most depression treatments. ECT requires a hospital stay, while tricyclics commonly have side effects such as blurred vision, dry mouth, orthostatic hypotension and abnormal electrocardiograms in the elderly. Lithium can cause gastrointestinal upset, tremors, and poor appetite. Because it is a salt, lithium can also complicate medical conditions of the heart, kidneys, and thyroid gland (Shamoian, 1983). These side effects of drugs make exercise an attractive treatment alternative in some instances. But, determining the efficacy of exercise requires an understanding of depression's origins.

The roots of depression are often viewed as a disregulation of either cognitive (Beck, 1976) or neurobiological processes (Post and Ballenger, 1984). Akiskal and McKinney (1975), however, have proposed that depressive illness is best conceptualized as an impairment of the reinforcement function of the diencephalon (the mood and reward center of the brain) due to lowered catecholamine (e.g., norepinephrine or dopamine) or indoleamine (e.g., serotonin) levels, or to production of faulty neuronal transmitters, or to sodium accumulation. In this model, depression is viewed as the final common pathway for various chemical, experiential, and behavioral processes; both reactive and endogenous depression is explained by genetic disposition and developmental, physiological, or psychosocial stressors. These etiological (origins) and nosological (diagnostic) definitions are important, because they provide a clinical framework for viewing the potential role of exercise as a theapeutic adjunct or alternative in treating depressive illness. In many cases, the usefulness of exercise is likely to depend on the *cause* of the depression as much as its symptoms.

Table 1
Ten Models of Depression

School	Model	Mechanism
Psychoanalytical	Aggression-turned-Inward	Conversion of aggressive instinct into depressive affect
	Object loss	Separation: disruption of an attachment bond
	Loss of self-esteem	Helplessness in attaining goals of ego-ideal
	Negative Cognitive set	Hopelessness
Behavioral	Learned helplessness	Uncontrollable aversive stimulation
	Loss of reinforcement	Rewards of "sick role" substitute for lost sources of reinforcement
Sociological	Sociological	Loss of role status
Existential	Existential	Loss of meaning of existence
Biological	Biogenic amine	Impaired monoaminergic neurotransmission
	Neurophysiological	Hyperarousal secondary to intraneuronal sodium accumulation
		Cholinergic dominance
		Reversible functional derangement of diencephalic mechanisms of reinforcement

From Akiskal, H.S. & McKinney, W.T., Jr. (1975, March). Overview of recent research in depression. *Archives of General Psychiatry, 32,* 286.

Various hypotheses have been put forth to explain why exercise might have antidepressant properties (Greist, Klein, Eischens, Faris, Gurman, & Morgan, 1979). These include (a) generalizable feelings of achievement, (b) feelings of self-control or competence, (c) symptom relief or distraction, (d) substitution of good habits for bad ones (i.e., those that are self-edifying replace those that are self-destructive), (e) development of patience, and (f) consciousness alterations. These concepts apply mainly to nonpsychotic depression. That is, when the illness is primary and reactive, exercise or its setting might permit a generalized management of several client-specific origins of depression.

Physical activity is also an incompatible behavior when compared with the passivity that characterizes many depressions. It might counter-condition depressive mood by mimicking the behavior that has been restricted by the disorder; this was a common theory held by the ancient Greeks (Ryan, 1984). But, it probably is not feasible to motivate severe depressives for exertion.

An antidepressant effect might also stem from neurobiological changes with exercise, for example, regulation of sympathetic-parasympathetic balance in the autonomic nervous system or changes in the release or uptake of neurotransmitters such as norepinephrine, dopamine, serotonin, GABA, endorphins and enkephalins. These hormones help regulate mood and nervous system functions (Hippius & Winokur, 1983; Post and Ballenger, 1984). After exercise, several are elevated in the plasma of human beings and are altered in the brains of rats and mice. Altered cerebral circulation and metabolism have also been implied as a mood elevator (Dishman, 1985).

Exercise might also be effective for reducing depression that is superimposed on medical or surgical illness by rehabilitating the physical disorder (e.g. cardiac rehabilitation) and rebuilding physical self-confidence for safe exertion and a return to normal life roles.

Exercise and depression. Studies confirm that chronic aerobic exercise can be associated with reductions in clinical and psychometric symptoms of non-psychotic depression. These can parallel increased fitness ($\dot{V}O_2$ max) (Doyne, Chambless, & Beutler, 1983; Greist, et al., 1979; Kavanaugh, Shepard, Tuck, & Quershi, 1977; McCann & Holmes, 1984), but can also occur when fitness changes are not measured or reported (Blumenthal, Williams, Needels & Wallace, 1982; Brown, Ramirez, & Taub, 1978; Conroy, Smith & Felthous, 1982; Folkins, 1976; Klein, Greist, Gurman, Neimeyer, Lesser, Bushnell & Smith, 1985; Morgan, Roberts, Brand, & Feinerman, 1970; Morgan & Goldston, in press; Stern & Cleary, 1981). The MMPI depression scale discriminated between middle aged men who are highly fit and active and those who are unfit and sedentary (Lobstein, Mosbacher, & Ismail, 1983). But cross-sectional contrasts like this cannot determine if low depression precedes, follows, or interacts with exercise training or fitness. There is no relationship between fitness and depression among sedentary psychiatric patients (Morgan, 1970). Also, fitness has been unrelated to depression (MMPI) and urinary metabolites of catecholamine neurotransmitters during resting conditions and occupational stress (Sothmann & Ismail, 1984). However, a recent controlled experiment from Norway reported by Martinsen (Morgan & Goldston, in press) has shown a direct, though small, correlation between increased aerobic fitness (Åstrand-Ryhming) and symptom abatement for patients suffering major depressive episode (DSM III). This was strongest for males and appeared to reflect real fitness gains moreso than changes in the autonomic nervous system. Whether fitness contributed to the antidepressant effect or merely accompanied increases in activity as the depression subsided is unknown.

Although several exercise training studies of healthy adults and college students show significant decreases in psychometric depression, this is not a reliable result among individuals that begin exercise within the normal range on standard depression tests. Randomized experimental trials across 20 weeks (Morgan & Pollock, 1978) and two years (Stern & Cleary, 1982) show no change from initially normal scores. This suggests that when changes are seen for normal subjects in non-randomized studies they reflect an expectancy effect, a self-selection bias, or a mood elevation that is not part of psychiatric depression or cannot be measured by psychiatric scales.

Exercise effects can, however, be comparable to conventional psychotherapy or counseling and meditation-relaxation techniques (Greist et al., 1979; Jankowski, 1976; Klein et al., 1985; Morgan & Goldston, in press) used for treating moderate psychiatric depression. In fact, in one 12-month followup of randomly assigned psychiatric outpatients (Greist et al., 1979), 11 of 12 effectively treated with running therapy were still asymptomatic, while one-half of those who had received traditional psychotherapy had returned for treatment. In a replication study (Klein et al., 1985), treatment gains after 12 weeks were comparable between running therapy and meditation training; in each case gains were greater than in group psychotherapy and remained so nine months following treatment.

Uncontrolled clinical trials (Kavanagh et al., 1977; Shephard, Kavanagh & Klavora, 1985; Stern & Cleary, 1981) have also shown that depression is alleviated among cardiac patients following chronic exercise rehabilitation. In a randomized trial (Stern et al., 1983), however, improvements seen after three months were lost by one year. Fitness training does, however, contribute to exertional self-confi-

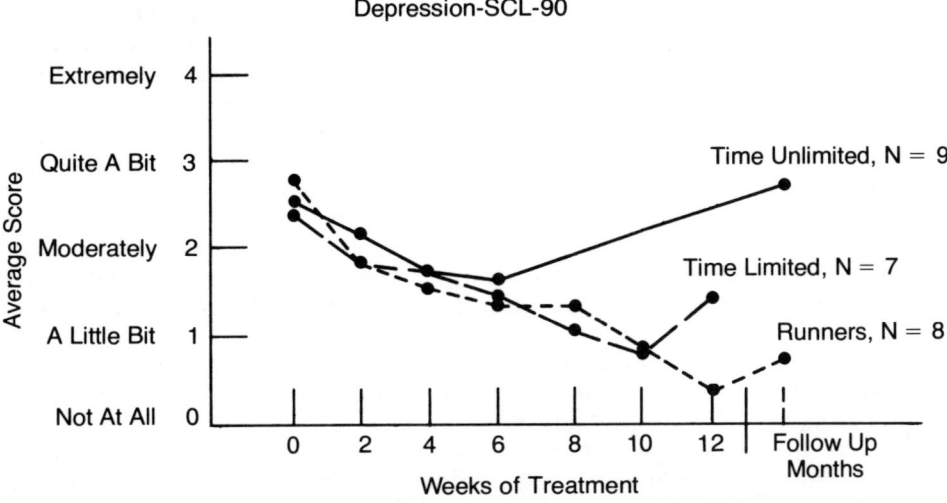

Fig. 3. From Greist, J., Klein, M., Eischens, R., Faris, J., Gurman, A., & Morgan, W.P. (1978). Running through your mind. *Journal of Psychosomatic Research, 22,* 278.

dence among cardiac patients, and this is consistent with symptom reduction in depressive disorders that are secondary to medical/surgical illness. Because these findings occur reliably in group outpatient programs, but not in physician encouraged home rehabilitation (Mayou, 1983; Erdman & Duivenvoorden, 1983), social reinforcement within an exercise setting may be equally or more important than exercise training. Studies of cardiac patients scoring within the normal range on psychometric tests of depression at the outset of training show no change following cardiopulmonary exercise programs of three-month (Roviaro, Holmes, & Holmsten, 1984), six-month (Naughton, Bruhn, & Lategola, 1968), and two-year (Stern & Cleary, 1982) durations or following neuromuscular training for three months (Prosser, Carson, & Phillips, 1981).

None of the biochemical or social psychological speculations for the antidepressant effects of exercise have been confirmed, but it apears likely that the effects depend largely on graded mastery and feelings related to competence, self-control, and symptom distraction or substitution. Biochemical influences are likely but unproved, and the role of fitness remains unclear. There is presently no evidence that exercise training can be an effective intervention with endogenous depressions. Moreover, Morgan (1982) has reported that overtrained "stale" endurance athletes present a clinical profile that mimicks reactive depression. This reveals that there can be a paradoxical dosage effect with exercise, but little is now known about the optimal volume or mode for symptom abatement. Though not well studied, there seem to be no medical complications with exercise for patients using lithium or tricyclic antidepressants (Morgan & Goldston, in press). Because three of ten who suffer depression will not seek professional treatment (Shapiro et al., 1984), the potential usefulness of exercise is enhanced by the search for effective self-help strategies.

Mental Stress Tolerance

Because many people experience mental stress but are not clinically depressed or anxious, exercise might also offer an effective means for coping with normal life events and daily hassles. The aforementioned research suggests that exercise can help manage stress by changing thoughts, feelings, or symptoms that contribute to emotions such as anxiety, depression, and anger. Whether an increased ability to tolerate the metabolic stress of exercise (i.e. increased VO_2 maximum) can generalize to a diminished physiological response to mental or emotional stress remains unclear. This is important for public health because several chronic diseases are linked to behavior through stress emotions such as anxiety and the repression of hostility.

Exercise and mental stress tolerance. Although neurologic and neuroendocrine responses to cold and sound stressors diminish after a training run among experienced runners (Dienstbier et al., 1981), EMG,HR, and skin conductance responses to mental arithmetic in the sedentary have not differed when arousal levels were manipulated by a drug (smoking), perceptual conflict (a vigilance task), or bicycle exercise at 60% of maximum heart rate (Russell, Epstein, & Erickson, 1983).

The optimal exercise intensity for stress coping mechanisms is not known, however (McGowan, Robertson, & Epstein, 1985). The method of choice for manipulating exercise and mental stress interactions is also not clear because of the known dissociation of cortical, spinal, and muscular indices of neurologic activation from neuroendocrine response under various stress conditions (Hull, Young, Ziegler, 1984). There are also large individual differences in response to a standard mental stressor. Furthermore, acute studies do not examine the effects that chronic exercise training may have. Highly fit, trained individuals show an earlier and larger initial climb in plasma catecholamines and prolactin in response to mental stress and a more rapid recovery to baseline than do the untrained. This is indicative of better stress adaptability. Although heart rate and subjective anxiety appear similar during mental stress, high fit subjects have faster heart rate recovery and lower state anxiety after it is removed. High self-reported weekly aerobic activity has also been associated with lower heart rate, systolic blood pressure, and myocardial pre-ejection period in response to a shock-avoidance task (Light, Obrist, & James, 1984). Studies consistently show quicker cardiovascular and electrodermal recovery from psychological stress among metabolically fit subjects (Cox, Evans, & Jamieson, 1979; Hull et al., 1984; Keller, 1980; Keller & Seraganian, 1984; Sinyor, Schwartz, Peronnet, Brisson, & Seraganian, 1983). Cross-sectional study with intact groups also suggests aerobic fitness may interact with personality (e.g. Type A) to influence physiological response (e.g. blood pressure) to behavioral or psychological stress (Lake et al., 1985). Experimental study, however, has not confirmed these results (Roskies, Seraganian, Oseasohn, Hanley, Collu, Martin, & Smilga, 1986). Training studies with initially unfit individuals have only recently appeared, and they provide mixed findings (Roskies et al., 1986; Keller & Seraganian, 1984; Sinyor, Golden, Steinert, & Seraganian, 1986). However, training gains have not been documented by an increase in measured $\dot{V}O_2$ max; studies that rely on heart rate changes to measure fitness may confound fitness with dependent measures of psychophysiological reactivity that also are based on heart rate. It is important in mental stress tolerance studies to induce changes in metabolic variables because cross-sectional differences between existing fitness categories may stem from intrinsic sources other than activity history.

To determine the mechanisms of generalized stress adaptations from exercise it is necessary to distinguish between metabolic, subjective, and cortical/spinal arousal responses and their neural and endocrine pathways within the sympathetic nervous sytem. Because accomplishing this with human beings may exceed current experimental techniques, comparative studies of stress in animals can be informative. For example, corticosterone levels are higher than normal in rats who suffer stress-induced gastric lesions (Starzec, Berger, Hess, & Alperson, 1983), while 5-HT (serotonin) levels in the midbrain, cortex, and hippocampus are lower compared with non-lesion controls (Hellhammer, Hingtgen, Wade, Shea, & Aprison, 1983). Both cases seem to reveal biochemical markers of neuroendocrine stress that are sensitive to exertion. For example, acute swimming (Barchas & Freedman, 1963) and chronic running (Brown, Payne, Kim, Moore, & Krebs, 1979) elevate rat brain 5-HT in non-lesioned rats, while chronically exercised rats suffer less progressive ulceration than sedentary cohorts following reserpine induced gastric lesions (Johnson & Tharpe, 1974). Also, rats that spontaneously run after exposure to unpredictable, uncontrollable electric shock showed lower plasma corticosterone and cholesterol than their sedentary cohorts (Starzec et al., 1983). Collectively, these findings are indicative of psychoendocrine adaptations to exercise that might generalize across stress modalities.

Self-concept and Self-esteem

As described in more detail by Sage in Chapter 12, self-concept is our ordered awareness of personal experiences, behaviors, and social interactions. It defines us in comparison with others and with our past behaviors and future goals. We form specific self-concepts for major roles and abilities in life (e.g. academic, social, emotional, and physical), while our overall or global self-concept is a weighted composite of these specific self-concepts.

Self-esteem is that aspect of self-concept that provides a feeling of value or worth. Self-esteem has significance for mental health because it is a generalized indicator of psychological adjustment. Symptoms of anxiety, depression, and schizophrenia often are associated with low self-esteem or disordered identity of self.

Exercise and self-esteem. Studies of the effects of acute exercise on self-esteem are too limited for conclusions (Sonstroem, 1984), but it appears self-esteem is relatively enduring or stable rather than transitory. Thus, measurable changes with exercise are likely to be seen after prolonged involvement (e.g. training) more than during or following an acute period. Research indicates that chronic exercise cannot be expected to reliably enhance global self-esteem in adults (Sonstroem, 1984). This is probably because the components of self-esteem become more multidimensional by adulthood; many behaviors and skills weigh heavily in the global self-esteem of adults. But the degree to which the relative importance of exercise or fitness abilities changes as we age is unknown.

Changes in body image or self-perceptions of physical abilities are, however, associated with chronic exercise when actual increases in fitness or ability occur (Dishman & Gettman, 1981; Kowal, Patton, & Vogel, 1978; Pauly, Palmer, & Wright, 1982; Sidney & Shephard, 1976). These perceptions approximate objective fitness levels among both typical (Koocher, 1971) and atypical (Gary & Guthrie, 1972; Rohrbacher, 1973) groups, and this relationship does not appear to change following aerobic training with schizophrenic outpatients (Gimino & Levin, 1984). Because body image is related to overall self-concept, enhanced body image or physical competence can contribute to global self-esteem in individuals for whom physical attributes are highly valued relative to other aspects of self-concept. Both increases and decreases in self-esteem can also occur without actual changes in fitness or ability depending upon whether reinforcing feedback of a positive or negative nature is provided by the exercise setting (Sonstroem, 1984).

Physical activities and their settings typically are as effective as other social/behavioral settings that influence feelings of competence. The potential effectiveness of physical activity appears to depend, however, on facilitating self-perceptions of personally valued attributes either directly, by inducing biological or behavioral change, or indirectly by augmenting social reinforcement (Collingwood, 1972; Collingwood & Willett, 1971; Erdman & Duivenvorden, 1983; Hilyer & Mitchell, 1979). The greatest gains in self-esteem can be expected for individuals with low initial levels (Folkins, Lynch, & Gardner, 1972; Tucker, 1983) and for whom physical attributes are valued as a part of global self-concept.

Little is known about exercise and self-esteem among older persons, but it appears that positive changes among adults are less common than in children and youth. From his recent meta-analysis, Gruber (1986) concluded that the effects of physical activity programs on the self-esteem of children are greater (1) for those with disabling conditions (e.g. mental retardation or obesity) compared with normal children, (2) under clinically oriented rather than typical classroom conditions, and (3) using fitness activities (running or weight training) rather than motor or sport skills or creative movement. These findings reinforce for children the mental health importance of fitness actvities already believed to be related to cardiovascular health and reduced anxiety and depression among adults.

Schizophrenia

Certain types of depression, (e.g. manic-depressive disorder) are psychotic and prevalent in the population, but schizophrenia is the most severe and widespread diagnostic category of psychosis. It is a group of severe disorders that appear to stem from diverse causes and manifest a wide range of signs and symptoms (Najem, Lindenthal, Louria, & Thind, 1980). The most common clinical features of schizophrenia include all or some of the following: delusions, hallucinations, thought disorder, apathy, antisocial or aberrant behavior, hyperarousal, and breakdowns of normal affect, volition, and intellect (Liberman, 1982). There are wide differences among schizophrenics in the severity and periodicity of episodes, and schizophrenic-like symptoms are possible in many of us if environmental strain is sufficient (e.g. lack of sleep, abuse of stimulants, and social stress). It is believed that schizophrenia, like most mental disorders, develops from complex interactions between behavior, environment, and biological disposition. Schizophrenics can prompt, exacerbate, or conversely diminish, episodes by seeking or avoiding high risk situations. Antipsychotic medication (e.g. phenothiazines) is at the core of treatment, but the overall goal of therapy is usually to avoid episodes and manage symptoms rather than to cure the disease. Typically included are cognitive-behavior interventions designed to increase family cohesion and graded mastery at social skills.

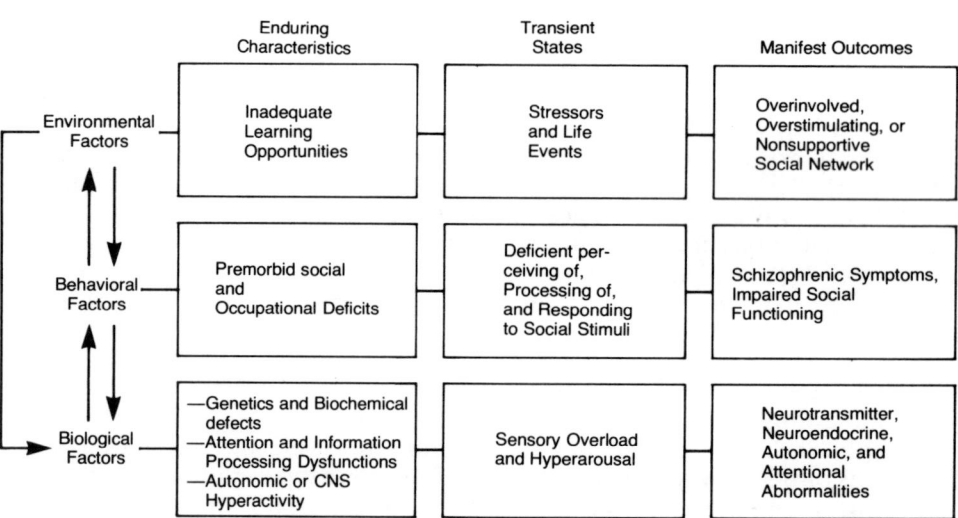

Fig. 4. An interactional model for understanding the nature of schizophrenia. From Strauss, J., Bowers, M.B., Keith, S.J., Meltzer, H.V., & Liberman, R.P. (1982). What is Schizophrenia? *Schizophrenia Bulletin,* 8(3), 436.

Exercise, fitness, and psychotic disorders. There is no convincing evidence that exercise directly influences psychotic disorders. Uncontrolled study (Dodson & Mullens, 1969) has shown changes in scales of the Minnesota Multiphasic Personality Inventory (MMPI) following a jogging program for hospitalized psychiatric patients, and improvements in psychiatric states after fitness training have been seen in geriatric mental patients (Powell, 1974; Stamford, Hanbacher, Fallica, 1974). None of these effects appear greater than those that will occur from increasing social interaction among psychiatric patients.

Other descriptive data suggest a role for fitness in defining certain psychoses (Morgan, 1974). Some chronic schizophrenics have neuromuscular dysfunction, elevated resting creatine kinase and abnormalities in muscle structure. Also, psychiatric patients consistently demonstrate low muscle strength and endurance. The relationships between fitness variables and symptoms, however, may reflect sedentary lifestyles and motivational deficits rather than etiology of the disorder. Length of hospitalization has, on the other hand, been shown to be shorter for psychiatric patients who show relatively high muscular strength at entry (Morgan 1970).

Two recent non-randomized trials with schizophrenic outpatients (Gimino & Levin, 1984) have shown that enhanced self-concept can accompany a cardiovascular training program, but isometric strength training did not alter MMPI profiles of chronic schizophrenics (Smith & Figetakis, 1970). The generalizability of these findings is difficult to evaluate because of inadequate control comparisons and problems with reliable diagnosis of schizophrenia (Liberman, 1982). They are noteworthy, however, because symptom management is important in the prognosis of schizophrenia. And, it is known that certain types of schizophrenic disorder do not respond to either neuroleptic medication or psychotherapy (Buckley, 1982). Moreover, one-half of the sufferers of schizophrenia do not seek or receive professional services (Shapiro et al., 1984).

The interpersonal interactions, concrete perceptual events, and the unambiguous goal and reinforcement structure typical of non-competitive group exercise programs might assist in symptom management and skill development in the social, perceptual, and cognitive areas of deficit which characterize certain schizophrenic disorders (Liberman, 1982).

Table 2
Some Possible Mental Health Benefits of Exercise

Increases	Decreases
Assertiveness	Absenteeism from work
Confidence	Alcohol abuse
Emotional Stability	Anger
Independence	Anxiety
Internal locus of control	Confusion
Mood	Depression
Body image	Premenstrual Syndrome
Self-concept	Phobias
Subjective well-being	Psychotic behavior
Self-control	Mental Stress
Work efficiency	Tension
Mental stress tolerance	Type A behavior

Adapted from Hughes, J.R. (1984). Psychological effects of habitual aerobic exercise: A critical review. *Preventive Medicine, 13,* 74; and Taylor, C.B., Sallis, J.A., & Needles, R. (1985). The relation of physical activity and exercise to mental health. *Public Health Reports, 100*(2), 199.

Eating Disorders, Exercise Abuse, and Exercise Neurobiology

Eating disorders. Anorexia nervosa, nervous loss of appetite, is principally an adolescent disease, predominately affecting females 12 to 25 years of age. About one in 250 young women over 15 will be diagnosed as a severe case, although 1% of the total population will show anorectic symptoms (McSherrey, 1984). The prevalence rate is ten times higher in females than males. Episodes of bulimia (binge eating followed by self-purging) are one manifestation of the disease, but bulimia can exist independently and presents its own health risks. The origin of anorexia is unknown, but like many disorders, it is believed to stem from psychological interactions between biological predisposition and social stress.

Anorexia involves a compulsive quest for weight control by extreme reductions in calorie intake, purging by vomiting and laxatives, and excessive activity. Clinical study (Yates, Leehey, & Shisslak, 1983) has suggested that excessive exercisers, particularly runners, present symptoms analagous to the anorectic: a common family history, socioeconomic class and pressures; preoccupation with food and leanness; and personality traits of anger suppression, asceticism, denial of medical risk, introversion, and perfectionism. Although exercise is promoted as a healthy alternative to restrictive dieting among weight conscious females, the concern raised is the possibility that exercise commitment could lead to anorexia for some personalities or could exacerbate an existing eating disorder.

While there are undoubtedly anorectics who are compulsive exercisers, controlled research (Blumenthal, Rose, & Chang, 1985; Dishman, 1985) reveals for the vast majority that exercise commitment and anorexia nervosa are separate entities. In fact, there are case reports (Kostrubala, 1976) of effective treatment of anorexia by combining psychotherapy with running. Although anorectics often boost the impact of food restriction by hyperactivity, their fitness ($\dot{V}O_2$ max) is very low compared to committed exercisers, while stress hormone profiles differ between the groups. Anorectics often have elevated scores on standard tests of psychopathology, while habitual runners usually score in the normal range of the same tests and show mood profiles that indicate positive mental health.

Although some studies of small samples of ballerinas, gymnasts, and wrestlers show higher than expected rates of eating problems, how long they persist and whether they represent goal-appropriate behaviors for the sport, rather than medical or psychological pathology, is not established (Dishman, 1985). In most cases the eating behaviors of athletes do not appear to signal anorexia nervosa or bulimia.

Exercise abuse. There are case reports, however, of excessive involvement or dependence with exercise training. Morgan (1979) described eight cases of "running addiction", when commitment to running exceeded prior commitments to work, family, social relations, and medical advice. Similar cases have been labeled as positive addiction, runner's gluttony, fitness fanaticism, athlete's neurosis, and obligatory running (Dishman, 1985). However, little is understood about the origins, diagnostic validity, or the mental health impact of abusive exercise. For most, the benefits of exercise exceed the risks of abuse.

However, the inability or unwillingness to interrupt and taper one's involvement in an exercise training program or replace a preferred form of exercise with an alternative, when this decision is indicated by medical exigency or vocational or social responsibilities, may reveal an emotional disturbance of clinical meaning. The few studies that show psychopathology in habitual runners (Sacks & Sachs, 1981), indicate that exaggerated emphasis on exercise roles or fitness abilities (as can happen for other areas of life) can reflect a pre-existing proneness to problems of an imbalanced and insecure self-concept.

Exercise neurobiology. Early speculations held that the increases in plasma monoamines (norepinephrine, serotonin, and dopamine) and endorphins (beta-

Table 3
Anorexic vs. Athletic Female

Shared features

Dietary faddism
Controlled calorie consumption
Specific carbohydrate avoidance
Low body weight
Resting bradycardia and low blood pressure
Increased physical activity
Amenorrhea or oligomenorrhea
Anemia (may or may not be present)

Distinguishing features

Athlete

Purposeful training
Increased exercise tolerance
Good muscular development
Accurate body image
Body fat level within defined normal range

Anorexic

Aimless physical activity
Poor or decreasing exercise performance
Poor muscular development
Flawed body image (patient believes herself to be overweight)
Body fat level below normal range
Biochemical abnormalities if abusing laxatives and/or diuretics

From McSherry, J.A. The diagnostic challenge of anorexia nervosa. *American Family Physician,* 29(2), 144.

endorphin and leucine-enkephalin) which accompany vigorous exercise could contribute to exercise euphoria ("runner's high") and subsequently to dependence because of the role of these hormones as neurotransmitters for mood, pain analgesia, and neuroendocrine stress (Morgan, 1985). A biochemical basis for exercise commitment or dependence has not been supported, however.

Acute endurance exercise does consistently increase plasma levels of monoamines, beta-endorphin, and leu-enkephalin in human beings (Harber & Sutton, 1984). One study found that naloxone (a drug that blocks endorphins from receptor binding) increased the perception of pain after running (Haier, Quaid, & Mills, 1981). However, a smaller naloxone dose in another study did not block mood elevation from a running session (Markoff, Ryan & Young, 1982).

If endorphins regulate exercise moods, blockade of their chemical action by a competing drug should prevent the mood swing. It did not. Although the dose of naloxone may have been too small, other studies that have measured mood and endorphins in experienced runners show that each are elevated after acute exertion, but mood is not predicted by the levels of endorphins present (Farrell, Gates, Maksud, & Morgan, 1982; Farrell, Gates, Morgan, & Pert, 1983). Endorphin levels also vary greatly across individuals at the same relative exercise intensity. Thus, they apparently cannot be predicted by prescribing workout intensity according to a percentage of aerobic fitness ($\dot{V}O_2$ max) in the same way as can many other stress responses to exercise. Moreover, levels found in the blood of exercising humans can come from several tissues other than the brain (e.g. the pituitary gland) and their importance for brain function and mood is unknown. Plasma levels also do not distinguish between changes in neuronal release, reuptake, or site of action.

On the other hand, exercise-related stress has influenced monoamine levels and endorphin receptor occupancy in rats and mice (Barchas & Freedman, 1963; Barta, Yashpal, & Henry, 1981; Bliss & Ailion, 1971; Pert & Bowie, 1979; Olson & Morgan, 1982; Wardlow & Frantz, 1980). The relevance of altered levels or regional distributions of neurotransmitters in animals for the regulation of human mood is not established, however. For these reasons, advances in human exercise neurobiology will likely depend on newer imaging technologies (e.g. nuclear magnetic resonnance or positron emission tomography) to determine the origin, direction, and psychological meaning of neurotransmitter changes during exercise. Comparative research using animal models of exercise neurobiology also represents a promising approach (Morgan, Olson, & Pedersen, 1982).

Some runners and swimmers report subjective elation during workouts (Sacks & Sachs, 1981), but exercise euphoria is an unpredictable phenomenon with no established biochemical cause; it is as likely to reflect a relaxation effect or acute feelings of competence. If chronic exercise helps a person manage somatic symptoms, these can return when training is interrupted, but it is not clear that this can be regarded as a "withdrawal" effect in the context of dependence (Robbins & Joseph, 1985; Thaxton, 1982). Moreover, the prevalence of psychopathology is no greater among habitual exercisers than in the population, while tension, anxiety, and depression levels are more favorable. Thus, there is no reason to believe that habitual exercise will lead to unhealthy dependence, addiction or self-abuse for a mentally healthy person; it can, in fact, be an adaptive behavior for many who suffer mental disorders.

Table 4
Proposed Psychological Harms of Exercise

Addiction to exercise
Compulsiveness
Decreased involvement in job, marriage, and so on
Escape or avoidance of problems
Exacerbation of anorexia nervosa
Exercise deprivation effects
Fatigue
Overcompetitiveness
Overexertion
Poor eating habits
Preoccupation with fitness, diet, and body image
Self-centeredness

From Taylor, C.B., Sallis, J.A., & Needles, R. (1985). The relation of physical activity and exercise to mental health. *Public Health Reports, 100*(2), 199.

Sleep Disorders

Problems with sleep (too much, too little, or disrupted) are a component of several mental health disorders, and they are particularly telling symptoms of anxiety and depression. Insomnia is a common complication of medical pain. Otherwise healthy individuals can also be unaware of sleep disturbances but feel unrefreshed. People who use alcohol or caffeine to excess, or who take physician-prescribed medications, can also have their sleep disturbed. Although prevalent, only about one in five people who suffer sleep disturbances will seek a physician's care, and only one-half of these individuals will be treated by a drug (usually a hypnotic or antianxiety agent) (Hollister, 1983). Many, however, who do not seek treatment probably purchase over-the-counter sleep aids. Because drugs often do not address the source of the sleep problem and can create a behavioral dependence, other interventions such as psychotherapy and cognitive-behavior modification are often recommended.

Exercise is also believed to have sleep promoting effects. Exercise may regulate sleep by increasing the need for energy conserving rest or restorative tissue repair due to increased metabolic demands. It is also believed that exercise can regulate the sympathetic nervous system in ways that offset the hyperarousal that can characterize anxiety or depression.

Sleep patterns are measured by cyclical changes in the frequency and amplitude of brain electroencephalograms (EEG), by observation, and by self-report. Sleep cycles typically include rapid eye movement (REM) sleep, where dreaming occurs, and four stages of non-REM sleep: the first two are light sleep, while stages 3 and 4 indicate slow wave sleep (SWS) believed to represent deep, restorative sleep. There is controversy about measuring body restoration, however, and it is most accepted that changes in EEG during sleep can only assure brain activity, not necessarily bodily rest.

Exercise and sleep. Many studies show that acute exercise is followed by increased SWS on the exercise evening (Horne, 1981). When the exercise is of vigorous intensity (e.g. 50-70% $\dot{V}O_2$ max) and continued to exhaustion, the increase in SWS occurs early in the night's sleep and is accompanied by a decrease in REM sleep (Bunnell, Bevier, & Horvath, 1983). While these effects can occur for untrained, but moderately active individuals, the most consistent SWS changes are seen for trained athletes (Horne, 1981).

Table 5
Processes Hypothesized to Mediate the Psychological Benefits of Exercise

Psychological
  Anxiety
    Diversion
    Social reinforcement
    Mastery experience
    Changes in the somatic symptoms of anxiety
  Depression
    Diversion
    Social reinforcement
    Mastery experience
Physiological
  Anxiety
    Improved response to stress
      Muscle tension
      Heart rate
      Skin conductance
      Catecholamines
      Glucocorticoids
      Lactate
  Depression
    Increased neurotransmission of catecholamines
    Increased endogenous opiates

From Hughes, J.R. (1984). Psychological effects of habitual aerobic exercise: A critical review. *Preventive Medicine, 13,* 74.

These modifications in SWS are believed to result from the greater energy expenditure in an exercise session by athletes. The few acute studies of ultra-endurance runs, however, show mixed results (Shapiro, Bortz, Mitchell, Bartel, Jooste, 1981; Torsvall, Åkerstedt, & Lindbeck, 1984). Although the SWS of trained athletes, under typical conditions, seems consistently to benefit from acute exercise, and the trained can experience disrupted sleep when they abstain from training (Baekeland, 1970), it is not established that these effects are due to habitual activity history rather than to intrinsic personality or biological characteristics that might predispose athletes both to chronic exercise and to enhanced SWS after acute exercise. Acute comparisons of fit and unfit subjects show that differences in sleep cycles between the groups are not dependent on daily exercise (Paxton, Trinder, & Montgomery, 1983; Trinder, Stevenson, Paxton, & Montgomery, 1982; Trinder, Paxton, Montgomery, & Frasier, 1985). This implies that sleep is more responsive to chronic changes in energy expenditure than to daily variations. However, convincing prospective training studies of initially low fit individuals have not been conducted.

It has been proposed that SWS is more dependent on metabolic needs, while REM sleep is more a function of personality and lifestyle. If so, longitudinal studies of exercise effects should consider individual differences other than fitness alone. The question of mechanisms whereby exercise may facilitate sleep remains unresolved, but it is likely that both energy expenditure and central nervous system characteristics or changes are involved. Acute rhythmic exercise like running fits psychophysiologic criteria for a relaxation response, and recent evidence of an endogenous pyrogenic effect during vigorous running (Cannon & Kluger, 1983) is consistent with comparative research showing neuroleptic and serotonergic responses to heating of the hypothalamus. Each change has been implicated in aiding sleep. Recent study also suggests that body heating during exercise plays a key role in acute SWS changes among highly fit females who are normal sleepers (Horne & Moore, 1985). Findings collectively suggest the increased body temperature that accompanies running might facilitate sleep through a relaxation response.

Alcohol and Drug Abuse

Excessive use of alcohol or other drugs is a frequent complication of mental stress and disorders. Not only can it be a symptom of underlying problems (e.g. low self-esteem, life stress, anxiety, and depression), but substance abuse can precipitate or exacerbate a psychiatric episode in some instances. Amphetamine-induced psychosis, for example, has long been an experimental and theoretical model for the study of schizophrenia.

The etiology of substance abuse remains controversial, but it seems to stem from multiple biological and environmental causes. Ten million American adults are chronic abusers of alcohol and drugs, but less than 20% will seek professional treatment (Shapiro et al., 1984). Treatment for alcoholism can involve drug therapy, psychotherapy, and behavior modification, but social support seems to be crucial for maintaining abstinence once a commitment to change has been made. Because alcoholics can experience reversible neuropathology, hyperarousal, somatic complaints, and respond well to social reinforcement, exercise has frequently been mentioned as a treatment adjunct.

Exercise and alcohol abuse. There have been few studies reported, however, about the effects exercise programs can have on either the personality, symptoms, or behaviors of alcoholics. The typical study has been a chronic training program with hospital inpatients, so little is known about the role of exercise in the prevention of alcohol abuse and relapse after treatment or in the acute management of symptoms. In an uncontrolled case report, fitness increases were accompanied by reduced clinical signs of neuropathology for 25 male inpatients after a 10-month recreational basketball program was introduced (Tsukue & Shohoji, 1981). Because the fitness changes seen were based on performance tests and not physiological capacities, and no attempt was made to correlate them with clinical improvement, the outcomes seen can be equally attributed to a change in environment rather than exercise effects. Another uncontrolled case report of 214 men included aerobics and calisthenics, one hour daily, in an 84-day inpatient rehabilitation program (Frankel & Murphy, 1974). A relationship was seen between an increased score on Cureton's Illinois Test of Physical Fitness and decreases in the depression scale of the MMPI. Because the fitness test was again based on performance, these outcomes could also be attributable to a generalized motivation effect, rather than exercise. Another study randomly assigned 20 male inpatients to continued treatment in the alcoholic ward or to 20 miles of jogging over a 20 day period (Gary & Guthrie, 1972). A physiological increase in fitness (decreased post-exercise heart rate) was correlated slightly with changes in self-satisfaction and body-satisfaction, but only self-satisfaction increased. This pattern of change with fitness suggests the outcomes resulted from more than just a novel intervention, but they still could stem in part from an expectancy of benefits or altered autonomic nervous system arousal due to abstinence rather than increased metabolic fitness. None of these studies measured abstinence or maintenance of abstinence after leaving the treatment center.

More recently, however, Sinyor, Brown, Rostant, and Seraganian (1982) introduced a six-week program of stretching, calisthenics, and Cooper's 12-minute walk-run five days per week to 58 male and female inpatients. Decreases in resting pulse and body fat and increased $\dot{V}O_2$ maximum (Åstrand-Ryhming estimate) accompanied training. Cross-sectional comparisons conducted three months after treatment suggested a higher than expected abstinence rate for the exercise group compared to pretreatment rates. Because patients who had been medically screened from vigorous exercise, but participated at lower intensity, showed no change in fitness, the results were unlikely to stem only from expectations of benefit or novelty or from spurious changes in heart rate responsivity due to drug withdrawal. However, abstinence comparisons were not made beween low active and high active participants.

There are not enough studies from which conclusions can be drawn, but it seems that exercise programs might offer a useful adjunct for the rehabilitation of chronic alcohol abusers by (a) increased stress tolerance, (b) reduced anxiety or depression, (c) increased acceptability to change, (d) increased acceptability to ongoing treatments such as psychotherapy, (e) decreased somatic symptoms, or (f) restructuring and scheduling of leisure time in a way that may generalize to an easier transition to social roles outside the hospital (Sinyor et al., 1982).

Exercise, Prevention, and Wellness

A focus on clinical popluations is warranted because of the prevalence of mental disorders and the incomplete effectiveness of conventional treatments. An exclusively clinical view obscures, however, the potential that exercise may offer for helping *prevent* mental illness and emotional problems and for promoting the health of population segments who already are within normal parameters but wish to optimize mental or emotional development. This perspective has been endorsed by the World Health Organization in the definition of health as "a state of complete physical, mental, and social well-being and not merely the absence of infirmity." Regular physical activity seems intimately linked with modern day conceptions of high level *wellness*, defined by Halbert Dunn, former chief of the National Office of Vital Statistics, as "an integrated method of functioning which is oriented toward maximizing the potential of which the individual is capable, within the environment where he (sic) is functioning." According to Dunn (1959), high level wellness involves:

> (1) direction in progress forward and upward towards a higher potential of functioning, (2) an open-ended and ever-expanding tomorrow with its challenge to live at a fuller potential, and (3) the integration of the whole being of the total individual—body, mind, and spirit—in the functioning process (p. 447).

A view that encompasses optimal health, not just avoidance of illness, is equally important for describing the role of exercise for mental health in the public. It expands our focus in ways consistent with the over arching theme of this monograph, "well-being."

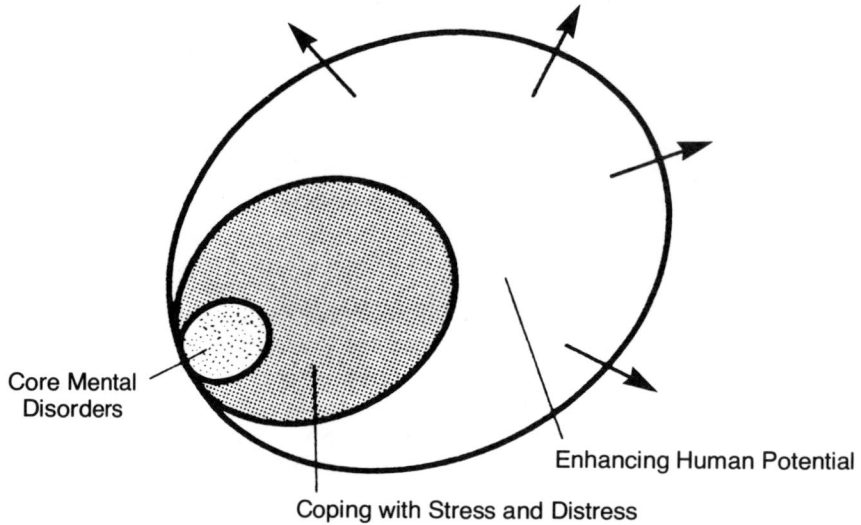

Fig. 5. Boundaries between mental illness and mental health. From Klerman, G.L. & Weissman, M.M. (1984). An epidemiologic view of mental illness, mental health, and normality. In *Normality and the Life Cycle: A Critical Integration,* edited by Daniel Offer and Melvin Sabshin. Copyright © 1984 by Basic Books, Inc., Publishers. Reprinted with permission of the publisher.

Population Studies

Cross-sectional population samples in the United States and Canada confirm an association between physical activity and feelings of subjective well-being. *The Perrier Study: Fitness in America* sampled 1,510 representative American adults 18 years and older in 1978 (Harris, 1979). Based on energy equivalence estimates from self-reported activity, 15% were classified as high actives in vigorous exercise and sports (about 1500 weekly Calories), 16% were moderately active, 28% were low active, while 41% were not active. In all instances where high actives were contrasted with non-actives, the highly active showed a greater rate of endorsement for positive mental health attributes: they usually (a) were not depressed (80% vs. 67%), (b) stood up well under pressure (68% vs. 52%), and were (c) optimistic (67% vs. 43%), (d) outgoing (61% vs. 48%) and (e) relaxed (60% vs. 47%). Non-actives reported more difficulty in sleeping, and were more likely than were the highly active to experience sleep problems at least one night a week (56% vs. 46%) and three or more nights a week (29% vs. 15%).

Because these results were based on self-perceptions and because the active vs. non-active distinction was confounded by age, sex, and income (i.e., high actives tended to be high income men under age 35, while inactives were mostly lower income women over 50), the mental health and exercise pattern is hard to evaluate. The psychological differences might come from characteristics other than activity level. However, when similar comparisons were made between the highly active and low active for whom age, gender, and income were more evenly distributed, mental health responses still favored the highly active. This comparison and the fact that it was based on the benefits people felt they had received, suggests the associations seen were not solely because of other characteristics of the highly active brought to exercise but, in part, stemmed from the activity.

Similar findings come from the *American Health* (1984) survey of more than 1,000 American adults 18 years and older. About 54% spent some time each week exercising and this differed little between gender. Gender also made little difference in psychological responses. About two in three who reported weekly exercise said it made them more relaxed, while 19% felt no difference. Twenty percent reported an improved relationship with a spouse or loved one, but 69% saw no change, while exercise was a source of conflict for 4%. Similarly, 45% felt those who exercise become more confident, while 16% believed exercisers become too self-involved and 29% perceived no change.

The more controlled *Canada Fitness Survey* (1983) sampled 22,000 Canadians aged 10 and above in 1981 and provides more compelling population evidence about activity patterns and mental health. A standardized test of overall happiness, Bradburn's Index of Psychological Well-being, was positively associated with activity level, and this did not differ for age or gender. The active (age 20 years and over) were more likely to rate their overall health as very good (23%) than were the moderately active (17%) and sedentary groups (14%), but the tendency of both the active and the moderately active to view their emotional well-being as positive (74% and 70%) was even more striking when contrasted with the sedentary (55%).

Associations between physical activity and mental health in the population assume added significance when they are viewed in the context of American attitudes toward mental health care. According to the General Mills *Amercian Family Report* (1979) which surveyed more than 1,200 households in 1978, 51% of adults felt that mental illness was a health problem, but 31% believed it was a personal emotional weakness. Six in ten adults agreed that people should try to solve their own problems, while saving a visit to a psychiatrist or psychologist as a last resort. In most cases for sleep disorders (76%), depression (59%), anxiety (55%), and alcohol abuse (48%), people reported they would handle the problem alone or would wait a while before seeing a doctor.

There seems to be an attitudinal climate receptive to alternative or preventive mental health care. Although this can undoubtedly represent an unhealthful view for many who need and would benefit from professional care, it also confirms that self-help behaviors such as exercise can be a preferred and useful coping strategy in many instances.

A Research Agenda

When representative surveys of the population are viewed with correlational and experimental studies of small self-selected samples, a positive association between chronic physical activity and mental health consistently emerges. And, it appears to exceed the known risks of exercise. However, evidence on clinically diagnosed populations is limited and not compelling. Only depression and self-esteem appear predictably enhanced, but the effects do not exceed other psychological or behavioral interventions. Individuals scoring in the normal range on standardized tests of mental disorders typically show no changes after exercise training. Only state anxiety and tension are predictably lowered after acute exercise. In several ways these facts seem to undermine a scientific evaluation of physical activity as an effective mental health behavior. At the same time they can misleadingly obscure the importance for the normal population of *feeling well* and the potential impact of exercise for coping with life stress in ways that prevent or buffer more dramatic disorders (Howard, Cunningham, & Rechnitzer, 1984; Kobasa, Maddi, & Pucetti, 1982; Kobasa, Maddi, Pucetti, & Zola, 1985; Roth & Holmes, 1985).

To resolve this confusion, future population descriptions must focus on important variables, while small sample experiments test more than one explanation at a time. Studies will have to pay more attention to specific definitions of mental health and physical activity. It seems unlikely that all types, volumes, and settings of exercise will affect all aspects of mental health for all people. While early taxonomies (Campbell & Davis, 1939-1940) for matching diagnosis with activity offer little help, they provide a startling illustration that we know little more today about tailoring exercise to the mental health needs of individuals than we knew 50 years ago when physical education programs were commonplace in psychiatric care.

Table 6
Table of Suggestive Activities For More Specific Application to Disease Entities[a].

Description	Informal Activities / Disease Entities
Baseball or Volleyball	For functional types particularly dementia praecox[b] cases and manic depressive cases.
Golf	For both organic and inorganic cases. An important type of activity serving as transitional activity to higher levels. One response activity, for those organic cases who can realize steps of motor improvement.
Handball	A one response type of activity for both functional and organic cases who are able to participate in a strenuous form of exercise.
Tennis	A combination of one and many response activity suitable for all types of the more alert categories; a valuable transitional form of exercise for the patient who is able to advance from one response to many response play.
Calisthenics	Mechanical forms of activity, especially adapted for those who cannot enter into more socialized game projects.
Swimming	(a) For both fundamental and organic types as a general conditioning exercise. (b) As an aid in differential diagnosis of distortion or restriction of movements due to hysteria or organic causes. (c) As a therapeutic aid in overcoming negativism.

[a]Adapted from Campbell & Davis (1939-40). *American Journal of Psychiatry.* 96, p. 931.
[b]Now diagnosed as Schizophrenia

More important than specifying exercise types and distinguishing between mental health variables based on cognitive, behavioral, or emotional *symptoms*, attention must be paid to causes: precipitating histories, premorbid personalities, and present day life events. The past focus on one-directional outcomes must grow to encompass processes and their paths. Initial test scores, exposure to exercise, and measurement of changes— the method of the past— describes an impact but cannot explain it or predict it for others. Determining the efficacy of exercise as a mental health behavior will minimally require experimental contrasts with other interventions and no-treatment controls, but exercise studies must more fully consider the etiology of the intervention target. This has been poorly done in the past, and the inclusion in this chapter of contemporary theoretical models for major disorders is an attempt to help resolve this shortcoming for future study and practical applications.

Health Status

The behavioral or psychiatric meaning is poorly established for many of the self-reports used in population surveys of exercise patterns. Likewise, most standardized tests of mental health were designed and validated for their ability to predict responses of a magnitude or frequency indicative of abnormal behaviors and extreme social or psychological adjustment. Their sensitivity is not well established for detecting thoughts and feelings that, while not disruptive in noticable ways, may diminish a productive and enjoyable life. Diagnostic categories (e.g. DSM-III) are useful to clinicians because they describe symptoms in an organized way and suggest treatments. But they usually have little theoretical basis for treatment and stem more from observational consensus among psychiatrists than from empirical evidence about underlying origins (etiology) of the behavioral and emotional syndromes seen (Eysenck, Wakefield, & Friedman, 1983). Although their reliability is comparable with medical diagnoses in general, forcing a mental health dichotomy upon a true continuum will unavoidably create borderline cases that do not fit neatly into categories of symptoms and treatments (Akiskal, 1981). People are usually not absolutely sick or healthy, they are sick or healthy relative to other people or other conditions that have their own continua, such as longevity. This is illustrated by neurobiology studies showing that the patterning of depressive personality with neurotransmitters seen in some types of clinically diagnosed depression is similar in form (though less in magnitude) for people diagnosed as normal (Post & Ballenger, 1984). These patterns can be positively influenced in normal adult males following an exercise program (Chodzko-Zjako & Ismail, 1984; Sothmann, Ismail, & Chodzko-Zjako, 1984).

Tests that measure or scale these continua in a way that is standardized across people allow abnormal extremes to be defined by contrasts with shared attributes and experiences. Only in this way can the origins of disorders be traced. For these reasons, studies of exercise outcomes with clinically diagnosed groups must be described by standardized scales as well as objective clinical categories, before their psychiatric meaning can be fully interpreted.

There also remains a question of self-selection bias in the exercise and mental health asociation seen in the population base. Are mentally or emotionally troubled people less able or less motivated to be physically active? If so, mental health might lead to activity rather than activity leading to mental health. While it is likely that each explanation is the case to some degree, the controlled longitudinal trial required to resolve the issue has not been conducted within a population sample.

The exertional and achievement components of physical activity must also be better quantified and distinguished from setting and social reinforcement effects if standardized explanations and applications are sought. The degree to which outcomes are due to expectations by participants of benefits or costs must be determined if the efficacy seen can be effectively delivered to others who could potentially benefit from physical activity.

Age and Gender

We also know little of how exercise effects may differ for gender and various age groups. There are not sufficient studies using similar methods, measures, and types of activity with males and females of different ages to allow comparisons (Blumenthal, Schocken, & Needles, 1982; Gruber, 1986). However, the prevalence rates of mental disorders and the sources of life stress vary according to gender and age (Aylward, 1985; Oakes, 1984; Offer & Sabshin, 1984). Self-comparisons with the standards of others and self-expectations vary with age and are important to psychological and social adjustment. It follows that their impact on mental health will vary across the age span. Life events and daily hassles also contribute to mental stress and may have different sources and impacts for males and females at various ages. Although the epidemiology of life stress is not well developed, it is believed that each stage in the life cycle includes risks for developing psychopathology. Transitions from stage to stage are frequently associated with acute episodes of depression, anxiety, alcohol and substance use, and visits to health care professionals (Offer & Sabshin, 1984).

Adjustment to these transitions or failure to develop behavioral and social skills or to accept the roles of vocational, familial, or social responsibilities can increase mental health risk. While the mental health outcomes may be similar across ages and gender, the origins of stress will likely vary and these may determine preferred strategies for coping or intervening. The clinical impact on individuals can be great even when overall group rates for age and gender do not differ. Failure to consider these patterns may obscure positive effects of exercise or prevent its appropriate use.

A national task force on women's mental health needs (American Psychological Association, 1985) recently concluded that the mental health needs of women are different from those of men. Although it has been suggested that the DSM-III categories for diagnosis and treatment falsely ascribe more mental illness to women because of social stereotypes, a recent analysis argues that meaningful differences exist between the genders at all age levels and must be considered in choosing effective treatment (Oakes, 1984). In childhood, for example, boys are as much as 10 times as likely as girls to show disorders relating to attention deficits, anxiety, and sleep. During adolescence, the prevalence of schizoid disorder is higher for boys, but 95% of anorexia cases are female. Females also experience more bulimia. Adult females have higher rates of depression, anxiety, and somatic complaints than males. But males show more alcohol abuse and personality disorders. Schizophrenia is equally prevalent in each gender but the time of onset differs. Males typically have episodes during childhood and adolescence, while the over-35 age group shows highest rates for women.

Table 7
Sex Differences in Schizophrenia

Male	Female
Occurs at earlier age	Better work record
Related to high adolescent stress	Better social skills
Higher relapse rate	Less chronicity
	Late onset
	Better response to neuroleptics

From Oakes, R. (1984). Sex patterns in DSM-III: Bias or basis for theory development? *American Psychologist,* 1320-1322.

Table 8
Schizophrenia Prevalence by Developmental Level and Sex

Level	Male to female ratio
Childhood	3:1
Adolescence	2:1
Early adulthood	1:1
Over 35 years	2:3

From Oakes, R. (1984). Sex patterns in DSM-III: Bias or basis for theory development? *American Psychologist,* 1320-1322.

Although it appears exercise outcomes are equally beneficial for males and females (Morgan & Goldston, in press), the reasons may differ and the role of exercise compared with other interventions may be more important for one gender at a certain age. If so, physical activity can be expected to exert its impact on mental health in different ways according to interactions between gender, age, and health status across the life span.

Summary

Two in ten American adults will experience a psychiatric episode during a year, yet only 20% of those who suffer will seek professional care. Although a costly decision for some, most people with mild to moderate problems prefer to handle them alone; they view a psychiatrist or psychologist as a last resort and usually seek first a primary care physician. This illustrates that people need to develop personal coping skills for life stress and some mental disorders.

Anxiety, alcohol and drug abuse, depression, and schizophrenia are our most prevalent disorders. Drug therapy, psychotherapy, and behavior modification can be effective for many, but recurrence is common. To cope with periodic stress, most people will also benefit from self-help skills such as exercise.

Many physicians prescribe physical activity for depression, tension, and chemical dependence, but they are just as likely to prescribe drugs which can have unpleasant or even dangerous side effects. For some, exercise is a low risk alternative.

Moderately intense, graduated aerobic exercise is a useful therapy for moderate depression and temporary reductions in state anxiety or tension. It can be as effective as psychotherapy, group counseling, or meditation. Distracting rest is also useful for anxiety and tension. Some types of non-aerobic exercise may also be effective, but they have not been well studied.

Fitness training conducted by qualified professionals offers little risk for psychiatric patients suffering from moderate depression, panic disorders, schizophrenia, or chemical dependence. How it works to enhance treatment is not well studied and is poorly understood, but in some instances aerobic fitness training is a useful adjunct to the primary therapy.

Self-esteem is important for mental health and low levels are often linked with anxiety, depression, and substance abuse. Fitness training and group exercise programs can increase self-esteem by social reinforcement or by fostering real or perceived gains in fitness or ability for those who value them highly.

Gains in self-esteem with exercise may be more likely in children than adults because attributes other than physical successes become more valued as we age. How much the importance of exercise and fitness to total self-esteem changes as we age is unknown, but it remains a strong influence for many middle-aged and elderly adults.

Habitual exercise can become abusive if it assumes a compulsive priority over one's adaptive roles in society and the family, over personal development in other areas, or over physical health. This happens infrequently, and probably signals a problem of an imbalanced self-identity. Commitment to exercise is a separate entity from eating disorders.

Mental health gains for children, particularly increased self-esteem, accompany fitness training with little risk. This reinforces the mental health importance of regular exercise habits already believed important for cardiovascular health.

The Public Health Service 1990 objective of 90% participation in regular health-related exercise by children and youth (with 60% daily participation in public school physical education classes) will likely not be met without intervention (Dishman, Sallis, & Orenstein, 1985). The association between physical activity and mental health is sufficiently strong to warrant a stronger emphasis by government agencies, schools, and physicians on childhood fitness and exercise skills that can motivate participation in adulthood.

According to the National Institute of Mental Health workshop on exercise (Morgan & Goldston, in press) available scientific evidence indicates:

1. Physical fitness is positively associated with mental health and well-being.

2. Exercise is associated with the reduction of stress emotions such as state anxiety.

3. Anxiety and depression are common symptoms of failure to cope with

mental stress, and exercise has been associated with a decreased level of mild to moderate depression and anxiety.

4. Long-term exercise is usually associated with reductions in traits such as neuroticism and anxiety.

5. Severe depression usually requires professional treatment, which may include medication, electroconvulsive therapy, and/or psychotherapy, with exercise as an adjunct.

6. Appropriate exercise results in reductions in various stress indices such as neuromuscular tension, resting heart rate, and some stress hormones.

7. Current clinical opinion holds that exercise has beneficial emotional effects across all ages and in both genders.

8. Physically healthy people who require psychotropic medication may safely exercise when exercise and medications are titrated under close medical supervision.

The mechanisms whereby mental health outcomes accompany exercise are not confirmed, and who will benefit under what circumstances remains poorly defined. Biological and cognitive-emotional changes through both exertional and social means are all likely contributors. It is also likely that some people are more prone than others to be active and to benefit, but the associations of activity and health are not merely due to the fact that mentally healthy people choose to be active while the unhealthy choose to be sedentary. Regular physical activity represents one effective, low-cost, low-risk behavior that can not only help prevent mental illness, but can promote mental health.

References

Akiskal, H.S. (1981). Subaffective disorders: Dysthymic, cyclothymic, and bipolar II disorders in the "borderline" realm. *Psychiatric Clinics of North America, 4,* 25-46.

Akiskal, H.S., & McKinney, W.T. (1975). Overview of recent research in depression: Integration of ten conceptual models into a comprehensive clinical frame. *Archives of General Psychiatry, 32,* 285-305.

American Health (1984). *Public attitudes and behavior related to exercise.* Princeton, NJ: The Gallup Organization, Inc.

American Psychological Association (1985). *Developing a national agenda to address women's mental health needs.* Washington, DC: author.

Aylward, G.P. (1985). Understanding and treatment of childhood depression. *The Journal of Pediatrics, 107,* 1-9.

Baekeland, F. (1970). Exercise deprivation. *Archives of General Psychiatry, 22,* 365-369.

Bahrke, M.S., & Morgan, W.P. (1978). Anxiety reduction following exercise and meditation. *Cognitive Therapy and Research, 2,* 323-333.

Balog, L. (1983). The effects of exercise on muscle tension and subsequent muscle relaxation training. *Research Quarterly for Exercise and Sport, 54,* 119-125.

Barchas, J.O. & Freedman, D.X. (1963). Brain amines: Response to physiological stress. *Biochemical Pharmacology, 12,* 1232-1235.

Barta, A., Yashpal, K., & Henry, J.L. (1981). Regional redistribution of B-endorphin in the rat brain: The effect of stress. *Proceedings of the Canadian College of Neuropsychopharmacology,* p. 44.

Beck, A. (1976). *Cognitive therapy and emotional disorders.* New York: International University Press.

Berger, B.G. & Owen, D.R. (1983). Mood alteration with swimming. *Psychosomatic Medicine, 45,* 425-433.

Berkman, L.F., & Syme, S.L. (1979). Social networks, host resistance, and mortality: A nine-year follow-up of Alameda county residents. *American Journal of Epidemiology, 109,* 186-204.

Bliss, E.L. & Ailion, J. (1971). Relationship of stress and activity to brain dopamine and homovanillic acid. *Life Sciences, 10,* 1161-1169.

Blumenthal, J.A., Rose, S., & Chang, J.L. (1985). Anorexia nervosa and exercise: Implications from recent findings. *Sports Medicine, 2,* 237-247.

Blumenthal, J.A., Williams, R.S., Needels, T.L. & Wallace, A.G. (1982). Psychological changes accompany aerobic exercise in healthy middle-aged adults. *Psychosomatic Medicine, 44,* 529-536.

Blumental, J.A., Schocken, D.D., & Needels, T.L. (1982). Psychological and physiological effects of physical conditioning on the elderly. *Journal of Psychosomatic Research, 26,* 505-510.

Branch, L.G., & Jette, A.M. (1984). Personal health practices and mortality among the elderly. *American Journal of Public Health, 74,* 1126-1129.

Brown, B.S., Payne, T., Kim, C., Moore, G., Krebs, P., & Martin, W. (1979). Chronic response of rat brain norepinephrine and serotonin levels to endurance training. *Journal of Applied Physiology, 46,* 19-23.

Brown, R.A., Ramirez, D.E., & Taub, J.M. (1978). The prescription of exercise for depression. *The Physician and Sportsmedicine, 6,* 34-45.

Buckley, P. (1982). Identifying schizophrenic patients who should not receive medication. *Schizophrenia Bulletin, 8,* 429-432.

Bunnell, D.E., Bevier, W., & Horvath, M. (1983). Effects of exhaustive exercise on the sleep of men and women. *Psychophysiology, 20,* 50-58.

Byrd, O.E. (1963a). The relief of tension by exercise: A survey of medical viewpoints and practices. *Journal of School Health, 33,* 238-239.

Byrd, O.E. (1963b). A survey of beliefs and practices of psychiatrists on the relief of tension by moderate exercise. *Journal of School Health, 33,* 426-427.

Califano, J.A. (1978). *Health, United States, 1978* (DHEW Publication No. PHS 78-1232). Washington, DC: U.S. Government Printing Office.

Califano, J.A. (1979). *Healthy People: The Surgeon General's Report on Health Promotion and Disease Prevention* (DHEW Publication No. 79-55071). Washington, DC: U.S. Government Printing Office.

Campbell, D.D., Davis, J.E. (1939-1940). Report of research and experimentation in exercise and recreational therapy. *American Journal of Psychiatry, 96,* 915-933.

Canada Fitness Survey (1983). *Fitness and Lifestyle in Canada.* Ottawa: Government of Canada, Fitness and Amateur Sport.

Cannon, J.G., & Kluger, M.J. (1983). Endogenous pyrogen activity in human plasma after exercise. *Science, 220,* 617-619.

Chodzko-Zajko, W.J., & Ismail, A.H. (1984). MMPI interscale relationships in middle aged male subjects before and after a eight month fitness program. *Journal of Clinical Psychology, 40,* 163-169.

Collingwood, T.R. (1972). The effects of physical training upon behavior and self attitudes. *Journal of Clinical Psychology, 28,* 583-585.

Collingwood, T.R., & Willett, L. (1971). The effects of physical training upon self-concept and body attitude. *Journal of Clinical Psychology, 27,* 411-412.

Collingwood, T.R., Bernstein, I.H., & Hubbard, D. (1983). Canonical correlation analysis of clinical and psychological data in 4,351 men and women. *Journal of Cardiac Rehabilitation, 3,* 706-711.

Conroy, R.W., Smith, K., & Felthous, A.R. (1982). The value of exercise on a psychiatric hospital unit. *Hospital and Community Psychiatry, 33*(8), 641-645.

Cox, J.P., Evans, J.F. & Jamieson, J.L. (1979). Aerobic power and tonic heart rate response to psychosocial stressors. *Personality and Social Psychology Bulletin, 5,* 160-163.

Daniels, F.S., & Fernhall, B. (1984). Continuous EEG measurement to determine the onset of a relaxation response during a prolonged run. *Medicine and Science in Sports and Exercise, 16* (abstract), 182.

Darabos, B.L., & Bulbulian, R. (1986). Motor neuron excitability: The Hoffman reflex following exercise at high and low intensity. *Medicine and Science in Sports and Exercise, 18*(2), Supplement (abstract) 221.

deVries, H.A. (1982). Tranquilizer effect of exercise. *The Physician and Sportsmedicine, 9,* 92-99.

deVries, H.A., & Adams, G.M. (1972). Electromyographic comparison of single doses of exercise and meprobamate as to effects on muscular relaxation. *American Journal of Physical Medicine, 51,* 130-141.

deVries, H.A., Simard, C.P., & Wiswell, R.A., (1982). Fusimotor system involvement in the tranquilizer effect of exercise. *American Journal of Physical Medicine, 61,* 111-122.

deVries, H.A., Wiswell, R.A., Bulbulian, R., & Moritani, T. (1981). Tranquilizer effect of exercise. *American Journal of Physical Medicine, 60,* 57-66.

deVries, H.A., Burke, R., & Hooper, R.T. (1977). Efficacy of EMG biofeedback in relaxation training. *American Journal of Physical Medicine, 56,* 75-81.

Dienstbier, R., Crabbe, J., & Johnson, G.U. (1981). Exercise and stress tolerance. In M.H. Sacks & M.L. Sachs (Eds.), *Psychology of Running* (pp. 192-210). Champaign, IL: Human Kinetics Publishers.

Dishman, R.K. (Ed.). (In press). *Exercise Adherence and Public Health.* Champaign, IL: Human Kinetics Publishers.

Dishman, R.K. (1985). Medical psychology in exercise and sport. *Medical Clinics of North America, 69,* 123-143.

Dishman, R.K., Sallis, J.F., & Orenstein, D. (1985). The determinants of physical activity and exercise. *Public Health Reports, 100,* 158-171.

Dishman, R.K., & Gettman, L.R. (1981). Psychological vigor and self-perceptions of increased strength. *Medicine and Science in Sports and Exercise, 13* (abstract), 75.

Dodson, L.L. & Mullens, W.R. (1969). Some effects of jogging on psychiatric hospital patients. *American Corrective Therapy Journal, 33,* 120-134.

Doyne, E.S., Chambless, D.L. & Beutler, L.E. (1983). Aerobic exercise as a treatment for depression in women. *Behavior Therapy, 14,* 434-440.

Driscoll, R. (1976). Anxiety reduction using physical exertion and positive images. *Psychological Record, 26,* 87-94.

Dunn, H.L. (1959). What high-level wellness means. *Canadian Journal of Public Health, 50,* 447-457.

Eisenberg, L., & Parron, D. (1979). *Strategies for the prevention of mental disorders* (DHEW Publication No. PHS 79-55071A). Washington, DC: U.S. Government Printing Office.

Erdman, R.A., & Duivenvoorden, H.J. (1983). Psychologic evaluation of a cardiac rehabilitation program: A randomized clinical trial in patients with myocardial infarction. *Journal of Cardiac Rehabilitation, 3,* 696-704.

Eysenck, H.J., Wakefield, J.A., & Friedman, A.F. (1983). Diagnosis and clinical assessment: The DSM-III. *Annual Review of Psychology, 34,* 167-193.

Eysenck, H.J., Nias, D.K.B., & Cox, D.N. (1982). Sport and personality. *Advances in Behavioral Research and Therapy, 4,* 1-55.

Farmer, P.K., Olewine, D.A., & Comer, D.W. (1978). Frontalis muscle tension and occipital alpha production in young males with coronary prone (type A) and coronary resistant (type B) behavior patterns. *Medicine and Science in Sports and Exercise, 10* (abstract), 51.

Farrell, P.A., Gates, W.K., Maksud, M.G., & Morgan, W.P. (1982). Increases in plasma B-endorphin/B-lipotropin immunoreactivity after treadmill running in humans. *Journal of Applied Physiology: Respiratory, Environmental, and Exercise Physiology, 52,* 1245-1246.

Farrell, P.A., Gates, W.K., Morgan, W.P., & Pert, C.R. (1983). Plasma leucine enkephalinlike radioreceptor activity and tension-anxiety before and after competitive running. In H.G. Knuttgen, J.A. Vogel, and J. Poortmans (Eds.), *Biochemistry of Exercise* (pp. 637-644). Champaign, IL: Human Kinetics Publishers.

Fernhall, B., & Daniels, F.S. (1984). Electroencephalographic changes after a prolonged running period: Evidence for a relaxation response. *Medicine and Science in Sports and Exercise, 16* (abstract), 181.

Folkins, C.H. (1976). Effects of physical training on mood. *Journal of Clinical Psychology, 32,* 385-388.

Folkins, C.H., Lynch, S. & Gardner, M.M. (1972). Psychological fitness as a function of physical fitness. *Archives of Physical Medicine and Rehabilitation, 53,* 503-508.

Folkins, C.H., & Sime, W.F. (1981). Physical fitness training and mental health. *American Psychologist, 35,* 373-389.

Frankel, A., & Murphy, J. (1974). Physical fitness and personality in alcoholism: Canonical analysis of pre- and post-treatment measures. *Quarterly Journal of Studies on Alcohol, 35,* 1272-1278.

Gary, V., & Guthrie, D. (1972). The effect of jogging on physical fitness and self-concept in hospitalized alcoholics. *Quarterly Journal of Studies on Alcohol, 33,* 1073-1078.

General Mills (1979). *American family report, 1978-1979: Family health in an era of stress.* New York: Yankelovich, Skelly, and White, Inc.

Gilman, A.G., Goodman, L.S., & Gilman, A. (Eds.). (1984). *Goodman and Gilman's: The Pharmacological Basis of Therapeutics,* (7th Edition). New York: Macmillan.

Gimino, F.A., & Levin, S.J. (1984). The effects of aerobic exercise on perceived self-image in post-hospitalized schizophrenic patients. *Medicine and Science in Sports and Exercise, 16* (abstract), 139.

Goff, D. & Dimsdale, J.E. (1985). The psychologic effects of exercise. *Journal of Cardiopulmonary Rehabilitation, 5,* 234-240.

Gorman, J.M., Levy, G.F., Liebowitz, M.R., McGrath, P., Appleby, I.L., Dillon, D.J., Davies, S.O., & Klein, D.F. (1983). Effect of acute *b*-Adrenergic blockade on lactate-induced panic. *Archives of General Psychiatry, 40,* 1079-1082.

Greist, J.H., Klein, M.H., Eischens, R.R., Faris, M. Gurman, A., & Morgan, W.P. (1979). Running as a treatment for depression. *Comprehensive Psychiatry, 20,* 41-54.

Gruber, J. (1986). Physical activity and self-esteem development in children: A meta-analysis. In G.A. Stull and H.M. Eckhardt (Eds.), *Effects of Physical Activity on Children: Papers of the American Academy of Physical Education, 19* (pp. 30-48). Champaign, IL: Human Kinetics Publishers.

Haier, R.J., Quaid, B.A., & Mills, J.S. (1981). Naloxone alters pain perception after jogging. *Psychiatry Research, 5,* 231-232.

Hamburg, D.L., Elliott, G.R. & Parron, D.L. (1982). *Health and behavior: Frontiers of research in the biobehavioral sciences, Institute of Medicine.* Washington, DC: National Academy Press.

Harber, V.J. & Sutton, J.R. (1984). Endorphins and exercise. *Sports Medicine, 1,* 154-171.

Harris, L. (1979). *The Perrier Study: Fitness in America.* New York: Perrier-Great Waters of France, Inc.

Harris, P. (1981). *Health, United States, 1980* (DHHS Publication No. PHS 81-1232). Washington, DC: U.S. Government Printing Office.

Hellhammer, D.H., Hingtgen, J.N., Wade, S.A., Shea, P.A., & Aprison, M.II. (1983). Serotonergic changes in specific areas of rat brain associated with activity-stress lesions. *Psychosomatic Medicine, 45,* 115-122.

Hilyer, J.C., & Mitchell, W. (1979). Effect of systematic physical fitness training combined with counseling on the self concept of college students. *Journal of*

Counseling Psychology, 26, 427-436.

Hippius, H., & Winokur, G. (Eds.). (1983). *Psychopharmacology 1: Clinical psychopharmacology.* Amsterdam: Excerpta Medica.

Hodgson, T.A., & Kopstein, A. (1984). *Health care expenditures 1981* (HCFA Publication No. 03146). Washington, DC: U.S. Government Printing Office.

Hollister, L.E. (1983). Insomnia: An introduction. *Journal of Clinical Psychopharmacology, 3,* 127-128.

Horne, J.A. (1981). The effects of exercise upon sleep: A critical review. *Biological Psychology, 12,* 241-290.

Horne, J.A. & Moore, V.J. (1985). Sleep EEG effects of exercise with and without additional body cooling. *Electroencephalography and Clinical Neurophysiology, 60,* 33-38.

Howard, J.H., Cunningham, D.A. & Rechnitzer, P.A. (1984). Physical activity as a moderator of life events and somatic complaints: A longitudinal study. *Canadian Journal of Applied Sport Sciences, 9,* 194-200.

Hughes, J.R. (1984). Psychological effects of habitual aerobic exercise: A critical review. *Preventive Medicine, 13,* 66-78.

Hull, E.M., Young, S.H., & Ziegler, M.G. (1984). Aerobic fitness affects cardiovascular and catecholamine responses to stressors. *Psychophysiology, 21,* 353-360.

Jankowski, K. (1976). Psychotherapic, Pharmocotherapic and sportherapic bei emotional gestorten Jugendicken: Eirne vergleichende analyse von Stationarer und Ambulanter Therapic mit hilfe Physiologischer and Psychologisher. *Methoden Klin Psychologia, Psychotherapie, 24,* 251-255.

Jasnowski, M.L. Holmes, D.S., Soloman, S. & Aguiar, C. (1981). Exercise, changes in aerobic capacity, and changes in self-perceptions: An experimental investigation. *Journal of Research in Personality, 15,* 460-466.

Johnson, T.H., & Tharp, G.D. (1974). The effect of chronic exercise on reserpine-induced gastric ulceration in rats. *Medicine and Science in Sports, 6,* 188-190.

Kavanagh, T., Shephard, R.J., Tuck, J.A., & Qureshi, S. (1977). Depression following myocardial infarction: The effects of distance running. *Annals of the New York Academy of Sciences, 301,* 1029-1038.

Keller, S. (1980). Physical fitness hastens recovery from emotional stress. *Medicine and Science in Sports and Exercise, 12* (abstract), 118.

Keller, S. & Seraganian, P. (1984). Physical fitness level and autonomic reactivity to psychosocial stress. *Journal of Psychosomatic Research, 28,* 279-287.

Klein, M.H., Greist, J.H., Gurman, A.S. Neimeyer, R.A., Lesser, D.P., Bushnell, N.J. & Smith, R.E. (1985). A comparative outcome study of group psychotherapy vs. exercise treatments for depression. *International Journal of Mental Health, 13* (3-4), 148-177.

Kobasa, S.C., Maddi, S., & Puccetti, M.C. (1982). Personality and exercise as buffers in the stress-illness relationship. *Journal of Behavioral Medicine, 5,* 391-404.

Kobasa, S.C., Maddi, S.R., Puccetti, M.C., & Zola, M.A. (1985). Effectiveness of hardiness, exercise, and social support as resources against illness. *Journal of Psychosomatic Research, 29,* 525-533.

Koocher, G.P. (1971). Swimming, competence, and personality change. *Journal of Personality and Social Psychology, 18,* 275-278.

Kostrubala, T. (1976). *The Joy of Running.* New York: J.B. Lippincott.

Kowal, D.M., Patton, J.F., & Vogel, J.A. (1978). Psychological states and aerobic fitness of male and female recruits before and after basic training. *Aviation, Space and Environmental Medicine, 49,* 603-606.

Kuyler, P.L., & Dunner, D.L. (1976). Psychiatric disorders and the need for mental health services among a sample of orthopedic inpatients. *Comprehensive Psychiatry, 17,* 395-400.

Lake, B.W., Suarez, E.C., Schneiderman, N. & Tocci, N. (1985). The type A behavior pattern, physical fitness, and psychophysiological reactivity. *Health Psychology, 4,* 169-187.

Levine, C.D., & Willmer, S.G. (1976). *Mental health statistical note no. 125* (DHEW Publication No. ADM 76-168). Washington, DC: U.S. Government Printing Office.

Liberman, R.P. (1982). What is schizophrenia? *Schizophrenia Bulletin, 8,* 435-437.

Lichtman, S. & Poser, E.G. (1983). The effects of exercise on mood and cognitive functioning. *Journal of Psychosomatic Research, 27,* 43-52.

Light, K.C., Obrist, P.A., & James, S.A. (1984). Self-reported exercise levels and cardiovascular responses during rest and stress. *SPR Abstracts, Psychophysiology, 21,* 586.

Lobitz, W.C., Brammell, H.L., & Stoll, S. (1983). Physical exercise and anxiety management training for cardiac stress management in a non-patient population. *Journal of Cardiac Rehabilitation, 3,* 683-688

Lobstein, D.D., Mosbacher, B.J. & Ismail, A.H. (1983). Depression as a powerful discriminator between physically active and sedentary middle-aged men. *Journal of Psychosomatic Research, 27,* 69-76.

Long, B.L. (1984). Aerobic conditioning and stress inoculation: A comparison of stress-management interventions. *Cognitive Therapy and Research, 8,* 517-522.

Margraf, J., Ehlers, A., & Roth, W.T. (1986). Sodium lactate infusions and panic attacks: A review and critique. *Psychosomatic Medicine, 48,* 23-51.

McCann, I.L. & Holmes, D.S. (1984). Influence of aerobic exercise on depression. *Journal of Personality and Social Psychology, 46,* 1142-1147.

McGowan, C.R., Robertson, R.J., & Epstein, L.H. (1985). The effect of bicycle ergometer exercise at varying intensities on the heart rate, EMG, and mood state responses to a mental arithmetic stressor. *Research Quarterly for Exercise and Sport, 56,* 131-137.

McSherry, J.A. (1984). The diagnostic challenge of anorexia nervosa. *American Family Physician, 29* (2), 141-145.

McPherson, B.D., Paivio, A., & Yuhasz, M.S. (1967). Psychological effects of an exercise program for post-infarct and normal adult men. *Journal of Sports Medicine and Physical Fitness, 7,* 95-102.

Markoff, R.A., Ryan, P., & Young, T. (1982). Endorphins and mood changes in long-distance running. *Medicine and Science in Sports and Exercise, 14,* 11-15.

Matarazzo, J.D., Weiss, S.M., Herd, J.A., Miller, N. & Weiss, S.M. (Eds.) (1984). *Behavioral Health: A handbook of health enhancement and disease prevention.* New York: Wiley Interscience.

Mayou, A. (1983). A controlled trial of early rehabilitation after myocardial infarction. *Journal of Cardiac Rehabilitation, 6,* 387-402.

Meyer, N. (1977). *Mental Health,* Statistical Note No. 138 (NIMH Publication). Washington, DC: U.S. Government Printing Office.

Morgan, W.P. (1974). Exercise and mental disorders. In A.J. Ryan & F.L. Allman (Eds.), *Sports Medicine* (pp. 215-242). New York: Academic Press.

Morgan, W.P. (1982). Psychological effects of exercise. *Behavioral Medicine Update, 4,* 25-30.

Morgan, W.P., & Goldston, S.N. (Eds.) (in press). *Exercise and Mental Health.* Washington, DC: Hemisphere Publishing.

Morgan, W.P. (1985). Affective beneficence of vigorous physical activity. *Medicine and Science in Sports and Exercise, 17,* 94-100.

Morgan, W.P. (1979). Anxiety reduction following acute physical activity. *Psychiatric Annals, 9,* 141-147.

Morgan, W.P. (1979). Negative addiction in runners. *The Physician and Sportsmedicine, 7,* 57-70.

Morgan, W.P. (1970). Physical fitness correlates of psychiatric hospitalization. In

G.S. Kenyon (Ed.), *Contemporary Psychology of Sport* (pp. 315-321). Chicago: Athletic Institute.

Morgan, W.P. (1980). The trait psychology controversy. *Research Quarterly for Exercise and Sport, 50,* 50-76.

Morgan, W.P., Olson, E.B., & Pedersen, N.P. (1982). A rat model of psychopathology for use in exercise science. *Medicine and Science in Sports and Exercise, 14,* 91-100.

Morgan, W.P., and Pollock, M.L. (1978). Physical activity and cardiovascular health: Psychological aspects. In F. Landry and A. Orban (Eds.), *Physical Activity and Human Well-being* (pp. 163-181). Miami: Symposium Specialists.

Morgan, W.P., Roberts, J.A., Brand, F.R., & Feinerman, A.O. (1970). Psychological effect of chronic physical activity. *Medicine and Science in Sports, 2,* 213-217.

Muller, B., & Armstrong, H.E. (1975). A further note on the "running treatment" for anxiety. *Psychotherapy: Theory, Research, and Practice, 12,* 385-387.

Myers, J.K., Weissman, M.M., Tischler, G.L., Holzer, C.E., Leaf, P.J., Orvaschel, H., Anthony, J.L., Boyd, J.H., Burke, J.D., Dramer, M., & Stoltzman, R. (1984). Six-month prevalence of psychiatric disorders in three communities. *Archives of General Psychiatry, 41,* 959-967.

Najem, G.R., Lindenthal, J.J., Louria, D.B., & Thind, I.S. (1980). Epidemiology of Schizophrenia. *Public Health Reviews, 19,* 113-137.

National Center for Health Statistics, H. Koch (1983). *Utilization of psychotropic drugs in office-based ambulatory care.* National Ambulatory Medical Care Survey, 1980 and 1981. Adv. Data from Vital and Health Statistics, No. 90 (DHHS Pub. No. PHS 83-1250). Hyattsville, MD: Public Health Service.

Naughton, J., Bruhn, J.G., & Lategola, M.T. (1968). Effects of physical training on physiologic and behavioral characteristics of cardiac patients. *Archives of Physical Medicine and Rehabilitation, 49,* 131-137.

Oakes, R. (1984). Sex patterns in DSM-III: Bias or basis for theory development? *American Psychologist,* 1320-1322.

Offer, D., & Sabshin, M. (Eds.) (1984). *Normality and the Life Cycle.* New York: Basic Books.

Olson, E.B., & Morgan, W.P. (1982). Rat brain monoamine levels related to behavioral assessment. *Life Sciences, 30,* 2095-2100.

Orwin, A. (1973). The running treatment: A preliminary communication on a new use for an old therapy (physical activity) in the agoraphobic syndrome. *British Journal of Psychiatry, 122,* 175-179.

Orwin, A. (1974). Treatment of a situational phobia—a case for running. *British Journal of Psychiatry, 125,* 95-98.

Pauly, J.T., Palmer, J.A., & Wright, C.C. (1982). The effect of a 14-week employee fitness program on selected physiological and psychological parameters. *Journal of Occupational Medicine, 24,* 457-463.

Paxton, S.J., Trinder, J., & Montgomery, I. (1983). Does aerobic fitness affect sleep? *Psychophysiology, 20,* 320-324.

Peronnet, F., Blier, P., Brisson, G., Diamond, P., Ledoux, M., & Volle, M. (1986). Plasma catecholamines at rest and exercise in subjects with high- and low-trait anxiety. *Psychosomatic Medicine, 48,* 52-58.

Pert, C.B., & Bowie, D.L. (1979). Behavioral manipulations of rats causes alterations in opiate receptor occupancy. In E. Usdin, W.E. Bunney, & N.S. Kline (Eds.), *Endorphins in Mental Health* (pp. 93-104). New York: Oxford University Press.

Poe, R.O., Lowell, F.M., & Fox, H.M. (1966). Depression: Study of 100 cases in a general hospital. *American Medical Association Journal, 195,* 345-350.

Post, R.M. & Ballenger, J.L. (Eds.) (1984). *Neurobiology of mood disorders.* Baltimore: Williams and Wilkins.

Powell, R.R. (1974). Psychological effects of exercise therapy upon institutionalized geriatric mental patients. *Journal of Gerontology, 29,* 157-161.

Prosser, G., Carson, P., & Phillips. (1981). Morale in coronary patients following an exercise program. *Journal of Psychosomatic Research, 25,* 587-593.

Regier, D.A., Myers, J.K., Kramer, M., Robins, L.N., Blazer, D.G., Hough, R.L., Eaton, W.W., & Locke, B.Z. (1984). The NIMH epidemiologic catchment area program. *Archives of General Psychiatry, 41,* 934-941.

Robbins, J.M., & Joseph P. (1985). Experiencing exercise withdrawal: Possible consequences of therapeutic and mastery running. *Journal of Sport Psychology, 7,* 23-39.

Robins, L.N., Helzer, J.E., Weissman, M.M., Orvaschel, H., Gruenberg, E., Burke, J.D., & Regier, D.A. (1984). Lifetime prevalence of specific psychiatric disorders in three sites. *Archives of General Psychiatry, 41,* 949-958.

Rohrbacher, R. (1973). Influence of a special camp program for obese boys on weight loss, self-concept, and body image. *Research Quarterly, 44,* 150-157.

Roskies, E., Seraganian, P., Oseasohn, R., Hanley, J.A., Collu, R., Martin, N., & Smilga, C. (1986). The Montreal Type A Intervention Project: Major findings. *Health Psychology, 5,* 45-69.

Ross, M.A., & Levin, S.J. (1981). The psychological responses of post-hospitalized psychiatric patients to exercise stress testing. In F.J. Nagle & H.J. Montoye (Eds.), *Exercise in Health and Disease* (pp. 276-290). Springfield, IL: C.C. Thomas.

Roth, D.L. & Holmes, D.S. (1985). Influence of physical fitness on determining the impact of stressful life events on physical and psychological health. *Psychosomatic Medicine, 47,* 164-173.

Roviaro, S., Holmes, D.S. & Homsten, R.D. (1984). Influence of a cardiac rehabilitation program on the cardiovascular, psychological, and social functioning of cardiac patients. *Journal of Behavioral Medicine, 7,* 61-81.

Russell, P.O., Epstein, L.H., & Erickson, K.T. (1983). Effects of acute exercise and cigarette smoking on autonomic and neuromuscular responses to a cognitive stressor. *Psychological Reports, 53,* 199-206.

Ryan, E.D. (1981). The emergence of psychological research as related to performance in physical activity. In G.A. Brooks (Ed.), *Perspectives on the academic discipline of physical education* (pp. 327-341). Champaign, IL: Human Kinetics Publishers.

Ryan, A.J. (1984). Exercise and health: Lessons from the past. In H.M. Eckert, & H.J. Montoye (Eds.), *Exercise and Health: American Academy of Physical Education Papers, 17* (pp. 3-13). Champaign, IL: Human Kinetics Publishers.

Sacks, M.H., & Sachs, M.L. (Eds.) (1981). *Psychology of running.* Champaign, IL: Human Kinetics Publishers.

Schwartz, G.E., Davidson, R.J., & Coleman, D. (1978). Patterning of cognitive and somatic processes in the self-regulation of anxiety: Effects of meditation versus exercise. *Psychosomatic Medicine, 40,* 321-328.

Schweiker, R.S. (1981). *Health, United States, 1981.* Washington, DC: U.S. Government Printing Office.

Shamoian, C.A. (1983). Psychogeriatrics. *Medical Clinics of North America, 67,* 361-378.

Shapiro, C.M., Bortz, R., Mitchell, D., Bartel, P., & Jooste, P. (1981). Slow wave sleep: A recovery period after exercise. *Science, 214,* 1253-1254.

Shapiro, S., Skinner, E.A., Kessler, L.G., VonKorff, M., German, P.S., Tischler, G.L., Leaf, P.J., Benham, L., Cottler, L., & Regier, D.A. (1984). Utilization of health and mental health services. *Archives of General Psychiatry, 41,* 971-978.

Shephard, R.J., Kavanagh, T., & Klavora, P. (1985). Mood state during postcoronary cardiac rehabilitation. *Journal of Cardiopulmonary Rehabilitation, 5,* 480-484.

Sidney, K.H., & Shephard, R.J. (1976). Attitudes towards health and physical activity in the elderly: Effects of a physical training program. *Medicine and*

Science in Sports, 8, 246-252.

Sime, W. (1977). A comparison of exercise and meditation in reducing physiological response to stress. *Medicine and Science in Sports, 9* (abstract), 55.

Sime, W. (1984). Psychological benefits of exercise training in the healthy individual. In J.D. Matarazzo, S.M. Weiss, J.A. Herd, & N.E. Miller (Eds.), *Behavioral Health: A handbook of health enhancement and disease prevention* (pp. 488-508). New York: Wiley Interscience.

Sinyor, D., Brown, T., Rostant, L., & Seraganian, P. (1982). The role of a physical fitness program in the treatment of alcoholism. *Journal of Studies on Alcohol, 43*, 380-386.

Sinyor, D., Golden, M., Steinert, Y., & Seraganian, P. (1986). Experimental manipulation of aerobic fitness and the response to psychosocial stress: Heart rate and self-report measures. *Psychosomatic Medicine, 48*, 324-337.

Sinyor, D.A., Schwartz, S.G., Peronnet, F., Brisson, G., & Seraganian, P. (1983). Aerobic fitness level and reactivity to psychosocial stress: Physiological, biochemical, and subjective measures. *Psychosomatic Medicine, 45*, 205-217.

Skinner, B.F., & Vaughan, M.E. (1983). *Enjoy old age*. New York: N.W. Norten.

Smith, W.C., & Figetakis, N. (1970). Some effects of isometric exercise on muscular strength in chronic schizophrenics. *American Corrective Therapy Journal, 24*, 100-107.

Sonstroem, R.J. (1984). Exercise and self-esteem. In R. Terjung (Ed.), *Exercise and Sport Sciences Reviews, 12*, 110-130.

Sothmann, M.S. & Ismail, A.H. (1984). Relationships between urinary catecholamines, metabolites, particularly MHPG, and selected personality and physical fitness characteristics in normal subjects. *Psychosomatic Medicine, 46*, 523-533.

Sothmann, M.S., Ismail, A.H., & Chodzko-Zajko, W.J. (1984). The influence of catecholamine activity on hierarchical associations involving physical fitness and personality. *Journal of Clinical Psychology, 40*, 1308-1317.

Stamford, B.A., Hanbacher, W., & Fallica, A. (1974). Effects of daily exercise on the psychiatric state of institutional geriatric mental patients. *Research Quarterly, 45*, 34-41.

Starzec, J.J., Berger, D.F., & Hesse, R. (1983). Effects of stress and exercise on plasma corticosterone, plasma cholesterol, and aortic cholesterol levels in rats. *Psychosomatic Medicine, 45*, 219-226.

Stern, M.J., Gorman, P.A., & Kaslow, K.L. (1983). The group counseling and exercise therapy study. *Archives of Internal Medicine, 143*, 1719-1725.

Stern, M., & Cleary, P. (1981). National Exercise and Heart Disease Project: Psychosocial changes observed during a low level exercise program. *Archives of Internal Medicine, 141*, 1463-1467.

Stern, J.J., & Cleary, P.J. (1982). The National Exercise and Heart Disease Project: long term psychosocial outcomes. *Archives of Internal Medicine, 142*, 1093-1097.

Sweeney, D.R., Maas, J.W., & Heninger, G.R. (1978). State anxiety, physical activity, and urinary 3-methoxy-4-hydroxphenethylene glycol excretions. *Archives of General Psychiatry, 35*, 1418-1423.

Taylor, C.B., Sallis, J.F., & Needle, R. 1985). The relation of physical activity and exercise to mental health. *Public Health Reports, 100*, 195-200.

Tharp, G.D., & Carson, W.H. (1975). Emotionality changes in rats following chronic exercise. *Medicine and Science in Sports, 7*, 123-126.

Thaxton, L. (1982). Physiological and psychological effects of short-term exercise addiction on habitual runners. *Journal of Sport Psychology, 4*, 73-80.

Torsvall, L., Åkerstedt, T., & Lindbeck, G. (1984). Effects on sleep stages and EEG power density of different degrees of exercise in fit subjects. *Electroencephalography and Clinical Neurophysiology, 57*, 347-353.

Trinder, J., Paxton, S.J., Montgomery, I., & Fraser, G. (1985). Endurance as opposed to power training: Their effect on sleep. *Psychophysiology, 22*, 668-673.

Trinder, J., Stevenson, J., Paxton, S.J., & Montgomery, I. (1982). Physical fitness, exercise, and REM sleep cycle length. *Psychophysiology, 19,* 89-93.

Tucker, L.A. (1983). Effect of weight training on self-concept: A profile of those influenced most. *Research Quarterly for Exercise and Sport,* 389-397.

Tuma, A.H., & Maser, J.D. (Eds.). (1985). *Anxiety and the anxiety disorders.* Hillsdale, NJ: Lawrence Erlbaum Associates.

Tsukue, I., & Shohoji, T. (1981). Movement therapy for alcoholics. *Journal of Studies on Alcohol, 42,* 144-149.

Vaillant, G.E. (1979). Natural history of male psychologic health. *New England Journal of Medicine, 201,* 1249-1254.

Waldo, D.R. & Gibson, R.M. (1982). *National Health Care Expenditures 1981: Health Care Financing Reviews* (HCFA Publication No. 03146). Washington, DC: U.S. Government Printing Office.

Wardlaw, S.L., & Frantz, A.G. (1980). Effect of swimming stress on brain B-endorphin and ACTH. *Clinical Research, 28* (abstract), 482.

Weber, J.C., & Lee, R.A. (1968). Effects of differing prepuberty exercise programs on the emotionality of male albino rats. *Research Quarterly, 39,* 748-751.

Weinstein, W.S., & Meyers, A.W. (1983). Running as treatment for depression: Is it worth it? *Journal of Sport Psychology, 5,* 288-301.

Wiese, J., Singh, M., & Yeudall, L. (1983). Occipital and parietal alpha power before, during, and after exercise. *Medicine and Science in Sports and Exercise, 15* (abstract), 117.

Yates, A., Leehey, K., & Shisslak, C.M. (1983). Running—an analogue of anorexia? *New England Journal of Medicine, 308*(5), 251-255.

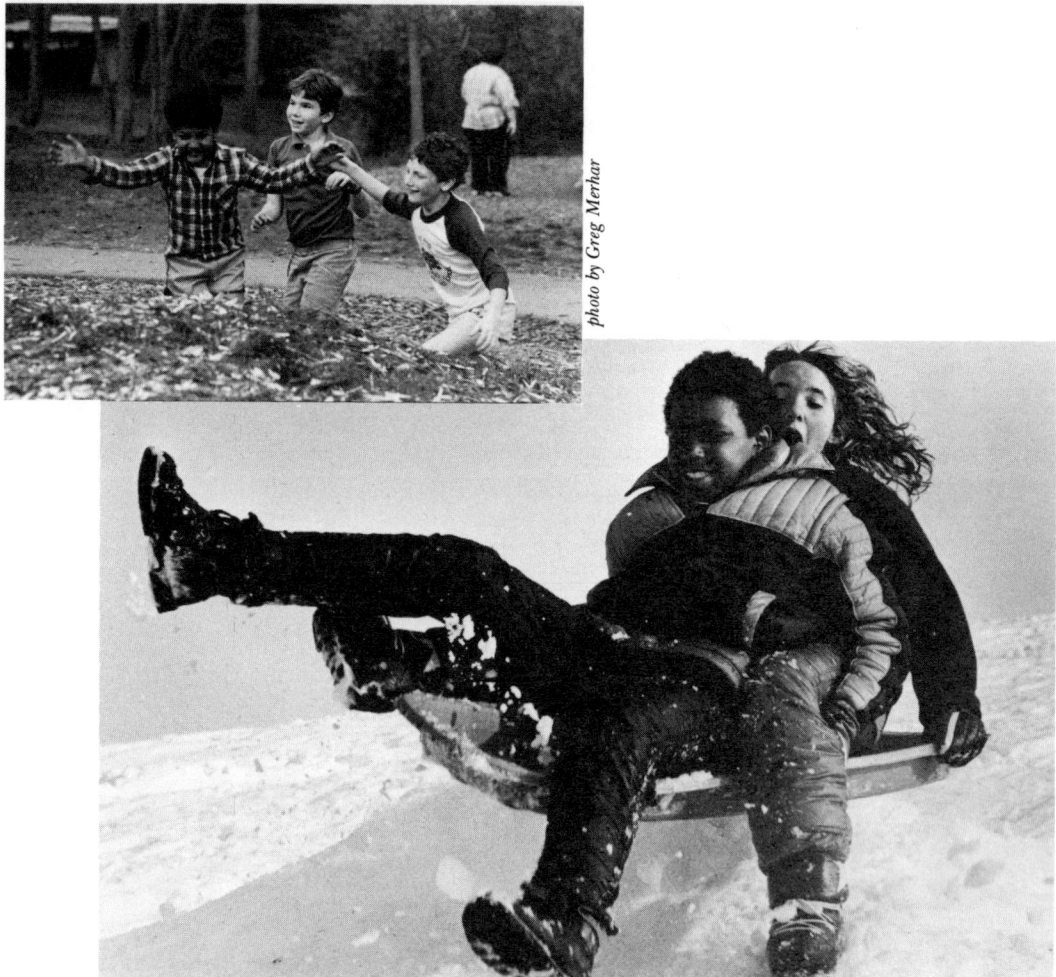

photo by Greg Merhar

photo by Jim Kirby

CHAPTER TWELVE

Social Development

George H. Sage
School of Health, Physical
Education, and Recreation
University of Northern Colorado
Greeley, Colorado

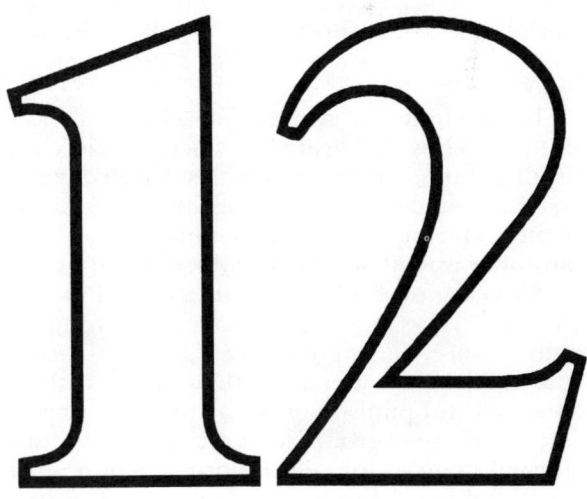

There is a deep-seated and pervasive belief that the effects of involvement in physical activities extend beyond the immediate fun and excitement of the moment. It is believed that physical activities, especially games and sports, provide an environment for acquiring culturally valued personal-social attitudes, values, and behaviors. Moreover, the lessons learned in the physical activity setting are thought to transfer to other spheres of life. Indeed, the well-known slogan that "sport builds character" is used time and again by community sports leaders, school officials, and parents when asked to justify the expenditure of vast amounts of time and money for organized sports programs.

This chapter summarizes what is known about the effects of involvement in physical activities on social development. Current research fails to provide definitive answers to many questions that have been raised about physical activity and its effect on social development. It does, however, throw considerable doubt upon the simplistic cliches and slogans about physical activity's presumed role in the socialization of the individual.

Social Development and Socialization

Definition of Social Development and Socialization

Social development refers to the acquisition of personal-social characteristics that enable an individual to function in society. The newborn infant is not a socialized being; only through interactions with various social agents and agencies does social development occur. The process that medicates social development is called socialization.

Socialization is the process by which persons learn the skills, attitudes, values, and behaviors that enable them to participate as members of the society in which they live. The systematic study of socialization has its roots in psychology, sociology, and anthropology. In the case of psychology, the focus has been on the development of individual characteristics involved in social behavior and on the basic processes through which these behavioral characteristics are acquired; sociology has concentrated on characteristics of social groupings or institutions in which socialization occurs and on the social skills learned by individuals in various social contexts; anthropology views socialization from the standpoint of a broader cultural perspective which helps determine the process of socialization (Goslin, 1969).

In the context of society, the activity of socialization is called cultural transmission, which is the means by which a society preserves its norms and perpetuates itself. A human being raised in isolation develops only its animal nature, while one raised in human society demonstrates the human aspects which derive from social living. The impact of an individual's society is illustrated by the wide variations in attitudes, values, and behaviors which are produced from one society to another.

Socialization begins at birth and continues throughout the life cycle, but the "critical" years in which primary and lasting socialization occurs are from birth to adolescence. During these years the basic cultural transmission takes place. Because of the frequency of their contact, their primacy, and their control over rewards and punishments, the primary agents and agencies for socialization are the family, peer group, school, community, and media. Regardless of the extent of formal agencies for cultural transmission, socialization depends to a large extent upon informal face-to-face contacts. Culture is not merely learned from the written or spoken word—it is conveyed through the activities of daily living.

Active and passive aspects of socialization

Much recent discussion has centered on the active and passive aspects of socialization. Giddens (1979) contends that "socialization is never anything like a passive imprinting by 'society' upon each 'individual.' From its very earliest experiences, the infant is an active partner in the double contingency of interaction and in a progressive 'involvement with society'" (p. 129).

Wentworth (1980) has criticized past approaches to the study of socialization and labeled them as "sociologistic" and "individualistic" orientations. The former approach stresses social structure, role learning through internalization by a passive "socializee", and conformity so that an "oversocialized" perspective prevails. The latter approach, according to Wentworth, is based on a view held by psychologists who are concerned with moral, cognitive, and ethical learning of personality.

Wentworth has proposed a socialization-as-interaction model which gives the socializee the role of coproducer of his or her own socialization contents. His model attempts to synthesize the micro and macro perspectives of socialization theory, and is most succinctly described by Wentworth's statement: "It seems that the person is both a function of society and relatively autonomous" (p. 60).

Agents of Social Development

Family

The family is the first and perhaps the most important social environment in a young person's life, and there is overwhelming evidence that the family—its social class, its structure, and its patterning of activities—has a significant influence on socializing youngsters into physical activities.

Participation in organized sports cuts across all socioeconomic strata; however, some sports are overrepresented with children from upper-middle class families because parents encourage their children to participate in physical activities that they deem appropriate for their socioeconomic status. For example, age group swimmers tend to come from upper-middle class homes. The same can be said for age-group skiing and gymnastics (Greenspan, 1983). On the other hand, baseball, boxing, and wrestling programs tend to attract youngsters for blue-collar families.

A positive relationship exists between parental encouragement and actual participation and sport involvement for both males and females (Greendorfer, 1977, 1979; Greendorfer & Lewko, 1978; McPherson, 1977; Sage, 1980a; Snyder and Spreitzer, 1973, 1976). Parents influence their children through their own attitudes, participation (the modeling influence), and through their interest in and encouragement of their offspring's involvement in sport (Melcher and Sage, 1978). A recent national survey of American families found that 40% of parents reported *frequently* engaging in some kind of sports activity with their children (the Miller Lite Report, 1983).

In addition to parents encouraging their offspring's participation, some parents are socialized into sport through their children's sport participation. Snyder and Purdy (1982) show that many parents learned about sports and became more involved in sport because of their children. The findings suggest that the socialization between parents and their children is often bidirectional. Thus, while parents may initiate their children into sports, the children's participation has behavioral and attitudinal consequences for the parents.

In the past decade a sizable body of theoretical and empirical research has suggested that participation in dangerous sports is a function of birth order, with later-borns being over-represented in dangerous sports (Casher, 1977; Landers, 1979; Nisbitt, 1968; Yiannakis, 1976a).

Peers

In addition to the influence of the family, the neighborhood and the peer group also serve as powerful socializing agents for sport involvement, especially as youngsters move into adolescence. During adolescence, less time is spent with one's family and more time is typically spent with peers. Interactions with peers almost force compliance with their interests and activities.

When peers are involved in sports there is frequently a great deal of pressure to become involved or give up one's cherished social relationships. In a study examining the influence of socializing agents on the process of socialization of women into sport, Greendorfer (1977) found that peers were the major influence through each life-cycle stage (childhood, adolescence, early adulthood).

School

The school, with its physical education classes and interschool sports programs, serves a significant socializing role for American youth. Most American children are taught the rudiments of a variety of sports as they pass through the grades, and six million participate in interscholastic athletics each year *(National Federation Handbook,* 1984).

Community

Community sponsored sports programs for children exist through the country, with 30 million annual participants. Programs such as Little League, Babe Ruth League, American Legion Baseball, Pop Warner League Football, Bittie Basketball, and age group swimming, soccer, wrestling, and track practically engulf young boys, and increasingly girls, from 7 to 16 years of age. These programs serve as another source of socializing youth into sports.

Mass Media

Finally, one must mention the mass media as a physical activity socializing agent. American youth are inundated with sports via newspapers, magazines, and television. Few boys and girls do not have idols among the current crop of professional and elite amateur athletes. The bedroom walls of many youngsters are plastered with sports posters of various types, demonstrating an abiding interest in sports of all kinds.

Play and Physical Activity in Childhood Socialization

The years from birth to adolescence are crucial in the psychosocial development of each individual. Active involvement in play and games has been said to constitute the work of childhood, and to prepare children for roles in adult life (Gilligan, 1982; Lever, 1978). There is a vast literature on the social developmental functions of play in childhood (Bruner, Jolly, & Sylva, 1976; Ellis, 1973; Erikson, 1963; Herron and Sutton-Smith, 1971; Mead, 1934; Millar, 1968; Piaget, 1962; Rubin, Fein, and Vanderberg, 1983) but space constraints preclude a detailed exposition of it here. Only a few of the most prominent ideas that have been proposed linking play and social development will be discussed.

Developmental and Cognitive Functions of Physical Activity

Developmental and cognitive scientists have emphasized the function of play in the cognitive development of children. Indeed, these scholars consider children's play to be the crucible of social development.

As part of his work on the cognitive development of children, Piaget (1962) analyzed play behavior. For Piaget, play forms an integral part of his theory of cognitive development; indeed, he believed that play and cognitive development are inseparable. According to Piaget, each cognitive stage exhibits a unique form of play. More importantly, as children pass through the developmental stages, each of the variations in play forms permit the child to interact in unique ways with the environment and its social participants. Social development, hence, occurs as the child assimilates various social roles. For Piaget, the consciousness and practice of rules, and the development of moral values—each associated with play and games in the last two developmental stages—are largely learned in the play environment and thus serve valuable functions in the larger social context (Piaget, 1965).

According to George Herbert Mead, the respected social psychologists whose work provided the inspiration for symbolic interactionism, play may serve as a powerful socializing agent in a child's life. A major concern of Mead was to determine how the individual obtains full development of self. It was his view that human beings are the product of social interaction. He said, "The self . . . is essentially a social structure, and it arises in social experience" (Mead, 1934, p. 140). Inferences from Mead's ideas suggest that play and games serve important functions in the development of self in both of his general developmental stages leading to self identity. Play may contribute to the first stage because in play, the child takes on and acts out roles which exist in the immediate, but also wider, social world. In the course of acting out such roles, the child learns to "stand outside himself," and thus develop a reflected view of him or herself as a social object, distinct from, but related to others. Games, on the other hand, may contribute to the second stage in the development of self. In a game, the child must take the role of every player, and must perceive what others are doing in order to make his or her own movements. As the child learns to take the attitude of the other, and permits that attitude to guide the choice of actions with reference to a common end, the child is becoming a contributing member of society.[1]

Erik Erikson (1963), whose work is generally considered within the psychoanalytic tradition, emphasized the functions of social growth that play may serve. Erikson proposed three stages of infantile play that are linked with his general theory of psychosexual development. In each stage, according to Erikson, the child is using play to acquire social skills. Through play the child gradually develops a sense of moral reasoning, insight into adult roles, and concern for others, as well as the ability to work cooperatively with others.

Jerome Bruner (Bruner, Jolly & Sylva, 1976) is well known for his prolific research on cognitive growth and the educational process. Bruner contends that random play is the main business of infancy and childhood, and is the precursor of adult competence. Play makes possible the practice of subroutines of behavior that later come together in problem solving and creativity, skills that contribute to social efficiency.

Mastery Function of Physical Activity

Sigmund Freud emphasized that children act out and repeat problematic situations in play in order to master them (Freud, 1959; 1963). According to this view, play enables children to deal with anxiety-evoking situations by allowing them to be the active masters of the situation, rather than the passive victims. Freud (1959;1963) believed that all children aspire to adult status. Through imitating adults in their play, children learn to master new or frustrating situations. Meanwhile, they acquire attitudes and dispositions about the social world of adults.

Games form a bridge between voluntary, spontaneous, informal play and formal, institutionalized sport. The studies of Roberts, Arth, and Bush (1959)

---

[1]Coakley (1984) has correctly pointed out that Mead (1934) does not suggest that play and games are necessary to the process of developing a self-concept.

comprise the most widely cited cross-cultural investigations of games, and their seminal work emphasizes the social function of games in cultural mastery. In their classic article "Games in Culture," Roberts and his colleagues constructed a classification of games based on how the game's outcome is determined. Three types of games are identified: games of physical skill, games of strategy, and games of chance. Based on their analysis of ethnographic data of 50 tribal societies, and applying their three-category classification of games, they concluded that games are expressive cultural activities similar to music and folktales; moreover, they are models of various cultural activities and thus exercises in cultural mastery. For example, games of physical skill are related to mastery of specific environmental conditions; games of strategy are related to the mastery of the social system; and games of chance are related to mastery of the supernatural.

Building on this work, Sutton-Smith and Roberts (1970) formulated a "conflict-enculturation" theory of games to explain relationships existing between types of games, child-training variables, and cultural variables. This theory proposed that conflict produced by specific child-rearing techniques in a culture lead to an interest and involvement in specific types of game activities which pattern this conflict in the role-reversals sanctioned by the game rules. According to Sutton-Smith, "Involvement over time in these rewarding game patterns leads to mastery of behaviors which have functional value or transfer to culturally useful behavior" (1974, p. 10).

Social Context and Socialization

Several social scientists have suggested that the social context in which sport activity takes place determines its social outcome. They have contrasted the peer-organized, spontaneous, free play of youngsters seen on playgrounds with the sport activity found in adult-organized youth sports programs. Two distinct social contexts and levels of sport activity emerge: peer group and adult-organized (Brower, 1979; Coakley, 1983; Devereux, 1976; Fine, 1979; Harris, 1984; Kleinman & Fine, 1979; Martens, Rivkin, & Bump, 1984; Podilchak, 1982; Polgar, 1976; Yiannakis, 1978).

Organization. Jay Coakley (1983) supervised a research project which studied spontaneous play, informal games, and organized teams sports of children. He concluded that "the most apparent aspect of the [organized team sports] was that both action and involvement were under adult control and the behavior of the players was strictly patterned by specialized rules and roles" (p. 440). Youth sport coaches are remarkably similar in the way that they organize practice sessions. Activities during practice tend to be very rule-bound. Coaches allow little flexibility in the executing of skills or in the carrying out of other tasks associated with practice. Most decisions are made by the coaches, and the participants are expected to carry them out obediently. The emphasis in the organized setting tends to be on the development of sport skills, not on the development of interpersonal skills.

Before the age of seven, children rarely play games with their peers spontaneously. If they do play them at all, it is usually on the initiative of adults or older children (Piaget, 1962). Thus, organized sports programs for youngsters under the age of seven are not organized extensions of what children of that age would be doing anyway. They are simply testaments to the power and influence adults have on young children.

When peer play is found—usually among youngsters over the age of seven—it is player controlled. Players relay on informal norms of conduct and informal rules to regulate the game. From her observations, Sylvia K. Polgar (1976) said: "The games children chose in free play generally had fewer rules and fewer specialized roles than the games [organized by adults] and children varied the rules in the process of play to suit the situation" (p. 267).

Process. Differences in the process of play in peer group sport and in adult-organized sport are also quite different. In the former, teams are chosen and the game usually begins quickly. Polgar (1976) reported that in the 22 sessions of peer play she observed, the average time from the entry into the playground until the start of the actual play was about two minutes. She also observed that play continued uninterrupted for up to 50 minutes. Play usually ended when one or more players had to leave or play was stopped by adults for one reason or another.

In the informal peer group games Coakley (1983) observed, "the primary focus in such activities was on the initiation and maintenance of a combination of action, personal involvement, a close contest, and the reaffirmation of friendships" (p. 438). The quest for victory, or a "win," is not one of the salient outcomes in peer play. Coakley observed that instead of focusing narrowly on winning the contest, "underlying the feelings and the imagination there was often an indication of a search for self-mastery, i.e., an attempt to create a situation or to perform an action up to some personal standard of satisfaction" (p. 437).

The play process in organized youth sports is quite different from informal play. There tends to be an emphasis on order, punctuality, respect for authority, obedience to adult directions, and a strict division of labor. Organized youth sport coaches typically insist on order, sometimes prohibiting participants from talking unless the coach speaks to them. Organizing the practice session or stopping practice to discuss mistakes or punish misbehavior sometimes takes up significant portions of the practice session. Since the participants become so accustomed to following orders in an organized sport setting, they frequently will cease to play the sport altogether if the coach is absent or not directly supervising it.

In organized youth sports programs, the participants have no say in the rules; the rules are made by adults. In the sports programs of national sport agencies (such as Little League Baseball), a national rules book is published to which all participants must conform. Thus, in this sport form, participants are merely followers of the rules, not makers or interpreters of the rules.

Winning, in formal youth sports programs, is frequently the overriding goal. By striving for league standings, by awarding championships, by choosing All Star teams, youth sports programs send the not-so-subtle message to the youngsters that the most important goal of sports is winning games.

Impetus. The impetus of peer play comes entirely from the youngsters; they play because they enjoy it. They are free to commence and terminate play on the basis of player interest. The impetus of play in organized sports progams comes from the coaches; they schedule the practices for a given time and end practices when they see fit. Games are scheduled by a league authority and are played in a very rigid time frame. The youngsters have no choice but to play in the way the adults wish them to play. Enjoyment of play appears to be of little concern to the adults. Table 1 summarizes the dimensions of the various forms of youth play.

Social implications. Adult-sponsored youth sports are basically an organized structure of groupings, activities, and rules that are imposed on the participants. Peer play, on the other hand, is a voluntary activity with a flexible process of social exchange based on consensus. Youngsters, therefore, are actually being exposed to very different experiences in what appear to be similar sport activities.

What are the social implications of these two different forms of organization of play activities for the socialization of youngsters? The application of adult-imposed rules in youth sports markedly contrasts with the spontaneous group-derived rules in peer-group play. The role of the peer group serves to bridge the gap between the individualistic world of children and the orientations of the wider society. The role of the organized team serves to emphasize the adult, universalist achievement orientations deemed appropriate by the society.

The differences between the goals of peer group play and of organized team effort becomes apparent in their emphasis on means and ends. In the peer

Table 1
Dimensions of Experience in Spontaneous Play, Informal Competitive Games, and Organized Team Sport Events

Dimensions of Experience	Spontaneous Play	Informal Games	Organized Team Sport Event
I. Basis of Action	A search for mastery, a use of imagination, and a coincidental meshing of personal interests and/or role playing activities	Prior experiences and existing social relationships coupled with the interpersonal and decision-making abilities of group members	Predesigned system of roles, adult leadership, and the collective role learning abilities of team members
II. Norms Governing Actions	Emergent and created to meet personal standards, interest, and/or to simulate imagined role relationships	Carried over from past experience with changes and qualifications based on individual needs and maintenance of uncertainty	Highly formalized and specific, serving both organizational needs and formal team goals
III. System of Social Control	Internally generated and dependent on individual role playing and role taking interests and abilities	Generally internal and dependent on the collective vested interests in the game at hand	Partially internal but heavily maintained by formal standards enforced by external agents and dependent on the compliance of players
IV. Types of Sanctions Used	Self-imposed on a token basis or informally administered when a scene is disrupted	Informal and primarily used to minimize threats to the maintenance of action, personal involvement, and uncertainty	Both informal and formal and used for the preservation of values as well as order
V. Basis of Group Integration	Generally coincidental and dependent on a continual commitment to and overlap of the roles played by each of the individuals involved	Generally based on the strength of personal relationships combined with a process of social exchange between group members	Based on a combination of collective satisfaction and an awareness of and compliance with a formal set of norms and role expectations
VI. Meanings Attached to Actions and Events	Emergent, nebulus, and vary with each individual's conception of what is or should be going on	Personal, situational, and related to the intensity of action and the social implications of the experience	Often serious, assuming relevance beyond the game itself, and frequently related to instrumental concerns
VII. Nature of Status Structure	Intrinsic and vary with each individual's personal experience	Primarily intrinsic and dependent on each individual's assessment of personal involvement and success	Both intrinsic and extrinsic; related to the experience itself, the quality of performance and/or game outcomes

Table 1 (cont.)
Dimensions of Experience in Spontaneous Play, Informal Competitive Games, and Organized Team Sport Events

Dimensions of Experience	Spontaneous Play	Informal Games	Organized Team Sport Event
VIII. Basis of Status Structure	Combination of age, individual creative abilities, and arbitrary situational distinctions	Age combined with interpersonal and physical abilities	Physical abilities, contributions to team success, and conformity to the coach's expectations
IX. Extent of Individual Freedom	Limited only by self-imposed restrictions with involvement voluntary at all times	Variable with restrictions related to individual physical skills and prior status within the group	Variable but restricted to the range of behavior accepted within the rules and expectations of the coach
X. Amount of Structural Stability	Variable and depends on the time span over which collective involvement can be maintained	Relatively high and grounded in prior group experiences and the anticipation of future games	Very high and grounded in the endorsement of adults and the formal goals of the team

Source: Jay Coakley, "Play, Games, and Sport: Developmental Implications for Young People," In *Play, Games and Sports in Cultural Contexts* eds. Janet C. Harris and Roberta J. Park (Champaign, IL: Human Kinetics Publishers, 1983), pp. 435-436.

context, play is not overly concerned with ends; the essence of the play is the play—its fun, decisions, ritual, and personal interactions. In contrast, in the organized sports process, play tends to be incidental. For the adults who organize sports programs, play is identified with ends. Adults want to develop in children certain values and attitudes toward social relationships and activities that reproduce the requirements of occupational life by emphasizing punctuality, periodicity, and performance. Coakley (1983) says:

> Arguments about judgements or the appropriateness of rules and procedures do not occur between players because of the universalistic applications and interpretations of norms by referees and coaches. Therefore, the experience in play and informal games emphasizes interpersonal skills (negotiations and compromise), while the experience in organized sport emphasizes a knowledge and dependence on strict rules and the acceptance of the decisions of others in positions of legitimate authority (p. 444).

Indeed, Sage has argued that the organized sport experience "is substantially influential in producing . . . the bureaucratic personality" (1978; see also Berlage, 1982).

Applying an empirically derived model of enjoyment of social experience—the Flow Model—to formal and informal sport settings, Chalip, Csikszenlmihalyi, Kleiber, and Larson (1984) found a high positive correlation between challenges and skills in informal sports settings, but not in adult-supervised settings. They observe that this finding "suggests that the flow experience is easier to achieve when adolescents are in control of the activity, probably because they can manipulate the balance between challenge and skills more easily in an informal setting" (p. 114).

In addition to the general differences in social context in which play takes place, there appear to be differences in the ways in which boys and girls play. The role of children's play in learning and practicing culturally specific gender roles has been studied by a number of scholars in several of the social sciences. The work of Sutton-Smith and Rosenberg (1961), and Sutton-Smith, Rosenberg and Morgan (1963) focused on the historical changes in the game preferences of American children and the development of gender differences in play choices during preadolescence. These studies illustrate how gender role differentiation is reflected in play activities of boys and girls and how changing cultural prescriptions of gender role behaviors are reflected in changes in play preferences.

Janet Lever (1978) studied play and games and how they serve as avenues for informal learning. Specifically, she looked at how social skills emerge as a consequence of a particular style of play. Her data show that there are significant differences in the organization of play between boys and girls, and that the primary difference is in the complexity of the social setting in which play occurs. Lever found that boys' play is more complex than girls' play. She suggests that the differences in the play forms engaged in by boys and girls may give males an advantage in the adult occupational world that shares structural features with complex games. Confirmation of Lever's findings about play preferences and the relationship between the structural complexity in games and preferences for structural complexity of adult roles was provided by Borman and Kurdek (1984). They found boys' play to be "more complex than that of girls" and that "boys had a stronger preference for more complex occupations than did girls" (p. 12).

Development of Personal-Social Attributes Through Physical Activities

Social experiences have consequences for the participants, and, as noted previously in this chapter, there is a popular belief that involvement in physical activities fosters the development of positive personal-social attributes. The Battle of Waterloo is supposed to have been won on the playing fields of Eton, and one of America's most famous generals, Douglas MacArthur, coined the slogan, "Upon the fields of friendly strife are sown the seeds that on other days on other fields will bear the fruits of victory." American physical educators uniformly include a "social development" objective in their statements of purpose, and athletic coaches universally claim that "sport builds character."

Actually, the personal-social effects of participation in physical activities is largely unknown. This is the case because well-controlled, experimental and/or longitudinal studies are scarce; moreover, of the completed research on this topic, one must fit alternative offerings of data together as in a jigsaw puzzle, with too many pieces missing or mismatched. Several reviews in recent years (Kenyon, 1968; McPherson, 1981, 1982; Staniford, 1979; Stevenson, 1975) have concluded that little empirical evidence exists to substantiate the claims that have been made for the contribution of physical activity to personal-social development. Loy and Ingham (1973) noted that:

> Socialization via play, games, and sport is a complex process having both manifest and latent functions, and involving functional and dysfunctional, intended and unintended consequences. Since research on the topic is limited, one must regard with caution many present empirical findings and most tentative theoretical interpretations of these findings (p. 298).

The personal-social attributes that have been most often studied in relation to physical activity are personality, self-concept, and social attitudes and values.

Personality

There is a consensus among behavioral scientists that personality is a product of both heredity and environment, although the actual contribution of each is a matter of continuing debate. Since personality is developed, to some extent, through a process of socialization, scholars interested in the contributions of physical activity to social development have frequently claimed that participation in physical activities influences the formation of personality. As a consequence, a massive research literature has been compiled in an effort to demonstrate how involvement in physical activities (mostly organized sports) produces personality differences between participants and nonparticipants (for reviews of the research, see (Cooper, 1969; Husman, 1969; Morgan, 1980; Ruffer, 1975, 1976; Stevenson, 1975).

Unfortunately, the typical research design that has been employed in the study of physical activity and personality development makes it impossible to determine whether the differences (when they were found) between participants and nonparticipants were actually *caused* by the physical activity experience. The research design upon which most studies have been based has taken an intact group of "athletes" and a group of "nonathletes" and assessed their personality structure, using one of the published personality instruments. Even the neophyte researcher will immediately realize that *causal* statements cannot be made from a design of this kind; but nevertheless this cross-sectional research design has been the typical approach to this topic.

Given the weakness of a cross-sectional design for making causal inferences, the findings of differences between physical activity groups and nonparticipants have been contradictive and inconclusive (Hardman, 1973). Worse, in the few studies that have used a longitudinal or quasi-longitudinal design, results indicated little or no changes in personality structure as a result of participation in sport over a particular time period (Arnold, and Straub, 1972; Rider, 1973; Rushall, 1972; Thomes, Young, and Ismail, 1973). These findings, however, should not be surprising because the athletic groups studied were high school or college age and the duration of the study was a few months. If personality psychologists are in agreement about anything, it is that personality structure is almost completely consolidated by late adolescence and it is not changed in a short period of time. Thus, realisticaly, changes in personality should not have been expected by the investigators, given the age group and the time span of the study.

While there is a belief that the achievement and expressive experiences of the kind found in physical activities have the potential to influence personality development, those developing physical activity programs would be wise to first identify the personality characteristics which they want to nurture. Only then can they set about creating physical activity environments that will most likely produce the desired personality attributes among those participating in the programs. Current programs of highly organized competitive athletics will probably not be the models one wishes to use for developing the desired personality characteristics.

Self-concept

One important aspect of social development is the formation of self-concept. The self-concept does not exist at birth; it is acquired through social experiences as the individual comes to perceive him or herself in relation to others. Throughout infancy and childhood, the self-concept is forming, and it typically becomes stabilized by adolescence (Campbell, 1984; Rosenberg, 1979; Wylie, 1979). The attitudes, values, and social behaviors one exhibits are, to a large extent, based upon one's self-concept, which is one of the results of one's social experiences. Mead (1934) said: "The self . . . is essentially a social structure, and it arises in social experience" (p. 140).

Self-concept is an organized set of perceptions one has of one's self. Morris Rosenberg, one of the most respected self-concept researchers, defines the self-concept as "the totality of an individual's thoughts and feelings having reference to himself as an object" (1979, p. 7).

Until recently, self-concept has been treated as a global construct that undergirds all aspects of one's social behavior. More recently, the emphasis has turned to a recognition of multiple conceptions of the self. In this view, persons have self-concepts of their academic ability, music ability, tennis ability, ability as a parent, etc. This linking of self-concept to specific roles and situations is supported by research demonstrating that people have different perceptions of their different attributes and roles (Brookover and Erickson, 1975; Gergen, 1971; Griffin, Chassin, and Young, 1981; Mintz and Muller, 1977; Shavelson and Bolus, 1982).

The view that self-concept is esentially a social construction, and that it arises from social experience, implies that successful involvement in activities demanding cognitive, social, and motor skills may foster the development of a positive self-concept. Positive self evaluations develop through self-efficacious behavior, and successful experiences are likely to result in the acquisition of a positive sense of self (Gecas and Schwalbe, 1983; Waters and Sroufe, 1983). For example, changes in self esteem have been linked to academic achievement (Scheier and Krout, 1979) and to feelings of competence (Kifer, 1975). Therefore, because self-concept is considered to be a directing influence in one's social behavior, physical activity experiences have the potential to influence social behavior through their influence on self-concept, and physical activity advocates have often speculated that involvement in physical activities contribute to changes in self-concept (Sonstroem, 1984).

Self-concept, physical fitness, and organized sport involvement: cross-sectional research.
That there is a positive relationship between physical fitness and self-concept has been demonstrated for elementary age children (Guyot, Fairchild, & Hill, 1981; Magill & Ash, 1979; Martinek, Cheffers & Zaichkowsky, 1978) and young adult males and females (Dishman, 1978; Dowell, Badgett, & Landiss, 1970; Leonardson, 1977). In spite of considerable evidence that physical fitness and self-concept are related, qualifications must be made. For example, Kay, Felker, and Varoz (1972) found no significant relationship between physical fitness and the self-concept of 9th grade boys, but they did find 2 of 6 tests of motor ability of 8th graders and 4 of 6 tests of motor ability of 7th graders were significantly related to self-concept. Sonstroem (1978) reported no significant relationships between self-esteem and physical ability of boys between 7 and 12 years of age in three separate studies using different measures of self-esteem. In addition, several investigators have reported no direct association between physical fitness and global self-concept, but they did find relationships between fitness and more specific forms of self-perception, especially concept of physical self (Heaps. 1978; Leonardson and Garguilo, 1978; Sonstroem, 1974, 1978).

Research on the relationship between participation in organized sports teams and self-concept does not display as consistent a pattern as does physical fitness and self-concept. Kay, Felker, and Varoz (1972) and Felker and Kay (1971) found that sports abilities and interests are related to a positive self-concept among junior high school boys, but the relationship differs by age; Morris, Vaccaro, and Clark (1979) reported similar results for age-group competitive swimmers. Wheeler (1981) reported similar results for a young adult population. On the other hand, some investigators have reported no significant differences between sports participants and non-participants among elementary school age children (Magill & Ash, 1979; Maul & Thomas, 1975) and high school and college age males and females (Ibraheim & Morrison, 1976; Vincent, 1976). In one study (Ibraheim & Morrison, 1976), the self concepts of high school and college athletes were lower than average.

Unfortunately, the design of the research in the studies cited makes it impossible to determine whether the differences found between athletic participants and nonparticipants are the *result* of participation or whether persons with certain personal or social characteristics are initially attracted to and remain involved in sports. Therefore, differences that exist between young athletes or skilled performers and the unskilled are not necessarily a consequence of sport involvement. Few persons dispute the potential contributions of competitive sports to the self-concept development of the participants, but causal designs are needed to provide direct and definitive evidence of a causal relationship.

Self-concept, physical fitness, and organized sport involvement: causal research. A few studies on this topic have employed causal research designs, and, in general, they indicate that involvement in physical activities enhances self-concept and self-esteem. Participation in physical activities, with the accompanying fitness, exhilaration, group identity, social affiliation, ego gratification, affective responses, and achievement, leads to positive self-conceputalization.

Several studies have focused on the effects of a physical fitness program on self-concept. In general, physical conditioning programs do lead to improved self-concept for both males and females (Folkins, 1976; Folkins & Sime, 1981; Henderson, 1974; Brown, Morrow, & Livingston, 1982; Pauly, Palmer, Wright & Pfeiffer, 1982; Tucker, 1982; Kowal, Patton, & Voegel, 1978). Increases in self-concept sometimes accompany exercise training even though there are no significant increases in actual fitness. Changes in how one views oneself may be associated with the exercise setting, and not necessarily the exercise itself (Morgan, 1981).

Several clinical psychologists have employed exercise programs in conjuction with counseling and have reported improvements in self-concept (Collingwood, 1976; Hilyer & Mitchell, 1979; Hilyer, Wilson, & Dillon, 1982). Self-concept enhancement tends to be more prevalent among the subjects initially low in self-concept. One obvious weakness of studies that combine treatments (exercise and counseling) is that the effects of one treatment are confounded by the other.

Sonstroem (1984) published an excellent review on research on exercise and self-concept. In addition to describing the research findings, he made a thorough methodological critique of the studies. He concluded:

> While it can be concluded that exposure to physical training programs is associated with increased self-esteem scores, it is not possible to certify that increased fitness influences these scores, or that these scores are related to enduring aspects of self-conception. Neither is it possible to identify the mechanisms responsible for change within these programs; therefore, one cannot reliably control or optimally promote them (p. 145).

A few investigators have assessed the *effects* of participation in organized sport on self-concept. While the studies are few in number and have important methodological flaws, they do suggest that self-concept can be modified through sport involvement for preadolescents (Hawkins & Gruber, 1981; Hershey, 1977). On the other hand, Ferrell (1977) and Hunsburger (1972) reported no significant change in self-concept among young adult females during a season of organized basketball; this finding is congruent with the self-concept theory that the self-concept becomes stabilized in adolescence.

Iso-Ahola (1976) studied the effects on self evaluation of Little League baseball players after winning and losing games. He found that degrees of winning and losing had distinctive effects on the players' evaluation of self immediately after a game. Zeigler (1972) reported that the won-loss record of teams affected the self-concept of basketball ability of female high school basketball players. A long term implication is that frequent winning or losing experiences will affect an individual's self-concept of ability.

Smoll and Smith carried out a unique two phase project over a seven year period that was designed to teach youth sport coaches instructional techniques for enhancing the self-esteem of the young athletes (Smith, Smoll, and Curtis, 1979; Smith, Zane, Smoll, and Coppel, 1983; Smoll and Smith, 1984). They designed a Coaching Effectiveness Training (CET) program that incorporated specific cognitive training strategies such as information processing, modeling, self-monitoring, and behavioral feedback, by which coaches could influence positive changes in self-esteem among the players. One group of youth sport coaches participated in preseason CET while a control group did not take part in the CET. Youngsters who played for the CET coaches exhibited a significant increase in general self-esteem compared with scores obtained a year earlier, while youngsters who played for the control group of coaches experienced no increase in self-esteem.

Attitudes and Values

A major function of socialization is the transmission of attitudes and values. Two fundamental assumptions undergird the understanding of attitudes and values. First, both are learned through social interaction; second, a great deal of social behavior is based on attitudes and values.

As was noted previously there is a widely held belief that physical activity is not merely physical exercise; it is also social experience and as such has the potiential to influence attitudes and values. As with attempts to assess the effects of physical activities experiences on other dimensions of social development, the research is not overwhelming in volume, and most of it is methodologically flawed for determining the effects of physical activity on attitudes and values.

Professionalization of attitude toward play. Undoubtedly the most widely cited work on attitudes and values and physical activity is Webb's 1969 study. Webb devised a scale for measuring value orientations toward competition. With this scale, respondents were asked, "What do you think is most important in playing a game?" They were then asked to rank three responses:
- to play fairly
- to play as well as you are able
- to beat your opponent

Webb found that as young boys and girls advance in age their fundamental attitudes toward play change. Webb stated that this change was represented by the "substitution of 'skill' for 'fairness' as the paramount factor in play activity, and the increasing importance of victory." He considered this attitudinal trend as a "professionalization of play." Webb suggested that there is a close relationship between values emphasized in the American economic sector and the orientations of youth sports programs.

Over the past 15 years several investigators have extended the work of Webb by assessing the orientations toward play of preadolescent and adolescent boys and girls (for a review and critique of this research, see Knoppers, 1985). Mantel and VanderVelden (1974) found preadolescent youth sport participants valued winning and skill to a greater extent than peers who were nonparticipants, who tended to more highly value fair play. Maloney and Petrie (1972) studied Canadian youth and reported that males and youth sport participants were more oriented toward winning than nonparticipants. Kidd and Woodman (1975) substituted "have fun" for "fair play" on the Webb instrument and found frequency of participation was directly related to winning orientations.

Loy, Birrell, and Rose (1976) extended this research tradition to college students and adults in the general population. Their findings replicated the previous research; that is, athletes rather than nonathletes were more likely to endorse a "professional" orientation toward sport. Using both the original Webb scale and the Kidd and Woodman variant of this scale, Snyder and Spreitzer (1979) replicated previous research in showing that athletes are more likely than nonathletes to manifest an extrinsic (winning) orientation toward sport. Finally, Sage (1980b), using intercollegiate athletes as subjects, employed the Webb scale and six other orientation-towards-sport items. Collegiate athletes displayed a "professional" orientation, but Sage noted that orientations toward sports are probably more complex than previously proposed by sport social scientists.

In all of the studies in which the Webb scale has been used, and in the studies in which variations of it have been used, females demonstrate lower professionalized sports attitudes than males. But females who have been involved in organized sports show higher professionalized attitudes than nonparticipants (Kane, 1982; Kidd & Woodman, 1975; Loy et al., 1976; Maloney & Petrie, 1972; Sage, 1980b; Snyder & Spreitzer, 1979; McElroy, & Kirkendall, 1980). Kane (1982) has suggested that "attitudes held toward play may be more a function of a level of athletic involvement and/or sex-role orientation than of gender" (p. 293). Using data from the International Project on Leisure Role Socialization sponsored by the International Committee on the Sociology of Sport, Theberge, Curtis, and Brown (1982) confirmed Kane's claim. They found sex differences toward winning among persons in the general population, but this was not true for top-flight athletes. Males and females among the elite athletes were similar in their orientations toward winning.

Although it is difficult to credit (or discredit) sports participation entirely for greater professionalized attitudes toward play, it seems that sport for fun, enjoyment, fairness, and equity are sacrificed at the altar of skill and victory as children move toward adulthood.

Sportsmanship. Sportsmanlike behavior—playing by the rules and not taking unfair advantage of competitors—is universally admired, but good sportsmanship sometimes conflicts with the quest for victory. Advocates contend that good sportsmanship attitudes and behaviors are promoted in sport, but on the other hand, victory in competition carries salient rewards. What attitudes do participants really acquire? The research in this topic is sparce, and it has glaring weaknesses, but it is consistent: persons who have had extended experience in organized sports display poorer sportsmanship attitudes than non-sportsmen (Kistler, 1957; Richardson, 1962; Allison, 1982; Kroll and Peterson, 1965; Lakie, 1964; Bovyer, 1963).

Rule violation in sport is complex and several scholars have commented on the inadequacy of research on this topic and have suggested new ways for analyzing this phenomenon (Allison, 1982; Silva, 1981). Silva (1981) has suggested that the normative rules of competitive sports are those of consensus, legitimized by peer decree. They frequently foster intentional violations of the formal rules of the sport, because such violations often increase the probability of a successful outcome, and result in social and personal rewards to offenders. He suggests that only when positive reinforcements for rule violating are replaced by salient personal and social punishment will normative rules encouraging illegal behavior become dysfunctional to success.

Character. The slogan that "sport builds character" is often heard but is rarely subjected to careful research. Character reflects culturally valued traits which reflect morally and ethically appropriate attitudes, values, and behaviors. Culturally valued traits in American society that reflect "character" are such prosocial behaviors as fairness, generosity, altrusim, and cooperation. Bryan (1977) has reported on a substantial body of literature showing that prosocial behavior may be undermined when achievement behavior is encouraged and rewarded through an emphasis on competitiveness. In one of the few studies to focus on the impact of sport experiences on the development of social character, Kleiber and Roberts (1981) sought to establish the actual effects of two specific aspects of prosocial behavior: cooperation and altruism. With male subjects, the sports experience actually seemed to inhibit prosocial behavior. The investigators noted that "to the extent that competition is allowed to dominate the interpersonal relationships in children's sports, their potential for actually facilitating the development of prosocial behavior is entirely lost" (p. 121).

Sport and Social Mobility

Some Assumptions and Realities

A common assumption about sport involvement is that it frequently serves as a means of social mobility. For example, in writing about college sports, Rudolph (1962) noted that "football would enable a whole generation of young men in the coal fields of Pennsylvania to turn their backs on the mines that employed their fathers" (p. 378). There are numerous "rags-to-riches" stories among past and present professional athletes which serve as visible examples of sport as an avenue of upward social mobility.

Questions need to be asked about professional athletics as a means of social mobility. How many individuals actually become professional athletes? How long do professional athletes remain at this level of sport? What happens when a professional athlete's career is over? Very few people realize that there are only about 3,600 total playing positions in professional sports. When that number is compared with the total number of 135,000,000 adults employed one can realize how few become professional athletes. Another way to make this point is that there are some 1,000,000 high school football players each year but only about 150 rookies are added to the National Football League rosters each year; approximately 7,000,000 boys play high school basketball each year and only about 30 first year players are included on the National Basketball Association roster each year. An average career in the professional team sports is about 5 years, and that is for the few who make it to the professional ranks.

Once a professional playing career is over, only a very few former professional athletes become sportscasters, coaches, or managers, nonwithstanding the popular impression that such jobs are readily available to former athletes. A few studies have examined the socio-economic status of professional athletes after retirement. The report of Roger Kahn (1971) about the 1953 Brooklyn Dodger players 15 years later is a bittersweet account showing that most the players drifted into occupations commensurate with their educational achievement. Others, using more appropriate research methods, have found essentially the same thing (Haerele, 1975a, and 1975b; Weinberg & Arond, 1952).

Although there are several potential means by which sport participation may serve as a social mobility conduit, there is actually very little empirical support for the notion that sports involvement leads to social mobility for large numbers of athletes. A prerequisite for ascertaining whether sport involvement actually influences social mobility would require a longitudinal research design, with subjects matched on original socioeconomic background and on educational attainment. Longitudinal studies, with subjects matched on important social variables, have not been done.

In recent years, investigators have used several different designs and groups of subjects in an effort to determine the effects of sport involvement on social mobility. Dubois (1978) attempted to determine whether participation in intercollegiate sports affects occupational achievement by comparing the post college business success of former athletes and former nonathletes. Using earnings and occupational prestige as his criteria for success, Dubois found, overall, there were no significant differences in occupation or earnings in the two groups.

Notre Dame University has one of the most renowned traditions in intercollegiate sports, and Sack and Thiel (1979) examined the social origins and occupational career mobility of football players who graduated from Notre Dame between 1946 and 1965. They found that both the former players and a comparison group of nonathletes had moved well beyond their family socioeconomic background, but the players tended to have come from lower social class origins than nonathletes. Players who had been starters on the football team experienced more mobility than reserves, but as a group players had earned fewer advanced degrees than nonathletes. The investigators concluded that the athletic experience itself did not seem to contribute to occupational mobility.

An effort to ascertain the effects of high school sports participation on socioeconomic attainment was undertaken by Howell, Miracle, and Rees (1984) using the five-wave Youth in Transition panel based on a national sample of males. The subjects were surveyed several times during their high school years; they were followed one year after high school graduation and again five years after graduation. No effects of athletic participation on occupational status were found. Moreover, for three measures of individual earnings, there was no economic payoff favoring the former high school athletes. The investigators noted that any economic payoff owing to participation in athletics may begin to accrue at a later time in the occupational career cycle or may only occur for those also subsequently attending college.

The findings of these studies suggest that social mobility is not one of the salient outcomes of organized sport involvement. This is not to deny that a few athletes transcend the almost insurmountable odds to raise their social station in the economic structure.

Physical Activity and Social Behavior

Educational Achievement

There is a consistent literature extending back over several decades showing a positive relationship between participation in interscholastic sports and academic achievement (Bend & Petrie, 1977; Landers, Feltz, Obermeier, & Brouse, 1978). Most studies on this topic prior to 1970 dealt with the overall comparison (zero-order association) between a single independent variable (athletic participation) and a single dependent variable (academic achievement). Studies during the past decade have gone beyond the simple exploration of relationships between one independent and one dependent variable, and have examined the impact of a number of antecedent and intervening variables. Control variables that have frequently been introduced include socioeconomic status, student IQ, course of study (college preparatory vs. noncollege preparatory), previous school grade point average, and race.

Schafer and Armer (1968) conducted one of the first studies on this topic in which important social variables were controlled. To isolate the effects of sport participation, they used five control variables: father's occupational rank, student IQ, year in school, curriculum, and junior high school academic records. Each athlete was matched with a nonathlete on all control variables. With these controls, the investigators found a positive association between academic performance and athletic participation. Moreover, they found that athletic participation made a greater positive contribution to the grade point average of those athletes "less disposed" toward high academic achievement (that is, blue collar, low IQ, noncollege preparatory students) than it did to the averages of those athletes "more disposed" toward high academic achievement (that is, white collar, high intelligence, college preparatory students).

More recent research has questioned the causal interpretation of the effects of high school athletics on academic achievement, since most studies rest upon cross-sectional evidence. Using a quasi-longitudinal design, Lueptow and Kayser

(1973) failed to find greater increases in grades over the high school years among athletes than nonathletes. More recently, Hauser and Lueptow (1978), utiltizing data that permits true longitudinal analysis, found that while athletes have higher GPAs at the end of their high school career than at the start, they do not gain as much as nonathletes over the years of high school, thus experiencing a relative decline in academic achievement.

Another strand of research weaves its way through the 1970s and suggests that the athletic participation-educational attainment issue is not a simple matter of whether athletes have higher GPAs than nonathletes. In 1970, William Spady published an article entitled, "Lament for the Letterman" in which he assessed the relative effects of athletic participation as compared with other forms of extracurricular activities having service or leadership functions on actual college attainment, that is, the completion of one or more years of college. He reported that the athlete was significantly underrepresented as compared to students who participated in service-leadership activities while in high school. Indeed, the athlete-only group fared no better than those having no form of extracurricular involvement at all. Spady concluded that there was only "lament" for the letterman who did not become involved in other phases of extracurriculum.

Spady's work has been corroborated by Rehberg and Cohen (1975) who divided the athlete group into "Pure Athletes" and "Athlete-Scholars," and Landers & Landers (1978), who divided athletes into an athlete-only and athlete-service groups categories. In both cases athletes-only fared poorly when compared with their classmates, suggesting that high school students who limit their interest and participation only to athletics will lack the academic and social skills necessary for higher educational attainemnt.

A 15-year study of male high school athletes led Otto and Alwin (1977) to conclude that participation in sports becomes relevant to academic achievement only when it is linked to academic encouragement by parents and friends. Their findings have been supported by subsequent research (Hanks, 1979; McElroy, 1979). Picou and his colleagues reported that white athletes transformed the prestige received by high school sport participation into positive academic attitudes but black athletes did not (Picou, 1978; Picou and Hwang, 1982; Wells and Picou, 1980).

Education Expectations

The influence of sport participation on academic achievement has another dimension, in addition to grades. Over the past 15 years investigators have focused on educational expectations, reasoning that this represents an educational achievement that may be as important in the long-run as grade point average. The research that has accumulated on this topic suggests that participation in high school sports is positively associated with high educational aspirations.

The pioneer study on this topic was carried out by Rehberg and Schafer (1968). They reported the first study to deal exclusively with the linkage between sports participation and aspirations for higher education, while controlling for important antecedent and intervening variables. They used socioeconomic status, academic performance, and parental encouragement as control variables and found that the effect of athletic participation on educational aspirations was greatest among those athletes who were initially less disposed to go to college (athletes from working class families). In a subsequent study (Schafer & Rehberg, 1970), using different control variables, these same investigators again found that athletes not predisposed to attend college actually aspired to college to a significantly greater extent than nonathletes with the same predispositions. Others have replicated and extended the original Rehberg and Schafer study and reported similar results (Otto & Alwin, 1977; Picou, 1978; Picou & Curry, 1974; Spreitzer & Pugh, 1973).

Although there has been little research with black and female athletes, recent studies by Hanks (1979) and Hartzell and Picou (1978) found that white and black athletes and white female athletes exhibited significantly higher educational aspirations and actual college-going behavior than corresponding nonathletes, but they report that the overall process through which educational aspiration relates to athletic participation appears to differ for these subpopulations of students. Snyder and Spreitzer (1977) reported that "successful" female athletes tend to hold higher educational aspirations than "less successful" athletes and nonathletes.

At the high school level, then, sport participation has a greater influence upon educational aspirations than it does upon grades. The findings on grades are contradictory, but there are few exceptions to the patterns of aspiration.

Sport Involvement and Delinquent Behavior

The idea that organized sports may serve as a deterrent to delinquent behavior appears to have originated in the public secondary schools of Britain in the nineteenth century (McIntosh, 1971). This notion was taken up and enthusiastically endorsed by the social and educational reformers in the United States in the early twentieth century, and proposals for expanded municipal recreational programs and the creation of interscholastic athletic programs frequently implied that such programs would thwart the growing problem of juvenile delinquency (Addams, 1974; Goodman, 1979; Hardy, 1982). Faith that participation in sports would effectively reduce delinquency is found in a resolution adopted in 1954 by AAHPERD: "The Association sincerely believes that sound programs of health, physical education, and recreation can help lessen dilinquency" (AAHPER, 1954, p. 3).

Belief in sports ability to "keep kids out of trouble" was generally taken for granted and solid empirical study of this issue has been underway for less than 20 years. The first major study of this topic was undertaken by Schafer (1969). He collected data on nearly 600 high school boys and found that, overall, athletes were less delinquent than nonathletes. However, when grade point average and social class background were controlled, the differences remained only for lower social class athletes. More recently, Segrave and Chu (1978) reported similar findings.

During the past few years there have been several important studies on this subject (Buhrman, 1977; Hastad, Segrave, Pangrazi, and Peterson, 1984; Landers and Landers, 1978; Purdy and Richard, 1983; Segrave and Hastad, 1984). There is now a substantial literature, and in a recent review of this research Segrave (1983) said that several conclusions are warranted:

> The first conclusion is that athletes tend to be less delinquent than comparable nonathletes.... The second conclusion is that the overall relationship between athletics and delinquency appears to be a function of an association among lower socio-economic groups.... The greatest differences in the delinquent behavior of athletes and nonathletes occur among lower-class youth.... The third conclusion is that the overall relationship between athletics and delinquency appears to be a function of the seriousness of the offense.... Delinquent behavior among athletes decreased when the type of offense is classified as more serious.... The final conclusion is that the profiles of deviants and athletes are different (pp. 191-195).

While the research has shown consistent evidence that delinquency among athletic groups tends to be significantly lower than among nonathletic groups, it is not possible at this time to declare with certainty that involvement in sports actually serves as a deterrent to delinquent behavior. Because the data are mostly descriptive and correlational, several explanations for the findings are possible.

For example, some investigators contend that the negative association between sport and delinquency is a result of a self-selection process; delinquent or youth predisposed to delinquent behavior are less attracted to organized sports (Straub and Felock, 1974; Yiannakis, 1976b).

Cooperative Behavior

One of the objectives of sports and physical activity programs is to teach participants cooperative behavior—to get along well with others and to share with one another. In a society that stresses competitive behavior and that provides many rewards for winning, the typical person may come to value winning over cooperation. Indeed, research by Kagen and his colleagues (Kagen and Madsen, 1972; Knight and Kagen, 1977) suggest a tendency for American children to become more competitive, even irrationally competitive, with age. According to these researchers, winning is so culturally emphasized that it is the "rational" behavior.

In a series of studies over the past decade, Orlick has experimented with play and games as a means of developing positive cooperative behavior among children. Cooperatively structured games were effective in producing cooperative social interaction among elementary school children, kindergarten children, and pre-school children (Orlick, 1978; 1981; Orlick & Foley, 1976; Orlick, McNally, & O'Hara, 1978).

Summary

There is a deep-seated belief that involvement in physical activity contributes to social development. Social development refers to the acquisition of personal-social characteristics that enable one to function in a society. Social development begins at birth and continues through life, but the "critical" years are from birth to adolescence, because in this period the basic cultural transmission takes place.

The family is the first and most important social environment, and its social class, its structure, and its patterning of activities have a significant influence on socializing youngsters into physical activities. Peers also serve as powerful socializing agents for sport involvement, especially during adolescence. Physical education classes, interscholastic athletics, and community youth sports programs are significant means by which many youngsters are introduced to sports and provided sport experiences. Finally, the mass media virtually inundate American youth with information about college and professional sports.

There is vast literature on the social developmental functions of play in childhood. For many developmental psychologists, children's play is considered to be the crucible of social development. Cross cultural investigations of physical activity emphasize the social functions of play and games in cultural mastery.

Social scientists have suggested that the social context in which physical activity takes place determines its outcomes. Spontaneous play and informal games have quite different structure and social processes than organized competitive sports. As a consequence, participants in these two forms of physical activity are being exposed to quite different social experiences.

It is frequently claimed that participation in physical activities influences the formation of personality. While there is an intuitive belief about physical activity involvement producing favorable personality characteristics, unfortunately most of the research on this topic is correlational and not causal in design, and, moreover, the findings are extremely equivocal.

There is considerable evidence suggesting positive relationships between physical fitness and self-concept; the relationship between participation in organized sport teams and self-concept is mixed. As with personality research, most of the investigations have used cross-sectional designs rather than causal designs.

A major aspect of social development is the acquisition of attitudes and values. It appears that involvement in organized competitive sports produces a professionalization of attitude, meaning that greater emphasis is given to performance outcomes and the quest for victory while less concern is held for playing fairly. Indeed, persons who have had extended experiences in organized sports display poorer sportsmanship attitudes than nonsport participants.

While the slogan "sport builds character" is often used to support organized sports programs, this notion has rarely been subjected to careful research. The little research done on this topic certainly does not lead to a confirmation of the slogan. It appears that a key ingredient in the character forming potential of physical activities is the leadership displayed by sports leaders.

A common assumption about sport involvement is that it frequently serves as a means of upward social mobility. Although there are several potential ways by which sports participation may serve as an avenue of social mobility, there is actually very little empirical support for this for large numbers of athletes. This is not to deny that a few athletes do raise their social station in the economic structure.

There is a consistent tradition of research showing a positive relationship between participation in interscholastic sports and academic achievement, even when important social variables are controlled. Recent studies have suggested that there are complexities to this topic that need further study before any definitive causal conclusions can be drawn.

At the high school level, it appears that sport participation does enhance educational aspirations, especially for youth from working class families.

Sport participants tend to be less delinquent than nonsport participants, and the greatest differences in the delinquent behavior of athletes and nonathletes occurs among lower social class youth. It is not possible, however, to claim with certainty that involvement in sport actually serves as a deterrent to delinquent behavior.

Cooperatively structured games have been found to be effective in producing cooperative social interactive behavior. More frequent use of cooperation in physical activities and a greater emphasis on cooperative processes will likely lead to a greater use of cooperative behavior.

References

Addams, J. (1909). *The spirit of youth and the city streets.* New York: McMillan.

Allison, M.T. (1982). Sportsmanship: Variations based on sex and degree of competitive experience. In A.O. Dunleavy, A.W. Miracle, and C.R. Rees (Eds.), *Studies in the sociology of sport* (pp. 153-165). Ft. Worth, TX: Texas Christian University Press.

American Association for Health, Physical Education, and Recreation. (1954). *Resolutions, 58th National Convention.* Washington, D.C.: AAHPER Publications.

Arnold, G.E. and Straub, W.F. (1972). Personality and group cohesiveness as determinants of success among interscholastic basketball teams. Unpublished manuscript.

Bend, E. and Petrie, B.M. (1977). Sport participation, scholastic success, and social mobility. In R.S. Hutton (Ed.), *Exercise and sport sciences reviews,* Vol. 5 (pp. 1-44). Santa Barbara, CA: Journal Publishing Associates.

Berlage, G.I. (1982). Are children's competitive team sports socializing agents for corporate America? In A.O. Dunleavy, A.W. Miracle, and C.R. Rees (Eds.), *Studies in the Sociology of Sport* (pp. 309-324). Ft. Worth, TX: Texas Christian University Press.

Borman, K.M. and Kurdek, L.A. (1984, August). *Children's game complexity as a predictor of later perceived self competence and occupational interest.* Paper presented at the annual meeting of the American Sociological Association, San Antonio, TX.

Bovyer, G. (1963). Children's concepts of sportsmanship in the 4th, 5th, and 6th grade. *Research Quarterly, 34,* 282-287.

Brookover, W.B. and Erickson, E.L. (1975). *Sociology of Education.* Homewood, IL: Dorsey.

Brower, J. (1979). The professionalization of organized youth sport: Social psychological impacts and outcomes. *Annals of the American Academy of Political and Social Science, 445,* 39-46.

Brown, E.Y., Morrow, J.R. Jr., and Livingston, S.M. (1982). Self-concept changes in women as a result of training. *Journal of Sport Psychology, 4,* 354-363.

Bruner, J., Jolly, A., and Sylva, K. (Eds.). (1976). *Play: Its role in development and evolution.* New York: Basic Books.

Bryan, J.H. (1977). Prosocial behavior. In H.L. Hom and P.A. Robinson (Eds.), *Psychological processes in early education* (pp. 233-259). New York: Academic Press.

Buhrman, H.G. (1977). Athletics and deviancy: An examination of the relationship between athletic participation and deviant behavior of high school girls. *Review of Sport and Leisure, 2,* 17-35.

Campbell, R.N. (1984). *The new science: Self-esteem psychology.* San Diego: University Press of America.

Casher, B.B. (1977). Relationship between birth order and participation in dangerous sports. *Research Quarterly, 48,* 33-40.

Chalip, L., Csikszentmihalyi, M., Kleiber, D., and Larson, R. (1984). Variations of experience in formal and informal sport. *Research Quarterly for Exercise and Sport, 55,* 109-116.

Coakley, J.J. (1983). Play, games, and sport: Developmental implications for young people. In J.C. Harris and R.J. Park (Eds.), *Play, Games, and Sports in Cultural Contexts* (pp. 431-450). Champaign, IL: Human Kinetics Publishers.

Coakley, J.J. (1984). *Mead's theory on the development of the self: Implications for organized youth sport programs.* Paper presented at the Olympic Scientific Congress, Eugene, OR.

Collingwood, T.R. (1976). Effective physical functioning: A precondition for the helping process. *Counselor Education and Supervision, 15,* 211-215.

Cooper, L. (1969). Athletics, activity, and personality: A review of the literature. *Research Quarterly, 40,* 17-22.

Devereux, E.C. (1976). Backyard versus Little League baseball: The impoverishment of children's games. In D.M. Landers (Ed.), *Social Problems in Athletics* (pp. 37-56). Urbana: University of Illinois Press.

Dishman, R.K. (1978). Aerobic power, estimation of physical ability, and attraction to physical activity. *Research Quarterly, 49,* 285-292.

Dowell, L.J., Badgett, J.L. Jr., and Landiss, C.W. (1970). A study of the relationship between selected physical attributes and the self-concept. In G.S. Kenyon (Ed.), *Contemporary Psychology of Sport* (pp. 657-672). Chicago: The Athletic Institute.

Dubois, P.E. (1978). Participation in sports and occupational attainment: A comparative study. *Research Quarterly, 49,* 28-37.

Ellis, M.J. (1973). *Why people play.* Englewood Cliffs, N.J.: Prentice-Hall.

Erikson, E.H. (1963). *Childhood and society.* New York: Norton.

Felker, D.W. and Kay, R.S. (1971). Self-concept, sports interests, sports participation and body type of seventh- and eighth-grade boys. *Journal of Psychology, 78,* 223-228.

Ferrell, D.T. (1977). Changes in self-concept between starters and substitutes during a basketball season. *Completed Research in Health, Physical Education, and Recreation, 19,* 177 (Abstract).

Fine, G. (1979). Small groups and culture creation: The idioculture of Little League baseball teams. *American Sociological Review, 44,* 733-745.

Folkins, C. and Sime, W. (1981). Physical fitness training and mental health. *American Psychologist, 36,* 373-389.

Freud, S. (1959). *Beyond the pleasure principle.* New York: Bantam Books.

Freud, S. (1963). *Jokes and their relation to the unconscious.* New York: Norton.

Gecas, V. and Schwalbe, M. (1983). Beyond the looking glass self: Social structure and efficacy-based self esteem. *Social Psychology Quarterly, 46,* 77-88.

Gergen, K.J. (1971). *The concept of self.* New York: Holt, Rinehart, and Winston.

Giddens, A. (1979). *Central problems in social theory.* Berkeley, CA: University of California Press.

Gilligan, C. (1982). *In a different voice.* Cambridge, MA: Harvard University Press.

Goodman, C. (1979). *Choosing sides: Playground and street life on the lower east side.* New York: Schocken.

Goslin, D.A. (1969). Introduction. In D.A. Goslin (Ed.), *Handbook of socialization theory and research* (pp. 1-21). Chicago: Rand McNally.

Greendorfer, S.L. (1977). Role of socializing agents in female sport involvement. *Research Quarterly, 48,* 304-310.

Greendorfer, S.L. (1979). Differences in childhood socialization influences of women involved in sport and women not involved in sport. In M. Krotee (Ed.), *The dimensions of sport sociology* (pp. 59-72). West Point: Leisure Press.

Greendorfer, S.L. and Lewko, J.H. (1978). Role of family members in sport socialization of children. *Research Quarterly, 49,* 149-152.

Greenspan, E. (1983). *Little winners: Inside the world of the child sports star.* Boston: Little Brown.

Griffin, N., Chassin, L. and Young, R.D. (1981). Measurement of global self-concept versus multiple role-specific self-concepts in adolescents. *Adolescence, 16,* 49-56.

Guyot, G.W., Fairchild, L. and Hill, M. (1981). Physical fitness, sport participation, body build, and self-concept of elementary school children. *International Journal of Sport Psychology, 12,* 105-116.

Haerle, R.K. (1975a). Career patterns and career contingencies of professional baseball players: An occupational analysis. In D.W. Ball and J.W. Loy (Eds.), *Sport and social order* (pp. 461-519). Reading, MA: Addison-Wesley.

Haerle, R.K. (1975b). Education, athletic scholarships, and the occupational career of the professional athlete. *Sociology of Work and Occupation, 2,* 373-403.

Hanks, M. (1979). Race, sexual status and athletics in the process of educational achievement. *Social Science Quarterly, 60,* 482-496.

Hardman, K. (1973). A dual approach to the study of personality and performance in sport. In H.T.A. Whiting, K. Hardman, L.B. Hendry, and M.G. Jones (Eds.), *Personality and performance in physical education and sport* (pp. 45-61). London: Henry Kimpton.

Hardy, S. (1982). *How Boston played: Sport, recreation, and community 1865-1915.* Boston: Northeastern University Press.

Harris, J.C. (1984). Interpreting youth baseball: Players' understanding of fun and excitement, danger, and boredom. *Research Quarterly for Exercise and Sport, 55,* 379-382.

Hartzell, M.J. and Picou, J.S. (1978, November). *Participation in interscholastic athletics and plans for college attendance: A comparison of males and females.* Paper presented at meeting of the Texas Association for Health, Physical Education, and Recreation, Houston, TX.

Hastad, D.N., Segrave, J.O., Pangrazi, R., and Peterson, G. (1984). Youth sport participation and deviant behavior. *Sociology of Sport Journal, 1,* 366-373.

Hauser, W.J. and Lueptow, L.B. (1978). Participation in athletics and academic achievement: A replication and extension. *Sociological Quarterly, 19,* 304-309.

Hawkins, D.B. and Gruber, J.J. (1981). *Influence of Little League baseball on player's self-esteem.* Unpublished manuscript.

Heaps, R.A. (1978). Relating physical and psychological fitness: A psychological point of view. *Journal of Sports Medicine and Physical Fitness, 18,* 399-408.

Henderson, J.M. (1974). *The effect of physical conditioning on self-concept in college females.* Unpublished doctoral dissertation, Washington State University, Pullman, WA.

Herron, R.E. and Sutton-Smith, B. (1971). *Child's play.* New York: Wiley.

Hershey, C.P. (1977). *The effects of participation in baseball programs conducted at different levels of competition on the self-concepts of elementary ages males.* Unpublished master's thesis, Pennsylvania State University.

Hilyer, J.C. Jr., and Mitchell, W. (1979). Effect of systematic physical fitness training combined with counseling on the self-concept of college students. *Journal of Counseling Psychology, 26,* 427-436.

Hilyer, J.C., Wilson, D.G., Dillon, C., Caro, L., Jenkins, C., Spencer, W.A., Meadows, M.E., & Booker, W. (1982). Physical fitness training and counseling as treatment for youthful offenders. *Journal of Counseling Psychology, 29,* 292-303.

Howell, F.M., Miracle, A.W. and Rees, C.R. (1984). Do high school athletics pay?: The effects of varsity participation on socioeconomic attainment. *Sociology of Sport Journal, 1,* 15-25.

Hunsberger, E.H. (1972). The study of the self-concept of church, college, and state university athletes and nonathletes. *Completed Research in Health, Physical Education, and Recreation, 14,* 165-166. (Abstract)

Husman, B. (1969). Sport and personality dynamics. *Annual Proceedings of the National College Physical Education Association for Men,* pp. 56-69.

Ibraheim, H. and Morrison, N. (1976). Self-actualization and self-concept among athletes. *Research Quarterly, 47,* 68-79.

Iso-Ahola, S. (1976). Evaluation of self and team performance and feelings of satisfaction after success and failure. *International Review of Sport Sociology, 11*(4), 33-44.

Kagen, S. and Madsen, M.C. (1972). Experimental analyses of cooperation and competition in Anglo-American and Mexican-American children. *Developmental Psychology, 6,* 49-59.

Kahn, R. (1971). *The boys of summer.* New York: Signet Books.

Kane, M.J. (1982). The influence of level of sport participation and sex-role orientation on female professionalization of attitudes toward play. *Journal of Sport Psychology, 4,* 290-294.

Kay, R.S., Felker, D.W. and Varoz, R.O. (1972). Sports interests and abilities as contributors to self-concept in junior high school boys. *Research Quarterly, 43,* 208-215.

Kenyon, G.S. (1968, November/December). Sociological considerations. *Journal of Health, Physical Education, and Recreation, 39,* 31-33.

Kidd, T.R. and Woodman, W.F. (1975). Sex orientations toward winning in sport. *Research Quarterly, 46,* 476-483.

Kifer, E. (1975). Relationships between academic achievement and personality characteristics: A quasi-longitudinal study. *American Educational Research Journal, 12,* 191-210.

Kistler, H.W. (1957). Attitudes expressed about behavior demonstrated in certain specific situations. *Proceeding College Physical Education Association, 60,* 55-58.

Kleiber, D.A. and Roberts, G.C. (1981). The effects of sport experience in the development of social character: An exploratory investigation. *Journal of Sport Psychology, 3,* 114-122.

Kleinman, S. and Fine, G. (1979). Rhetorics and action in moral organizations: Social control of little leaguers and ministry students. *Urban Life, 8,* 275-294.

Knight, G.P. and Kagen, S. (1977). Development of prosocial and competitive behaviors in Anglo-American and Mexican-American children. *Child Development, 48,* 1385-1394.

Knoppers, A. (1985). Professionalization of attitudes: A review and critique. *Quest, 37,* 92-102.

Kowal, D.M., Patton, J.F., and Vogel, J.A. (1978). Psychological states and aerobic fitness of male and female recruits before and after basic training. *Aviation and Space Environmental Medicine, 49,* 603-606.

Kroll, W. and Petersen, K.H. (1965). Study of values test and collegiate football teams. *Research Quarterly, 36,* 441-447.

Lakie, W.L. (1964). Expressed attitudes of various groups of athletes toward athletic competition. *Research Quarterly, 35,* 497-503.

Landers, D.M. (1979). Birth order in the family and sport participation. In M. Krotee (Ed.), *The dimensions of sport sociology* (pp. 140-167). West Point: Leisure Press.

Landers, D.M., Feltz, D.L., Obermeier, G.E. and Brouse, T.R. (1978). Socialization via interscholastic athletics: Its effect on educational attainment. *Research Quarterly, 49,* 475-483.

Landers, D.M. and Landers, D. (1978). Socialization via interscholastic athletics: Its effects on delinquency. *Sociology of Education, 51,* 299-303.

Leonardson, G.L. (1977). Relationship between self-concept and perceived physical fitness. *Perceptual and Motor Skills, 44,* 62.

Leonardson, G.R. and Garguilo, R.M. (1978). Self-perception and physical fitness. *Perceptual and Motor Skills, 46,* 338.

Lever, J. (1978). Sex differences in the complexity of children's play and games. *American Sociological Review, 43,* 471-483.

Loy, J.W. Birrell, S. and Rose, D. (1976). Attitudes held toward agonetic activities as a function of selected social identities. *Quest, 26,* 81-93.

Loy, J.W. and Ingham. A. (1973). Play, games, and sport in the psychosocial development of children and youth. In G.L. Rarick (Ed.), *Physical activity: Human growth and development* (pp. 257-302). New York: Academic Press.

Lueptow, L.B. and Kayser, B.D. (1973). Athletic involvement, academic achievement and aspiration. *Sociological Focus, 7,* 24-35.

Magill, R.A. and Ash, M.J. (1979). Academic, psycho-social, and motor characteristics of participants and nonparticipants in children's sports. *Research Quarterly, 50,* 230-240.

Maloney, T. and Petrie, B. (1972). Professionalization of attitudes toward play among Canadian school pupils as a function of sex, grade, and athletic participation. *Journal of Leisure Research, 4,* 184-195.

Mantel, R. and Vander Velden, L. (1974). The relationship between the professionalization of attitudes toward play of preadolescent boys and participation in organized sport. In G.H. Sage (Ed.), *Sport in American society* (2nd ed.) (pp. 172-178). Reading, MA: Addison-Wesley.

Martens, R., Rivkin, F. and Bump, L. (1984). A field study of traditional and nontraditional children's baseball. *Research Quarterly for Exercise and Sport, 55,* 351-355.

Martinek, T.J., Cheffers, J.T., and Zaichkowsky, L.D. (1978). Physical activity, motor development and self concept: Race and age differences. *Perceptual and Motor Skills, 46,* 147-154.

Maul, T. and Thomas, J.R. (1975). Self-concept and participation in children's gymnastics. *Perceptual and Motor Skills, 41,* 701-702.

McElroy, M.A. (1979). Sport participation and educational aspirations: An explicit consideration of academic and sport value climates. *Research Quarterly, 50,* 241-248.

McElroy, M.A. and Kirkendall, D.R. (1980). Significant others and professionalized sport attitudes. *Research Quarterly for Exercise and Sport, 51,* 645-653.

McIntosh, P.C. (1971). An historical view of sport and social control. *International Review of Sport Sociology, 6,* 5-13.

McPherson, B.D. (1977). The process of becoming an elite hockey player in Canada. In J. Taylor (Ed.), *Post-Olympic Games symposium* (pp. 170-179). Ottawa: Coaching Association of Canada.

McPherson, B.D. (1981). Socialization into and through sport involvement. In G. Luschen and G.H. Sage (Eds.), *Handbook of social science and sport* (pp. 246-273). Champaign, IL: Stipes.

McPherson, B.D. (1982). The child in competitive sport: Influence of the social milieu. In R.A. Magill, M.J. Ash, and F.L. Smoll (Ed.), *Children in sport* (2nd ed.) (pp. 247-278). Champaign, IL: Human Kinetics.

Mead, G. (1934). *Mind, self, and society.* Chicago: University of Chicago Press.

Melcher, N. and Sage, G.H. (1978). Relationship between parental attitudes toward physical activity and the attitudes and motor competence of their daughters. *International Review of Sport Sociology, 13*(3), 75-87.

Millar, S. (1968). *The psychology of play.* Baltimore: Penguin Books.

The Miller Lite Report on American Attitudes Toward Sports. (1983). New York: Research & Forecasters, Inc.

Mintz, R. and Muller, D. (1977). Academic achievement as a function of specific and global measures of self concept. *Journal of Psychology, 97,* 53-57.

Morgan, W.P. (1980). The trait psychology controversy. *Research Quarterly for Exercise and Sport, 51,* 50-76.

Morgan, W.P. (1981). Psychological benefits of physical activity. In F.J. Nagle and H.J. Montoye (Eds.), *Exercise in health and disease* (pp. 299-314). Springfield, IL: Charles C. Thomas.

Morris, A., Vaccaro, P. and Clark, D.H. (1979). Psychological characteristics of age-group competitive swimmers. *Perceptual and Motor Skills, 48,* 1265-1266.

National Federation Handbook (1984). Kansas City, MO: National Federation of State High School Associations.

Nisbitt, R.E. (1968). Birth order and participation in dangerous sports. *Journal of Personality and Social Psychology, 8,* 351-353.

Orlick, T. (1978). *The cooperative sports and games book.* New York: Pantheon Books.

Orlick, T.D. (1981). Positive socialization via cooperative games. *Developmental Psychology, 17,* 426-429.

Orlick, T. and Foley, C. (1976). Pre-school cooperative games: A preliminary perspective. In A. Yiannakis, T.D. McIntyre, M.J. Melnick, & D.P. Hart (Eds.), *Sport sociology: Contemporary themes* (2nd ed.). Dubuque, IA: Kendall/Hunt.

Orlick, T., McNally, J. and O'Hara, T. (1978). Cooperative games: Systematic analysis and cooperative impact. In F.L. Smoll and R.E. Smith (Eds.), *Psychological perspectives in youth sports* (pp. 203-225). Washington, D.C.: Hemisphere.

Otto, L.B. and Alwin, D.F. (1977). Athletics, aspirations, and attainments. *Sociology of Education, 42,* 102-113.

Pauly, J.T., Palmer, J.A., Wright, C.C., and Pfeiffer, G.J. (1982). The effect of a 14-week employee fitness program on selected physiological and psychological paramaters. *Journal of Occupational Medicine, 24,* 457-463.

Piaget, J. (1962). *Play, dreams, and imitation in childhood.* New York: Norton.

Piaget, J. (1965). *The moral judgment of the child.* New York: Free Press.

Picou, J.S. (1978). Race, athletic achievement, and educational aspiration. *The Sociological Quarterly, 19,* 429-438.

Picou, J.S. and Curry E.W. (1974). Residence and the athletic participation-educational aspiration hypothesis. *Social Science Quarterly, 55,* 768-776.

Picou, J.S. and Hwang, S. (1982). Educational aspirations of academically-disadvantaged athletes. *Journal of Sport Behavior, 5,* 59-76.

Podilchak, W. (1982). Youth sport involvement: Impact on informal game participation. In A.O. Dunleavy, A.W. Miracle, and C.R. Rees (Eds.), *Studies in the sociology of sport* (pp. 325-348). Fort Worth, TX: Texas Christian University Press.

Polgar, S.K. (1976). The social context of games: Or when is play not play? *Sociology of Education, 49,* 265-271.

Purdy, D.A. and Richard, S.F. (1983). Sport and juvenile delinquency: An examination and assessment of four major theories. *Journal of Sport Behavior, 6,* 179-193.

Rehberg, R.A. and Cohen, M. (1975). Athletes and scholars: An analysis of the compositional characteristics and images of these two youth culture categories. *International Review of Sport Sociology, 10,* 91-106, Number 1.

Rehberg, R.A. and Schafer, W.E. (1968). Participation in interscholastic athletics and college expectations. *American Journal of Sociology, 73,* 732-740.

Richardson, D. (1962). Ethical conduct in sport situations. *Proceedings of the National College Physical Education Association for Men, 66,* 98-103.

Rider, R.H. (1973). *The influence of basketball coaches on their players' personalities.* Unpublished doctoral dissertation, University of Utah, Salt Lake City.

Roberts, J., Arth, M.J. and Bush, R.R. (1959). Games in culture. *American Anthropologist, 61,* 597-605.

Rosenberg, M. (1979). *Conceiving the self.* New York: Basic Books.

Rubin, K.H., Fein, G.G., and Vanderberg, B. (1983). Play. In E.M. Hetherington (Ed.), *Handbook of child psychology: Socialization, personality and social development* (4th ed.) (pp. 693-774). New York: Wiley.

Rudolph, R. (1962). *The American college and university.* New York: Random House.

Ruffer, W.A. (1975, 1976). Updated bibliographies: Personality traits of athletes, *The Physical Educator, 32* (2, 3, 4), *33* (1, 2, 3).

Rushall, B.S. (1972). Three studies relating personality variables to football performance. *International Journal of Sport Psychology, 3,* 12-24.

Sack, A.L. and Thiel, R. (1979). College football and social mobility: A case study of Notre Dame football players. *Sociology of Education, 52,* 60-66.

Sage, G.H. (1978, October). American values and sport: Formation of a bureaucratic personality. *Journal of Physical Education and Recreation, 49,* 42-44.

Sage, G.H. (1980a). Parental influence and socialization into sport for male and female intercollegiate athletes. *Journal of Sport and Social Issues, 4* (Fall/Winter), 1-13.

Sage, G.H. (1980b). Orientations toward sport of male and female intercollegiate athletes. *Journal of Sport Psychology, 2,* 355-362.

Schafer, W.E. (1969). Some social sources and consequences of interscholastic athletics: The case of participation and delinquency. In G.S. Kenyon (Ed.), *Aspects of contemporary sport sociology* (pp. 29-44). Chicago: Athletic Institute.

Schafer, W.E. and Armer, M.J. (1968, November). Athletes are not inferior students. *Trans-Action, 6,* 21-26, 61-62.

Schafer, W.E. and Rehberg, R.A. (1970). Athletic participation, college aspirations, and college encouragement. *Pacific Sociological Review, 13,* 182-186.

Scheier, M.A. and Krout, R.E. (1979). Increasing educational achievement via self concept change. *Review of Educational Research, 49,* 131-150.

Segrave, J.O. (1983). Sport and juvenile delinquency. In R.L. Terjung (Ed.), *Exercise and Sport Sciences Reviews,* Vol. 11. (pp. 181-209). Philadelphia: Franklin Institute.

Segrave, J.O. and Chu, D. (1978). Athletics and juvenile delinquency. *Review of Sport and Leisure, 3,* 1-24.

Segrave, J.O. and Hastad, D.N. (1984). Interscholastic athletic participation and delinquent behavior: An empirical assessment of relevant variables. *Sociology of Sport Journal, 1,* 117-137.

Shavelson, R.J. and Bolus, R. (1982). Self-concept: The interplay of theory and methods. *Journal of Educational Psychology, 74,* 3-17.

Silva III, J.M. (1981). Normative compliance and rule violating behavior in sport. *International Journal of Sport Psychology, 12,* 10-18.

Smith, R.E., Smoll, F.L., and Curtis, B. (1979). Coach effectiveness training: A cognitive-behavioral approach to enhancing relationship skills in youth sport coaches. *Journal of Sport Psychology, 1,* 59-75.

Smith, R.E., Zane, N.W.S., Smoll, F.L. and Coppel, D.B. (1983). Behavioral assessment in youth sports: Coaching behaviors and children's attitudes. *Medicine and Science in Sports and Exercise, 15,* 208-214.

Smoll, F.L. and Smith, R.E. (1984). Leadership research in youth sports. In J.M. Silva III and R.S. Weinberg (Eds.,), *Psychological foundations of sport* (pp. 371-386). Champaign, IL: Human Kinetics.

Synder, E.E. and Spreitzer, E. (1973). Family influences and involvement in sports. *Research Quarterly, 44,* 249-255.

Snyder, E.E. and Spreitzer, E. (1976). Correlates of sports participation among adolescent girls. *Research Quarterly, 47,* 804-809.

Synder, E.E. and Spreitzer, E. (1977). Participation in sport as related to educational expectations among high school girls. *Sociology of Education, 50,* 47-55.

Snyder, E.E. and Spreitzer, E. (1979). Orientations toward sport: Intrinsic, normative and extrinsic. *Journal of Sport Psychology, 1,* 170-175.

Snyder, E.E. and Purdy, D.A. (1982). Socialization into sport: Parent and child reverse and reciprocal effects. *Research Quarterly for Exercise and Sport, 53,* 263-266.

Sonstroem, R.J. (1974). Attitude testing examining certain psychological correlates of physical activity. *Research Quarterly, 45,* 93-103.

Sonstroem, R.J. (1978). Physical estimation and attraction scales: Rationale and research. *Medicine and Science of Sports, 10,* 97-102.

Sonstroem, R.J. (1984). Exercise and self-esteem. In R.L. Terjung (Ed.), *Exercise and Sport Sciences Reviews* (Vol. 12) (pp. 123-155). Lexington, MA: Collamore Press.

Spady, W.G. (1970). Lament of the letterman: Effects of peer status and extra curricular activities on goals and achievement. *American Journal of Sociology, 75,* 680-702.

Spreitzer, E. and Pugh, M. (1973). Interscholastic athletics and educational expectations. *Sociology of Education, 46,* 171-182.

Staniford, D.J. (1979). *Play and physical activity in early childhood socialization.* (Sociology of Sport Monograph Series). Vanier City, Ontario: CAHPER.

Stevenson, C.L. (1975). Socialization effects of participation in sport: A critical review of the research. *Research Quarterly, 46,* 287-301.

Straub, W.F. and Felock, T. (1974). Attitudes toward physical activity of delinquent and nondelinquent junior high school girls. *Research Quarterly, 45,* 21-27.

Sutton-Smith, B. (1974, Fall). Toward an anthropology of play. *The Association for the Anthropological Study of Play Newsletter, 1,* 10.

Sutton-Smith, B. and Roberts, J.M. (1970). The cross-cultural and psychological study of games. In G. Luschen (Ed.), *The cross-cultural analysis of sport and games* (pp. 100-108). Champaign, IL: Stipes.

Sutton-Smith, B. and Rosenberg, B.G. (1961). Sixty years of historical change in the game preferences of American children. *Journal of American Folklore, 74,* 17-46.

Sutton-Smith, B., Rosenberg, B.G., and Morgan, E.F. (1963). Development of sex differences in play choices during preadolescence. *Child Development, 34,* 119-126.

Theberge, N., Curtis, J., and Brown, B. (1982). Sex differences in orientations toward games: Tests of the sport involvement hypothesis. In A.D. Dunleavy, A.W. Miracle, and C.R. Rees (Eds.), *Studies in the sociology of sport* (pp. 285-308).

Ft. Worth, TX: Texas Christian University Press.

Thomes, T.D., Young, R.J., and Ismail, A.H. (1973, April). The effect of a football season on the personality of high school athletes. Paper presented at the annual convention of the American Association of Health, Physical Education, and Recreation, Minneapolis, MN.

Tucker, L.A. (1982). Effect of a weight-training program on the self-concepts of college males. *Perceptual and Motor Skills, 54,* 1055-1061.

Vincent, M. F. (1976). Comparison of self-concept of college women: Athletes and physical education majors. *Research Quarterly, 47,* 218-225.

Waters, E. and Sroufe, L.A. (1983). Social competence as a developmental construct. *Developmental Review, 3,* 79-97.

Webb, H. (1969). Professionalization of attitudes toward play among adolescents. In G.S. Kenyon (Ed.), *Aspects of contemporary sport sociology* (pp. 161-178). Chicago: Athletic Institute.

Weinberg, S.K. and Arond, H. (1952). The occupational culture of the boxer. *American Journal of Sociology, 57,* 460-469.

Wells, R.H. and Picou, J.S. (1980). Interscholastic athletes and socialization for educational achievement. *Journal of Sport Behavior, 3,* 119-128.

Wentworth, M.W. (1980). *Context and understanding: An inquiry into socialization theory.* New York: Elsevier.

Wheeler, D.A. (1981). The self-concept of participants in kayaking, skydiving and hang gliding. Unpublished master's thesis, Brigham Young University, Provo, UT.

Wylie, R.C. (1979). *The self-concept: Theory and research on selected topics,* Vol. 2, (rev. ed.). Lincoln: University of Nebraska Press.

Yiannakis, A. (1976a). Birth order and preference for dangerous sports among males. *Research Quarterly, 47,* 62-67.

Yiannakis, A. (1976b). Delinquent tendencies and participation in an organized sports program. *Research Quarterly, 47,* 845-849.

Yiannakis, A. (1978). Formal and informal play settings: A discussive analysis of processes and outcomes for children. In *Proceedings of the National College Physical Education Association for Men/National Association of Physical Education for College Women* (pp. 175-182).

Zeigler, S.G. (1972). Changes in self-perception of high school girls toward themselves and their coaches during a basketball season. Unpublished master's thesis, Pennsylvania State College, PA.

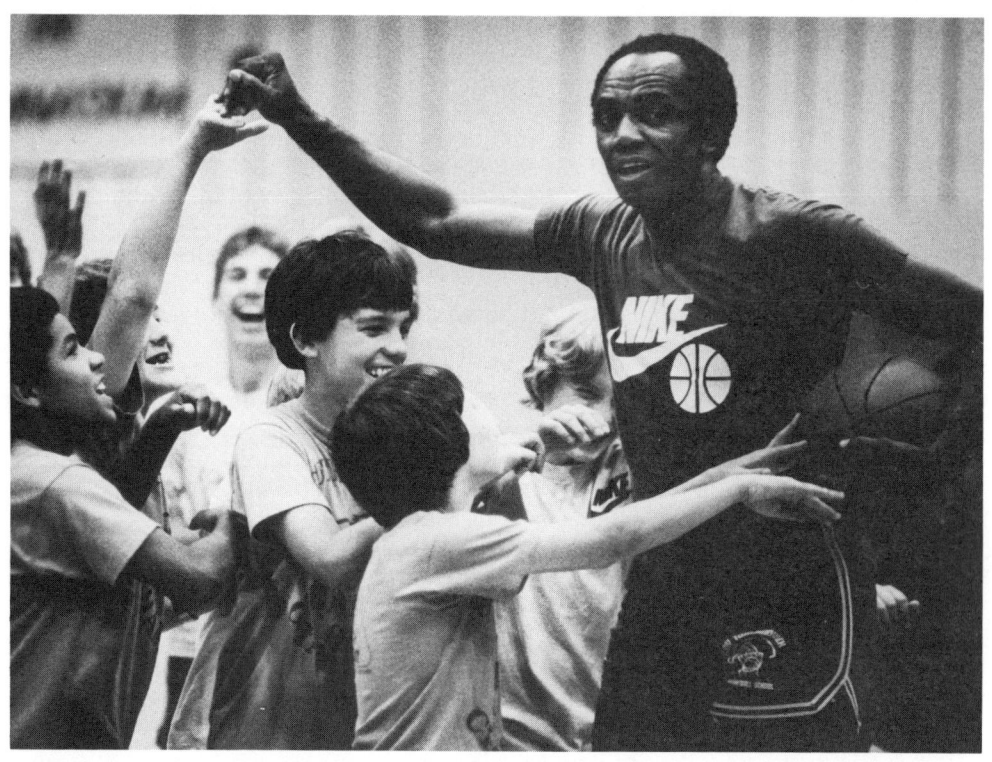
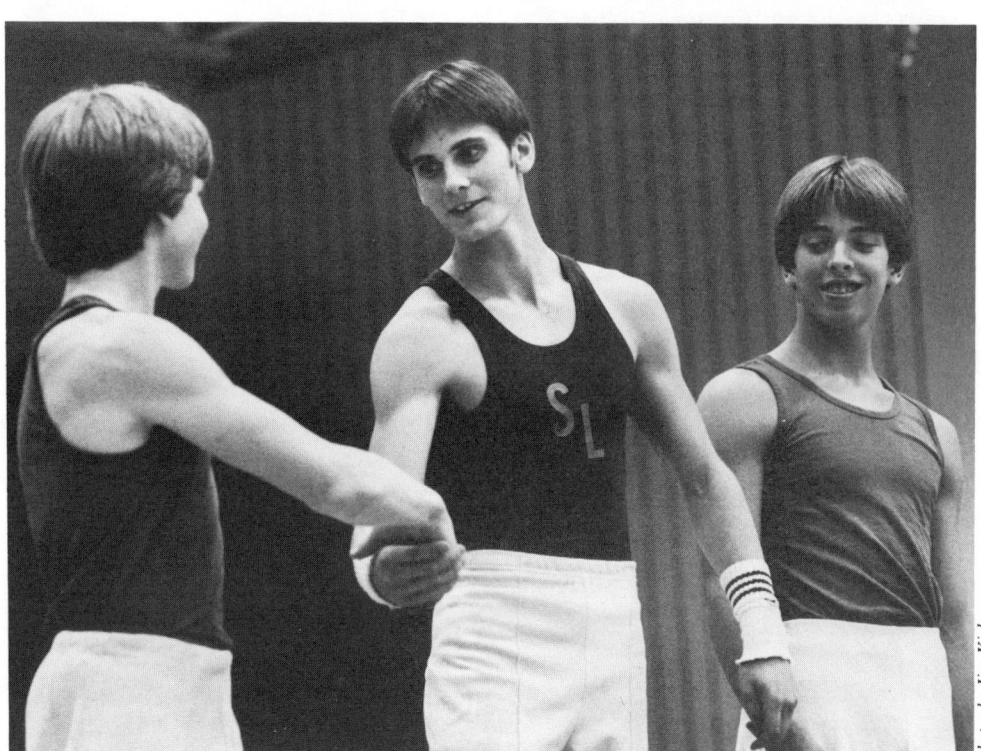

photos by Jim Kirby

CHAPTER THIRTEEN

Moral Development

Maureen R. Weiss
College of Human Development and Performance
University of Oregon
Eugene, Oregon

Brenda Jo Bredemeier
Department of Physical Education
University of California
Berkeley, California

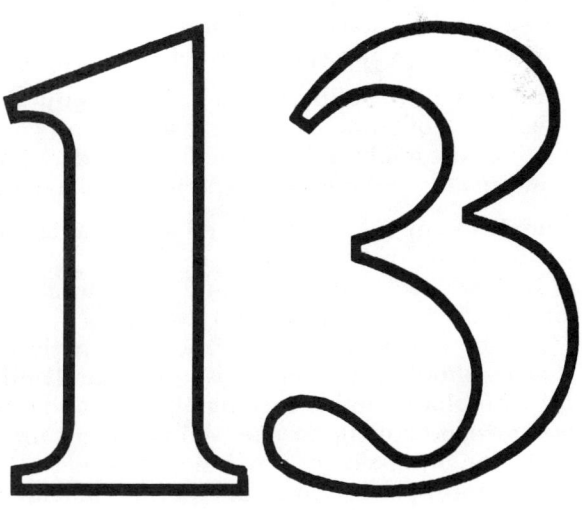

Many have claimed that moral development is one of the most important social psychological outcomes of participation in physical education and sport. Numerous experiences that occur in gymnasiums and on playing fields provide opportunities for enhancing moral growth. The contention that these experiences actually promote moral development, however, is not without a great deal of controversy.

We have all heard the adage "sport builds character" and yet it seems that a day does not go by without some unethical sport practice finding its way into the news. This paradoxical situation is one source for the divergent perspectives held in our culture about the role of physical activity. Tom Landry, successful coach of the Dallas Cowboys, contends that, "the greatest contribution that sports can make to young athletes is to build character. The greatest teacher of character is on the athletic field" (Smith, Smith & Smoll, 1983, p. 9). Yet Russell Baker (1984), eminent journalist of the New York Times, claims, "For the young, the lesson from the field is that rotten manners, greed and determination to win at any cost to body and soul are virtues . . . save the children. Stamp out sports."

Each of these divergent perspectives has, in its own way, functioned to impede physical educators' efforts to maximize moral development among their students. Those who challenge the contention that sport can build morals as well as muscles do not attempt to employ moral education programs. Those who believe sport builds character tend to assume that this process is automatic. They do not consciously construct moral education programs, but relegate moral development to the "hidden curriculum" (Jackson, 1968), assuming that moral growth will occur automatically as a natural response to experience in organized physical activity (Jewett & Bain, 1985). McIntosh (1979) and others (Bredemeier & Shields, 1983; Figley, 1984; Kroll, 1975; Park, 1983) have cautioned that if moral education is to be effective, it must be explicit and not part of a hidden curriculum. It is, perhaps, this point above all others that has eluded many of those who recognize the potential for facilitating moral development through physical education and sport.

In recognition of the potential influence of physical education on students' moral growth, the American Academy of Physical Education recently drafted a position statement designed to take moral development out of the hidden curriculum and emphasize it as an explicit goal of the profession:

> Because of the opportunities to teach ethical values and to influence moral behavior of students through sports and games, it is thought that physical educators might well place an increased emphasis on the problems of ethical judgments and morally responsible behavior in sports (Park, 1983, p. 53).

The Academy urged physical educators to consider, deliberate upon, and act on the following recommendations:

1. The development of moral and ethical values should be among the stated aims of the physical education program.

2. The educational preparation of physical education teachers and athletic coaches should place emphasis upon moral and ethical values.

3. Emphasis on the teaching of moral and ethical values by physical education teachers and athletic coaches should be encouraged.

4. The profession of physical education should establish criteria for the selection of appropriate ethical and moral values, develop formal plans of instruction, and develop methods for the assessment of results (p. 53).

Physical educators have been charged by the American Academy of Physical Education to work together to enhance the positive experiences that children may have in physical education and sport. The experience of practitioners, the conceptualization of theorists, and the findings of researchers can be pooled to develop sound physical education programs designed to promote moral growth.

This chapter summarizes what we know about how moral development is related to physical education and sport experiences. The chapter begins with a brief overview of the major theoretical approaches to moral development; this provides a framework for the subsequent critical review of empirical studies of moral growth among physical education and sport participants. Finally, theoretically-grounded instructional strategies are offered as possible alternatives for those physical educators who seek to facilitate their students' moral growth.

A Question of Terminology

A necessary starting point in reviewing the contributions of physical activity to moral development is to define the term "morality." Often, morality in the realm of sport is equated with "sportsmanship," a term with a variety of meanings. For example, when Martens (1978) asked children to define sportsmanship, they responded with the following descriptions: playing by the rules; being a good winner and loser; being even-tempered; respecting the decisions, requests, and opinions of others; and taking turns, letting others play.

A closer look at this list reveals that much of what children are defining as sportsmanship are social conventional behaviors. For our purposes, it will be important to distinguish that which is "moral" from what is "conventional." Social-conventional behaviors are those which conform to prescribed social norms and are intended to maintain social organization. Examples of such behavior include shaking an opponent's hand before or after a contest, not swearing at the referee, or wearing certain prescribed clothing (white shorts in tennis). In contrast, moral behaviors are those which are concerned with the physical or psychological welfare of others and the protection of rights and responsibilities (Bredemeier & Shields, 1983). Examples of moral behaviors in sport might include not physically intimidating an opponent by sliding with spikes up, and not lying about a game score when there are no referees.

Recently, Haan (1977) defined morality as a process in which individuals work to achieve agreement about the rights and responsibilities of involved parties. Using this as our basic definition, related terms can also be defined (Bredemeier & Shields, in press). Sportsmanship, for our purposes, will refer to the tendency to behave in accordance with one's most mature moral reasoning patterns, even when conventional dictates or success strategies would encourage alternative behaviors. Moral education, as we shall use the term, refers to the systematic effort to provide experiences intended to promote maturity of moral reasoning, deepen affective commitment to moral responsibility, and encourage the union of moral thought and action.

A common question in the study of moral development is, "What is the relationship between moral reasoning and moral behavior?" Moral reasoning refers to the thought processes or cognitions used to make decisions about the rightness/wrongness or goodness/badness of an act. Moral behavior, as noted earlier, is any action which has impact on another's well-being.

Many social scientists have documented the difficulty in assessing moral thought-action relationships (Blasi, 1980; Hartshorne & May, 1928). The consistency between reasoning and behavior is evaluated in light of each individual's rationale for his or her own behavior. Thus, teachers cannot determine whether an individual is acting in a morally mature way without assessing that individual's reasoning about the act. Reasoning and behavior go hand in hand, and both must be considered in any educational program of moral development.

Theories of Moral Development

Over the years, several theories have been formulated to explain the process of moral development and to offer prescriptions for facilitating its growth in various educational settings. The discussion in this section is drawn from social learning and structural developmental approaches.

Social Learning Approach

Social learning theorists (Aronfreed, 1968; Bandura, 1969; 1977) contend that moral development occurs as a product of modeling and reinforcement from others within the larger process of socialization. Moral behaviors, operationally defined by social learning theorists as action which conforms to social norms and regulations, are learned through interaction with socializing agents. Children are assumed to internalize the accepted behaviors of their society or culture through the powerful effects of models who are nurturant, warm, or high in status and power, and through differential reinforcement, especially the giving and withholding of affection.

The focus of social learning theory is on behavior as it approximates or fluctuates from social norms. In essence, the extent to which social norms are accepted and expressed reflects the relative moral development of an individual. Advocates of the social learning approach have not elaborated on theoretical constructs which would enable researchers to investigate the cognitive and affective dimensions of moral development (Aronfreed, 1976). Thus, structural developmental approaches, which emphasize cognitive and affective components of morality, complement the social learning approach.

Structural Developmental Approaches

Structural developmentalists focus primarily on the cognitions that individuals use to determine the legitimacy of particular behaviors. These theorists contend that all individuals go through an age-related progression in which representational thought becomes more sophisticated and integrated. Moral development occurs as a product of the child's active structuring of his or her experiences with the social environment.

Structural developmental theories distinguish between the *content* of moral knowledge and the *structure* of moral thought. The content of knowledge refers to what a person believes and is dependent upon culturally variable influences. As an individual matures, the content of knowledge increases in *quantity* as more and more experiences are internalized by the individual. Structure, however, refers to *how* a person organizes the contents of his or her thoughts and behaviors. Moral growth, according to structural developmentalists, involves *qualitative* changes in the way individuals organize moral experiences. Transformations in reasoning structure, referred to as stages or levels of reasoning, occur in an age-related sequence. Through these changes, one's interpretation of the content of the social environment, such as social definitions of rightness or wrongness of particular acts, is transformed.

For social learning theorists, a moral behavior is one in which the content of the act is consistent with society's norms. For structural developmentalists, morality is defined by the reasoning structure which underlies behavior. Changes in moral reasoning structures have been described and explained in two different structural developmental models: the cognitivist model and the interactionist model.

Cognitivist model. Moral development, according to this model, is related to the reasoning abilities and the cognitive role-taking abilities of individuals. Jean Piaget (1932) was the first to study moral thought and behavior from this perspective. He was not as interested in the actual expression of moral behavior as he was in the reasons children gave for behaviors that were considered to go against the grain of social norms and regulations. One set of Piaget's observations and assessments centered on children's participation in the game of marbles. He focused on how they adhered to or changed the rules as they negotiated with one another on what was fair in the game.

Piaget identified two major stages of morality: a morality of constraint, and a morality of cooperation. In the stage of constraint, the child submits to and accepts adult commands. What is "right" is what conforms to these demands. One important dimension of this stage of morality is the child's "objective" concept of responsibility. That is, children at this stage judge actions as right or wrong based on observable physical consequences rather than in terms of the actor's intent. For example, a girl in a kickball game who tries to kick a homerun but instead injures the pitcher by kicking the ball into her knee would be judged as naughtier than a baseball player who tries to hit the ball at the pitcher but misses, so no one gets hurt.

Piaget's second stage of morality is known as the morality of cooperation. When reasoning at this stage, the child does not rigidly adhere to rules commanded by adults, but engages in reciprocal social interaction with peers to construct mutual agreements. The conditions of cooperation are motivated by mutual respect for peers rather than by unilateral respect for adult authority. In this stage of morality, the child changes from a focus on "objective" responsibility for actions to "subjective" responsibility. That is, the individual at this more mature stage of moral development views the rightness and wrongness of actions based on the *intentions* underlying the observable action. Thus, the girl who had good intentions of kicking a home run but nonetheless injured the pitcher would be judged as less naughty than the baseball player whose bad intentions did not result in injury.

Piaget viewed the structural change from a morality of constraint to a morality of cooperation as being determined by two major sources: cognitive disequilibrium and peer interaction. The notion of cognitive disequilibrium follows from Piaget's discussions of cognitive development in that all cognitive structures are forms of organizing experiences and actions. When new experience cannot be assimilated into existing structures, the person is said to be in a state of disequilibrium. Thus, a child who cannot explain his or her interactions in a given situation using a morality of constraint "searches" for a new cognitive structure to reestablish equilibrium. The new cognitive structure provides a more adequate way of conceptualizing moral experience.

Piaget also suggested that moral growth occurs through social interaction with peers who negotiate and bargain with each other for arranging mutually beneficial experiences. This give-and-take among peers, he contended, fosters a recognition of the reciprocity of cooperation and facilitates role-taking opportunities which are critical for enhancing moral growth processes.

Lawrence Kohlberg (1981, 1984) extended and modified Piaget's cognitivist approach. The significance of Kohlberg's contribution to this field is demonstrated by the fact that his theory of moral stages is in some way taken into account by almost every other theory of moral development (Lickona, 1976). Kohlberg's primary goal was to continue what Piaget had begun: to chart the developmental changes in thinking about moral issues, to search for sequential and universal stages of moral growth, and to understand how conceptions of morality are related to the overall growth of the human mind (Lickona, 1976).

Unlike Piaget, who used forced choice story formats (i.e., "which child is naughtier?"), Kohlberg employed open-ended questions to probe individual's reasoning about how to resolve hypothetical moral dilemmas. Through his analyses of underlying thought structures, Kohlberg distinguished six stages of moral reasoning. These six stages, in turn, have been classified into three levels of moral growth, proceeding from an egocentric through a societal to a universal perspective in judging behaviors as right or wrong. The moral reasoning levels are labeled preconventional, conventional, and postconventional.

At the preconventional level (typical of children younger than 9 and some adolescents), individuals are most concerned with their personal welfare. They have yet to understand and uphold the rules and expectations of society. At this level, decisions tend to be based on whether or not one will get punished for engaging in a particular behavior. In other words, the physical consequences of action determine its goodness or badness, regardless of the human value inherent in the consequences.

For example, in a recent tennis tournament, John McEnroe threw his racket in disgust after losing his temper over a controversial line call. The racket head became dislodged from the handle and catapulted toward the crowd. It barely missed hitting one of the spectators. When asked by media personnel, "If this has happened before, why do you keep doing it?", McEnroe replied, "I might consider changing because it's not worth being fined for . . . and everyone in the crowd started booing after that and people like you ask me questions" (Boswell, 1984). McEnroe's response was limited to concern for the consequences he might experience as a result of such an action. If we were to assume that this response reflected McEnroe's considered moral opinion, then the statement would reflect a preconventional moral understanding.

The conventional level of morality is concerned with maintaining the norms of an individual's family, group, or society. According to Kohlberg, most adolescents and adults occupy this level of moral reasoning. Had McEnroe reconsidered his racket throwing because he perceived it to be in violation of tennis etiquette or civil law, he may have been employing conventional reasoning.

At the postconventional level of reasoning (engaged in by a minority of adults over the age of 20), individuals understand and generally accept society's rules, but on the basis of general moral principles that underlie societal rules. For Kohlberg, these moral principles are encompassed by justice, the most adequate of all moral principles. The principle of justice sometimes conflicts with society's rules; in these cases, the postconventional reasoner makes judgments guided by the justice principle, not by the social norm. McEnroe may have been using principled reasoning if, in his reconsideration of racket throwing, he had appealed to the rights of spectators to be protected from physical and psychological harm during athletic contests. Reasoning is principled when guided by prescriptive, abstract, and universalizable principles, rather than by a simple recognition of etiquette or laws.

Kohlberg has claimed that these six stages in his model are sequential, invariant, and universal for all human beings. While not everyone may reach a principled level of moral reasoning (stages 5 or 6), he has posited that each individual proceeds from stage 1 to stage 2, etc., with no skipping of stages.

Kohlberg's moral education programs encourage cognitive disequilibrium and role taking opportunities, both of which have been shown to enhance levels of moral reasoning (Kohlberg, 1984; Rest, 1983; Selman, 1976). It is believed that children who are exposed to reasoning one stage above their own will not be able to assimilate the experience with their existing structures, and consequently, will experience cognitive disequilibrium. Moral growth will occur when the children attempt to integrate higher level reasoning about hypothetical stories in their cognitive repertoire.

Role-taking opportunity, according to Kohlberg, is similar to cognitive disequilibrium in that it is a necessary but insufficient experience for attaining higher stages of moral reasoning. Role-taking refers to the capacity of a person to understand the relationship between his or her own perspective and that of others. This includes understanding and interpreting other's thoughts and feelings, and their role in society.

While Kohlberg has undisputedly made significant contributions to the area of moral development, his model has been criticized for a number of reasons. First, critics have been concerned about gender and cultural biases (Gilligan, 1982;

Haan, Smith, & Block, 1968), and have challenged the claim of a universal, invariant stage sequence. In addition, by reducing all morality to the virtue of justice, a philosophical bias may exist. Critics have charged that the use of hypothetical stories as opposed to actual moral dilemmas seriously limits an understanding of the moral reasoning-moral behavior relationship. Finally, Kohlberg's model does not take into account the role of affect in moral growth except to say that it disrupts the "true" emergence of the moral self (Haan, 1977).

Interactionist model. Norma Haan has proposed an alternative structural developmental model of morality. According to her scheme, morality is best understood by analyzing individuals' reasoning within specific social contexts. Haan's model of moral development (Haan, 1977; Haan, Aerts, & Cooper, in press) shares many features with Kohlberg's, but can be distinguished from his better known model in several important ways: (a) it defines moral reasoning as embodied in moral *action* rather than abstracted from a specific context; (b) it reflects the development of capacities for *inductive* moral construction, as opposed to Kohlberg's emphasis upon deductive reasoning used to determine moral judgments; (c) it is not grounded in a universal principle of justice which defines rights; rather, Haan's moral ground of respect for persons pertains to the procedures employed in negotiating about situational issues; and (d) it represents a more flexible interpretation of structuralism that is not based on a view of invariant, sequential, cognitively-based moral stages.

According to Haan, morality pertains to decisions about any act that has physical or psychological consequences for the well-being of one's self and others. Morality involves a process of constructing moral balance or agreement among parties involved in some relationship. The way in which moral balance is achieved is through dialogue which allows all participants to be aware of each viewpoint involved. Thus, dialogue and balance become the guiding principles for constructing morality. This contrasts with Kohlberg's notions of deductive reasoning based on the principle of justice which guides moral judgment. Thus, Haan contends that in each situational context, individuals must enter into moral dialogue in order to reach consensus about a solution to moral dilemmas that arise so that moral balance is achieved. Through this process, Haan's focus is on equalization through interpersonal processes.

There are five levels of interactional morality. Self-interest is the predominant characteristic in the first two levels. At the first level, moral balances result from the use of differential power; they entail complying with others when forced and compelling others when possible. An example of moral balancing at this level would be, "You have to let me go first in this game because I am older than you."

At the second level, moral balances which provide an advantage for oneself are sought, but the necessity of trade-offs or compromises is recognized. An example might be, "If you let me go first in this game, I'll let you go before me in the cafeteria line."

In contrast to the egocentric focus of the first two levels, the person at level three sees himself or herself as part of the human family, and acts morally by being altruistic in response to the needs and desires of others. Trust is an important characteristic at this level as individuals seek to create moral balance by making harmonious exchanges for the good of others. An example of moral reasoning at this level is "I'll let her go before me in line since she really loves this game."

At the fourth level of interactional morality, experience with people of "bad faith" lead to the seeking of objective and impartial external rules as a basis for balances. Individuals support rules and regulations that serve the common interest of all. As an illustration, a person reasoning at level four may state that "The rule is that we go in order according to how we get in line. We've all agreed to go by the rules and that should hold true for you and me, too."

At the highest developmental level, individuals seek situationally-specific moral

Table 1.
Reasoning Illustrations and Growth Prescriptions for Each Developmental Level

Moral Level	Reasoning Illustration	Prescription for Moral Growth
Level One: Power Balancing	"Of course it was fair. I got away with it, didn't I?"	Growth results from the person's discovery that: a) one is not completely dependent on the whims of others, and b) one can negotiate with others. Sport can aid growth by providing experiences of autonomy and use of such negotiation-oriented procedures as "taking turns" at doing things.
Level Two: Egocentric Balancing	"She elbowed me on a rebound, so I made sure I got her back the first chance I got."	Growth results as a person experiences the negative implications of egocentric behavior, such as the dissolution of friendships or the disruption of cooperation from others. Sport experience can encourage the recognition that one becomes isolated if others' interests are not taken into account. The disputes that naturally arise in sport become grist for growth if they are not prematurely resolved by authorities, but are allowed to highlight the consequences of self-interested action. Promoting images of good sportspersonship can also be helpful.
Level Three: Harmony Balancing	"I passed off to Tom because his parents were there and he really wanted a chance to play. So what if we lost."	Movement toward the next level is stimulated by experiences of "bad faith" and by disruptions in interpersonal relationships resulting from the desire to please more than one group. Sport experiences can encourage growth when participants recognize rather than rationalize about instances where opponents and others have taken advantage of naive trust. An emphasis on the need for "impartial" regulators (such as referees) can be useful.
Level Four: Common Interest Balancing	"Win or lose, you've got to go by the rules. We've all agreed to play the game and that means following the rules, doing what your coach tells you and accepting the opinion of the officials."	A moral transition may occur as one becomes aware that impartial regulation is inadequate to fully prescribe one's rights and duties given the complexities and particularities found in human life. Moral growth may be encouraged when dialogue among all participants, including opponents, is advocated. Sport dialogue can focus on such topics as unequal distribution of skills, differing motivations for play, lopsided scores, rule maintenance, etc.
Level Five: Mutual Interest Balancing	"Let's forfeit the meet. If she tries that dive in an effort to catch up with us, she could get hurt. We're all in this together."	Level five reasoning can be reinforced by providing opportunities to dialogue and participate in decision-making about real moral issues that arise. Focusing on the particularities of the situation and emphasizing how the rule structure is valuable but inadequate for all situations can be helpful.

balances which optimize the interests of all parties involved. At this level, moral balance is much more differential, sensitive, and flexible than that at level four. An example here would be, "You can go ahead of me this time because you have to leave in a few minutes." See Table 1 for Haan's five levels of morality with examples.[1]

These five moral levels chart the developmental course for understanding moral exchange from early self-centered through mature interpersonal interaction. Haan's conception of interactional morality seems to be the most appropriate for implementation into physical education programs because it includes affective and cognitive components in an action setting. Few investigators, however, have explored the usefulness of interactional morality in the physical education domain.

A summary chart of the social learning and structural developmental (cognitivist and interactional) approaches to moral development, including their basis for ethical practices, source of moral growth, and definition of morality can be found in Table 2 (Coakley & Bredemeier, in press).

Table 2.
Two Approaches to Moral Development

	Basis for Ethical Practices	Source of Moral Growth	Definition of Morality
I. Social Learning Approach	socialization & internalization of conventional social mandates	clear, consistent, & reinforcing feedback from significant others	action in accordance with social definitions of prosocial behavior
II. Structural Developmental Approach			
A. Cognitivist Model	role taking & the application of abstract moral principles	cognitive disequilibrium resulting when moral reasoning at current stage does not resolve moral conflicts	making individual judgments about the intrinsic merits and consequences of behaviors
B. Interactionist Model	interpersonal exchanges and the development of consensual agreements	social disequilibrium leading to dialogue & negotiation to achieve moral balance in relationships & groups	using interpersonal skills to optimize everyone's mutual interest in a particular setting

---

[1] Stage/level typing is a difficult process. While these illustrations are typical of the level indicated, one quotation is inadequate for stage/level typing.

Moral Development Research in Physical Education and Sport

For decades, physical educators have contended that there is a character-building function of physical activity, but empirical evidence substantiating such a claim has been lacking. More commonly, anecdotes abound that suggest that physical activity trains students, "to respect the rules, to play fairly, to be thorough and dependable—to be in other words, a good sportsman" (McCloy, 1941, p. 5). Recently, a few studies have been conducted to clarify the relationship between moral development and physical activity. These studies and their implications for moral education through physical education programs are discussed in this section.

Developing Character: A "Bag of Virtues" Approach

Many researchers who have investigated the relationship between moral development and physical education have adopted what might be called a "bag of virtues" approach to understanding this relationship. The term "bag of virtues" (Kohlberg, 1981) refers to the idea that morality can be defined by a list, or "bag" of character traits or virtues that are arbitrarily selected by the researcher. A sport psychologist using the "bag of virtues" strategy might, for example, define sportsmanship as honesty, sharing, peer encouragement, or not fighting. Such an approach fails to relate moral growth to an integrated and philosophically defensible definition of morality. Consequently, any conclusions drawn from the findings of such studies are confined to the selected characteristics as exhibited within the parameters of the study.

The moral growth-physical activity literature can be characterized by three types of "bag of virtues" studies: those which focus on personality characteristics, value orientations, and prosocial behavior. Researchers investigating personality characteristics have been interested in dispositional traits thought to represent the substance of moral character. Sportsmanlike and unsportsmanlike individuals were believed to be distinguished by these traits (McCloy, 1941).

A study by Blanchard (1946) is illustrative of personality trait research. Blanchard was interested in the impact of physical education on character development in boys and girls over a two-year period. Character was defined in terms of cooperation, self-control, and sociability. Behavioral measures were taken prior to and after the two-year period, with increases in positive character traits found to be associated with participation in physical education activities. Blanchard concluded that physical education activities do "build character" and claimed this to be especially true for girls as compared to boys.

Blanchard's study contains three problems which characterize most of the attempts to determine the influence of physical activity on personality traits. First, the selection of characteristics was based on the arbitrary preferences of the researcher. Because several expressive or interpersonal-oriented traits were chosen, it is not surprising that females showed greater gains than did males. Second, in saying that physical activity involvement *caused* changes in moral growth, Blanchard neglected the possibility that changes were a result of maturation or factors apart from involvement in physical education; she did not include a control group in her study. Finally, investigations such as Blanchard's lack a strong theoretical foundation, one that would solve definitional problems and suggest viable intervention techniques. In summary, personality studies, though the first empirical tests of the moral development-physical activity relationship, have not provided clear insights to this relationship.

A number of social scientists have examined participants' value orientations toward their sport (Kroll, 1975; Webb, 1969). According to Webb (1969), attitudes toward sport tend to evolve from a play orientation to a professional orientation.

The play orientation consists of a value hierarchy of *fairness, skill,* and *success* in that order; these priorities are reversed in a professional orientation so that success is most highly valued and fairness least valued. Webb found that as children get older and as they become more involved in organized sport, they tend to move from a play to a professional orientation.

The professionalization approach, while adding to our knowledge about sport experiences, also has severe limitations as an approach to moral growth through sport. While noting changes in value hierarchies, it does not inform us about how participants conceptualize the various values. Because participants' understanding of fairness, for example, is likely to change with age, the relationship between this value and other values is more complex than can be assessed by simply identifying relative value positions. Also, it is difficult to determine whether professionalization refers to a change in content of thought only, or a change in both the content and underlying structure of thought. The possibility exists that the professionalization of attitudes merely reflect children's conformity to the differing social norms of competitive sport rather than depicting structural development. Finally, the lack of an articulated definition of morality makes it very difficult to interpret findings from value orientation studies. Does professionalization reflect a change for the better or worse? Is it moral growth, moral retardation, or neither?

A third type of "bag of virtues" approach has been to define and observe prosocial play behaviors. This approach, favored by social learning theorists, has been the most enlightening of the "bag of virtues" approaches. Rather than focus on personality traits or value preferences, researchers operating within this framework operationalize morality in terms of identifiable behaviors such as altruism, taking turns, and cooperation with peers. Studies of prosocial play behavior have been conducted in order to establish relationships between a particular measure of moral behavior (e.g., cooperation) and participation in physical education and sport.

Kleiber and Roberts (1981) used this approach to investigate the impact of sport competition on the development of social character, operationally defined as the prosocial behaviors of cooperation and altruism. Fourth and fifth grade children were randomly assigned to a control or experimental group; the experimental group competed in a kickball tournament during a twenty minute recess period, for eight days. Before and after the tournament, prosocial behaviors were assessed using a valid paper and pencil scale. Analyses revealed that boys in the experimental group showed significantly less altruistic behavior after the experimental treatment as compared to boys in the control group.

The investigators concluded that sport competition can have the effect of diminishing prosocial tendencies. However, these results should be viewed with caution in light of using the single quality of altruism as the measure of morality, a very short experimental duration (two weeks), and the assertion that the kickball tournament resembles "organized sport."

Orlick (1981) also employed a prosocial behavior approach to investigate the relationship between physical activity and moral development. He was specifically interested in examining the effects of an 18-week cooperative games program on the willingness to share among 5-year-old children. All activities in the cooperative games program were designed to be conducted in partners or groups; activities in the traditional games program were similar to the cooperative program with regard to physical demands but stressed individual pursuits in which children could work independently of the group.

Willingness to share was assessed using a candy sharing task. Children were given five pieces of candy and asked to indicate how many pieces they would share with children in another class by putting these pieces in a designated brown bag. Orlick found conflicting results in that a cooperative games program in one school showed a significant increase in willingness to share while the other school showed no change. In one traditional games program, willingness to share significantly declined from pre- to post-test, while children in the other school's traditional program showed no difference. Again, a single measure of morality (willingness to share) provided important information about one moral variable, but offered limited insight into our general understanding of physical activity and moral development.

Finally, in a recent study, Giebink and McKenzie (1985) employed instructional strategies based on social learning and reinforcement theories to teach sportsmanship in physical education and recreation settings. Specifically, a behavioral contingency design was used with four target boys, with sportsmanlike behavior defined as positive social interaction related to game play. Unsportsmanlike behaviors were defined as negative social interaction during game play.

Intervention strategies included instructions and praise, modeling, and a point-reward system. Results revealed that the effects of the interventions varied considerably for all four boys, but all three strategies increased sportsmanship and decreased unsportsmanlike behaviors. Attempts to demonstrate generalization to a recreation setting, however, were unsuccessful.

Some weaknesses of this study are readily apparent. First, behavioral change was the only assessment made with regard to the development of sportsmanship. As other physical educators have strongly suggested (Bredemeier & Shields, 1983; Figley, 1984), it is the rationale behind the choice of behavior that determines the morality of the behavior. The increase in sportsmanlike and decrease in unsportsmanlike behavior may have occurred for a variety of reasons, including avoidance of points taken away, receiving a desirable prize, or merely complying with social convention.

Secondly, due to the research design in which instructions/praise, modeling, and point system followed baseline, it is impossible to determine which of the strategies in and of themselves affected behavior and which were the accumulation of previous strategies. The use of only four subjects also limits considerably the generalization of the results. Finally, the arbitrary selection of certain sportsmanlike behaviors and the lack of a fuller definition of morality make it hardly surprising that generalization did not occur from one setting to another.

Developing Character: Structural Developmental Approaches

In contrast to the "bag of virtues" approach, a number of investigators have based their research designs on the structure of moral reasoning. Jantz (1975) was the first to conduct a sport study based on the structural developmental theory of moral development. Specifically, he modified Piaget's marble experiment to test children's knowledge of the rules of basketball. Results revealed that children in grades 1 and 2 interpreted rules using a morality of constraint, while children in grades 3 through 6 primarily viewed rules using a morality of cooperation. The results of this study supported Piaget's developmental stages. Jantz suggested that knowledge of moral stages could be very helpful to teachers who wish to facilitate moral development during instruction and supervision of games.

Recently, Bredemeier and her colleagues (Bredemeier, 1985a, 1985b; Bredemeier, Weiss, Shields, & Shewchuk, 1985) have employed an interactionist approach to explore the potential of physical education in enhancing moral growth. Bredemeier et al. (1985) conducted a field experiment to examine the effects of structural strategies on children's moral reasoning. Children ages 5 to 7 attending a summer sports program were matched and assigned to either a structural developmental, social learning, or control group. During the six week intervention program, groups were provided the same physical education curriculum and the same weekly moral themes of fair play, sharing, verbal aggression, physical aggression, and righting wrongs.

Instructors in the control group employed traditional physical education pedagogy, encouraging conformity to game- or teacher-set rules. In the social learning class, instructors provided reinforcement for appropriate prosocial behavior and modeled these behaviors often. In the structural developmental group, strategies were based on Haan's interactional morality: children were provided opportunities and encouraged to engage in dialogue about the themes and related actions in the class. In addition, children in this group were encouraged to reach a consensus regarding appropriate interpersonal behaviors.

Moral reasoning levels were determined using Piagetian-type story pairs and a test for distributive justice (Enright, 1981). Analyses indicated that children in the social learning and structural developmental groups improved significantly in their moral reasoning; no change occurred for the control group. Differences between the groups only approached significance, however. Generally, these results were encouraging, suggesting that moral growth is possible in a physical education setting using theoretically-based instructional prescriptions.

Romance, Weiss, & Bockoven (1986) conducted a follow-up study of the Bredemeier et al. investigation to control for some of the factors that may have precluded stronger between-group findings. They employed older subjects (fifth graders) in an attempt to elicit more frequent and meaningful dialogue, and devised specific game strategies based on guidelines from Haan's interactional theory. Two groups of children participated in this study: a structural developmental group and a control group, which was not exposed to these particular game strategies. Before and after an eight-week intervention, children were asked to respond to four hypothetical moral dilemmas; two were sport-specific and two were non-sport related. Sport, non-sport, and overall moral reasoning levels were calculated.

The results indicated significant between-group differences on all three moral reasoning scores: sport, non-sport, and overall. In all cases, the experimental group demonstrated significant gains in comparison to the control group. Additionally, within-group analyses showed that the experimental group made significant pre- to post-moral reasoning gains on sport and overall scores but not non-sport scores. No significant changes were found in the control group.

Two features of the Romance et al. study are particularly noteworthy. First, the study was conducted in actual physical education classes in the time and manner that these children normally had physical education. More importantly, the careful design and procedures produced results that demonstrated that physical education experiences can promote moral development.

In an ongoing line of research, Bredemeier (1985a, 1985b) conducted two studies to derive a better understanding of children's moral development in physical activity settings. IQ ONE STUDY (Bredemeier, 1985a), the differential effects of sport and everyday life contexts on the moral reasoning of fourth through seventh grade children were explored. Results demonstrated that sixth and seventh grade children's sport reasoning was more egocentric than their everyday life reasoning, a pattern similar to that found among high school and college students (Bredemeier and Shields, in press). In addition, the amount of divergence in sport and non-sport moral scores was significantly greater for the sixth and seventh graders than for the fourth and fifth grade children who did not demonstrate conteyt-specific reasoning patterns.

The purpose of the second study (Bredemeier, 1985b) was to investigate the relationship between children's moral reasoning about sport and everyday life and their tendencies to behave assertively, aggressively, and submissively in sport and daily life contexts. The results of this study indicated that moral reasoning scores were predictive of self-reported assertive and aggressive action tendencies in the contexts of sport and daily life. Children who were relatively mature in their moral reasoning described themselves as more assertive and less aggressive in response to conflict situations than children who exhibited lower levels of reasoning. These results are meaningful in light of scientists' interest in the moral reasoning-moral behavior relationship.

In summary, there are only a few investigators that have examined the relationship between moral development and physical education. Recent studies, however, have demonstrated the potential to enhance moral growth in physical education curricula.

Facilitating Moral Growth Through Physical Education

In this section, specific suggestions for facilitating moral development in physical education settings are offered, based both on the theoretical and empirical efforts of social learning and structural developmental scientists.

Structural Developmental Propositions

Several propositions grounded in structural development can be tentatively offered as strategies designed to enhance moral growth in the gymnasium. The essential elements of any program of moral development, according to structural developmentalists, are provision of (a) role-taking opportunities, (b) actual experiences of moral conflict, and (c) opportunities for moral dialogue and negotiation. In addition to these general principles, several more specific strategies might be suggested. In this section, four strategies will be offered together with illustrations.

One strategy for enhancing moral growth is to *allow for disorganizing experiences to occur* in the gymnasium. That is, unless moral dilemmas are allowed to surface within class, the opportunity for dialogue, and thus augmented moral growth, are not likely to occur. All too often, the teacher is responsible for and does a very good job of avoiding dilemmas in the gym by selecting fair teams, distributing equipment equally and not allowing situations that may encourage unequal opportunities for play (e.g., ball hogging). However, building dilemmas into the various activities encountered in physical education provides the vehicle through which we can become moral educators in the gym. Some possible dilemmas include not sharing equipment, unequal opportunities for practice, unfair play, hurting with words, hurting with actions, and admitting and righting wrongs.

In their moral development program, Romance et al. (1986) employed a teaching strategy called Built-in Dilemma/Dialogue (BIDD). In this situation, students participate in a game or drill which has a built-in dilemma such as a conflict between one's interest in performing well on a task and being considerate of other's needs. The game or drill is stopped and the dilemma is discussed. Finally, the game is replayed with changes made to reduce the conflict. An example of a BIDD strategy would be a "score ten" basketball shooting game where students (in pairs) are asked to make ten baskets as a two-person team. The first team to make ten baskets is the winner. After the activity, adequate time for dialogue is allowed with discussion focused on how each team decided who was to shoot how many shots and also how their decisions were related to individual needs and interests. Thus, a strategy such as BIDD is easily adapted from the teacher's normal repertoire of activities; it allows for moral dilemmas to occur in the gymnasium, and provides for student dialogue and the creation of moral balances.

A second major strategy is to *allow students to design group experiences*. Recent literature on developmental levels of motor control (Bressan & Woollacott, 1982) suggest a specific sequencing of instructional strategies for optimal skill acquisition. The sequencing proceeds from children exploring qualities for moving, to demonstrations and practice of single skill or skill combinations, to child-designed sequences or games using given parameters, to demonstrations and practice of more complex skills. It is the third developmental level, formally called the accommodating level, that has especially exciting possibilities for moral development. In addition to the children having opportunities to design sequences or routines using given parameters, they also make decisions on when and how to use the skills and qualities in their sequence or routine. Since the problem-solving style of teaching is used with this developmental level, it affords excellent opportunities for children to experience moral dilemmas, take the role of others, engage in dialogue and negotiation, and ultimately reach consensus.

An example from the Romance et al. (1986) program that illustrates these ideas is Built-in Dilemma/Problem-Solve (BID-PS). This technique entails student participation in a game or drill in small groups using certain guidelines provided by the teacher. The game or drill has a built-in moral dilemma. The students are encouraged to change the game at any time they want to, as long as there is consensus among group members. After sufficient time for play and dialogue, students discuss the moral dilemma and the accommodations that were made. A specific example is the game of "pickle in the middle" (basketball passing). Students (in threes) are instructed to play pickle in the middle as follows: "Try to pass the basketball back and forth between two players while a third player (in the middle) tries to touch it. Passers must stand on the red lines and if the middle person touches a pass, that person changes places with the passer. If, during the drill, your group feels that the game would be improved by adding or changing the rules, then do so immediately." Post-game discussions can focus on rule changes which the group makes and how those changes relate to individual needs and interests.

Another specific strategy illustrative of child-designed sequences and decision-making is "Create Your Own Game" (Romance et al., 1986). In this strategy, students are asked to make up games in small groups, keeping in mind the following rules: everyone plays, everyone enjoys, and everyone has a chance for success. For example, children are asked to create their own basketball dribbling game in groups of three. The games are played and discussion follows regarding game rules and organization and the opportunity for equalization.

A third teaching strategy stemming from structural developmental approaches is to *link sport moral issues to general life situations*. Teachers can highlight the commonalities between sport and everyday life through specially-designed learning activities. For example, in the activity called "Two Cultures" (Romance et al., 1986), students were instructed to play a competitive four-square game in which students were eliminated or moved to more desirable squares according to their performance. After playing this way, students were taught to play the game cooperatively by trying to get as many consecutive passes as possible and even sharing squares with extra players. Post-game discussions involved comparison of the two games with respect to needs for challenge and playing time.

Finally, a strategy to maximize moral growth is the use of *inductive discipline*. Inductive discipline incorporates the use of explaining and discussing *why* a rule must be followed or why activities must proceed in a certain way. This type of discipline is contrasted with the traditional "time out" procedure often used in physical education classrooms. The inductive technique is preferred because it is deemed most effective in long-term control and is especially suited to moral education because it facilitates role taking and social disequilibrium.

Social Learning Propositions

Although the authors believe that instructional prescriptions based on structural developmental theory are most appropriate for maximizing moral development through physical education, social learning strategies such as differential reinforcement and modeling cannot be ignored. In studies where both social learning and structural developmental experimental groups have been employed (Bredemeier et al., in press; McCann & Prentice, 1981), both conditions have been found to promote moral growth. Thus, strategies for enhancing sportsmanship such as those outlined by Gould (1984) are also considered viable. For example, Gould suggests adopting a "sportsmanship code" in which sportsmanlike and unsportsmanlike behaviors are identified, and strategies for controlling these behaviors are suggested. Specifically, the modeling of good sportsmanship by teachers, rewarding sportsmanlike and penalizing unsportsmanlike behaviors, and providing explanations when teaching sportsmanship are all strategies stemming from a social learning perspective.

Conclusion

This chapter presented evidence that moral development *can* be fostered through physical education programs. In order to enhance sportsmanship, however, curricular strategies based on structural developmental and social learning theories must be implemented.

The moral psychology of physical education experience is in its infancy. Only in recent years have psychological and philosophical keys been used to unlock the moral dimensions of physical education activity. Researchers and practitioners must continue to share insights and resources in order for the potential of physical education settings to promote moral growth to mature.

Children's games and physical activities are unique among educational contexts. The learning of physical and psychological game skills provides an ideal setting for role taking and the coordination of various interests and perspectives in an ongoing joint activity.

Fairness is a salient issue in games and sports, and participants often engage in negotiation about appropriate behavior within a rule-defined structure.

Children in physical education settings can gain confidence in their ability to engage in cooperative enterprises, while incorporating and adapting to the specific needs created by the heterogeneity of skills and interests among participants.

Physical education *can* and *should* be an integrated part of the curricular program of the school, not only for its obvious benefits in the areas of health and physical development, but also for the important and unique contributions it can make to students' moral development.

References

Aronfreed, J. (1968). *Conduct and conscience: The socialization of internalized control over behavior.* New York: Academic Press.

Aronfreed, J. (1976). Moral development from the standpoint of a general psychological theory. In T. Lickona (Ed.), *Moral development and behavior: Theory, research, and social issues* (pp. 54-69). New York: Holt, Rinehart, & Winston.

Baker, R. (1984, April). Kids corrupted by organized sports. *New York Times.*

Bandura, A. (1969). *Principles of behavior modification.* New York: Holt, Rinehart, & Winston.

Bandura, A. (1977). *Social learning theory.* Englewood Cliffs, NJ: Prentice-Hall.

Blasi, A. (1980). Bridging moral cognition and moral action: A critical review of the literature. *Psychological Bulletin, 88,* 1-45.

Blanchard, B. (1946). A comparative analysis of secondary school boys' and girls' character and personality traits in physical education classes. *Research Quarterly, 47,* 33-39.

Boswell, T. (1984, January 14). A disaster just waiting to happen. *The Register-Guard,* Eugene, OR.

Bredemeier, B.J. (1985a). *Divergence in children's moral reasoning about issues in daily life and sport specific contexts.* Manuscript submitted for publication.

Bredemeier, B.J. (1985b). *Children's moral reasoning and action tendencies in sport and daily life contexts.* Manuscript submitted for publication.

Bredemeier, B.J., & Shields, D.L. (1983). *Body and balance: Developing moral structures through physical education.* Eugene, OR: Microform Publications, University of Oregon.

Bredemeier, B.J., & Shields, D.L. (in press). Moral growth among athletes and non-athletes: A comparative analysis. *Journal of Genetic Psychology.*

Bredemeier, B.J., Weiss, M.R., Shields, D.L., & Shewchuk, R.M. (in press). Promoting moral growth in a summer sport camp: The implementation of theoretically grounded instructional strategies. *Journal of Moral Education.*

Bressan, E.S., & Woollacott, M.H. (1982). A prescriptive paradigm for sequencing instruction in physical education. *Human Movement Science, 1,* 155-175.

Coakley, J.J., & Bredemeier, B.J. (in press). Youth sports: Development of ethical perspectives. In J. Thomas (Ed.), *Ethical practices in competitive sports.* Champaign, IL: Human Kinetics.

Enright, R. (1981). *A user's manual for the Distributive Justice Scale.* Unpublished manuscript, University of Wisconsin-Madison.

Figley, G. (1984). Moral education through physical education. *Quest, 36,* 89-101.

Giebink, M.P., & McKenzie, T.L. (1985). Teaching sportsmanship in physical education and recreation: An analysis of interventions and generalization effects. *Journal of Teaching in Physical Education, 4* (3), 167-177.

Gilligan, C. (1982). *In a different voice: Psychological theory and women's development.* Cambridge, MA: Harvard University Press.

Gould, D. (1984). Psychosocial development and children's sport. In J. Thomas (Ed.), *Motor development during childhood and adolescence* (pp. 212-234). Minneapolis: Burgess.

Haan, N. (1977). *Coping and defending: Processes of self-environment organization.* San Francisco, CA: Academic Press.

Haan, N., Aerts, E., & Cooper, B. (in press). *On moral grounds.* New York: New York University Press.

Haan, N., Smith, M., & Block, J. (1968). Moral reasoning of young adults: Political-social behavior, family background and personality correlates. *Journal of Personality and Social Psychology, 10,* 183-201.

Hartshorne, H., & May, M. (1928). *Studies in the nature of character: Vol. 1. Studies in deceit.* New York: MacMillan.

Horrocks, R. (1979). *The relationship of selected prosocial play behaviors in children to moral reasoning, youth sports participation, and perception of sportsmanship.* Unpublished doctoral dissertation, University of North Carolina-Greensboro.

Jackson, P.W. (1968). *Life in the classroom.* New York: Holt, Rinehart, & Winston.

Jantz, R.K. (1975). Moral thinking in male elementary pupils as reflected by perception of basketball rules. *Research Quarterly, 46* (4), 414-421.

Jewett, A.E., & Bain, L.L. (1985). *The curriculum process in physical education.* Dubuque, IA: Wm. C. Brown.

Kleiber, D.A., & Roberts, G.C. (1981). The effects of sports experience in the development of social character: An exploratory investigation. *Journal of Sport Psychology, 3,* 114-122.

Kroll, W. (1975, April). *Psychology of sportsmanship.* Paper presented at the American Alliance of Health, Physical Education, Recreation, & Dance National Convention, Atlantic City, NJ.

Kohlberg, L. (1981). *The philosophy of moral development: Moral stages and the idea of justice.* San Francisco: Harper & Row.

Kohlberg, L. (1984). *Essays of moral development: Vol. 2. The psychology of moral development.* San Francisco, Harper & Row.

Lickona, T. (1976). *Moral development and behavior: Theory, research, and social issues.* New York: Holt, Rinehart, & Winston.

Martens, R. (1978). *Joy and sadness in children's sports.* Champaign, IL: Human Kinetics.

McCann, D., & Prentice, N. (1981). Promoting moral judgment of elementary school children: The influence of direct reinforcement and cognitive disequilibrium. *The Journal of Genetic Psychology, 139,* 27-34.

McIntosh, P. (1979). *Fair play: Ethics in sport and education.* London: Heinemann.

McCloy, C.H. (1941). What is modern physical education? *University of Iowa Extension Bulletin* (No. 505). Iowa City, IA: State University of Iowa.

Orlick, T. (1981). Positive socialization via cooperative games. *Developmental Psychology, 17* (4), 426-429.

Park, R. (1983, January). Three major issues: The Academy takes a stand. *Journal of Physical Education, Recreation, & Dance, 59,* 52-53.

Piaget, J. (1965). *The moral judgment of the child.* New York: Free Press. (Original work published in 1932).

Rest, J.R. (1983). Morality. In P.H. Mussen (Ed.), *Handbook of child psychology: Vol. III. Cognitive development* (pp. 556-629). New York: Wiley.

Romance, T.J. (1984). *A program to promote moral development through elementary school physical education.* Unpublished doctoral dissertation, University of Oregon, Eugene.

Romance, T.J., Weiss, M.R., & Bockoven, J. (1986). A program to promote moral development through elementary school physical education. *Journal of Teaching Physical Education, 5,* 126-136.

Selman, R.L. (1976). Social-cognitive understanding: A guide to educational and clinical practice. In T. Lickona (Ed.), *Moral development and behavior: Theory, research, and social issues* (pp. 299-316). New York: Holt, Rinehart, & Winston.

Smith, N.J., Smith, R.E., & Smoll, F.L. (1983). *Kidsports: A survival guide for parents.* Reading, MA: Addison-Wesley.

Webb, H. (1969). Professionalization of attitudes toward play among adolescents. In G.S. Kenyon (Ed.), *Aspects of contemporary sport sociology* (pp. 161-168). Chicago: The Athletic Institute.

Section IV

SPECIAL APPLICATIONS

- Disabling and Handicapping Conditions
- Cardiorespiratory Diseases
- Metabolic Disease: Diabetes Mellitus

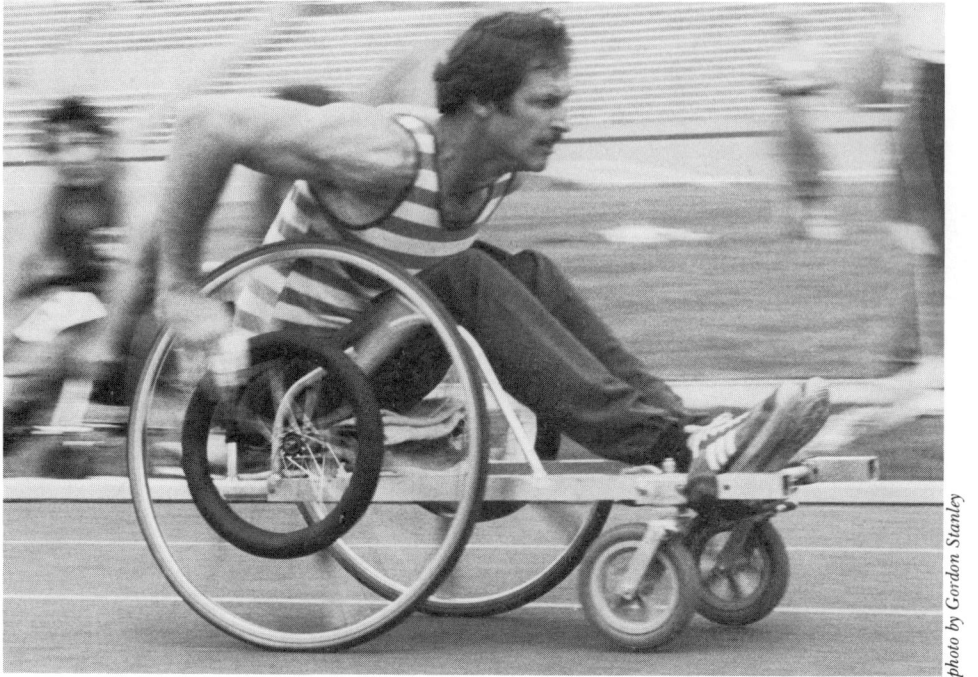

photo by Gordon Stanley

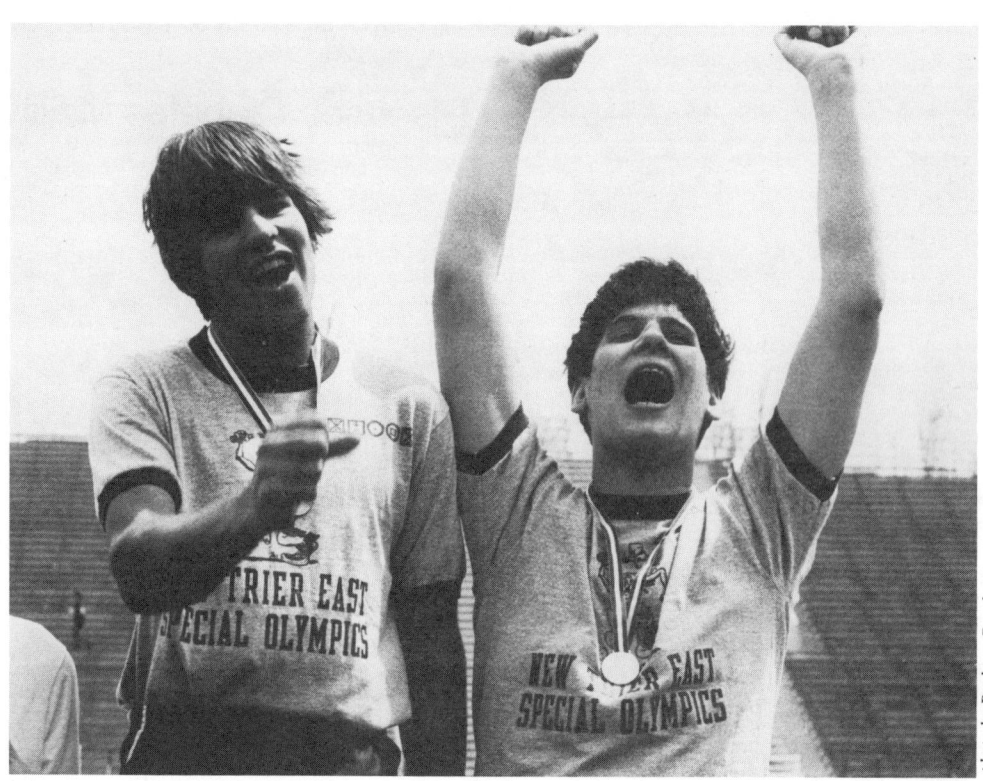

photo by Barbara Beach

CHAPTER FOURTEEN

Disabling and Handicapping Conditions

Alfred F. Morris
Director, Health and Fitness Programs
Armed Forces Staff College
Norfolk, Virginia

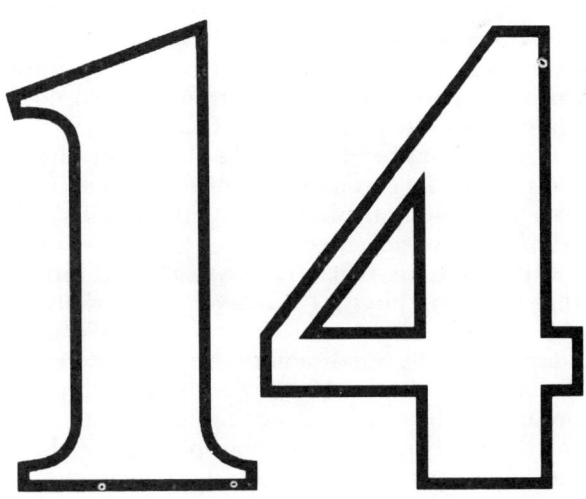

Introduction

We "normal," "typical," "representative" people face a dilemma as we journey through life. We want to excel in our professional and personal lives, yet we also try to "fit in." We constantly monitor our lapels or skirt lengths to see how we do fit in. Then we strive to become average, very good, even outstanding in our professional, family, social, love, or athletic lives. When we do this striving, we face the prospect of being assertive, obsessive, aggressive, compulsive, and risk the stresses inherent in that personality (Greenberg, 1984). All human beings must resolve this "fitting in" and "standing out" conflict. Most people somehow manage this dilemma (Lemaire, 1984).

People with disabling and handicapping conditions[1] have a related dilemma. They want first and foremost to "fit in." People with disabilities seek normalcy. This concept regarding average people striving for uniqueness and disabled people striving for normalcy is important to remember when we work with individuals who are disabled. If we display intelligence and understanding in our contact with people who are disabled, then we can help them to lead more productive lives. In fact, certain people with disabilities can develop their other remaining abilities to an exceptional level. People with disabilities can also strive for distinction, and feel the need to be unique.

Individuals with disabilities comprise about 10% of the total U.S. school age population (Auxter & Pyfer, 1985; Seaman & DePauw, 1982). Both able-bodied individuals and people with disabilities express their thoughts, feelings, and eventually their actions, through the *physical* medium. Therefore, physical activity, sport, and physical education (Morris, 1985a) are important to both able-bodied individuals and people with disabling and handicapping conditions.

Physical activity is a sign of life. In fact, when one loses the ability to move or to speak (and speech involves moving musculature), we often think that their quality of life has fallen to such a degree that life may no longer seem worth living. To be fully functioning and productive, one must move!

Since physical activity is so crucial to human well-being, this chapter will explore and evaluate how physical activity and sports can contribute to the total health and well-being of people with disabling and handicapping conditions.

Physical activity has been advocated for individuals with disabling and handicapping conditions. Because they are people first and foremost, they too, need physical activity (Buell, 1983; Guttman, 1976; Morris, 1982b, 1984a, 1985a). In fact, a case may be made that because some disabling and handicapping conditions tend to restrict certain forms of movement, it may be *more* important for individuals with mental, physical or emotional disabilities to pursue appropriate or adapted physical activity.

Often parents, teachers, physical educators, coaches, and athletic trainers think that vigorous physical activity benefits only athletes or other physically gifted individuals. This is not the case. Almost any type of physical activity can be adapted for a given disability (Auxter & Pyfer, 1985; Buell, 1983; Guttman, 1976; Seaman & DePauw, 1982). Enough thought and effort must be put forth by the organizer, the coach, or the teacher of the activity to make the proper adaptations for disabled people. For example, many able-bodied individuals train for and participate in road races, including the Boston Marathon. However, how often do we realize that blind, deaf, wheelchair, and cerebral palsied athletes can also compete successfully in such long distance road races? People compete on

---

[1] Disability and handicapping condition will be used in this chapter to mean any dysfunction from normal, typical, representative human function, whether it be physical, mental, or emotional.

crutches, and amputees compete on artificial limbs in many vigorous athletic events. The world record for an athlete competing in a wheelchair over the Boston Marathon course is about one and three-quarter hours, while the record for able-bodied men running the same course is well over two hours!

Organization of the Chapter

This chapter will be organized in the following way. First, the disabling and handicapping conditions that affect school age children will be listed. This will enable the reader to relate physical activity to individuals of a specific age with a specific disability or handicap. A partial description of each disability or handicap will be provided.

The second major thrust of this chapter will be to show how intelligently planned, conducted, and evaluated physical activity programs may help youngsters with disabilities and handicaps.

Because there are numerous psycho-social benefits of exercise for people who participate in physical activity, a third section dealing with the benefits of physical activity in the social domain for disabled and handicapped individuals will be presented.

In the fourth section, the physiological benefits of exercise and physical activity for individuals with specific physical impairments will be discussed. The effects of training and long-term conditioning for people with disabling and handicapping problems will be noted.

Finally, an integration and summary to this chapter will be given, in which parallels between the benefits of physical activity for non-handicapped individuals and benefits for disabled and handicapped people will be discussed, with regard to life quality and optimal human well-being. The question of how much good health and optimal functioning one can achieve will also be addressed.

Who Are the Disabled School Age Children?

The United States Department of Education (1984) periodically lists numbers and types of disabilities and handicaps among school age children. Some recent figures are shown in Table 1 and Figure 1.

Table 1
Percentage of School Enrollment Served as Handicapped (in all states)
1981-82 and 1982-83 School Years

Handicapping Condition Rank	Years	
	1981-82	1982-83
1. Learning disabled	4.04	4.40
2. Speech impaired	2.83	2.86
3. Mentally retarded	1.96	1.92
4. Emotionally disturbed	.85	.89
5. Physically disabled	.32	.30
6. Hard of hearing/deaf	.19	.18
7. Visually impaired/blind	.07	.07
8. Other	.01	.01

Source: United States Department of Education, Office of Education of Handicapped Children. Washington, DC, 1984.

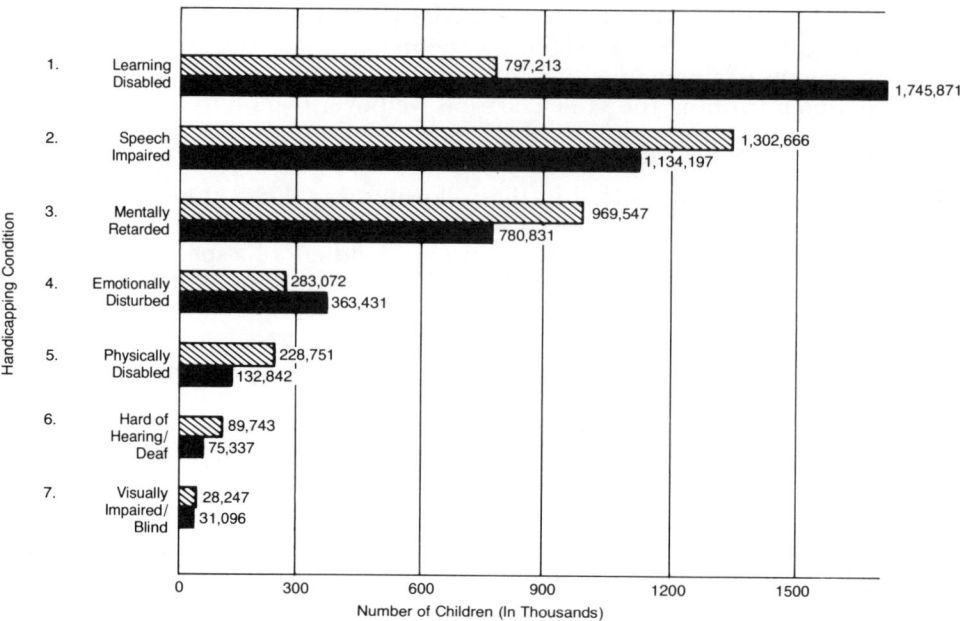

Fig. 1. Population of school children ages 3-21 served by handicapping condition for school years 1976-77 and 1982-83. *Note.* Adapted from: *Percentage of school enrollment served as handicapped (in all states) 1981-82 and 1982-83 school years,* United States Department of Education, Office of Education of Handicapped Students, 1984, Washington, DC.

Note that different tabulations often provide different numbers for the various disabling and handicapping conditions of school age children. The reason for this is that various methods of identifying children and then classifying them into specific groups are being used throughout the United States. An analogous situation would be to identify the gifted children in a specific school district. One could give an I.Q. test or achievement test and take the top 5 or 10%. This then would theoretically yield the potentially academically "gifted." But if, in fact, there are no truly gifted students in a certain school, or there are more than 10% gifted in another school, using an overall percentage of gifted children could be misleading. Similar pitfalls in determining disabled and handicapped students may occur when one tries to identify "slow learners," the emotionally disturbed, or students with speech impediments. The problem of how to define and then establish "cut-off" limits for these different disability categories remains (Morris, 1982a). Recognizing that there are inherent limitations in forming categories and numbers of students in each category of disabling and handicapping conditions, Table 1 and Figure 1 are presented.

Figure 1, which shows changes in the school age population of handicapped students from the school year 1976-77 to the year 1982-83, again underscores the difficulties in establishing numbers of persons with handicapping conditions. Note in Figure 1 that the percentages of learning disabled individuals rose to a much greater percentage than those with speech impairments. This different tabulation should have little effect on the types of physical activity suggested for these school children, because as the next section indicates, proper physical activity can aid most students in their psycho-social development (Morris, 1985).

Some Psycho-Social Benefits of Physical Activity

Most people, regardless of their particular disability or handicapping condition, can derive positive psycho-social and mental health benefits from proper physical activity (Morgan, 1985a; Morris, 1984a, 1985a; Shangold & Mirkin, 1985; Van Andel & Austin, 1984; Vargo, 1978). It may be more difficult to pinpoint psychosocial benefits accruing to people with disabilities, because one has to consider not only the many factors related to their present disability, but also differences which may have existed in the pre-morbid state of the disabled individual (Katz, Shurks, & Florian, 1978). Various factors must be considered, such as age, gender, personal development (educational level), the age of the person *at the time of the disability,* and the nature and severity of the disability (Harper, 1978; Shontz, 1978; Simon, 1971). A group of Canadian investigators (Davis, Kofsky, Shephard, & Jackson, 1981) showed that current, self-reported personality attributes and attitudes toward physical activity discriminated well between disabled adults with high level versus low level spinal cord injured people. The significant predictors of lesion level included Cattell's Personality Attributes, the Nowicki-Strickland Locus of Control Inventory, and Kenyon's Physical Activity Questionnaire (Davis et al., 1981; Lazar, Demos, Gaines, Rogers, & Stirnkorb, 1978).

It is interesting to note that Davis et al. (1981), and Morris, Vaccaro, and Clark (1979) also found that young swimmers were higher on the locus of control construct if they participated in age-group swimming.

Several authors have shown that improvements in self-concept and self-acceptance in disabled students can be made by those who participated in sports, physical activity, and/or recreational programs (Ankerbrand, 1972; Croucher, 1976; Dendy, 1978; Guttman, 1976; Van Andel & Austin, 1984). When physical activity programs significantly elevate cardiovascular functioning, they may also improve mental health (Feltz & Weiss, 1982; Morgan, 1985a; Van Andel & Austin, 1984).

In some instances, athletes with disabilities may compete on an equal status with their able-bodied colleagues. Given that the objectives of social integration and physical development may occur through physical activity and sports, then optimal benefits may result from activities in which people with disabilities compete against healthy individuals on an equal basis (Buell, 1983; Guttman, 1976; Humphrey, 1975; Jones, 1984; Shontz, 1978; Vargo, 1978).

Life Quality and Disability

Many medical researchers and scientists have established life quality scales which relate to the severely disabled or institutionalized patients, as well as to normal adults (Dalkey, Lewis, & Snyder, 1972; Morris, 1984a; Morris, Lussier, Vaccaro, & Clarke, 1982; Pflaum, 1973). However, there are other simpler life quality scales which have been used and deemed appropriate with both the able-bodied and disabled (Morris, 1984a; Morris et al., 1982; Morris & Husman, 1978). In a series of studies using the life quality construct, Morris (1985a), Morris et al. (1982), Morris and Husman (1978), Morris, Layman, Stone, Creswell, and Figoni (1985), and Morris, Vaccaro, and Harris (1983) have suggested that individuals who are more active physically may benefit psychologically and socially through improved self-concept when they engage in long-term physical activity programs (Ankerbrand, 1972). Physical benefits also accrue to participants in these programs (Morris, 1984a, 1985a).

In a recent unpublished work, Morris and Figoni (1985) indicated that life quality was enhanced in a group of women athletes playing wheelchair basketball. These young adult women were participating in a national wheelchair basketball tournament. Evidently, this physical training and associated activities (travel, social contacts) enabled these wheelchair athletes to report higher life quality than other individuals who were not handicapped. Granted that this was a cross-sectional study and mechanisms of self-selection can be cited as deficiencies in this line of research; however, the results are positive in that they suggest reported life quality increases with active physical fitness and sports.

The above data and comments relating to positive psycho-social attributes and increases in life quality may accrue to nearly all disabled and handicapped individuals who engage in sustained physical activity programs (Hedrick, 1984). Some improvements in mental health and self-concept can be attributed in part to increased physical fitness (Fox, Corbin, & Couldry, 1985; Morgan, 1985a; Van Andel & Austin, 1984).

Let us now examine some specific disabilities and see how physical activity may aid human well-being. Once again, not much research evidence is available on certain disabilities. Again, it must be pointed out that each person with a disability is unique, and therefore, grouping subjects for experimental purposes is difficult (Surburg, 1985). Controlled experiments are nearly impossible. However, some evidence indirectly suggests or is teleologically indicative of improvements in total well-being when disabled individuals participate in appropriate physical activities or sports (Henschen, Horvat, & French, 1984).

Physical Activity and Students with Learning Disabilities

Learning disabled students represent a major category when considering disabling and handicapping conditions in any school age population. From Table 1 and Figure 1 note that learning disabled students represent the largest category of disabled and handicapped children in our schools. Closer scrutiny of this disability may indicate how physical activity may help learning disabled students enjoy better health and well-being.

What is a "Learning Disability"?

"Learning disability" is a term currently used oh educators to describe a handicap that interferes with someone's ability to store, process, or produce information (Hartzell & Compton, 1984; Levine, 1984). This results in a discrepancy between intellectual ability and academic achievement, due to a deficit in one or more psychological processes such as attention, memory, or perception (Hartzell & Compton, 1984). Such disabilities affect mostly children, but they may also affect adults. The learning disability may be subtle, and go undetected throughout the child's early scholastic career. However, a learning disability generally creates a gap between the person's true capacity to learn and their day-to-day productivity and performance. Learning disabilities occur in a number of areas, including attention, language, spacial orientation, memory, motor control, and sequencing.

Attention. Perhaps the most common kind of learning disorder involves difficulty in attending to a task. In such situations teachers must plan activities with minimal directions and quickly involve all students with activity (Ashlock & Humphrey, 1976; Auxter & Pyfer, 1985; Humphrey, 1975). As a child gets older, he or she may outgrow this lack of attention. Parents and teachers must have patience with such individuals, and try to focus their attention with simple directions on basic, concrete, specific tasks, constantly providing supervision and reinforcement as they go through the learning process. Specific physical tasks and assignments may aid the learning disabled student's progress in the academic sphere (Ashlock & Humphrey, 1976; Humphrey, 1975; Humphrey & Sullivan, 1970; Prager, 1968).

Language disabilities. Some school children are very good at understanding things, but have difficulty interpreting complicated verbal instructions, remembering instructions, and then expressing them in a language of their own. Sometimes these individuals develop behavior problems because they are embarrassed about their disorientation.

Spacial orientation. Other children have a learning disability regarding spacial orientation. They may look at letters and confuse similar script letters, such as p and g, or b and d.

Memory. Another group of school children has difficulty retrieving information from memory. Again, if rapid recall of much information is necessary, these youngsters may have difficulty remembering and acting upon that information.

Motor control. Some children have difficulties with coordination of gross and fine muscular movements (Clark, 1984). It is important to remember that gross muscular movements tend to mature more quickly than fine motor control (Auxter & Pyfer, 1985; Humphrey, 1975; Humphrey & Sullivan, 1970; Rarick, Dobbins, & Broadhead, 1977). Recognizing this, teachers and physical activity instructors can properly plan programs which will contribute to gross motor control (walking, running, jumping, throwing), and then lead to some fine motor control activities (Humphrey, 1975, 1976).

Sequencing. Children with this type of learning disability become confused about sequences, and may only be able to keep one or two, or perhaps three things in order before any task disintegrates. They too, have difficulty following instructions.

Can Learning Disabilities and Disorders be Treated?

Yes. There are many educational offerings that are of benefit to children with learning disabilities. However, behind all of these strategies there must be one overriding principle, and that is, all of the interventions attempted, and all of the special instructions given prior to any physical activity must insure that the youngster will not endure any humiliation or embarrassment as a result of participating (Levine, 1984). Instruction frequently must be custom fitted to the child's learning style (Humphrey, 1976) to emphasize a particular strength, and possibly avoid a weakness (Levine, 1984). Special professionals, such as speech and language therapists, physical therapists, counselors, and other trained professionals may be a part of the regular or auxiliary school staff, and can be brought in to assist with the management and counseling of these children. Occasionally a physician will be asked to examine the child to see if any medication should be prescribed.

Physical Activity and the Learning Disabled Child

It has been difficult to do carefully controlled studies in this area, because each individual manifests his or her own signs and symptoms of disability. However, physical activity programs have been successful with the learning disabled child (Fidler, 1984; Hartzell & Compton, 1984; Humphrey, 1976). Recently, Hartzell and Compton (1984) reported on 114 learning disabled students who increased self-perception and academic success as a result of organized sport programs. Although the primary focus of their study was to evaluate, in a longitudinal fashion, self-perception, these researchers noted that there was a significant correlation between sports participation and social success. Individuals who had been diagnosed as learning disabled for 7 to 14 years, and ranged in age from 16 to 30 years at the time of the study, showed significant improvement as a result of their sport experience when evaluated in a follow-up study ten years later (Hartzell & Compton, 1984). Table 2 shows that participation and interest in sports significantly correlated with academic and social success in learning disabled children.

Hartzell and Compton suggested three possible reasons why sports and physical activity participation may benefit the learning disabled child. First, an organized

Table 2
Factors Correlated with High Academic, Social and Job Success in Learning Disabled Students

	Academic	Social	Job
Verbal IQ	.40§ (86)	.34§ (85)	
Performance IQ	.30† (86)	.28† (85)	
Full-scale IQ	.42§ (88)	.35§ (87)	
Current age			.38§ (109)
Age at diagnosis			.25† (109)
Psychosocial functioning	.41§ (112)	.44§ (111)	
Occupational level	.23‡ (111)		
Education of mother	.20† (104)	.21† (103)	
Family functioning	.46§ (112)	.33§ (111)	
Family support	.41§ (109)	.19† (108)	
Private tutoring	.28‡ (114)	.35§ (113)	
Interest in sports	.25† (112)	.38§ (111)	
Other interests	.19† (112)	.27‡ (111)	

†$P < .05$.
‡$P < .01$.
§$P < .001$.
Source: Hartzell & Compton, 1984.

time schedule was necessary for sports and physical activity participation. Second, physical activity, the researchers postulated, helped drain anxiety and tension, thus increasing concentration in school and other tasks. Finally, friendships in the physical activity and sport arenas were not based upon classroom expertise. Studies of this type indicate that if a child achieves success on the playground or in a sporting activity, some components of this success may be carried over into the classroom and other social learning environments. Any ten year follow-up study is difficult to complete, so these significant findings regarding physical activity and sport for the learning disabled students are extremely important.

Chapters 11, 12, and 13 of this monograph have discussed the psychological and affective benefits of vigorous physical activity and exercise. Morgan (1985a) reported the following benefit of vigorous physical activity: "clinical opinion would indicate that exercise has beneficial emotional effect for all ages and in both sexes." Since achieving success is critical for any school aged youngster who displays a learning disability, proper physical activity and sport participation may aid in the total development of the student.

Physical Activity and Speech Impaired Students

The second major category of people with disabilities and handicaps in schools are those with speech impairments (refer to Table 1 and Figure 1). However, there are approximately 1½ times as many children classified as learning disabled as there are speech impaired. Speech impairment is categorized as "a communication disorder, such as stuttering, impaired articulation, a language impairment, or voice impairment, which adversely affects a child's educational performance" (Seaman & DePauw, 1982). Many elementary school age children have speech difficulties in their early school years because their first teeth become loose and fall out. A recent publication on necessary or recommended medical tests indicated that after puberty it is probably not necessary to have yearly physical exams of speech in older adolescents (Langone, 1985). This indicates that as children mature and develop, their speech patterns improve and the number of students in the category of speech impaired decreases as they reach high school.

Many sports and physical activities can be presented to school age children which do not affect speech or articulation (Ashlock & Humphrey, 1976, Humphrey, 1976). Many sports and games can be played with little speech required (Auxter & Pyfer, 1985). The quarterback in football must be articulate, speak clearly and constantly, but many other individual and team sport activities do not require much speech production (Seaman & DePauw, 1982). On the other hand, some research indicates that students in early elementary school with speech impairments can improve speech patterns and articulation if they are properly guided in good physical activity (Humphrey, 1976; Humphrey & Sullivan, 1970).

Physical Activity and Students with Mental Retardation

The third major handicapping condition among school age children is the category of mental retardation. A definition of mental retardation indicates mental subnormalcy, as measured on a standardized I.Q. test (Grossman, 1977). There are several categories of this dysfunction, and Table 3 indicates the types and numbers of the different mental retardation categories.

Table 3
Types and Severity of Mental Retardation as Reflected in I.Q. Scores*

	Stanford-Binet I.Q.	WISC-R I.Q.	Educational Classification
Mildly Retarded	68-52	69-55	Educable Mentally Retarded
Moderately Retarded	51-36	54-40	Educable Mentally Retarded
Severely Retarded	35-20	39-25	Trainable Mentally Retarded
Profoundly Retarded	20	25	Mostly Custodial Care

*Adapted from H.J. Grossman. *Manual on Terminology in Mental Retardation.* Washington, DC: American Association on Mental Deficiency, 1977.

There have been several review papers and an excellent text by Rarick, Dobbins and Broadhead (1977) relating the motor domain and its correlates in educationally handicapped children. This text identifies basic physical components of the motor behavior of educable mentally retarded children. Rarick's was the largest, most comprehensive assessment of "the role of educational physical activity in the modification of the motor, strength, intellectual, social and emotional development of the educable mentally retarded and minimally brain injured child of elementary school age." Previous research had indicated that physical improvements and increases in motor performance can occur in young, educable mentally retarded children. Also, changes in measured intelligence may occur when proper physical activity lessons were *added* to the daily school schedule of mentally retarded and typical elementary school children. Such authors as Humphrey (1975, 1976), Humphrey and Sullivan (1970), Prager (1968), and Rarick et al. (1977) have indicated that when academic lessons are supplemented with physical activity, academic learning in math, social science, and biological science can be significantly improved (Fidler, 1984).

In Rarick's study (1977), the range of chronological ages of the children was from 6 to 13, the majority being in the 7 to 12 year age range. This landmark study, involving hundreds of children with disabilities of mild mental retardation and minimal brain damage resulted in the following four major conclusions:

1. Special treatment in the form of well-designed programs of physical education and physical activity elicited greater changes in motor, intellectual, and emotional development of retarded and brain injured children than occurred from the usual classroom instructional program.

2. Of the specifically planned experimental programs, the physical education programs demonstrated a superior role in modifying motor performance.

3. The physical education program which was oriented toward the individual rather than the group was more successful in eliciting change in the motor, intellectual, and emotional parameters of the development of the child.

4. Positive changes in development were shown more by the older than by the younger children.

There are several important recommendations that physical education teachers and physical activity instructors can gain from the conclusions of this report (Rarick et al., 1977). The major finding is that all children, even those with deficits in mental functioning, can improve their motor performance, as well as their intellectual and emotional development, by participating in a physical activity program. These programs should be oriented toward the individual or for small groups. When changes and improvements in physical fitness and sport skills occur in school age children, these positive physical improvements may also elicit positive changes in intellectual and social growth (Clark, 1984; Feltz & Weiss, 1982, & Van Andel & Austin, 1984). This overall growth and maturation can occur in all ages and to members of both genders. Younger school age people may, in fact, display the greater gains in intelligence, when contrasted with older mentally retarded individuals (Rarick et al., 1977). This finding indicates that proper physical activity programs be available for young, mentally retarded people. Research data suggests that all ages and both sexes can profit from exemplary physical activity programs. It is especially important that the early elementary school youngster who may be somewhat mentally retarded have successful experiences in physical education and physical activity programs.

Another study involving mentally retarded students evaluated strength and flexibility in children with Down's Syndrome (Morris, Vaughan, & Vaccaro, 1982). Twenty-eight children with Down's Syndrome were contrasted with 33 normal children for muscle tone as measured by patellar tendon reflex and muscle strength (grip). All subjects were between 4 and 17 years of age, indicating a wide population of school age subjects. Results indicated that children with Down's Syndrome had a less brisk reflex tendon response and inferior grip strength; neuromuscular tone was diminished and grip strength lower in these students. These authors suggested that increased physical education and physical activity programs might aid this special population in improving muscular strength and overall neuromuscular tone.

Recently, DePauw (1984) evaluated total body mass centroid in 40 subjects with Down's Syndrome (DS) who varied in age from youngsters (6 to 10 years old) to adults. DePauw reported that DS children had a center of mass located within the range noted for non-handicapped children, but that adult DS subjects had consistently lower centers of mass than non-DS adults. DePauw speculated that since older DS children and adults tend to become overweight and assume a pear-shaped (protruding) abdomen, this tendency may result in the lowering of the body center of mass. If this is so, then proper physical activity programs stressing physical fitness and weight control would be beneficial to DS school children (Morris, 1984b).

Physical Activity and Students with Emotional Disturbances

Emotionally disturbed youngsters are defined according to Public Law 94-142, Section 121a, 5(b), (8) as individuals who have: (a) inability to learn which cannot be explained by intellectual, sensory or health factors; (b) an inability to build or maintain satisfactory interpersonal relationships with peers and teachers; (c) inappropriate types of behavior or feelings under normal circumstances; (d) a general pervasive mood of unhappiness or depression; (e) a tendency to develop physical symptoms or fears associated with personal or school problems (Auxter & Pyfer, 1985; Seaman & DePauw, 1982).

The above characteristics are portrayed to a marked degree in emotionally disturbed school children over a long period of time. These inappropriate characteristics adversely affect educational performance. The category of autistic (extreme aloneness and inability or refusal to communicate) and schizophrenic (personality disorganization with reality) school children are also included in the population of emotionally disturbed (Seaman & DePauw, 1982).

Children with emotional disturbances, although presenting unique and different challenges to the physical education teacher, can improve physical, social and intellectual skills through proper physical activity (Fidler, 1984; Humphrey, 1975, 1976). It is necessary, however, for the teacher to understand these individuals and the conditions that cause these students to behave in atypical ways. Proper knowledge of these disabling conditions, together with a keen understanding of physical activity, can greatly enhance well-being in emotionally disturbed school children (Auxter & Pyfer, 1985; Seaman & DePauw, 1982).

Educators have suggested that active games, sports, and vigorous physical activity can aid children with emotional disturbances (Auxter & Pyfer, 1985; Humphrey, 1976; Seaman & DePauw, 1982). Recently, two studies have shown that physical activity can aid institutionalized juvenile delinquents (Munson, Baker, & Lundegren, 1985), and that good physical education programs can help behaviorally disordered students (Jeltma & Vogler, 1985). Munson et al. (1985) conducted an eight week strength training program in a Pennsylvania Youth Development Center for three groups of institutionalized juvenile delinquents. After this program of strength conditioning, results indicated that attitudes toward treatment programs improved.

Jeltma and Vogler (1985) tested individual contingency programs on behaviorally disordered students and reported that individual programs worked better with students who could be categorized as emotionally and behaviorally disturbed. Their results suggest that physical education and physical activity programs should provide for individual instruction strategies and opportunities to increase physical fitness in students with emotional disturbances.

Physiological Benefits of Physical Activity and Exercise for Students with Physically Disabling and Handicapping Conditions

Thus far, the major non-physically handicapping conditions of the learning disabled, speech impaired, mentally retarded, and emotionally disturbed have been discussed, and the possible psycho-social benefits of activity for youngsters with these disabling and handicapping conditions have been documented. This final section considers some of the physiological benefits of exercise. These physiological benefits of physical activity might benefit the physically, as well as the non-physically handicapped.

First, certain methods of fitness assessment in the individual with physical disability will be considered. Secondly, the three components of fitness, as noted by Morris (1985a), will be examined. Benefits of physical activity and exercise, as they relate to increases in physical fitness in the areas of cardiorespiratory fitness, strength fitness, and improvements in flexibility, will be enumerated.

Physiological Benefits of Physical Activity

Of all the benefits that can accrue from long term physical activity and sports participation, perhaps the easiest to document is physiological changes occurring in the human organism (Basmajian, 1984; Morris, 1985a). There are many studies and textbooks which show improvement in both the able-bodied and the physically disabled as a result of proper physical exercise (Dresden, DeGroot, Mesa Menor, & Bouman, 1985; Morris, 1984a, 1984b, 1985a; Pollock, Miller, Linnerud, Laughridge, Coleman, & Alexander, 1974; Shephard, 1978; Winnick, 1984). All individuals engaging in proper physical exercise and activity programs can improve their physiological fitness (Morris, 1985a). Details regarding the benefits of physical activity in the physiological improvement of disabled and handicapped students will be provided in a subsequent section.

Methods of Fitness Assessment in Individuals With Physically Disabling and Handicapping Conditions

When assessing energy expenditure and cardiorespiratory fitness in individuals with physical disabilities, certain precautions must be taken. Morgan (1985b) has shown that metabolism may be increased, even as the individual anticipates impending physical activity.

Initially, a complete physical examination and medical evaluation prior to the fitness test is advised. This examination should include a drug history and complete documentation of the nature and treatment of the physical disability. Second, the utmost safety of the individual being tested must be assured at all times. Finally, the test should not only provide accurate information about the current state of fitness of the individual, but also should be suggestive, in terms of providing guidelines for exercise prescription (Shephard, 1978).

Numerous motor and fitness tests have been suggested for evaluating the fitness of individuals with disability (Auxter & Pyfer, 1985; Seaman & DePauw, 1982). Recently, Winnick and Short (1984) suggested different test item selections to be used as a physical fitness test for the physically disabled. In any complete test of physical fitness it is important to include evaluations of cardiorespiratory function, muscular strength and flexibility (Morris, 1985a; Winnick & Short, 1984). Table 4, by Winnick and Short (1984), demonstrates that their Project Unique physical fitness test items evaluate all three components of fitness. Winnick and Short's fitness test is an extension and modification of the original Health Related Fitness test proposed in 1980 (American Alliance for Health, Physical Education, Recreation and Dance, 1980). The Project Unique physical fitness test was established after testing 1,192 normal, 1,468 auditory impaired, 649 visually impaired, and 605 orthopedically impaired school age children, ages 10-17.

There are several field tests that one can use to test the disabled individual (Auxter & Pyfer, 1985; Seaman & DePauw, 1982). In addition, several laboratory tests have recently been used. There are several arm-cranking devices and wheelchair ergometers which can be used in the laboratory evaluation of fitness (Davis et al., 1981; Davis et al., 1984; Lundberg, 1980). Some of these laboratory methods are new, and norms and standards have not yet been provided. This lack of norms

Table 4
Project UNIQUE Physical Fitness Test Items According to Major Participant Groups

Test items	Normal, auditory, impaired, visually impaired[a]	Cerebral Palsy[a]	Wheelchair paraplegic Spinal neuro-muscular[a]	Congenital anomaly/ amputee[a]
Body composition skinfolds	X	X	X	X
Muscular strength/ endurance grip strength (strength)	X[b]	X[c,f]	X[g,h]	X[b,j]
50-yard dash (power/speed)	X	X[d]	X[d]	X
sit-ups (power-strength)	X	—	—	X[i]
softball throw for distance (power/strength)	—	X[e]	—	—
Flexibility sit-and-reach	X	X	—	X
Cardiorespiratory endurance long-distance run	X	X	X	X

[a] Items may require modification or elimination for selected group subclassifications.
[b] The broad jump may be substituted for grip strength tests as a measure of strength for these groups.
[c] Grip strengths measure power-strength for males with cerebral palsy.
[d] The dash measures power-endurance for individuals in this group.
[e] The softball throw is recommended for females only as a measure of power-strength.
[f] The arm hang may be substituted for grip strength tests for males.
[g] The arm hang or softball throw for distance may be substituted for grip strength measures (strength factor) for males.
[h] The softball throw may be substituted for grip strength measures (strength factor) for female participants.
[i] The softball throw for distance may be substituted for sit-ups (as a power-strength factor) when the sit-up would be considered inappropriate.
[j] Males may substitute the arm hang for grip tests (strength factor).
Adapted from Winnick & Short, 1984.

for comparative purpose is common of a non-traditional group of individuals. Earlier in our exercise physiology history, we did not have adequate norms for testing girls and young women. Later, we did not have adequate physical fitness norms for testing older people. However, as more of these subject populations become available to exercise physiologists, we will gain more normative values regarding their physiological and cardiorespiratory functions.

The Arm Cycle Ergometer

The arm cycle ergometer (see Figure 2) has proved to be a satisfactory mode for evaluating responses of the cardiorespiratory system in people who cannot be tested on a treadmill or on a bicycle ergometer (Davis et al., 1981, 1984). One can place a cycle ergometer on a raised table and have a subject with disability

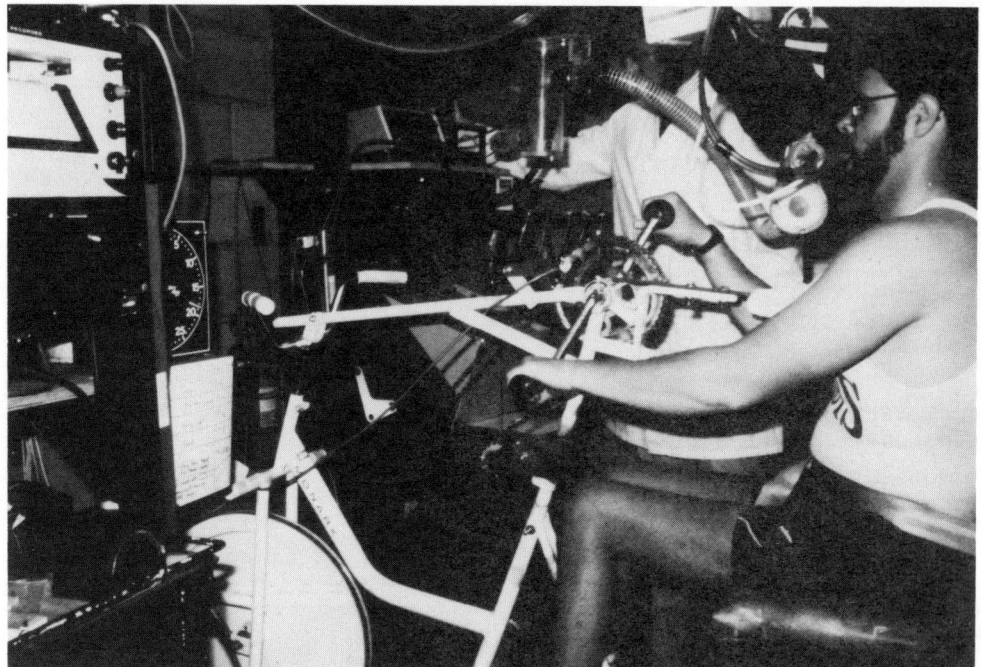

Fig. 2. This figure presents a person with a lower limb disability getting a total body aerobic workout via arm ergometry.

arm-crank the cycle ergometer to evaluate their fitness level (Davis, Shephard, & Jackson, 1981).

By standardizing arm-crank rates and resistance applied, investigators can obtain an accurate assessment of heart rate, oxygen intake and respiratory function (Davis et al., 1981, 1984). During maximal arm-cranking effort, there are differences in the physiological responses to exercise when these same responses are compared to leg exercise (Franklin, 1985). In a major review paper, Franklin (1985) has indicated that max $\dot{V}O_2$ and heart rate responses are different. $\dot{V}O_2$ max is generally lower in arm, as contrasted with leg (treadmill) exercise or leg pedaling exercise tests. This factor must be kept in mind when evaluating physiological responses in individuals with different body masses and with different amounts of functional skeletal musculature (Lussier, Knight, Bell, Lohman, & Morris, 1983; Morris, 1982b, 1985b).

Muscular Strength Tests

Muscular strength and endurance are important components of fitness (Morris, 1984a, 1985a; Shephard, 1978). Muscular strength is also important in people who have neuromuscular diseases, such as Cerebral Palsy, Poliomyelitis, Muscular Dystrophy, Multiple Sclerosis, and Spinal Cord Injury. Various individuals have tried to examine muscle strength in individuals with disabilities (Davis, Kofsky, Shephard, Keene, & Jackson, 1980; Davis et al., 1981; Morris, 1974). Static hand grip has been a good predictor of general muscle function in healthy, able-bodied subjects. Davis et al. (1980) have indicated that a single measure of dominant hand grip forces correlated .79 with an index of total upper body isokinetic strength. One can readily observe that hand grip strength may be a significant predictor in overall body strength in individuals using wheelchairs. However, there is significant variation in predictive ability based on a single test such as this. Davis et al. (1980), and Morris and Figoni (1984) evaluated strength in certain individuals with lower limb disabilities and found wide individual variations that were often not related to body mass.

Recently, isokinetic strength testing has become more prominent (Davis et al., 1984). Several individuals have used isokinetic devices to measure strength. As more isokinetic testing devices become available in the laboratory, more investigators will use this mode for assessing muscular strength, thus leading to the development of norms for special populations.

Identification of some parameters of physical fitness in disabled individuals, and suggestions about how to interpret these evaluations leads us to the next section which will discuss some of the responses to different training programs.

Training Responses to Physical Activity in the Physically Disabled

Muscle wasting and body fat accumulation will occur during prolonged periods of hospitalization and restriction of physical activity (Engel & Hillebrandt, 1973; Morris, 1985a; Shephard, 1978). If continued inactivity is present in individuals with severe physically handicapping conditions, then very low levels of cardiorespiratory fitness will result. In fact, when endurance fitness levels in athletes competing in wheelchairs are compared with those of sedentary, non-disabled individuals of a similar age, it has been noted by several investigators that fitness levels are similar (Davis et al., 1981; Gass & Camp, 1979). Lundberg (1980) has noted that $\dot{V}O_2$ max of some disabled basketball players were the same as able-bodied controls, using the same wheelchair ergometer. This would indicate that there is room for physiological improvement in individuals with disabilities and handicapping conditions.

Some reports have indicated, in a cross-sectional fashion, that elite wheelchair athletes have higher levels of fitness if their conditioning activities are different. Zwiren and Bar-Or (1975) indicated that there were different responses to exercise in paraplegics who participated in different conditioning programs. In 11 elite wheelchair athletes, they noted a lower body fat value than in nine sedentary non-athletic wheelchair users. However, they also reported that the cardiorespiratory fitness of the elite wheelchair athletes, expressed as a percent of body mass, was only 9 percent below that of a group of able-bodied athletes. This max $\dot{V}O_2$ was fully 90 percent below that of a group of able-bodied athletes. They also reported, however, that $\dot{V}O_2$ max, again expressed as a percent of body mass, was 50 percent higher than that of sedentary wheelchair athletes. This indicates that elite wheelchair athletes are far superior, physiologically, when compared to sedentary wheelchair users, but they fall within the range of normal, able-bodied athletes.

Davis et al. (1981) reported that habitual physical activity could be evaluated on the basis of measures of isokinetic strength and endurance. That is, as individuals engaged in proper fitness activities, improvements in strength and muscular endurance were reported.

There are some obstacles that must be overcome by the physically disabled in their training programs (Davis et al., 1984). These include:
1. A fear of exercise.
2. Poor balance and upper body control in individuals wtih lower limb disabilities.
3. Activation of only a small total muscle mass.
4. Pooling of blood in the active regions.
5. Lack of vision or hearing.
6. Poor comprehension of exercise instructions.
7. Associated disorders, such as diabetes and vascular disease, these mostly affecting older subjects.

Cardiorespiratory Training Devices

The arm-crank ergometer, or bicycle ergometer raised on an elevated platform, can be used as a rehabilitation, as well as a training device. Generally, power output can be controlled and monitored precisely, and evaluations in fitness and exercise programs can be quantified for the individual with disability. Pollock et al. (1974) noted that wheelchair users were able to increase their $\dot{V}O_2$ max, as measured by forearm ergometry, by 19 percent via a 20 week program of arm ergometer training. Non-disabled and age matched controls who underwent equivalent arm exercise demonstrated a much larger gain. Pollock et al. (1974) speculated as to why these gains might have occurred:

1. A higher intensity of effort (that is, the non-disabled and age matched controls may have been using some associated trunk and leg muscles for their ergometer training).

2. A greater habituation of the subjects who were intitially unfamiliar with vigorous exercise for the disabled.

3. A lower baseline peripheral oxygen extraction occurred in the paralytic group.

As more sports and athletic opportunities become available for athletes in wheelchairs, there will be greater training improvements in overall performance, as measured by times on a track (Morris, 1984b, 1985b). An analogous situation may be drawn here between other individuals who were not exposed to many opportunities for training and participation (i.e., older men and women athletes). One only has to realize the dramatic improvements seen in the women's world record time for the marathon run to realize that as more and more women participate in this type of athletic event, times will continue to fall at a faster rate than those of men. As more athletes with disabilities are allowed to compete in different and longer distance events, we can also expect that their improvements in performance, as well as cardiorespiratory fitness, will increase (Morris, 1985b).

Physical Activity, Physiological Improvements and Increases in Life Quality

Several authors have alluded to the fact that physical activity plays an important role in the total health, fitness and well-being of the individual (Ankerbrand, 1972; Morris, 1984a, 1985a; Morris & Figoni, 1985; Morris & Husman, 1978; Morris et al., 1979, 1982, 1983, 1985; Morgan, 1985a). Morris has expressed this concept in what he describes as a health/fitness continuum (Morris, 1984a, 1985a). This relationship between physical activity and human wellness is portrayed in Figure 3. This figure indicates that individuals with average health (no sickness) occupy a middle point on a health/fitness continuum. If individuals of average, typical, or representative human functioning participate in proper physical conditioning programs, while at the same time they pay attention to other good health habits (like diet, proper rest, and relaxation), then above normal human functioning and human well-being may occur. If one looks at the higher end (right ride) of the spectrum, one can see the athlete and person displaying high levels of fitness and wellness.

Alternatively, with periods of de-training, injury or inactivity, individuals who do not or cannot persist in their physical activity will likely regress from this high level of wellness. Inactivity and injury cause regression back through the middle portion of the continuum to lower fitness levels (left side of Figure 3), according to Morris' model. In inactivity continues, or further injury or illness is present, or perhaps a severe, permanent, physical disability occurs, then that person may catapult to the far left of the continuum. When this happens, they are then in a state of ill health, or low level of human functioning. The athlete who is injured

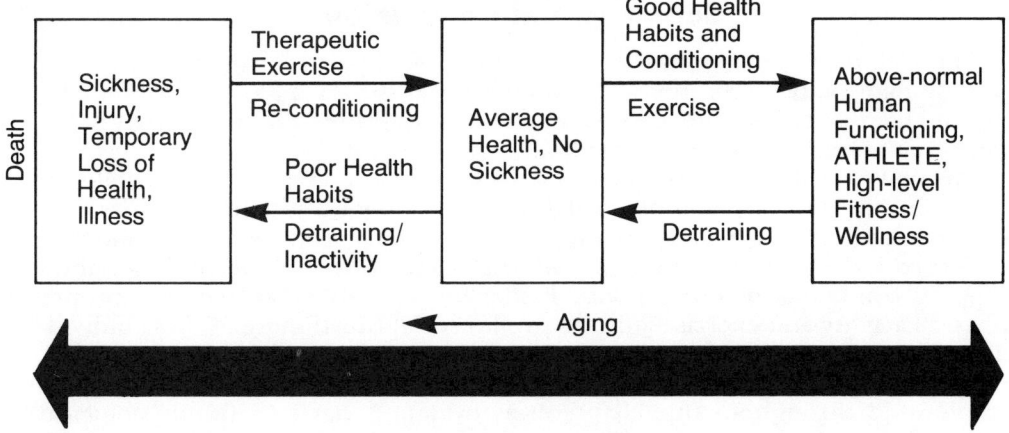

Fig. 3. A proposed Health/Fitness Continuum indicating that individuals displaying average health and no sickness can move to more optimal human functioning by participating in physical activity and exercise classes, while maintaining good health habits. It also shows that individuals who are injured, sick, or have a temporary loss of health or human function can, with proper therapeutic exercise, move to a more average and finally, to a higher level of human wellness and fitness. Finally, aging tends to move all individuals along the Continuum to the left, that is, less optimal functioning.

can, through therapeutic and reconditioning exercises over a long period of weeks and months, begin to move back into average or typical human health and well-being. With even more work and proper physical activity, anyone should be able to move to the right along the continuum (Morris, 1984a).

The disabled athlete can also be portrayed, together with the average individual, on this continuum. After recovery from injury or surgical procedure necessary to stabilize the handicapping condition, that individual may, with good health habits and proper physical activity, approach higher levels of human functioning and positive well-being.

Aging Affects Life Quality

A final point to consider in studying Figure 3 is that all living individuals, once they become adults, face the problem of competing with the aging process. While this specific chapter does not deal itself with aging (the reader is referred to chapter 5 on aging by W. Spirduso for a complete discussion), the effects of aging tend to move all adults to the left side of this continuum. The physiological results of aging occur whether the individual is disabled or able-bodied. Once again, research has shown that individuals who display good health habits and proper physical activity and exercise may retard, postpone, or delay this aging process.

Van Aaken (1972), a prominent German physician, has noted that therapeutic exercise is similar to training exercises for all people. Even individuals with severe, permanent, physical disabilities may engage in therapeutic or physical training exercises. Van Aaken (1972) reported that the only things which have to be modified in physical exercise programs for individuals with disabilities may be the *mode* of exercise, that is, an arm-crank ergometer or a bicycle ergometer. Also, Van Aaken noted that the *dosages* of physical activity or of exercise must be modified, in terms of intensity and duration. Principles of training (Morris, 1984c) must be followed in any physical activity program. Once physical activity accommodations are met for the person with disability, then the physiological, as well as psychosocial benefits of exercise, are likely to accrue to the disabled individual.

Summary and Conclusion

This chapter has explored the contributions of physical activity to individuals with disabling and handicapping conditions. It was shown that people with disabling and handicapping conditions may benefit from proper physical activity in the same manner as able-bodied individuals.

The first part of the chapter discussed the numbers and types of school children displaying the different non-physical disabilities. School population statistics indicate that learning disabled, speech impaired, mentally retarded and emotionally disturbed individuals represent the largest groups of people displaying handicapping conditions in our schools. Evidence was also presented that proper physical activity and exercise aids the psycho-social functioning of these individuals. That in itself would be reason enough to promote proper physical activity programs for individuals with disabling and handicapping conditions. However, emphasized throughout this chapter was evidence that specific physiological improvements in human functioning and human well-being can occur with proper physical activity and exercise programs. Lastly, it was shown that improvements in life quality and a high level of health and wellness can occur to individuals who practice good health habits and engage in proper physical activity and exercise programs.

References

American Alliance for Health, Physical Eduction, Recreation and Dance. (1980). *Lifetime health related physical fitness test manual.* Reston, VA: Author.

Ankerbrand, L.J. (1972). *The self-concept of students physically handicapped and non-handicapped related to participation in an individual sport.* Unpublished doctoral dissertation, University of Missouri, Columbia.

Ashlock, R.B., & Humphrey, J.H. (1976). *Teaching elementary school mathematics through motor learning.* Springfield, IL: Charles C. Thomas.

Auxter, D., & Pyfer, J. (1985). *Principles and methods of adapted physical education and recreation.* St. Louis: C. V. Mosby.

Basmajian, J.V. (1984). *Therapeutic exercise* (4th ed.). Baltimore: Williams & Wilkins.

Buell, C.E. (1983). *Physical education for blind children* (2nd ed.). Springfield, IL: Charles C. Thomas.

Clark, D.F. (1984). Body image and motor skills in normal and subnormal subjects. *International Journal of Rehabilitation Research, 7,* 207.

Croucher, N. (1976). Sport and disability. In J.G.P. Williams & P.N. Sperryn (Eds.), *Sports medicine* (pp. 523-538). London: Arnold.

Dalkey, N.C., Lewis, R., & Snyder, D. (1972). *Studies in life quality.* Boston: D.C. Heath.

Davis, G.M., Jackson, R.W., & Shephard, R.J. (1984). Sports and recreation for the physically disabled. In R. Strauss (Ed.), *Sports medicine* (pp. 286-304). Philadelphia: W.B. Saunders.

Davis, G.M., Kofsky, P.R., Shephard, R.J., & Jackson, R.W. (1981). Classification of psycho-physiological variables in the lower limb disabled. *Canadian Journal of Applied Sport Science, 6,* 4.

Davis, G.M., Kofsky, P.R., Shephard, R.J., Keene, G.C.R., & Jackson, R.W. (1980). Muscular strength in the lower limb disabled. *Canadian Journal of Applied Sport Science, 5,* 4.

Davis, G.M., Shephard, R.J., & Jackson, R.W. (1981). Cardiorespiratory fitness and muscular strength in the lower limb disabled. *Canadian Journal of Applied Sport Science, 6,* 159.

Dendy, E. (1978). Recreation for disabled people. *Physiotherapy, 64,* 290.

DePauw, K.P. (1984). Total body mass centroid and segmental mass centroid locations in Down's Syndrome individuals. *Adapted Physical Activity Quarterly, 1,* 221.

Dresden, M.H.W., DeGroot, G., Mesa Menor, J.R., & Bouman, L.N. (1985). Aerobic energy expenditure of handicapped children after training. *Archives of Physical Medicine and Rehabilitation, 66,* 302.

Engel, P., & Hillebrandt, G. (1973). Long term spiro-ergonometric studies of paraplegics during the clinical period of rehabilitation. *Paraplegia, 11,* 105.

Feltz, D.L., & Weiss, M.R. (1982). Developing self-efficacy through sport. *Journal of Physical Education, Recreation and Dance, 53,* 4.

Fidler, D.A. (1984). *Effects of daily physical education on the physical fitness scores of special education and non-special education students.* Unpublished master's thesis, George Mason University, Fairfax, VA.

Fox, K.R., Corbin, C.B., & Couldry, W.H. (1985). Female physiological estimation and attraction to physical activity. *Journal of Sport Psychology, 7,* 125.

Franklin, B.A. (1985). Exercise testing, training, and arm ergometry. *Sports medicine, 2,* 100.

Gass, G.C., & Camp, E.M. (1979). Physiological characteristics of trained paraplegic and tetraplegic subjects. *Medicine and Science in Sports, 11,* 256.

Greenberg, J.S. (1984). *Managing stress.* Dubuque, IA: Wm. C. Brown.

Grossman, H.J. (1977). *Manual on terminology in mental retardation.* Washington, DC: American Association on Mental Deficiency.

Guttman, L. (1976). *Textbooks of sport for the disabled.* London: HM & M Publishers.

Harper, D.C. (1978). Personality characteristics of physically impaired adolescents. *Journal of Clinical Psychology, 34,* 636.

Hartzell, H.E., & Compton, C. (1984). Learning disability: 10-year follow-up. *Pediatrics, 74,* 1058.

Hedrick, B.N. (1984). *The effect of wheelchair tennis participation and mainstreaming upon the perceptions of competence of physically disabled adolescents.* Unpublished doctoral dissertation, University of Illinois, Urbana-Champaign.

Henschen, K., Horvat, M., & French, R. (1984). A visual comparison of psychological profiles between able-bodied and wheelchair athletes. *Adapted Physical Activity Quarterly, 1,* 118.

Humphrey, J.H. (1975). *Education of children through motor activity.* Springfield, IL: Charles C. Thomas.

Humphrey, J.H. (1976). *Improving learning ability through compensatory physical education.* Springfield, IL: Charles C. Thomas.

Humphrey, J.H., & Sullivan, D.D. (1970). *Teaching slow learners through active games.* Springfield, IL: Charles C. Thomas.

Jeltma, K., & Vogler, E.W. (1985). Effects of an individual contingency on behaviorally disordered students in physical education. *Adapted Physical Activity Quarterly, 2,* 127.

Jones, J.A. (Ed.). (1984). *Training guide to cerebral palsied sports* (2nd ed.). New York: The National Association of Sports for Cerebral Palsy.

Katz, S., Shurks, E., & Florian, V. (1978). The relationship between physical disability, social perception and psychological stress. *Scandinavian Journal of Rehabilitation Medicine, 10,* 109.

Langone, J. (1985, June). The annual physical re-examined. *Healthline Newsletter,* pp. 20-22.

Lazar, A.L., Demos, G.D., Gaines, L., Rogers, D., & Stirnkorb, M. (1978). Attitudes of handicapped and non-handicapped university students on three attitude scales. *Rehabilitation Literature, 38,* 49.

Lemaire, L. (1984, January). Redline. *Ultrasport,* p. 4.

Levine, M. (1984, September). Learning abilities and disabilities. *The Medical Forum Newsletter,* pp. 3-6.

Lundberg, A. (1980). Wheelchair driving: Evaluation of a new training outfit. *Scandinavian Journal of Rehabilitation Medicine, 12,* 67.

Lussier, L., Knight, J., Bell, J., Lohman, T., & Morris, A.F. (1983). Body composition comparison in two elite female wheelchair athletes. *Paraplegia, 21,* 16.

Miles, B.H. (1985). Competitions for special populations: Personal perspectives. *Adapted Physical Activity Quarterly, 2,* 15.

Morgan, W.P. (1985a). Affective beneficence of vigorous physical activity. *Medicine and Science in Sports and Exercise, 17,* 94.

Morgan, W.P. (1985b). Psychogenic factors and exercise metabolism: A review. *Medicine and Science in Sports and Exercise, 17,* 309.

Morris, A.F. (1974). Myotatic reflex effects on bilateral reciprocal leg strength. *American Corrective Therapy Journal, 28,* 24.

Morris, A.F. (1982a, March/April). The track athlete needs medical classification. *Sports 'n Spokes,* p. 3.

Morris, A.F. (1982b, November). *Wheelchair sports for the athlete with severe, permanent, physical disability.* Paper presented at UNESCO International Symposium on Physical Education and Sport Programs for the Physically and Mentally Handicapped, Washington, DC.

Morris, A.F. (1984a). *Sports medicine: Prevention of Athletic injuries.* Dubuque, IA: Wm. C. Brown.

Morris, A.F. (1984b). A philosophy of sports and recreation at a comprehensive rehabilitation center. *Rehabilitation World, 8,* 30.

Morris, A.F. (1984c). General sports training for individuals with cerebral palsy. In J.A. Jones (Ed.), *Training guide to cerebral palsy sports* (2nd ed.), (pp. 36-39). New York: The National Association of Sports for Cerebral Palsy.

Morris, A.F. (1985a). *Sports medicine handbook.* Dubuque, IA: Wm. C. Brown.

Morris, A.F. (1985b, in press). An analysis of racing wheelchairs used at the 1980 Olympic Games for the Disabled. *Research Quarterly for Exercise and Sport.*

Morris, A.F., & Figoni, S.F. (1984, June). Strength measures of men and women wheelchair athletes. Paper presented at the International Medical Society of Paraplegia Meetings, Denver, CO.

Morris, A.F., & Figoni, S.F. (1985, May). Life quality characteristics of women athletes who participate in wheelchair basketball. Paper presented at The American Spinal Injury Association Annual Meeting, Atlanta, GA.

Morris, A.F., & Husman, B.F. (1978). Life quality changes following an endurance conditioning program. *American Corrective Therapy Journal, 32,* 3.

Morris, A.F., Layman, D.P., Stone, D., Creswell, W., & Figoni, S.F. (1985). *Long distance running and life quality in male master runners.* Manuscript submitted for publication.

Morris, A.F., Lussier, L., Vaccaro, P., & Clarke, D.H. (1982). Life quality characteristics of national class women masters long distance runners. *Annals of Sports Medicine, 1,* 23.

Morris, A.F., Vaccaro, P., & Clarke, D.H. (1979). Psychological characteristics in age group competitive swimmers, *Perceptual and Motor Skills, 48,* 1265.

Morris, A.F., Vaccaro, P., & Harris, R. (1983). Life quality changes of older adults during various physical activity programs. *Medicine and Science in Sports and Exercise* (abstract), *15,* 117.

Morris, A.F., Vaughan, S.E., & Vaccaro, P. (1982). Measurements of neuromuscular tone and strength in down syndrome children. *Journal of Mental Deficiency Research, 26,* 41.

Morris, V. (1985, May). Lament for the scholar-athlete. *The Graphic,* Amherst, MA, p. 4.

Munson, W.W., Baker, S.B., & Lundegren, H.M. (1985). Strength training and leisure counseling as treatments for institutionalized juvenile delinquents. *Adapted Physical Activity Quarterly, 2,* 65.

Pflaum, J.H. (1973). *Development of a life quality inventory.* Unpublished doctoral dissertation, University of Maryland, College Park.

Pollock, M., Miller, H., Linnerud, A., Laughridge, E., Coleman, E., & Alexander, E. (1974). Arm pedaling as an endurance training regimen for the disabled. *Archives of Physical Medicine and Rehabilitation, 55,* 418.

Prager, I.J. (1968). *The use of physical education activities in the reinforcement of selected first grade science concepts.* Unpublished master's thesis, University of Maryland, College Park.

Rarick, G.L., Dobbins, D.A., & Broadhead, G.D. (1977). *The motor domain and its correlates in educationally handicapped children.* Englewood Cliffs, NJ: Prentice-Hall.

Seaman, J.A., & DePauw, K.P. (1982). *The new adapted physical education.* Palo Alto, CA: Mayfield Publishing Co.

Shangold, M., & Mirkin, G. (1985). *The complete sports medicine book for women.* New York: Simon & Schuster.

Shephard, R.J. (1978). *Human physiological work capacity.* London: Cambridge University Press.

Shontz, F. (1978). Psychological adjustment to physical disability: Trends in theories. *Archives of Physical Medicine and Rehabilitation, 59,* 251.

Simon, J.I. (1971). Emotional aspects of physical disability. *American Journal of Occupational Therapy, 25,* 408.

Surburg, P.R. (1985). Basic problems in motor learning research. *Adapted Physical Activity Quarterly, 2,* 98.

United States Department of Education, Office of Education of Handicapped Students. (1984). *Percentage of school enrollment served as handicapped (in all states) 1981-82 and 1982-83 school years.* Washington, DC: author.

Van Aaken, E. (1972). *The Van Aaken method.* Mountain View, CA: World Publications.

Van Andel, G.E., & Austin, D.R. (1984). Physical fitness and mental health: A review of the literature. *Adapted Physical Activity Quarterly, 1,* 207.

Vargo, J. (1978). Some psychological effects of physical disability. *American Journal of Occupational Therapy, 32,* 31.

Winnick, J.P. (1984). Recent advances related to special physical education and sport. *Adapted Physical Activity Quarterly, 1,* 197.

Winnick, J.P., & Short, F.X. (1984). Test item selection for the project unique physical fitness test. *Adapted Physical Activity Quarterly, 1,* 296.

Zwiren, L., & Bar-Or, O. (1975). Responses to exercise of paraplegics who differ in conditioning level. *Medicine and Science in Sports, 7,* 94.

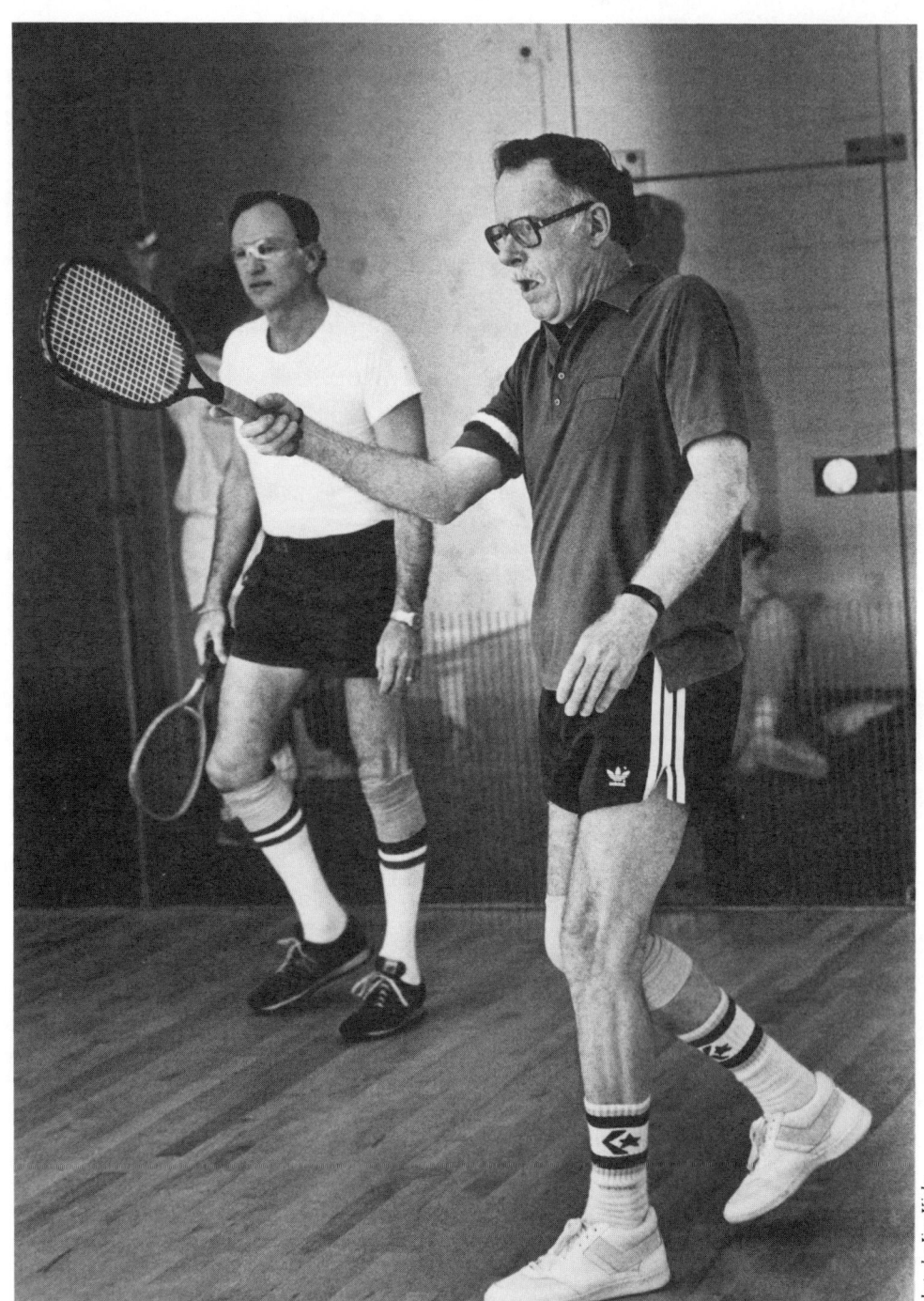

photo by Jim Kirby

CHAPTER FIFTEEN

Cardiorespiratory Diseases

Patty S. Freedson
Department of Exercise Science
University of Massachusetts
Amherst, Massachusetts

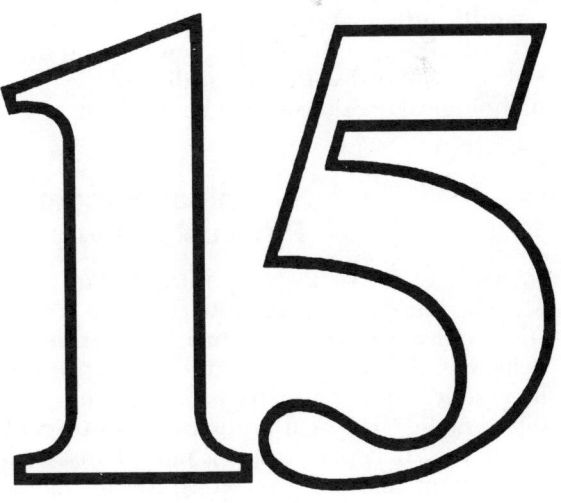

Introduction

Chronic degenerative cardiovascular disease (CVD) is a primary health care problem and is one of the leading causes of death in the United States. In 1978, CVD accounted for nearly 1,000,000 deaths, with 40% of all deaths among white males over the age of 55 being a direct result of coronary heart disease (CHD) (Levy, 1981). Moreover, each year over 1,250,000 Americans have heart attacks, with nearly one quarter of these individuals dying prior to receiving long term medical rehabilitation (Levy, 1981). In addition to these staggering morbidity and mortality statistics, CVD ranks among the highest medical economic burdens in terms of direct medical costs ($6 billion per year) and indirect costs ($20 billion per year) resulting from lost work hours, and early death (Levy, 1981).

On the positive side, however, this country has experienced a decline in CHD mortality over the least 15 years. For example, the death rate from CHD has decreased at least 20% among white and nonwhite males and females between the ages of 35-75 years (Levy, 1981).

The factors suggested to be associated with this decline in CHD mortality are improved medical treatment and lifestyle modification, including such factors as decreased smoking, dietary alterations, and an increase in physical activity. For example, in 1984, results of a Gallup Poll indicated that the number of adult Americans involved in "daily exercise" was nearly double the participation rate observed in 1961.

Interestingly, the important role of physical activity for health maintenance was recognized as early as 400 B.C. by Hippocrates (Simri, 1977). The value of exercise in preventive medicine applications was also identified during the 12th century by Maimonides, a famous theologian, philosopher, and physician. He viewed exercise as the best way to prevent disease, and noted that a lack of physical activity causes disease.

While these early writings were simply opinions, the observations are supported by the contemporary research literature. This review will summarize the available scientific information concerning the beneficial effects of physical activity in terms of cardiovascular disease prevention and therapeutic rehabilitation from selected cardiovascular diseases. In addition, the deleterious effects of exercise in certain pathological conditions will be summarized.

Epidemiological Studies: Physical Activity and CHD Risk

In one of the first survey studies of its kind published more than 30 years ago, Morris, Heady, Raffle, Roberts, and Parks (1953) reported that the London conductors who collected bus fares on double decker buses and postmen who delivered mail were at a reduced risk for CHD and sudden death compared to their sedentary counterparts (bus drivers and postal clerks). In a follow-up investigation, the CHD death rate for the more active conductors was 50% less than that of the bus drivers (Morris, Kagan, Patison, Gardner, & Raffle, 1966). Although subsequent analyses revealed that at the beginning of the study, waist girth, blood pressure and blood lipids were higher among the bus drivers (Morris, 1975), suggesting a confounding self-selection effect, this information led to the hypothesis that differences in physical activity were associated with differences in the risk for the development of CHD.

The application of the occupational activity model to differentiate low and high levels of physical activity has been used in numerous other epidemiological studies to further investigate the physical activity/CHD risk interaction. Studies of farm and non-farm workers (Pomrehn, Wallace & Burmeister 1982; Zukel, Lewis, Enterline & Painter, 1959; Cassel, Heyden, Bartel, Kaplan, Tyroler & Cornoni, 1971), utility company employees (Stamler, Lindberg, Berkson, Shaffer, Miller & Poindexter, 1960), railroad laborers and clerks (Menotti & Puddu, 1976; Taylor, Klepetar & Keys, 1962), kibbutz members (Brunner, Manelis, Modan & Lewis, 1974) and longshoremen (Paffenbarger & Hale, 1975; Paffenbarger, Hale & Brand, 1977) generally confirm the findings of Morris et al. (1953). However, several of these investigations failed to control for the potential confounding effects of smoking, body weight, stress, alcohol consumption and diet.

The retrospective study of the kibbutz inhabitants in Israel is noteworthy since the confounding effects of body weight, blood lipids, environmental factors and socioeconomic status did not dilute the results (Leon, 1985). The CHD risk was 2.5 times greater for the sedentary male kibbutz workers, in contrast to the active workers ($N = 5288$) (Brunner et al., 1974). Similarly, a 3-fold greater CHD risk was observed for inactive female kibbutzniks ($N = 5229$) (Brunner et al., 1974).

In an effort to quantify activity level more precisely than had been previously done, an evaluation of kilocalorie expenditure among 3686 longshoremen was related to the risk of fatal CHD (Paffenbarger, Hyde, Jung & Wing, 1984). They reported that weekly work-time caloric expenditure in excess of 8500 kcal was related to a significantly lower relative risk (44%) of death associated with CHD (Paffenbarger et al., 1984).

In a study of leisure time exercise among Harvard male alumni between 1962 and 1972, individuals who expended at least 2000 kcal/week in leisure time activity had nearly a 40% reduced risk of CHD (Paffenbarger et al., 1984). A 10-year follow up of men aged 35-69 from the Framingham study support these findings, as it was reported that the CHD risk was 46% lower for individuals whose activity index was greater than 37 (high activity) versus those whose activity index was less than 29 (low activity) (Kannel & Sorlie, 1979).

Although these types of studies do not propose mechanisms by which either occupational or leisure time activities protect against CHD, the epidemiological evidence supports an apparent association between relatively high levels of energy expenditure and reduced risk of CHD.

Physical Fitness and CHD Risk

In contrast to the multitude of epidemiological studies reporting that high levels of physical activity are associated with a reduced risk of CHD, relatively few data are available that examine the physical fitness-CHD relationship. Bruce and colleagues (1980) studied the CHD incidence among 2365 healthy 30-64-year old males who five years earlier had performed maximal exercise tests. Maximal treadmill testing, the measure of physical fitness employed, was only a significant predictor of CHD when it was considered along with other risk factors. Thus, it could not be concluded that poor cardiovascular fitness was an *independent* predictor of CHD risk over a five year follow up period. In contrast, a large prospective study ([$N = 2779$] healthy males, 55 years old or younger) of Los Angeles firefighters and police officers revealed a 2.2 relative risk for a myocardial infarction in individuals who scored below the median on a physical work capacity test after a 4.8 year follow-up period (Peters, Cady, Bischoff, Bernstein, & Pike, 1983). Moreover, those men with at least two other risk factors (high cholesterol, smoking, high blood pressure) and a below median physical work capacity had a relative risk of 6.6. These data led the investigators to conclude that men, particularly those with multiple CHD risk factors, should participate in regular physical activity to promote or maintain better than average fitness and perhaps reduce CHD risk.

The paucity of data relating specifically to the independent association between physical fitness and CHD risk and/or mortality prevents any conclusions from being drawn. More research in this area over a longer period of follow-up time is indicated.

To date there are no conclusive studies that directly implicate physical activity and/or physical fitness as providing an independent favorable effect on CHD. As presented earlier, there are numerous studies suggesting that regular physical activity is *associated* with a reduced risk for CHD. However, direct evidence confirming this link is not available.

The basic underlying factor responsible for CHD is atherosclerosis. The blood lipid/lipoprotein environment generally determines the degree of atherosclerosis. Several cross sectional and longitudinal studies have supported the hypothesis that individuals who are physically active and physically fit have a "healthier" blood lipid environment including a higher concentration of high density lipoproteins (HDL-C), lower concentration of low density lipoproteins (LDL-C), and increases in apolipoprotein A-1 and lipoprotein lipase (Oberman, 1985). Nevertheless, this favorable blood lipid pattern, apparently influenced by regular physical activity, has never been separately associated with a reduction in atherosclerosis. However, Kramsch, Aspen, Abramowitz, Kreimendahl, and Hood (1981) directly studied the effects of moderate exercise training in monkeys on the development of occlusive coronary artery disease. The results of their study clearly show that hypercholesterolemic monkeys (serum cholesterol = 600 mg/dl) who exercised at a moderate intensity for 1 hour, 3 times per week over a 36-42 month period developed significantly less atherosclerosis than a control group. In addition, the exercise group had higher high density lipoprotein levels and lower very low density lipoprotein and triglyceride levels than their untrained counterparts who were matched for total cholesterol. Although a study of this type is difficult to perform in human subjects, these data certainly support the notion of a direct association between physical activity and/or fitness and reduced atherogenesis. These data provide a strong complement to the epidemiological evidence which support the physical activity/reduced CHD risk association.

Physical Activity as a Therapeutic Modality for the Treatment of Coronary Artery Disease

Exercise training has become a popular and effective component of the multifaceted treatment of coronary artery disease. Numerous positive physiological adaptations occur in the CHD patient consequent to exercise training. These adaptations include a decrease in resting heart rate, a decrease in submaximal exercise heart rate and systolic blood pressure, a decrease in submaximal exercise myocardial oxygen consumption, an increased peripheral utilization of oxygen and an increase in aerobic work capacity ($\dot{V}O_2$ max). A detailed discussion of the cardiovascular adaptations to exercise training was provided in Chapter 10.

Until recently, the primary mechanism associated with the increase in $\dot{V}O_2$ max and the decrease in myocardial oxygen requirement at a given submaximal $\dot{V}O_2$ in cardiac patients was believed to be an enhanced peripheral utilization of oxygen (increased arterio-venous oxygen difference) (Detry, Rousseau, Vandenbroucke, Kusumi, Brasseur & Bruce, 1971) rather than an improved heart pump (central adaptation). However a recent study by Hagberg, Ehsani, & Holloszy (1983) revealed that 12 months of intense physical training, four to five times per week in cardiac patients ($\dot{V}O_2$ max increase of 42%) elicited significant improvements in myocardial function and an increase in stroke volume at a fixed submaximal workload. Of course, all cardiac patients will not have the capacity to train as intensely (85-90% of $\dot{V}O_2$ max) as these patients. However, the results from this study suggest that the mechanisms responsible for inducing an improvement in physical work capacity may be more similar in health and disease than previously recognized.

The value of regular physical activity following a cardiac event for improvement of morbidity and mortality rates has been studied via randomized clinical trials (Wilhelmsen, Sanne, Elmfeldt, Grimby, Tibblin, Wedel, 1975; Kallio, Hamalainen, Hakkila, Luurila, 1979; Kentala, 1972; Naughton, 1984; Rechnitzer, Cunningham, Andrew, Buck, Jones & Kavanagh, 1983). Post myocardial infarction patients were randomly assigned to either a control or a treatment group. Treatment either consisted of regular physical activity exclusively or in combination with group therapy sessions on smoking cessation and diet education. These longitudinal interventions generally were two to four years in duration. Although mortality rates were reduced from 28 to 37% in three of the five studies, only the results reported by Kallio et al. (1979) were statistically significant. The results concerning the effect of physical activity intervention on cardiac event recurrence are less impressive, with no observable difference evident between control and treatment groups. More randomized clinical trials are needed, with particular attention towards large samples, longer study duration, multifactor intervention, and improved compliance to intervention programs.

Physical Activity and Hypertension

The role of chronic physical activity for treatment of hypertension has been reviewed by Tipton (1984) and by Seals and Hagberg (1984). Although most intervention studies reported decreases in blood pressure ranging from 9 to 28 mm for systolic blood pressure and 5 to 14 mm for diastolic blood pressure, the long term consequences of such reductions in hypertensive individuals, with regard to morbidity and mortality, is not known. Moreover, it is difficult to definitively interpret these studies because they are inadequately controlled from a methodological perspective. These limitations include study design, sample size, blood pressure measurement techniques, exercise training programs, and the confounding effects of other factors such as body weight reduction and diet modification.

In a very well designed study that included a control group, Hagberg, Goldring & Ehsani (1983) examined the effects of six months of running, 30-40 minutes per session (60-65% of $\dot{V}O_2$ max), five times per week on 25 adolescent essential hypertensives whose resting blood pressure values were all above the 95th percentile for age and sex. The 10% improvement in $\dot{V}O_2$ max was accompanied by a 6% ($P < .01$) reduction in resting systolic and diastolic blood pressure and a 7% ($P < .05$) reduction in submaximal exercise blood pressure responses. It should be noted that body weight did not change during the course of this investigation. The results of their study support the notion that the exercise training, which stimulated a 10% increase in aerobic capacity, positively influenced blood pressure in these adolescent hypertensives. Further research is indicated, however, before any conclusions can be made regarding physical activity as an independent therapeutic modality for the treatment of hypertension.

Physical Activity as a Therapy for the Treatment of Pulmonary Disease

Although the mortality rate associated with cardiovascular heart disease has declined over the last 15 years, the death rate from pulmonary disease during that same period of time rose by almost 30%. However, the influence of physical activity on pulmonary disease has not been studied as extensively as cardiovascular disease. Attention should be focused on this problem where clinical trials are designed to study the effectiveness of exercise training as a modality for treatment of pulmonary disease.

The first observation that an exercise walking program resulted in an improvement in exercise capacity in two pulmonary patients was reported by Barach, Bickerman, and Beck (1952). Subsequent investigations have reported similar positive improvements in more quantitative terms. For example, a 24% increase in a 12 minute walk/run test was observed consequent to a 10 month exercise program in chronic bronchitis patients (Sinclair & Ingram, 1980).

Nevertheless, while exercise training reportedly increases exercise endurance capacity, resting pulmonary function tests and maximum oxygen consumption have not been shown to improve with exercise training (Weg, 1985). The factors that appear to be associated with the increased endurance capacity are an improved efficiency in the exercise ventilation pattern and enhanced economy of whole body movement attributed to an acquisition of better mechanical skills (Paiz, Phillipson & Masngkay, 1967). Thus, although the mechanisms underlying an improved exercise capacity are not from significant physiological and hemodynamic improvements, it appears that regular physical activity has a very positive influence on the quality of life in pulmonary patients and may facilitate maintenance of *independent* participation in activities of daily living.

Detrimental Effects of Physical Activity

An alarming survey study by Thompson, Stern, William, Duncan, Haskell & Wood (1979) reported that the CHD death rate of older Rhode Island joggers was seven times the CHD death rate of Rhode Island residents who spent their leisure time in more sedentary activities. Although these deaths seemed to be precipitated by exercise, there was some type of underlying cardiovascular pathology that resulted in death. While CHD is usually implicated as the cause of exercise-related sudden death in older individuals, the autopsy findings among young athletes who died suddenly include hypertrophic cardiomyopathy, anomalous origin of the left coronary artery, aortic stenosis or a ruptured aorta (Maron, Roberts, McAllister, Rosing & Epstein, 1980). In selected cases cardiac anatomy in sudden death victims is normal and no significant atherosclerosis is evident in the coronary arteries. It has been speculated that transient coronary artery spasm (McLaughlin, Dohery, Martin, Goris & Harrison, 1977) or myocardial bridging over the coronary artery (Morales, Romanelli & Boucek, 1980) may be related to the sudden death. In all conditions of sudden death, it appears that ventricular fibrillation, which occurs as a result of the myocardial ischemia, is the ultimate cause of death.

It should be noted that the incidence of sudden death, particularly in young athletes, is quite rare. The beneficial effects of physical activity far outweigh the sudden death phenomenon. Perhaps through more complete medical screening practices, the identification of those individuals who are susceptible to this phenomenon can be made.

The final negative consequence of physical activity is in exercise induced asthma (EIA). However, the bronchoconstriction that is produced by exercise, particularly in cold dry environments, can be prevented by inhaling a bronchodilator (Rossing, Weiss & Breslin, 1982). The mechanisms by which airway cooling causes bronchoconstriction is not known and has been a focus of research in this area (Bleecker, 1984).

Exercise induced asthma is usually easily controlled with pharmacological agents. Individuals with EIA should be encouraged to exercise, but forewarned that they must be prepared to handle an exercise induced asthmatic episode.

Summary

Moderately intense regular leisure time and occupational activity is associated with reduced coronary heart disease related morbidity and mortality.

The evidence does not clearly indicate that a high level of physical fitness will reduce the risk of cardiovascular disease.

High levels of aerobic fitness have been associated with a favorable blood lipid profile, particularly with regard to high density lipoprotein levels.

Regular physical activity has been shown to improve aerobic capacity in individuals with coronary heart disease via increasing peripheral utilization of oxygen.

Long term, high intensity exercise rehabilitation in cardiac patients may elicit central (heart pump) adaptations similar to the adaptations observed for healthy individuals.

Two to four year cardiac rehabilitation intervention is associated with reduced coronary heart disease mortality, but no apparent beneficial effect of reducing the risk for another cardiac event can be claimed.

Regular physical activity appears to have a beneficial influence on reducing blood pressure in individuals who have hypertension.

The positive effects of regular physical activity in pulmonary disease are not the result of physiological adaptations, but rather reflect an improvement in ventilatory patterns and mechanical efficiency.

Sudden death associated with exercise has been related to atherosclerosis, a variety of cardiac anatomy anomalies or transient coronary spasm.

Exercise induced asthma causes bronchoconstriction, but is easily controlled by pharmacological intervention.

References

Barach, A.L., Bickerman, H.A., & Beck, G. (1952). Advances in the treatment of non-tuberculosis pulmonary disease. *New York Academy of Medicine, 28,* 353-384.

Bleecker, E.R. (1984). Exercise-induced asthma: Physiologic and clinical considerations. In J. Loke (Ed.), *Clinics In Chest Medicine, 5,* 109-119.

Bruce, R.A., De Rouen, T.A., Hossack, K.F., Blake, B., & Hofer, V. (1980). Value of maximal exercise tests in risk assessment of primary coronary heart disease events in healthy men. *American Journal of Cardiology, 46,* 371-378.

Brunner, D., Manelis, G., Modan, M., & Lewis, S. (1974). Physical activity at work and the incidence of myocardial infarction, angina pectoris and death due to ischemic heart disease: An epidemiological study in Israeli collective settlements (kibbutzim). *Journal of Chronic Diseases, 273,* 217-233.

Cassel, J., Heyden, S., Bartel, A.C., Kaplan, B.H., Tyroler, H.A., & Cornoni, J.C. (1971). Occupation and physical activity and coronary heart disease. *Archives of Internal Medicine, 128,* 920-928.

Detry, J.M.R., Rousseau, M., Vandenbroucke, G., Kusumi, F., Brasseur, L.A., & Bruce, R.A. (1971). Increased arteriovenous oxygen difference after physical training in coronary heart disease. *Circulation, 44,* 109-118.

Hagberg, J.M., Ehsani, A.A., & Holloszy, J.O. (1983). Effect of 12 months of intense exercise training on stroke volume in patients with coronary artery disease. *Circulation, 67,* 1194-1199.

Hagberg, J.M., Goldring, D., & Ehsani, A.A. (1983). Effect of exercise training on blood pressure and hemodynamics of adolescent hypertensives. *American Journal of Cardiology, 52,* 763-768.

Kallio, V., Hamalainen, H., Hakkila, J., & Luurila, O.J. (1979). Reduction in sudden death by a multifactorial intervention programme after acute myocardial infarction. *Lancet 2,* 1091-1097.

Kannel, W.M. & Sorlie, P. (1979). Some health benefits of physical activity: The Framingham Study. *Archives of Internal Medicine, 139,* 857-861.

Kentala, E. (1972). Physical fitness and feasibility of physical rehabilitation after myocardial infarction in men of working age. *Annals of Clinical Research, 9* (suppl), 1-84.

Kramsch, D.M., Aspen, A.J., Abramowitz, B.M., Kreimendahl, T., & Hood, W.B. (1981). Reduction of coronary atherosclerosis by moderate conditioning exercise in monkeys on an atherogenic diet. *New England Journal of Medicine, 305,* 1483-1489.

Leon, A.S. (1985). Physical activity levels and coronary heart disease: Analysis of epidemiologic and supporting studies. *Medical Clinics of North America, 69,* 3-19.

Levy, R.I. (1981). Declining mortality in coronary heart disease. *Arteriosclerosis, 1,* 312-325.

McLaughlin, P.R., Dohery, P.W., Martin, R.P., Goris, M.L., & Harrison, D.C. (1977). Myocardial imaging in a patient with reproducible variant angina. *American Journal of Cardiology, 39,* 126-129.

Maron, B.J., Roberts, W.C., McAllister, H.A., Rosing, D.R., & Epstein, S.E. (1980). Sudden death in young athletes. *Circulation, 62,* 218-229.

Menotti, A., & Pudda, V. (1976). Death rates among the Italian railroad employees with special reference to coronary heart disease and physical activity at work. *Environmental Research, 11,* 331-342.

Morales, A.R., Romanelli, R., & Boucek, R.J. (1980). Transmural left anterior descending coronary artery, strenuous exercise and sudden death. *Circulation, 62,* 230-237.

Morris, J.N. (1975). *Uses of epidemiology* (3rd ed). New York: Churchill Livingstone.

Morris, J.N., Heady, J.A., Raffle, P.A.B., Roberts, C.G., & Parks, J.W. (1953). Coronary heart disease and physical activity of work. *Lancet, 2,* 1053-1057, 1111-1120.

Morris, J.N., Kagan, A., Patison, D.C., Gardner, M.J., & Raffle, P.A.B. (1966). Incidence and prediction of ischaemic heart disease in London busmen. *Lancet, 2,* 552-559.

Naughton, J. (1984). Contributions of exercise clinical trials to cardiac rehabilitation. *Clinics in Sports Medicine, 3,* 545-557.

Oberman, A. (1985). Exercise and the primary prevention of cardiovascular disease. *American Journal of Cardiology, 55,* 10D-20D.

Paiz, P.N., Phillipson, E.A., Masngkay, M. (1967). The physiologic basis of training patients with emphysema. *American Review of Respiratory Diseases, 95,* 944-953.

Paffenbarger, R.S., Jr., & Hale, W.E. (1975). Work activity and coronary heart mortality. *New England Journal of Medicine, 292,* 545-550.

Paffenbarger, R.S., Jr., Hale, W.E., & Brand, R.J. (1977). Work-energy level, personal characteristics, and fatal heart attack: A birth-cohort effect. *American Journal of Epidemiology, 105,* 200-213.

Paffenbarger, R.S., Jr., Hyde, R.T., Jung, D.L., & Wing, A.L. (1984). Epidemiology of exercise and coronary heart disease. *Clinics in Sportsmedicine, 3,* 297-318.

Peters, R.K., Cady, L.D., Bischoff, D.P., Bernstein, L., and Pike, M.C. (1983). Physical fitness and subsequent myocardial infarction in healthy workers. *Journal of the American Medical Association, 249,* 3052-3057.

Pomrehn, P.R., Wallace, R.B., & Burmeister, L.F. (1982). Ischemic heart disease mortality in Iowa farmers: The influence of lifestyle. *Journal of the American Medical Association, 248,* 1073-1076.

Rechnitzer, P.A., Cunningham, D.A., Andrew, G.M., Buck, C.W., Jones, N.L., & Kavanagh, T. (1983). Relation of exercise to the recurrence rate of myocardial infarction in men. Ontario exercise-heart collaborative study. *American Journal of Cardiology, 51,* 65-69.

Rossing, T.H., Weiss, J.W., & Breslin, F.J. (1982). Effects of inhaled sympathomimetics on obstructive response to respiratory heat loss. *Journal of Applied Physiology, 52,* 1119-1123.

Seals, D.R., and Hagberg, J.M. (1984). The effect of exercise training on human hypertension: A review. *Medicine and Science in Sports and Exercise, 16,* 207-215.

Simri, V. (1977). The role of exercise in arabic medicine in the 12th century. In D. Brunner and E. Jokl (Eds.), *The Role of Exercise in Internal Medicine* (pp. 174-179). New York: S. Karger.

Sinclair, D.J.M., & Ingram, C.G. (1980). Controlled trial of supervised exercise training in chronic bronchitis. *British Medical Journal, 280,* 519-521.

Stamler, J., Lindberg, H.A., Berkson, M.D., Shaffer, A., Miller, W., & Poindexter, A. (1960). Prevalence and incidence of coronary heart disease in strata of the labor force of a Chicago industrial corporation. *Journal of Chronic Diseases, 11,* 405-420.

Taylor, H.L., Klepetar, E., & Keys, A. (1962). Death rates among physically active and sedentary employees of the railroad industry. *American Journal of Public Health, 52,* 1697-1707.

Thompson, P.D., Stern, M.P., William, P., Duncan, K., Haskell, W.L., & Wood, P.D. (1979). Death during jogging or running: A study of 18 cases. *Journal of the American Medical Association, 242,* 1265-1267.

Tipton, C.M. (1984). Exercise, training and hypertension. In R.L. Terjung (Ed.), *Exercise and Sport Sciences Reviews,* (Vol. 12) (pp. 245-306). Toronto: The Collamore Press.

Weg, J.G. (1985). Therapeutic exercise in patients with chronic obstructive pulmonary disease. In N.K. Wenger (Ed.), *Exercise and the Heart* (2nd ed) (pp. 261-275). Philadelphia: F.A. Davis Company.

Wilhelmsen, L., Sanne, H., Elmfeldt, D., Grimby, G., Tibblin, G., & Wedel, H. (1975). A controlled trial of physical training after myocardial infarction. *Preventive Medicine, 4,* 491-508.

Zukel, W.J., Lewis, R.H., Enterline, P.E., & Painter, R.C. (1959). A short term community study of the epidemiology of coronary heart disease: A preliminary report on the North Dakota Study. *American Journal of Public Health, 49,* 1630-1639.

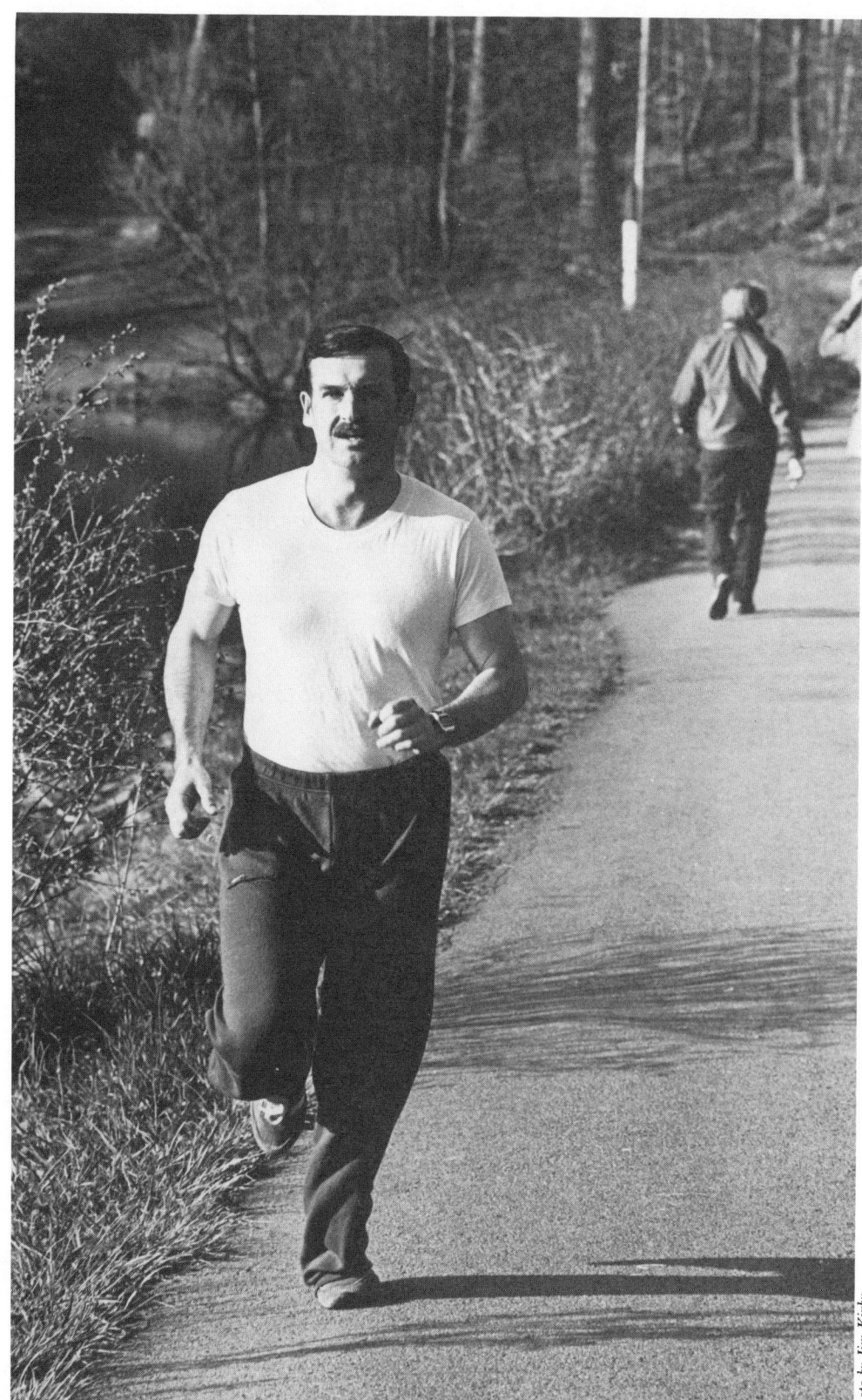
photo by Jim Kirby

CHAPTER SIXTEEN

Metabolic Disease: Diabetes Mellitus

Kris Berg
Department of Health, Physical
Education, and Recreation
University of Nebraska at Omaha
Omaha, Nebraska

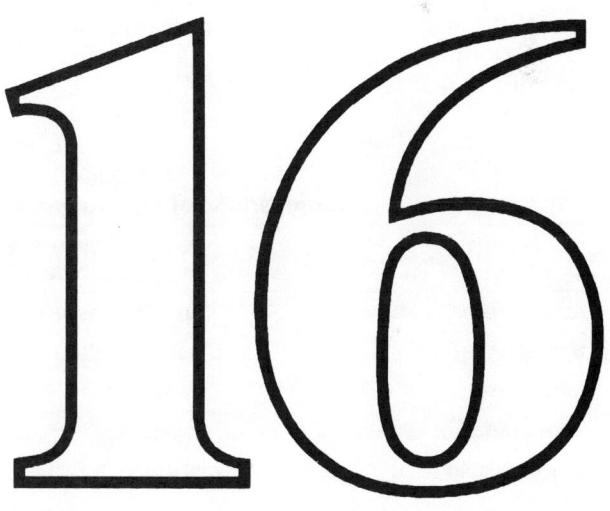

Introduction

Even before the discovery of insulin in 1921, exercise was used in the treatment of diabetes. Standard therapy, in fact, has traditionally included physical activity. While the acute effects of exercise in diabetics have been studied widely and are relatively well understood, the chronic effects of training are difficult to assess and have not received nearly as much attention (Berger, 1983). Much of the information regarding the chronic effects of training are anecdotal and theoretical. However, the implications are meaningful because they suggest a number of benefits to both type 1 and type 2 diabetics. Today newly diagnosed diabetics receive education not only in insulin or drug therapy and diet, but also in the use of exercise. Current medical opinion holds that physical activity can be beneficial to diabetics and that its place in the total management of the disease is important (Cantu, 1982; Vranic and Berger, 1979).

Types of Diabetes

Diabetes mellitus is a chronic condition which affects some 10 million Americans. About 10 percent of these have type 1 diabetes, also referred to as insulin-dependent diabetes mellitus (IDDM). This type was formerly called juvenile-onset diabetes because the disease is usually, but not always, contracted in children and adolescents. The great majority of diabetics have type 2 diabetes and are not necessarily dependent on insulin. Therefore, type 2 diabetes is also called non-insulin dependent diabetes mellitus (NIDDM). Type 2 diabetes was previously called adult-onset diabetes.

The two types of diabetes are compared in Table 1. Type 1 diabetes is characterized by an absence or marked reduction of insulin production, while in type 2 diabetes insulin production is generally normal or even above normal, but insulin effectiveness is reduced. Type 1 diabetics are usually diagnosed before age 20 with acute symptoms of extreme rise in blood sugar, thirst, sudden weight loss, frequent urination, and ketoacidosis. In type 2 diabetics symptoms typically appear gradually at age 40 or later. A family history of the condition is often found to exist in NID (non-insulin dependent) diabetics, while the opposite is true for ID (insulin-dependent) diabetics. As the nomenclature suggests, juveniles with dia-

Table 1
Comparison of the two types of diabetes.

	type 1 or insulin dependent	type 2 or non-insulin dependent
former nomenclature	juvenile-onset	adult-onset
age at onset	usually before 20	usually after 40
family history	infrequent	frequent
appearance of symptoms	rapid	slow
use of insulin	always	common but not always required
proneness to ketoacidosis	prone	not prone; rarely occurs
production of insulin by pancreas	absent or greatly reduced	usually normal or elevated
body fatness	usually normal or lean	usually obese

betes require insulin by injection, while many adults do not require insulin. As a matter of fact, adult diabetics who use insulin after diagnosis of the conditon are frequently able to be taken off insulin once they become physically active and lose body fat. ID diabetics are prone to excess ketone production, while this condition rarely occurs in NID diabetics. Although the majority of NID diabetics are overweight, ID diabetics are typically of normal fatness and body weight or even slender.

Medical Problems Common to Diabetics

Diabetics are at greatly increased risk of suffering cardiovascular disease, eye problems, nerve disorders, and kidney failure. Diabetes is presently the fifth leading cause of death in the United States and third if all of its complications are included. Diabetics are 25 times more prone to blindness, 2-3 times more prone to cardiovascular disease, and 17 times more likely to incur kidney disease (Crofford, 1975). Current research suggests that the sequelae of diabetes are caused by chronic blood sugar elevation. Excess glucose from the blood penetrates tissues and alters their function. The walls of capillaries are damaged, leading to a reduced effectiveness of the microcirculation called microangiopathy. This chronic reduction in blood flow can lead to hypoxia and eventually necrosis of tissues.

Damaged nerves due to neuropathy reduce sensory perception to the point that diabetics often suffer injury to the feet without feeling any discomfort. Consequently, an untreated injury, when accompanied by reduced blood flow and reduced immune function, can lead to serious infections. Damage to nerves regulating cardiovascular function alters the response of the heart and blood vessels to exercise. Nerve conduction velocity is impaired, which affects the overall neuromuscular function. Reaction time, movement time, and strength and power may, consequently, be reduced.

Kidney function is impaired as damage occurs to the nephron. Urinary tract infections are common because elevated blood sugar encourages bacterial growth. As glucose accumulates within the lens of the eye, cataracts are formed. Damage to the blood vessels in the eye and retina produce diabetic retinopathy. Vessels enlarge, rupture and hemorraging within the eye can occur.

Heart and blood vessel disease are two to three times more frequent in diabetics than in the non-affected population. Diabetes, in itself, is considered an independent cardiovascular disease risk factor, but it is also related to other risk factors such as obesity, elevated cholesterol and triglycerides, hypertension, reduced fibrinolysis, and low levels of circulorespiratory fitness.

The frequency and severity of these problems make the treatment goal of of this disease clear: to achieve normal blood sugar levels as frequently as possible. Because blood sugar level is reduced during physical activity if the diabetic is in a controlled metabolic state (i.e., a functional level of insulin is present in the blood and ketone production is normal), exercise can be of value in treatment of diabetes.

All diabetics should be evaluated by their physician before beginning an exercise program. If heart and blood vessel or specific tissue impairment exists, physicians may recommend that the exercise be supervised. Many cardiac rehabilitation programs have diabetics as clients. Even if cardiovascular disease is not evident, diabetics are often included in these programs because of their high risk for circulatory problems. Also, modification of insulin and diet are usually necessary adjustments to the energy expenditure associated with the exercise program.

Benefits of Exercise

Consistent, long-term maintenance of normal blood glucose reverses, to some degree, nearly every medical problem previously discussed. Furthermore, diabetics today are trained to measure their blood sugar at home and make necessary corrections in insulin, diet, and exercise. Until recently, diabetics attempted to strive for good glucose control without the aid of even knowing what their blood sugar level was each day. Consequently, there was only a limited basis for achieving appropriate glucose levels. Today, multiple insulin injections, direct measurement of blood glucose at home, and use of insulin infusion pumps to release small boluses of insulin periodically throughout the day increase the likelihood of achieving effective blood sugar control. To a large extent, successful treatment of diabetes depends directly on the degree that each diabetic carefully monitors his or her blood sugar one or more times daily and then makes adjustments with insulin, medication, and diet. Because of these advances in technology and knowledge, diabetics should find initiating an exericse program easier and safer than it was years ago. The benefits of exercise can consequently be made available to nearly all diabetics.

The psychological effects of exercise may be just as important as the more readily measured physical and physiological effects. The realization that participation in physical activity, including vigorous sport, can be engaged in safely and even beneficially may do much to create a positive feeling about life. Physically active diabetics may even be encouraged to maintain a higher degree of control of their condition so that they can maintain a vigorous lifestyle.

If diabetics are reasonably well controlled metabolically, their blood sugar and ketone levels well-balanced, then exercise appears to provide the same benefits enjoyed by non-diabetics. While research on the trainability of diabetics as compared to non-diabetics is far from complete, it appears that diabetics are capable of experiencing significant improvement in fitness and physical performance. In some instances these training effects have not been experimentally tested in diabetics, but it is presumed that they would occur with appropriate conditioning. Many of the training changes, however, have been verified with diabetic subjects and are so noted. The following paragraphs outline some of the benefits of physical activity to the diabetic patient.

1. *Improved circulorespiratory fitness.*
    a. Greater pulmonary function
       Greater maximum ventilation and frequency
    b. Greater cardiovascular function
       1) Increased maximum stroke volume, cardiac output and oxygen pulse
       2) Increased oxygen-carrying capacity of the blood
       3) Increased dissociation of oxygen from hemoglobin so that more oxygen is delivered to the tissues (Dietzel, 1976)
       4) Increased capillarization of lungs and trained muscle fibers
    c. Greater ability to use oxygen
       Increased mitochondrial size and number as well as enzymes to facilitate oxidation within muscle cells. Costill, Cleary, Fink, Foster, Ivy and Witzmann (1979) concluded that ID diabetics experience the same magnitude of change from endurance training as do non-diabetics. These results substantiate those of Larsson, Persson, Sterky, and Thoren (1964). Costill et al. (1979) compared $\dot{V}O_2$ max, lactic acid, and enzyme levels (malate dehydrogenase, succinate dehydrogenase, hexokinase, lipoprotein lipase, and carnitine palmityltransferase) in diabetics and non-diabetics. The only difference in training response occured in carnitine-palmityl CoA oxidation capacity, which was 41% greater in the diabetics,

but was still within the normal range. This latter measure is an index of the ability of muscle tissue to oxidize fatty acids.
   d. Greater $\dot{V}O_2$ max (Costill et al., 1979)
2. *Greater muscle fitness.*
   Increased strength and muscle mass (Miller, Sherman and Ivy, 1984) and increased power and muscle endurance
3. *Greater joint flexibility.*
4. *Reduced risk factors for cardiovascular disease.*
   a. Weight reduction
   b. Decreased blood pressure
   c. Reduced cholesterol and triglyceride levels (Costill et al., 1979; Ruderman, Ganda, and Johansen (1979)
      1) Increased high density lipoprotein cholesterol (HDL-C) and HDL-C/total cholesterol ratio
      2) Reduced low density lipoprotein cholesterol (LDL-C) and total cholesterol
   d. Improved $\dot{V}O_2$ max (Costill et al., 1979)
   e. Increased fibrinolysis (dissolving of clots)
   f. Reduced tendency to form clots
   g. Reduced uric acid
   h. Enhanced ability to cope with stress
   i. Increased joie de vivre
5. *Improved blood sugar control and therefore reduced complications such as retinopathy, neuropathy, nephropathy, and microangiopathy.*
   Better blood sugar regulation with exercise occurs only in diabetics in a reasonable state of metabolic control. If exercise is performed when an inadequate level of insulin is in the blood and/or when ketones are elevated, the blood glucose and ketone levels tend to rise during exercise. This is an important qualifier because exercise should be avoided when either of these conditions exists. Daily exercise which expends a large number of calories provides a margin of tolerance which facilitates blood sugar regulation. Because carbohydrate as well as fat is combusted during prolonged exercise if blood insulin level is adequate, muscle tissue becomes somewhat depleted of glycogen each day of exercise. Therefore, some blood glucose is transported into the exercised muscle mass, thereby reducing the tendency for the blood sugar to become elevated.
6. *Reduced likelihood of hypoglycemia during exercise.*
   Endurance training provides greater reserves of glycogen in both the trained muscle fibers and liver. Hence, a trained diabetic can work or exercise longer before glycogen levels are depleted to the point of allowing hypoglycemia to occur. Consequently, severe hypoglycemia or insulin reaction is less likely because of the extra supply of glycogen in the liver. Furthermore, endurance training allows trained muscles to depend to a greater extent on the oxidation of fat as an energy substrate rather than glucose and glycogen. This is reflected in a lower respiratory exchange ratio during any level of submaximum work. Trained muscles also produce more alanine during work. This amino acid is a precursor of glucose formation in the liver and provides an additional source of glucose for uptake by muscles during exercise, which reduces the chance of hypoglycemia during exercise.
7. *Enhanced efficiency for fat metabolism and/or enhanced capacity to clear ketones from the blood.*
   Costill, Miller, and Fink (1980) found that trained diabetic distance runners who took no insulin 24 hours before running experienced no significant elevation in ketones during or after a 90 minute treadmill run. The highest ketone level in any athlete was 107 mM. Berger, Berchtold, Cuppers, Drost,

Kley, Miller, Wiegelmann, Zimmerman, Telschow, Gries, Kruskemper, and Zimmerman (1977) observed higher ketone levels under similar conditions in untrained diabetics. These results indicate that trained diabetics can perform safely in long duration events without undue fear of either hypoglycemia or ketosis occurring.

8. *Reduced requirement for insulin for ID diabetics, and reduced amount or elimination of insulin or medication to control blood sugar in NID diabetics.*

   Chronic activity increases the sensitivity of the insulin receptors, which reduces the need for insulin and may obviate the need for insulin or oral medication (Becker-Zimmerman, Berger, Berchtold, Gries, Herberg, & Schwenen, 1982; Berger et al., 1979; Bjorntorp, De Jounge, Stostrom, & Sullivan, 1970). Receptors for insulin line the cells of nearly all tissues; they serve to attach the insulin circulating in the blood to the outer cell membrane so that insulin can facilitate the uptake of glucose. With chronic endurance training, the insulin receptors increase in number and sensitivity so that less insulin or medication is needed to regulate blood sugar. ID diabetics who become physically active typically reduce the amount of injected insulin about 20-40% (A Round Table, 1979). Some NID diabetics who use oral medication are often able to eliminate their medication. Part of the physical training effect which allows for reduced insulin or medication occurs because of the reduction in body fat. Insulin sensitivity is highly correlated to body fatness. Conversely, sedentary living accompanied by weight gain (i.e., fat) results in increased insulin production in non-diabetics and some NID diabetics. Even sudden change in exercise habits such as experienced by astronauts confined to limited space and activity has resulted in hyperinsulinemia. Recently, weight training has been found effective in reducing plasma insulin levels. The reduction was highly correlated with the increased lean body mass ($r = .89$, $p < .05$) (Miller et al., 1984). Because some type 2 diabetics are able to be taken off medication and still maintain metabolic control, exercise is possibly of greater value to them as comred to type 1 diabetics.

9. *Reduced body weight.*

   As previously discussed, weight reduction, specifically fat loss, increases insulin sensitivity.

10. *Reduced stress.*

    Stress stimulates the adrenal medulla to secrete the catecholamines epinephrine and norepinephrine and the adrenal cortex to secrete a group of hormones called the glucocorticoids. The catecholamines stimulate the liver to split stored glycogen into glucose in a process known as glycogenolysis. The glucocorticoids also enhance glycogenolysis and inhibit the action of insulin. The net result of these secretions is an elevation of blood sugar in some diabetics. However, some diabetics respond to stress with a decrease in blood sugar. Whatever the response, a reduction in stress would assist in normalizing blood sugar. A number of studies have reported that exercise has a stress-reducing effect (Morgan, Roberts, Brandy, & Feinerman, 1970; Morgan, 1979) which should reduce the secretion of the catecholamines and glucocorticoids. Also, exercise increases the rate at which catecholamines are degraded. Some evidence supports the idea that a pituitary secretion called B-endorphin is secreted during physical activity (Appenzeller, Standefer, Appenzeller, & Atkinson, 1980; Gambert, Garthwaite, Hagen, Tristani, & McCarty, 1981; and Fraioli, Moretti, Paolucci, Alicicco, Crescenzi, & Fortunato, 1980). This hormone has even been proposed to explain the "runner's high" which is a feeling of unlimited energy and an exaggerated feeling of well-being (Callen, 1983). However, the measurement of B-endorphin is complex and variable, and it is not agreed on by researchers as to whether or not the hormone is able to penetrate the blood-brain barrier to enter the brain (Rapoport, Klee, Pettegrew, Ohno, 1980; Nakao, Nakai, Oki, Matsubara, Konishi, Nishitiani, & Imura, 1980). Furthermore, during exercise some research subjects have demonstrated large increases in B-endorphin levels without demonstrating changes in behavior (Catlin, Gorelick, Gerner, Hui, & Li, 1980). Several investigators believe that adequate evidence does not now exist to support the hypothesis that B-endorphin causes "runner's high" (Moore, 1982).

The calming effect of repetitive rhythmic movement still appears to be valid, although it is difficult to specify the regulatory mechanisms. However, anecdotally, exercise is used by some psychiatrists for its calming as well as anti-depressant effects (Kostrubala, 1976). So, for whatever the cause, exercise which promotes relaxation would seem to be a useful adjunct to the diabetic who wishes to achieve better control of blood sugar.

11. *Improved self-image and self-concept.*
Many studies have clearly shown improved ratings of self-image and self-concept after several months of physical training (Sonstroem, 1982; Morgan et al., 1970). Although no supporting evidence exists, it is plausible that diabetics with good self-image and self-concept should be more likely to take better care of themselves. Also, good diabetic care should minimize diabetic complications and even demonstrate that diabetics can live quite normal lives in all respects. Thus, diabetics who control their condition should experience enhanced self-image and self-concept simply because of the good health they can maintain. Also, diabetics who are well-controlled can largely avoid fluctuations in metabolism such as hypo- and hyperglycemia, and ketosis. The symptoms of these conditions all include feeling anxious and irritable. The symptoms themselves then are stressing nd do not contribute to a sense of feeling good. Conversely, however, when blood sugar levels are within the normal range, diabetics tend to feel better emotionally.

Management of Diabetes

The treatment of both types of diabetes is aimed at maintaining blood sugar levels close to the normal range. If blood sugar drops below a critical point, symptoms such as sweating, blurred vision, reduced coordination, tingling around the mouth, and elevated pulse rate occur. If blood sugar rises much beyond 250 mg%, acidosis occurs. A further rise in blood sugar is usually accompained by an elevation of ketones to produce a condition called ketosis or ketoacidosis, which often necessitates hospitalization to prevent coma. Skyler, Skyler, and O'Sullivan (1981) consider ideal glucose values for ID diabetics to range from 60-140 mg% depending on when the measurement is taken (e.g., fasting or before or after meals). To achieve tight control over blood glucose, diet, exercise and insulin or medication to reduce blood are manipulated. In ID diabetics, insulin is required to control blood sugar whereas it is not always needed in type 2 diabetes (NID).

Insulin

Insulin is classified by the time that is required to exert a blood sugar-lowering effect and the duration of this effect. Short acting insulin such as Regular exerts its peak effect about one to two hours after being injected and the peak effect is sustained for about six hours. Intermediate type insulins such as Lente and NPH have a peak effect about 6 to 12 hours after injection, with a reduced action 12 to 24 hours later. Long acting insulin such as Ultralente does not demonstrate an effect on blood sugar for about 12 hours but the effect lasts for about 36 hours.

Many ID diabetics administer insulin several times daily and mix two types of insulin with each injection. This muliple injection-mixed dosage regimen is advantageous because it provides a fairly constant supply of insulin to the blood yet provides several insulin peaks to coincide with the major meals. Figure 1 displays the insulin levels over a 24 hour period using this regimen. The fast acting Regular insulin taken at 7 a.m. and 5 p.m. is designed to cover the calories consumed at breakfast and dinner, respectively. The intermediate insulin administered at these times provides a longer duration insulin base to cover ongoing metabolic needs throughout the 24 hour cycle. Because most the calories are typically consumed during the day and because more insulin is needed in the morning than later in the day to exert the same decrease in blood sugar, most ID diabetics on a multiple injection regimen take about two-thirds of their total day's insulin in the morning (Skyler et al., 1981).

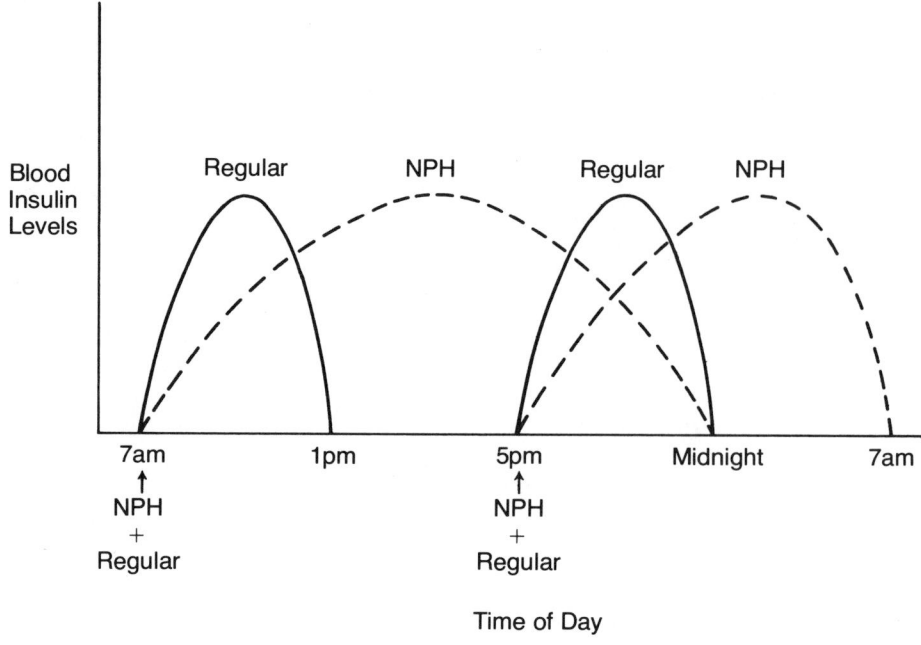

Fig. 1. Blood insulin levels over 24 hours using a multiple injection, mixed-dosage regimen (Regular +NPH).

Food intake should be related to the various peak levels of insulin. For example, many diabetics take their morning insulin 30 to 60 minutes before eating breakfast. As blood glucose begins to rise an hour or two after breakfast, it should coincide with the beginning of the peak effect of the regular insulin taken before breakfast. At lunch the intermediate type insulin should begin to peak. An afternoon snack is commonly used to accommodate the intermediate insulin which peaks 6 to 12 hours after injection. Similarly, an evening snack provides coverage for the intermediate insulin taken before dinner. This snack is often comprised of a mix of protein, fat and carbohydrate because the digestion and rise of blood sugar associated with protein and fat are fairly slow and sustained. Consequently, it provides a relatively steady source of energy while sleeping.

Diet

The major dietary guidelines for diabetics are related to factors which prevent the blood sugar from being too low or too high. First, diabetics must eat meals of a fairly consistent composition from day to day. That is, the insulin needed to cover a particular feeding is affected by the speed with which the food can be digested and absorbed through the gut into the bloodstream. Obviously, consumption of simple carbohydrates such as candy and soft drinks undergo these processes fairly fast, 30 minutes or less, while fats take about 1.5 hours and protein about 3 hours. Such foods can be selected at times when hyperglycemia may otherwise be likely to occur.

The time at which feedings are taken should coincide with insulin intake. If a meal is delayed, the insulin which peaks to cover that meal will cause a fall in blood sugar, leading to insulin reaction or hypoglycemia. Similarly, a skipped meal will usually produce marked hypoglycemia. Excess total calories at a feeding will obviously cause hyperglycemia, as will consumption of foods which lead to an abrupt rise in blood sugar. So, for diabetics, the timing as well as composition of meals is important.

Beyond these special dietary guidelines, diabetics are currently urged to follow a diet similar to that recommended for the general population. The American Diabetes Association (1979) suggests a diet which is 12 to 20 percent protein, 25 to 38 percent fat, and 50 to 55 percent carbohydrate the majority of which should be fruits, vegetables, and grains. Because the preponderance of diabetics are type 2 and generally overweight, the intake of fat should probably be closer to 30 percent or even less because of the high caloric value of fats. Also, because of the increased incidence of cardiovascular disease in diabetics, a reduction of dietary fat, particularly saturated fat, may be beneficial in some diabetics by reducing serum cholesterol.

Exercise

Diabetics can exercise at any time during the day, but as with eating, the timing of the various insulin peaks should be considered. Exercising in the mid-afternoon when intermediate insulin peaks will invite a hypoglycemic reaction. To prevent this, the exercise session could be switched to a different time of day, such as an hour of so after a major meal, or the quantity of intermediate insulin taken in the morning could be reduced, or extra food could be consumed in an afternoon snack preceding the exercise session. Surveys of active diabetics indicate that the great majority of ID diabetics supplement their snacks or meals to provide extra glucose for strenuous exercise (Costill et al., 1980; a Round Table, 1979). In the first several months after beginning an exercise program, most diabetics reduce their insulin intake by about 20 to 40 percent (A Round Table, 1979). Further reductions in insulin are usually unnecessary because endurance-trained muscles store and utilize more fat (Felig & Wahren, 1971; Hagenfeldt & Wahren, 1971), and the store of glycogen in the liver and muscle are substantially greater (Bergstrom, Hermansen, & Saltin, 1967). Consequently, although exercise can involve considerable energy expenditure and increases insulin sensitivity, training also enhances fat metabolism with the result that the need for insulin is unchanged after a certain amount of training. However, the effects of training provide a greater buffer against exercise leading to hypoglycemia. NID diabetics using oral medication also must reduce or even eliminate medication to avoid hypoglycemia as a result of training. While the dosage of insulin is typically within a range of .5 to 1.0 units per kg of bodyweight (Skyler et al., 1981), this guideline does not necessarily apply to highly active diabetics (Berg, 1983).

The best means of determining insulin intake or dosage of oral medication is by determining the effect of exercise on the blood sugar level. Most diabetics today are advised to assess their blood sugar daily, using a whole blood sample. This technique involves puncturing a finger tip or ear lobe to obtain a single drop of whole blood. The blood is placed on a chemically treated strip which reacts with the sugar in the blood. The blood sugar level can then be estimated by comparing the color of the strip indicator with colors on the container which represent varying ranges of blood sugar. A more precise measure can be determined by placing the strip indicator into a reflectance photometer which provides a digital reading. The degree which insulin and/or food need to be altered to accommodate for exercise can be determined by measuring the blood sugar before and after exercise. If the pre-exercise blood sugar is low, then a snack can be taken beforehand. If the blood sugar is moderately elevated, then a snack may not be needed. If ketones are elevated or the blood sugar is excessively high before exercise, the diabetic must not exercise because this will result in a further rise in ketone production, as well as blood sugar. If a diabetic consistently performs a specific physical activity most days, then the effect of this activity on the blood sugar level can be studied. Daily blood sugar testing before and after the activity will indicate the extent to which the blood sugar is decreased. This procedure is helpful when beginning an exercise program or participating in a new activity. Such testing allows exercise to be performed so that it can be done safely and enjoyably, and so that it contributes to overall better care for the diabetic.

With prolonged exercise such as backpacking and running a marathon, the diabetic is advised to consume some carbohydrate every 20 to 30 minutes or so to prevent hypoglycemia (A Round Table, 1979). One diabetic athlete has combined this procedure with periodic blood sugar measurement during activity to complete the rugged Iron Man Triathlon held in Hawaii. This event epitomizes endurance sport because it involves swimming two miles in the ocean, bicycling more than 100 miles, and running a 26.2 mile marathon. Unusual levels of physical activity, lasting beyond several hours, usually require a decrease of the morning insulin in order to avoid hypoglycemia. Periodic snacking, however, will still be needed. Etzwiler (1974) has recommended reducing the insulin dosage by 50 percent on days where activity is continuous such as hiking and canoeing. It is advised that some insulin should be taken even on days of unusually high physical activity because some insulin must be present in the blood to enhance glucose absorption into the muscle, liver, and adipose tissue (Berger et al., 1977).

Costill et al. (1980) compared the metabolism of ID diabetics who ran for 90 minutes with and without insulin. When exericse was performed 24 hours after the last insulin injection, perception of fatigue, using the Borg scale, was greater in the last 30 minutes of the run and the respiratory exchange ratio was markedly lower than when insulin had been administered several hours prior to exercise. The ketone level was elevated, but not significantly, when no insulin had been given. Ahlborg and Felig (1976) noted that the administration of 200g of glucose 50 minutes before 4 hours of exercise enhanced work capacity. The blood glucose level and carbohydrate utilization were increased, while lipolysis and hepatic gluconeogenesis were decreased. Sanders, Levinson, Abelmann, and Freinkel (1964) and Wahren, Felig, Hendler, and Ahlborg (1973) found that peripheral glucose utilization was similar in ID diabetics to that of normal control subjects when exercise was performed 24 hours after the last insulin injection, while gluconeogenesis was significantly greater in diabetics. Berger et al. (1977) observed that a 3 hour bicycle ride 18 hours after the last injection of insulin with Semilente insulin reduced initial glucose values of 150 to 200 mg% to the normal range.

On days of normal activity, surveys of active diabetics such as runners indicate that the majority make no alteration in insulin (Flood, 1979). This is probably true particularly if exercise is done daily. A fairly consistent expenditure of energy each day associated with exercise may facilitate regulation of blood sugar. The more consistent the diabetic's diet and exercise, the more amenable is the blood sugar to regulation. This consistency requires less adjustment of insulin and food, which tends to promote normoglycemia.

When departure from the normal day's routine occurs, such as when sick or traveling, direct blood sugar measurement is valuable. Skyler et al. (1981) recommend checking blood sugar levels several times daily under such conditions and at times when blood sugar control is lacking. Instruments to measure blood sugar are typically about $1 \times 4 \times 8$ inches in size or less, and weight less than a pound. Even with accessories such as alcohol pads, lancets, and strip indicators, the equipment and supplies can be easily transported to and from school or work and can even be used in the field because the units are battery operated.

Because the absorption of injected insulin into the blood is affected by the activity of the underlying muscle (Vranic and Berger, 1979), diabetics sometimes adjust the injection site. For example, in exercise requiring extensive use of the legs such as running, cycling and backpacking, injection into the thigh may result in a faster than normal peak effect of the insulin because absorption rate into the blood is accelerated. To counter this effect, the injection could be made in the abdomen, arm or shoulder. Similarly, for activities using the arms such as weight training and the crawl stroke in swimming, the abdomen would be a preferential injection site.

Capacity of Diabetics to Exercise

The ability of diabetics to participate safely and effectively in physical activity is limited primarily by the state of metabolic control and presence of pathologies including retinopathy, neuropathy, nephropathy and cardiovascular disease. Where reasonable metabolic control is lacking, diabetics will not experience the drop in blood sugar seen in well-controlled diabetics (Klachko, Lie, Cunningham, Chase, and Burns, 1972). If the blood insulin level is low enough, exercise causes the blood sugar to rise markedly and ketone production to be accentuated. The existence of organ disease to the eyes, nerves, kidneys and cardiovascular system limits the type, as well as intensity, of exercise in many diabetics. However, diabetics have run marathons, completed triathlons, and compete in intercollegiate and professional sports, so the notion that diabetics are too fragile to engage in vigorous physical activity is false.

Metabolic Differences Between Diabetics and Non-Diabetics

Exercise performance in poorly regulated diabetics is inhibited metabolically in three ways: (a) lack of insulin accelerates the degradation of protein and encourages muscle atrophy; (b) lack of insulin can produce hyperglycemia and ketosis; and (c) excessive insulin produces hypoglycemia because it limits the exogenous supply of glucose, FFA, and glycerol to muscle tissue and enhances glucose uptake and utilization. Consequently, it should be emphasized that in ID diabetics, exercise can only be performed effectively and safely if the metabolism is in a relatively normal state, that is, a functional level of insulin is in the blood and no ketones are present in the urine. Should exercise be done while ketotic, hepatic glucose production is accelerated and exceeds the rate of muscle glucose utilization, with the result that the blood sugar rises. Thus, exercise can be of value to diabetics only if they are willing to maintain good metabolic control and frequently measure the extent of control.

In a summary of the literature regarding diabetics and exercise, Vranic and Berger (1979) concluded that below a certain blood insulin level, liver glucose production and muscle utilization are equal, with the result that plasma glucose does not change with exercise. If insulin is absent or below this threshold level, then muscle glucose utilization is not stimulated while liver glucose production is. Consequently, blood sugar will rise during exercise. Even in well-controlled subjects, gluconeogenesis is more pronounced than in non-diabetics. This tendency limits the capacity for exercise to have a blood sugar-lowering effect. If exercise follows insulin injection, insulin will be absorbed more quickly. The resulting increase in circulating insulin inhibits or prevents glucose production by the liver but enhances peripheral glucose utilization. The combined effect decreases the blood sugar level. For these reasons diabetics who participate in long duration endurance activities are advised to use a long-lasting insulin and dramatically reduce the dosage of short-acting insulin. The long-lasting insulin provides a basis for promoting glucose utilization and the reduction in fast-acting insulin minimizes the inhibition of lipolysis and gluconeogenesis. This insulin regimen maximizes the utilization of both fat and carbohydrate as muscle substrates.

The importance of the diabetic exercising while in reasonable metabolic control is further substantiated from studies which show that after hours of cycling, the levels of blood FFA, ketone bodies, amino acids, growth hormone, glucagon, cortisol, and thyroid hormones of diabetics in moderate control are nearly the same as in non-diabetics (Berchtold, Berger, Cuppers, Herrmann, Nieschlag, Rudorff, Zimmerman, & Krushemper, 1978; Berger et al., 1977). However, diabetics in several studies have been found to have higher lactate levels during exercise. The difference has been observed even when the work is performed at the same relative intensity (Berger et al., 1977; Murray, Zimmerman, McClean, Denoga, Albisser, Leibel, Nakhooda, Stokes, & Marliss, 1977). However, other investigators have not observed this difference (Maehlum, Jervell, & Pruett, 1976; Wahren et al., 1973; Costill et al., 1980). It is difficult to determine, therefore, if the accumulation of more lactate during exercise accurately typifies the diabetic. The different findings regarding lactate levels in diabetics may be due to a lesser state of fitness in diabetics in some studies and to the blood sugar levels in the weeks preceding data collection. The release of oxygen to the tissues is known to decrease as glucose combines with erythrocyte hemoglobin to form hemoglobin A_{lc} (Ditzel, 1976). This may result in a greater reliance on anaerobic metabolism. This alteration of hemoglobin occurs readily when blood sugar is elevated.

In 40 minutes of exercise in diabetics, there occurs a net exchange of branched chain amino acids including valine, leucine, and isoleucine from the liver to the working muscles. These amino acids provide an additional fuel for muscles during exercise and likely reflect the limited glycogen storage in many diabetics. Also, alanine from muscle tissue serves as a precursor for liver gluconeogenesis. This increased exchange of amino acids does not occur in non-diabetics until two to four hours of exercise (Felig and Wahren, 1971).

Oxygen Transport

Ditzel (1976) found that the oxygen transport capacity of red blood cells in diabetics is defective. This defect is caused by the disruptive effect of glucose which binds to hemoglobin in red blood cells to form Hb A_{lc}. ID diabetics were found to have two to three times as much Hb A_{lc} as non-diabetics. The affinity of hemoglobin A_{lc} for oxygen is reduced because a hexose component of Hb A_{lc} impairs the binding of Hb and 2,3-diphosphoglycerate (2,3-DPG). Also, plasma inorganic phosphate level (Pi) was reduced in diabetics which limits the production of 2,3-DPG. In ketotic diabetics, inorganic phosphate and 2,3-DPG remained low for one week. These findings suggest that maintenance of good blood sugar control should enhance red blood cell 2,3-DPG and inorganic phosphate levels, which in turn should enhance the transport of oxygen into the tissues.

Hemodynamics

Gundersen (1974) observed that blood pressure, pulse rate, and body temperature were increased when ID diabetics were taken off insulin or when metabolic control was lacking. Blood flow to muscle, skin, and adipose tissues also increased. These changes normalized when insulin administration was resumed and the subjects regained metabolic control. Ditzel (1976) speculated that these blood flow changes may be a compensatory mechanism for the reduced oxygen release capacity in the erythrocytes of many diabetics.

The concentration of plasma norepinephrine is consistently elevated in ketotic diabetics (Christensen, 1972). This elevation increases lipolysis and blood flow. Gundersen (1974) stated that the extent of increased blood flow indicates a low total peripheral resistance in poorly controlled diabetics. To maintain blood pressure, heart rate must be raised. Because blood pressure was mildly high in these subjects, it was suggested that other factors such as increased sympathetic stimulation are involved.

Conflicting data exist in comparing the $\dot{V}O_2$ max of diabetics and non-diabetics. In studies reporting lower $\dot{V}O_2$ max in diabetics, the causes have been attributed to microangiopathy, decreased 2,3-DPG levels in red blood cells, increased blood viscosity, autonomic neuropathy, and lower levels of physical activity (Ditzel, 1976; McMillan, 1979). However, in several studies no differences in $\dot{V}O_2$ max have been found (Costill et al., 1979; Hagen et al., 1979). Larsson et al. (1964) found that adolescent ID diabetics had a lower $\dot{V}O_2$ max than normal control subjects. However, the response to training, that is, the gain in $\dot{V}O_2$ max, was typical of non-diabetics. Costill et al. (1979) reported the same results, while Eckel, McLean, Albers, Cheung, and Biermann (1981) found this to be true for diabetics who had no microvascular disease.

Neuropathy

Altered function of the autonomic nervous system changes the hemodynamic and metabolic adjustment to exercise. Autonomic neuropathy impairs the cardiovascular responses to graded exercise (Hilsted et al.,1979). When compared to diabetics with no evidence of autonomic neuropathy, diabetics with this condition had a higher resting heart rate, a lower maximum heart rate (157 vs. 181), performed less maximum work (125 vs. 161w), and had a lower $\dot{V}O_2$ max (25 vs. 38 ml · kg^{-1} · min^{-1}). The cardiovascular responses to graded exercise testing clearly suggested sympathetic as well as parasympathetic involvement. Others have suggested that nerve lesions could also involve muscle receptors, muscle afferents and the central nervous system.

Loss of tendon reflexes, reduced nerve conduction velocity, and loss of muscle mass are associated with lesions of the somatic nervous system (Ewing et al., 1976). These effects reduce overall neuromusclar function.

Summary

There are two types of diabetes mellitus: insulin-dependent or type 1 and non-insulin dependent or type 2.

Diabetics suffer a high incidence of cardiovascular disease, blindness, kidney disease, and nerve damage. However, long-term maintenance of controlled blood glucose and ketone levels may reverse each of these to some degree.

Diabetics who are metabolically well-controlled appear to experience the same training changes in a similar magnitude as non-diabetics. Of special value to diabetics who exercise appropriately are a reduced tendency for hypoglycemia or ketosis to occur during exercise, reduced requirement for insulin, and a reduced amount or elimination of medication used to regulate blood sugar.

The management of both types of diabetes is aimed at maintaining blood sugar levels reasonably close to the normal range. This requires manipulation of insulin, diet, and physical activity.

Diabetics typically snack before exercise to minimize the occurrence of hypoglycemia. If the activity is prolonged much beyond that usually undertaken, it is recommended that some form of rapidly digestible carbohydrate be taken every

20 to 30 minutes. In addition, the morning insulin dosage is usually reduced about 50 percent.

When beginning an exercise program, insulin dosage or oral medication to assist in blood sugar control is usually reduced about 20 to 40%. Further reductions in dosage are not typically needed due to enhanced lipolysis and increased insulin sensitivity associated with training.

The ability of diabetics to participate safely and effectively in physical activity is limited primarily by the state of metabolic control and the existence of medical problems associated with diabetes such as cardiovascular disease, retinopathy, kidney damage, and nerve damage.

Diabetics should not exercise if ketones are present in the urine or if the blood sugar level is unduly high. At these times exercise will increase ketone production as well as raise the blood sugar.

Excess insulin produces hypoglycemia because it limits the exogenous supply of glucose, FFA, and glycerol to muscle tissues while it enhances glucose uptake and utilization.

Chronic lack of insulin accelerates protein degradation and encourages muscle atrophy.

Maintenance of a well-controlled metabolic state in diabetics (i.e., adequate insulin, non-ketotic state, and blood sugar levels reasonably close to normal) normalizes the acute metabolic and cardiovascular responses to exercise. However, some data indicate that diabetics accumulate more lactic acid during submaximal work than non-diabetics. Other studies refute this.

In 40 minutes of exercise, the working muscle mass of diabetics receives a supply of amino acids from the liver which is used as a source of fuel. The muscle contributes a supply of the amino acid alanine to the liver which is used in the production of glucose. In non-diabetics, a transfer of amino acids between the liver and skeletal muscle to this extent does not occur until after several hours of activity.

Some of the hemoglobin in the red blood cells of diabetics is defective due to chronic blood sugar elevation. The result is a reduced oxygen transport into the tissues.

In poorly controlled diabetics, blood flow to the muscle and skin is increased in an apparent attempt to compensate for the reduced oxygen transport capacity associated with the alteration of hemoglobin.

While some studies have reported lower $\dot{V}O_2$ max values in diabetics, other investigators have found no difference in highly active diabetics who are well-controlled. If microangiopathy does not exist, their response to training appears to be typical of non-diabetics.

Neuropathy can alter the hemodynamic and metabolic responses to exercise. Such diabetics have a higher resting heart rate, lower maximum heart rate, and a lower $\dot{V}O_2$ max.

References

A Round Table. (1979). Diabetes and exercise. *The Physician and Sportsmedicine, 7,* 49-64.

Ahlborg, G., & Felig, P. (1976). Influence of glucose ingestion on fuel-hormone response during prolonged exercise. *Journal of Applied Physiology, 41,* 683-88.

American Diabetic Association. (1979). Principles of nutrition and dietary recommendations for individuals with diabetes mellitus. *Diabetes, 28,* 1027-1030.

Appenzeller, O., Standefer, J., Appenzeller, J., & Atkinson, R. (1980). Neurology of Endurance Training: B-Endorphins. (Abstract). *Neurology, 30,* 418-419.

Berchtold, P., Berger, M., Cuppers, H.J., Herrmann, J., Nieschlag, E., Rudorff, K., Zimmermann, H., & Kruskemper, H.L. (1978). Non-glucoregulatory hormones (T_3, T_4, rT_3, TSH and testosterone) during physical exercise in juvenile type diabetics. *Hormone and Metabolic Research, 10,* 269-73.

Becker-Zimmermann, K., Berger, M., Berchtold, P., Gries, F.A., Herberg, L., & Schwenen, M. (1982). Treadmill training improves intravenous glucose tolerance and insulin sensitivity in fatty Zucker rats. *Diabetologia, 22,* 468-474.

Berg, K. (1938). Blood glucose regulation in an insulin-dependent diabetic backpacker. *The Physician and Sportsmedicine, 11,* 101-104.

Berger, M. (1983). Metabolic diseases and exercise performance. In H.G. Knuttgen, J.A. Vogel, & J. Poortman, (Eds.), *Biochemistry of exercise: International series on sports sciences,* (Vol. 13), (pp. 97-110). Champaign, IL: Human Kinetics.

Berger, M., Berchtold, P., Cuppers, H.J., Drost, H., Kley, H.K., Muller, W.A., Wiegelmann, W., Zimmermann-Telschow, H., Gries, F.A., Kruskemper, H.L. & Zimmermann, H. (1977). Metabolic and hormonal effects of muscular exercise in juvenile type diabetics. *Diabetologica, 13,* 355-365.

Berger, M., Kemper, F.W., Becker, K. (1979). Effect of physical training on glucose tolerance and glucose metabolism of skeletal muscle in anesthetized normal rats. *Diabetologica, 16,* 179-181.

Bergstrom, J., Hermansen, L. & Saltin, B. (1967). Diet, muscle glycogen and physical performance. *Acta Physiologica Scandinavica, 71,* 140-150.

Bjorntorp, P., De Jounge, K., Stostrom, L., & Sullivan, L. (1970). The effect of physical training on insulin production in obesity. *Metabolism, 19,* 631-638.

Callen, K.E. (1983). Mental and emotional aspects of long-distance running. *Psychosomatics, 24,* 133-151.

Cantu, R. (1982). *Diabetes and Exercise.* New York: E.P. Dutton, Inc.

Catlin, D.H., Gorelick, D.A., Gerner, R.H., Hui, K.K., & Li, C.H. (1980). Clinical effects of B-endorphin infusions. In E. Costa, & M. Trabucchi, (Eds.), *Neural peptides and neuronal communication* (pp. 465-472). New York: Raven.

Christensen, N.J. (1972). Diabetic angiopathy and neuropathy. *Acta Medica Scandinavica,* Suppl. 541, pp. 1-60.

Costill, D.L., Cleary, P., Fink, W.J., Voster, C., Ivy, J.L., & Witzmann, F. (1979). Training adaptations in skeletal muscle of juvenile diabetics. *Diabetes, 28,* 812-822.

Costill, D., Miller, J.M., & Fink, W.J. (1980). Energy metabolism in diabetic distance runners. *The Physician and Sportsmedicine, 8,* 64-71.

Crofford, O. (1975). *Report of the National Commission on Diabetes.* (DHEW Publication no. NIH 76-1018). Washington, DC: U.S. Government Printing Office.

Ditzel, J. (1976). Oxygen transport impairment in diabetes. *Diabetes, 25* (suppl. 2), 832-838.

Eckel, R.H., McLean, E., Albers, J.J., Cleung, M.C. & Biermann, E. L. (1981). Plama lipids and micro-angiopathy in insulin-dependent diabetes mellitus. *Diabetes Care, 4,* 447-453.

Etzwiler, D.D. (1974). When the diabetic wants to be an athlete. *The Physician and Sportsmedicine, 2,* 45-50.

Ewing, D. J., Burt, A.A., Williams, I.R., Campbell, I.W., & Clarke, B.F. (1976). Peripheral motor nerve function in diabetic autonomic neuropathy. *Journal of Neurological Neurosurgery and Psychiatry, 39,* 453-60.

Felig, P. & Wahren, J. (1971). Amino acid metabolism in exercising man. *Journal of Clinical Investigation, 40,* 2703-2714.

Flood, T. (1979, March-April). Who's running? *Forecast, 22.*

Fraioli, F., Moretti, C., Paolucci, D., Alicicco, E., Crescenzi, F., & Fortunato, G. (1980). Physical exercise stimulates marked concomitant release of beta-endorphin and adrenocorticotropic hormone (ACTH) in peripheral blood in man. *Experientia, 36,* 987-989.

Gambert, S.R., Garthwaite, T.L., Hagen, T.C., Tristani, F.E., & McCarty, D.J. (1981). Exercise increases plasma beta-endorphin (EP) in untrained human subjects. (Abstract) *Clinical Research, 29,* 429A.

Gundersen, H.G.H. (1974). Peripheral blood flow and metabolic control in juvenile diabetes. *Diabetologica, 10,* 225-231.

Hagen, R.D., Marks, J.F., & Warren, P.A. (1979). Physiological responses of juvenile onset diabetic boys to muscular work. *Diabetes, 28,* 1114-1119.

Hagenfeldt, L. & Wahren, J. (1971). Metabolism of free fatty acids and ketone bodies in skeletal muscle. In B. Pernow & B. Saltin (Eds), *Muscle metabolism during exercise* (pp. 153-164). New York: Plenum Press.

Hilsted, J. & Christensen, N.J. (1979). Impaired cardiovascular responses to graded exercise in diabetes autonomic retinopathy. *Diabetes, 28,* 313-319.

Klachko, D.M., Lie, T.H., Cunningham, E.J., Chase, G.R., & Burns, I.W. (1972). Blood glucose levels during walking in normal and diabetic subjects. *Diabetes, 21,* 80-100.

Kostrubala, T. (1976). *The joy of running.* Philadelphia and New York: J.B. Lippincott.

Larsson, Y., Persson, B., Sterky, G., & Thoren, C. (1964). Functional adaptation to vigorous training and exercise in diabetic and nondiabetic adolescents. *Journal of Applied Physiology, 19,* 629-635.

Maehlum, S., Jervell, J., & Pruett, E.D. (1976). Arterial-hepatic vein glucose differences in normal and diabetic man after a glucose infusion at rest and after exercise. *Scandinavian Journal of Clinical Laboratory Investigations, 36,* 415-22.

McMillan, D.E. (1979). Exercise and diabetic microangiopathy. *Diabetes, 28* (suppl. 1), 103-106.

Miller, W.J., Sherman, W.M., & Ivy, J.L. (1984). Effect of strength training on glucose tolerance and post-exercise insulin response. *Medicine and Science in Sports and Exercise, 16,* 539-543.

Moore, M. (1982). Endorphins and exercise: a puzzling relationship. *The Physician and Sportsmedicine, 68,* 11-114.

Morgan, W.P., Roberts, J.A., Brand, F.R., & Feinerman, A.D. (1970). Psychological effect of chronic physical activity. *Medicine and Science in Sports, 2,* 213-217.

Morgan, W.P. (1979). Anxiety reduction following acute physical activity. *Psychiatric Annuals, 14,* 141-147.

Murray, F.T., Zinman, B., McClean, P.A., Denoga, A., Albisser, A.M., Leibel, B.S. Nakhooda, A.F., Stokes, E.F., & Marliss, E.B. (1977). The metabolic response to moderate exercise in diabetic man receiving intravenous and subcutaneous insulin. *Journal Clinical Endrocrinology and Metabolism, 44,* 708-720.

Nakao, K., Nakai, S., Oki, S., Matsubara, S., Konishi, T., Nishitani, H., & Imura, H. (1980). Immunoreactive beta-endorphin in human cerebrospinal fluid. *Journal of Endocrinology and Metabolism, 50,* 230-233.

Rapoport, S.I., Klee, W.A., Pettigrew, K.W., & Ohno, K. (1980). Entry of opiate peptides into the central nervous system. *Science, 207,* 84-86.

Ruderman, N.B., Ganda, O., & Johansen, K. (1979). The effect of physical training on glucose and plasma lipids in maturity-onset diabetes. *Diabetes, 28* (Suppl. 1), 89-92.

Sanders, C.A., Levinson, G.E., Abelmann, W.H., & Freinkel, N. (1964). Effect of exercise on the peripheral utilization of glucose in man. *New England Journal of Medicine, 271,* 220-25.

Skyler, J., Skyler, D. & O'Sullivan, M. (1981). Algorithms for adjustment of insulin dosage by patients who monitor blood glucose. *Diabetes Care, 4,* 311-318.

Sonstroem, R.J. (1982). Exercise and self-esteem: Recommendations for expository research. *Quest, 33,* 124-139.

Vranic, M. & Berger, M. (1979). Exercise and diabetes mellitus. *Diabetes, 28,* 147-163.

Wahren, J., Felig, P., Hendler, R., & Ahlborg, G. (1973). Glucose and amino acid metabolism during recovery after exercise. *Journal of Applied Physiology, 34,* 838-45.

Section V

ORGANIZED DELIVERY SYSTEMS FOR PHYSICAL ACTIVITY

- The Relation of Movement and Cognitive Function

- Effects of Physical Education Programs on Children

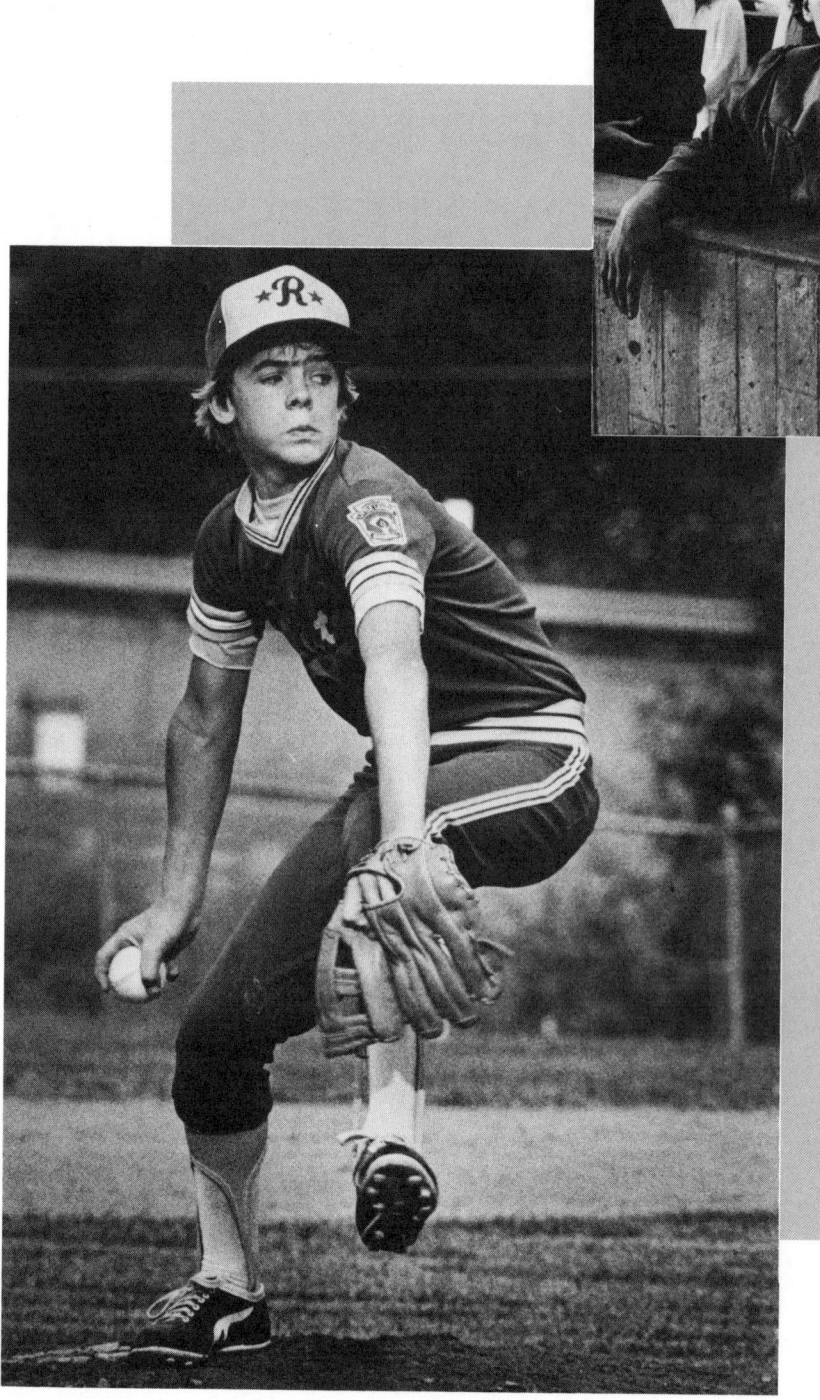

photos by Jim Kirby

CHAPTER SEVENTEEN

The Relation of Movement and Cognitive Function

Jerry R. Thomas
School of Health, Physical Education,
Recreation, and Dance
Louisiana State University
Baton Rouge, Louisiana

Katherine T. Thomas
Department of Physical Education
Southeastern Louisiana University
Hammond, Louisiana

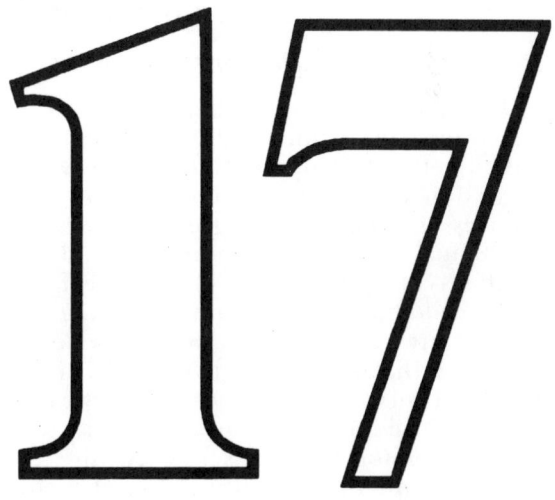

In evaluating the relation between movement and cognitive function, the term perceptual-motor development has frequently been used. This term has been used inconsistently in the physical education, special education, and psychological literature. In psychology, perceptual-motor development is used to refer to motor coordination skills that have a substantial cognitive component. For example, the skills required of pilots are frequently called perceptual-motor. These skills require coordination of hands and vision (and sometimes feet) when flying planes. This topic received a lot of attention from research psychologists during World War II because they were trying to aid in the training and performance of combat pilots. In special education, perceptual-motor development has generally referred to attempts to influence cognitive and intellectual performance through motor and perceptual skill training. Examples include Kephart's (1960) Purdue Perceptual Motor Training Program, Frostig and Horne's (1964) program and test of visual motor perception, and Delacato's (1959) Neurological Organization. These programs are based on earlier concerns about teaching children who had difficulty meeting age-related expectations in academic achievement (e.g., Montessori, 1966/1909). Physical education has adopted both uses, creating considerable confusion, and added its own—the use of perceptual-motor development as an interchangeable term for motor development.

The first part of this chapter focuses on perceptual-motor development as it is used consistently in special education and inconsistently in physical education—attempts to influence cognitive and intellectual function through movement. The discussion will cover several areas and age levels. Pertaining to preschool and elementary age children, the chapter will evalute the relations among motor, perceptual, cognitive, and intellectual functioning. In addition, approaches which attempt to influence cognitive and intellectual functioning through perceptual-motor training programs will be examined. The remainder of the chapter is devoted to the relation between movement (in particular, sports participation) and academic performance. Because there have been many studies and reviews of these topics previously, this discussion will focus on the general findings with references to the various reviews and a few representative studies.

Perceptual-Motor Development

Relation Between Perceptual-Motor and Cognitive Function

The fact that certain types of motor tasks at specific ages are related to cognitive functioning (academic readiness and performance, intelligence tests) has been the basis for the development of theories about how cognitive function can be improved by motor activity. There is little doubt that some types of motor performances are related to cognitive function. For example, a motor task with a substantial cognitive component would be expected to be related to academic readiness or performance, particularly for young or mentally impaired children. If the child has trouble counting, asking her/him to hop three times on the right foot and twice on the left foot will reflect the child's difficulties with numbers. However, that does not mean the child cannot hop. Of course, it is possible that the child will fail the test item because of the inability to hop, but it is just as likely that the child will fail because of an inability to count.

Other motor test items that require cognitive functions such as matching shapes, identifying differences, serial performance of movements, and decisions are also likely to relate to cognitive measures of performance in young or mentally impaired children. Asking a kindergarten child to perform the motor task of completing a shape puzzle as quickly as possible will be related to the child's academic readiness, because recognizing and discriminating among shapes is important for successful use of letters and numbers. Any motor task where mental rehearsal of a series of movements is helpful will be related to cognitive tasks for which rehearsal is useful. The cognitive skill of rehearsal involves the same memory and information processing functions, regardless of whether it is used with academic or motor skills (Thomas, 1980).

The relation between motor items, such as those just described, and early cognitive function decreases as children move through the elementary grades; most children master the simple cognitive skills required by the motor tasks. This relation between motor and cognitive functions is easily attenuated by increasing the complexity of the cognitive component of the movement (e.g., alternate hopping and jumping while counting backwards from 100 by threes), but what is the point of this experience? The cognitive requirement really has little to do with the nature of the movement. As a general principle, *movement and cognitive function are only related to the degree that the movement involves substantial cognition, or that success in the movement task underlies successful cognitive performance.* Of course, this principle only applies as long as children have not mastered the cognitive component of a movement task. Numerous reviews of the hundreds of studies that have evaluated the relation between perceptual-motor and cognitive performance are available (e.g., Kirkendall, 1985; Mann & Goodman, 1976; Seefeldt, 1974; Thomas, 1977), and generally reach the same conclusions summarized here.

Perceptual-Motor Training and Cognitive Function

The hypothesis that improving perceptual-motor function will improve cognitive function comes from the observation that the two areas are positively correlated. One must remember, however, that because two areas are related does not mean one causes the other; in fact, the relation between perceptual-motor and cognitive functions is a perfect example of that rule. An understanding of the reason for the correlation between perceptual-motor and cognitive function (explained in the previous section) also explains why improving movement skills has had no effect on cognitive performance. Yet, studies of these relations have persisted (nearly all of which show no significant effect) for over 25 years. These programs fall into three general types:

1. Programs which, by training some motor parameter, attempt to improve a specific curriculum area (for example, by practicing balance the child will read more proficiently).

2. Programs which, by practicing an underlying motor skill(s) related to some specific academic area, attempt to influence the academic area (for example, practicing fine eye-hand coordination in an attempt to improve handwriting).

3. Programs which use motor tasks to teach academic content (for example, throwing a ball into a numbered barrel which represents the correct answer for an addition problem).

All three types of programs have been justified and/or criticized in three ways: research done specifically to prove that the programs do or do not work, theoretical position papers for and against perceptual-motor programs, and reviews/ meta-analyses which synthesize the literature on perceptual-motor programs.

Intuitively, perceptual-motor interventions could be criticized due to weaknesses in the theories from which they evolve. Mann and Goodman (1976) summarize these weaknesses, beginning with the development of programs using diagnostic tests which identify that problems exist but which do not identify what the problem is. They suggest that low scores on the tests may be due to lack of motivation, short attention span, or poor perception. Perceptual-motor programs that reduce mature children to immature levels of activity under the guise of remediation may simply reinforce immature behavior. Perceptual training is too narrow in scope and oversimplifies the objective of the remediation. Reading is typically a target of the programs, yet reading is more than the sum of vision and perception—which are the activities of the programs. Finally, Mann and Goodman suggest that perceptual training is irrelevant, because everything we do is based on perception. If we train reading by training perception, we can train perception by training reading.

The numerous reviews and critiques of the experimental research on perceptual-motor programs (Hallahan & Cruickshank, 1973; Kirkendall, 1985; Meyers & Hammill, 1982; Rarick, 1980; Seefeldt, 1974; Thomas, 1977) all reach the same basic conclusions. However, one of the most comprehensive, thorough, and quantitative studies is a recent meta-analysis of perceptual-motor training studies by Kavale and Mattson (1983). This meta-analysis was based on 180 perceptual-motor training studies (the single criteria for elimination of a study from their analysis was the lack of a control group) which included 13,000 subjects. A summary of their findings indicated that perceptual-motor training has little benefit. If the programs are considered by the various categories, they may be summarized as, *training is ineffective for:*

1. Any outcome class—perceptual/sensory motor, academic achievement, cognitive aptitude, adaptive behavior.

2. Any specific type of program—Barsch, Cratty, Delacato, Frostig, Getman, Kephart, combination, or other.

3. Any specific subject group—normal, educable mentally retarded, trainable mentally retarded, slow learner, culturally disadvantaged, learning disabled, reading disabled, or motor disabled.

4. Any grade level—preschool, kindergarten, primary grades, middle grades, junior high school, or high school.

5. Any level of internal validity of the study (low, average, or high)—in fact, studies with the highest internal validity actually showed a negative effect for perceptual-motor training.

A substantial amount of space could be devoted to summarizing these studies, placing them into categories based on their theoretical underpinning, and citing the studies and their specific weaknesses. But since that has all been done before (Glass & Robbins, 1967; Hallaham & Cruickshank, 1973; Kavale & Mattson, 1983; Meyers & Hammill, 1982; Mann & Goodman, 1976), it does not seem necessary to repeat the process. Children's performances have been enhanced by perceptual-motor training, but the performance of those trained was no better than the control group who did not receive the training. In most studies the control group was likely to have continued in their regular activities. The point is, if the children are deficient in certain cognitive skills, the best solution to the deficiency is to work on the specific cognitive skills. Research on human movement has repeatedly confirmed that even very similar motor skills are task specific and require task specific practice for improvement (for a summary, see Schmidt, 1982, pp. 400-402). Thus, it seems even more unlikely that transfer from movement to cognitive performance would be expected, and the research uniformly supports this statement.

Children have very uneven rates of cognitive and motor development during the preschool, kindergarten, and primary grades. Thus, a child may lag behind in one area and a few months later perform at a normal or even above average level. This fact was reflected in a study by Thomas and Chissom (1974) where kindergarten children falling in the bottom quartile on academic and perceptual-motor development were spread over all four quartiles a year later in the first grade.

The authors are not suggesting that cognition is not involved in the performance of movement and sport skills; quite the contrary (see Thomas & Gallagher, Chapter 4, this volume). In particular, information processing skills are important for learning, controlling, and performing movements, as is the base of knowledge required to perform specific sports. However, attempts to improve or remediate cognitive function through the use of movement are not theoretically sound, nor does this approach have any empirical support in the research literature.

Why did Physical Education Jump on the Perceptual-Motor Bandwagon?

A few paragraphs will be devoted to a pseudo-psychological analysis of why physical educators have shown such persistent interest in and motivation for the area known as perceptual-motor development. Because physical education is not conducted in the classroom and is a "special" subject like art and music, many professional physical educators seem to have experienced some difficulty in accepting the value of their roles as educators. Math, science, language, reading, and social studies are important because they represent the "main" subjects of academic concern in the public schools. The advent of perceptual-motor programs provided physical education with an opportunity to make a contribution to the "mainstream" of education—children's academic achievement. Physical educators jumped on the bandwagon when the research evidence about the value of perceptual-motor programs was at best neutral and well before any reasonable decision about the value of these programs could be verified.

In some instances partially, and in some completely, programs that had a proven ability to contribute to the motor skill and physical fitness development of children were abandoned in favor of hopping on the numbers and letters, tracing shapes, and playing relays with numbers and letters. Further, physical educators lost sight of their real purpose, helping children develop quality movements; as long as the child correctly identified the number, letter, or shape the program was successful.

Of paramount concern is whether the profession of physical education has learned anything from this experience. Can physical educators accept that their role in the educational process is to develop movement and sport skills and enhance physical fitness? Have we learned that this function is valued by society if we do it well, and will assure physical education an important place in the educational system? Or will we fall for the next attractive way to enhance our "academic" image that comes along? Causing children to sweat and breathe hard and enhancing their movement skills so that they can enjoy participating and developing fitness is important. Physical educators have demonstrated that they are able to change the movement skills and physical fitness of children and adults (see the other chapters of this book). Helping children and adults move effectively and efficiently is an educational challenge, commensurate in importance to any in the public school curriculum.

Sport and Academic Achievement

There are two questions one might try to answer about the contribution that interscholastic sport makes toward academic achievement. First, is the influence of sport positive or negative? Second, if sport is beneficial, why is sport not required for all students by academic institutions? The response to the first question is often a result of personal bias, either the "dumb jock" syndrome, or the notion that athletics is so important that the athlete is *given* excellent grades (as opposed to earning them). Several factors must be controlled when addressing this question through research. Among these are:

1. Athletes must maintain a minimum grade point average, so comparisons to general populations of students (with no minimum G.P.A.) inflates the athletes' performance.
2. Athletes may be viewed differently by teachers ("dumb jock," or held in esteem) simply because they are athletes—again confounding the comparison to the general student population.
3. Athletes as a group may differ on factors other than just athletic participation—for example, athletes may be high achievers.
4. The findings on athletes do not typically apply to women athletes.

Each of these factors increase the risk of generalizing from the results of research, and further, makes the attribution of outcomes to athletics tenuous. Because the findings may be confounded by other factors, and since the two groups may differ on more than just athletic participation, many research studies have provided us with little conclusive evidence. Because the findings on women are very different from those on men involved in athletics—in general, women athletes are better students, who succeed in education—the influence of athletics on academic performance is also at question. The gender differences may be a result of research on women athletes, the relatively recent involvement of women in big-time sport (as a result of Title IX), or in fact, a difference attributable to gender.

Athletes as Students

Numerous studies (Eidsmoe, 1963; Schafer, 1968; Schafer & Armer, 1968; Spreitzer & Pugh, 1973) have reported that athletes have higher grade point averages (GPA) than non-athletes of equal intelligence. The problem with most of these studies is that the athletes had to maintain a minimum GPA in order to be athletes, so even if intelligence was equal between athletes and non-athletes, factors other than athletic participation could account for the GPA differences. High school athletes also enrolled in college-prep curricula more often than non-athletes. Athletes were found (Lueptow & Kayser, 1973-4; Otto, 1975; Rehberg & Schafer, 1968; Spreitzer & Pugh, 1973) to have higher educational expectations than non-athletes even when controlled for GPA, IQ, socio-economic status, and/or parental encouragement.

In a more recent study involving students (men and women) from two states, Landers et al. (1978) reported that male athletes who participated in a service-related extracurricular activity in addition to athletics were more successful on the Scholastic Aptitude Test (SAT) than athletes who had no other extracurricular activity. The male athlete-only groups were below the national average for the SAT, while the athlete-service groups were above the national average. The females were not different, based on the athlete-only or athlete-service criteria. An interesting point is that 17 to 36% of the students did not take any college entry examination, indicating a lack of interest in attending college.

Several years earlier Spady (1970) indicated that athletes may have a higher level of aspiration for education than their preparation warrants. His main criticism was that athletics encourages athletes to enter college, but athletics does not provide the necessary skills for academic success in college. Spady used the years of college completed to determine success, and did not take into account athletes dropping out for non-academic reasons. Athletes may have dropped out because they did not make the team, or because of injury, and not because they were not academically able.

These studies indicate that athletes may not be brighter than other students; however, their aspirations and expectations may exceed those of the general student population. In instances where athletes excel (when compared to non-athletes), the cause can not be attributed directly to athletics; the cause may in fact be some underlying characteristic which motivates these individuals to achieve in many areas. Athletics, then, does not cause these individuals to be better students; rather, some characteristic which influences athletic participation also influences academic performance. Perhaps athletes aspire to continue their athletic career (in college), and are forced to continue their academic education in order to have the opportunity to pursue their main interest in sport. There is considerable indirect evidence regarding this possibility as a motivation for minority athletes to continue attending school (Perkins, 1983, 1985).

If athletics had been conclusively shown to positively influence academic performance, school administrators would have insisted that athletics be a mandatory part of high school and college. Coaches and other proponents of athletics should be satisfied with the knowledge that athletics does not interfere with academic performance, nor with the curricular requirements and activities of most high schools. This will allow them to get on to the business of athletics, and to the unique contributions which athletics can make during development. Coaches, like physical educators, should emphasize the values of sport for sport's sake—not because of what sport can allegedly do for academics.

College Athletics—To Play or Learn?

While some may argue that intercollegiate athletics and quality education are mutually exclusive terms, the research indicates that athletics does not necessarily interfere with education. Purdy et al. (1982) found that athletes were slightly lower on measures of academic achievement than non-athletes, and male athletes' educational achievement was slightly less than females.

There are numerous dissertations which examine the academic performance and graduation rates of various universities, but these often have flaws in design and are rarely published in good refereed journals. Reports from sources using data from more than one university are conflicting, and often have weaknesses. Considerable research, resulting from the controversy surrounding NCAA Proposition 48[1], reports varying levels of academic success for athletes. Desruisseaux (1982) suggests that collegiate athletes are being exploited, rather than educated. He suggests that the universities benefit from the athletes' performance, but that the athletes are forced to sacrifice their education in the process. "Big time" athletics may be more guilty than the less intense programs, as exemplified by the graduation rates of basketball players for the various conferences as reported in the Chronicle of Higher Education (1982). The Ivy League, Big East and Southern conferences report relatively high graduation rates (100, 77 and 63 percent respectively), while conferences (SEC, Big Ten, Atlantic Coast, Pacific Ten) noted for "big time" athletics report lower rates, none above 50 percent (with the lowest ranked institution having one in three athletes graduating). Another study of graduation rates for all athletes indicated that athletes actually had a higher rate of graduation than non-athletes (Crowl, 1983). Approximately 55% of all students get their degrees on time, compared to 57% for athletes. A higher percent who required 5 years to graduate was also reported for athletes. The data reported in this NCAA-sponsored study were criticized (Monaghan, 1985) because the survey response rate was low, and because the analysis of the data was not appropriate. The American Association of Collegiate Registrars and Admissions Officers with the American Council on Education (Farrell, 1984) completed a study of 57 institutions and over 2,000 athletes which was less subject to bias. The results were similar to the NCAA study; athletes and non-athletes had similar freshmen grade point averages (2.5 of 4.0), with the athletes slightly higher. The results were attributed to three documented factors: tutors for athletes, increased motivation resulting from scholarship support, and attending summer school. A final factor was suggested, but not documented. The athletes may have enrolled in easier courses, and were not making progress toward degrees.

The general conclusion must be that athletes are not less competent academically than non-athletes, nor does being a good athlete exclude a student from academic success. However, situations exist where the education of athletes is deemed less important than his/her athletic career. This is evidenced by athletes

---

[1] A proposal which would raise academic standards for freshman athletes, including minimum GPA in high school core courses, and minimum scores on SAT or ACT.

being automatically enrolled in "jock majors," given grades which are not deserved based on performance, and situations where coaches, athletes and advisors break academic rules to keep athletes eligible.

University Presidents (through the American Council on Education and the NCAA President's Committee) have developed stricter eligibility rules for athletes, are encouraging the NCAA to enforce rules, and have shown a continuing interest in the academic life of athletes. The critical issues must be that these are student athletes, not just athletes. There is and will be life after intercollegiate athletics for these young people. The athlete, coach, and university must accept the responsibility for ensuring the right of each athlete to an education.

Minority Athletes and Academics

Eitzen (1975) stated that athletics held more prestige than scholarship—typically we pursue what is prestigous and spend little effort on that which is not. Eitzen further suggested that this problem is magnified in the non-white, lower socio-economic population.

There has been a growing concern for the disproportionate number of black athletes and black scholars. Harry Edwards (1979), a prominent black sociologist, expresses the frustration of many because of the overwhelming influence of sport on black youth. The problem is not with sport, but the fact that black youth tend to ignore all other aspects of development to concentrate on sport. The implication is clear—these youth invest their futures in sport, not in their educations. The high visibility of professional athletes as a method of upward mobility becomes the primary goal. Unfortunately, there are very few opportunities to become a professional athlete. Of one million high school athletes, only 23,000 receive college scholarships for athletics, and only 500 college athletes annually enter the ranks of the 4,000 professional athletes (Perkins, 1985). The tragedy of the black athlete (who make up nearly 50% of college athletes) is that only 25% graduate, and 75% of them have "jock majors"—degree programs designed to keep them eligible, but not necessarily employable. Perkins suggested that seeing sport and entertainment as "ways up and out" has caused a deficit of blacks in academics and the professions (medical doctors, dentists, etc.). The solution is to use athletic scholarships as a *means* to an education. But first, black athletes must perceive the need for and value of an education.

Summary

Physical education and sport each make valuable and unique contributions to the development, health, knowledge, and skill of children, youth and adults. The need to justify either one beyond their unique contributions is unnecessary and usually without cause. Statements that perceptual-motor development, physical education, or athletics enhance academic performance are without foundation. Neither sport nor physical education interferes with athletic performance—let us be satisfied with that fact and with our profession. Rather than trying to glorify physical education and sport with academic rationales, let us do an excellent job of promoting fitness and developing motor skill. As McIntosh (1984) suggests, "If physical education and physical recreation (sport) are pursued for their own sake and for their intrinsic appeal they may bring those social and personal benefits which we seek but which escape our grasp if we use physical education and recreation (sport) as little more than clincial, social, educational and political instruments to fashion those very benefits."

References

Crowl, J.A. (1983). President's view of athletics. *The Chronicle of Higher Education, 25* (Jan. 5), 21.

Delacato, C. (1959). *The treatment and prevention of reading problems.* Springfield, IL: Charles Thomas.

Desruisseaux, P. (1982, April 14). Colleges accused of exploiting student athletes. *The Chronicle of Higher Education,* p. 6.

Edwards, H. (1979, May 6). For blacks, a life in sport is no different from life. *New York Times,* p. 2s.

Eidsmoe, R.M. (1963). High school athletes are brighter. *School Activities, 35,* 75-77.

Eitzen, D.S. (1975). Athletics in the status system of male adolescents: A replication of Coleman's the adolescent society. *Adolescent, 10,* 267-276.

Farrell, C.S. (1984, November 21). Grades of freshman athletes are found the same as those of other students. *The Chronicle of Higher Education,* pp. 23, 28.

Frostig, M., & Horne, D. (1964). *The Frostig program for the development of visual perception.* Chicago: Follett.

Glass, G., & Robbins, M.P. (1967). A critique of experiments on the role of neurological organization in reading performance. *Reading Research Quarterly, 3,* 5-51.

Hallahan, D.P., & Cruickshank, W.M. (1973). *Psycho-educational foundations for learning disabilities.* Englewood Cliffs, NJ: Prentice-Hall.

Kavale, K., & Mattson, P.D. (1983). "One jumped off the balance beam": A meta-analysis of perceptual-motor training. *Journal of Learning Disabilities, 16,* 165-173.

Kephart, N. (1960). *The slow learner in the classroom.* Columbus, OH: Charles Merrill.

Kirkendall, D.R. (1986). Effects of physical activity on intellectual development and academic performance. In G.A. Stull (Ed.), *Academy papers* (pp. 49-63). Champaign, IL: Human Kinetics.

Landers, D.M., Feltz, D.L., Obermeier, G.E., & Brouse, T.R. (1978). Socialization via interscholastic athletics: Its effects on educational attainment. *Research Quarterly, 49,* 475-483.

Lueptow, L.B., & Kayser, B.D. (1973-4). Athletic involvement, academic achievement, and aspiration. *Sociological Focus, 7,* 24-26.

Mann, L., & Goodman, L. (1976). Perceptual training: A critical retrospect. In E. Schopler, & R.J. Reichler (Eds.), *Psychopathology and child development: Research and treatment* (pp. 271-289). New York: Plenum Press.

McIntosh, P.C. (1984, December 3). *Physical education and physical recreation—The great divide.* Prince Phillip Lecture of the Physical Education Association of Great Britain and North Ireland, Given in the House of Commons, London.

Meyers, P.I., & Hammill, D.D. (1982). *Learning disabilities: Basic concepts, assessment practices, and instructional strategies.* Austin, TX: Pro-Ed.

Monaghan, P. (1985, September 18). Flaws found in NCAA studies of athletes graduation rate. *The Chronicle of Higher Education,* p. 37.

Montessori, M. (1909/1966). *The Montessori method* (translated by A.E. George in 1912). New York: Schocken Books.

Otto, L.B. (1975). Extracurricular activites in the educational attainment process. *Rural Sociology, 40,* 162-176.

Perkins, H.D. (1985, May). *Academics and the black athlete.* A paper presented at the Conference on Ethics and Athletics, Louisiana State University, Baton Rouge.

Perkins, H.D. (1983, September). Higher academic standards for athletes do not discriminate against blacks. *The Chronicle of Higher Education,* p. 88.

Purdy, D.A., Eitzen, D.S., & Hafnagle, R. (1982). Are athletes also students: The educational process of college athletes. *Social Problems, 29,* 439-448.

Rarick, L. (1980). Cognitive-motor relationships in the growing years. *Research Quarterly for Exercise and Sport, 51,* 174-192.

Rehberg, R.A., & Schafer, W.E. (1968). Participation in interscholastic athletics and college expectations. *American Journal of Sociology, 73,* 732-740.

Schafer, W.E. (1968). Some social sources and consequences of interscholastic athletics: The case of participation and delinquency. In G. Kenyon (Ed.), *Aspects of Contemporary Sport Sociology* (p. 11). Chicago: Athletic Institute.

Schafer, W.E., & Armer, J.M. (1968). Athletes are not inferior students. *Trans-Action, 6,* 21-26.

Schmidt, R.A. (1982). *Motor control and learning: A behavioral emphasis.* Champaign, IL: Human Kinetics.

Seefeldt, V. (1974). Perceptual-motor programs. In J. Wilmore (Ed.), *Exercise and sport sciences reviews* (Vol. 2) (pp. 265-288). New York: Academic Press.

Sidelines. (1982, November 3). *The Chronicle of Higher Education,* p. 17.

Spady, W.G. (1970). Lament for the letterman: Effects of peer status and extracurricular activities on goals and achievement. *American Journal of Sociology, 75,* 680-702.

Spreitzer, E., & Pugh, M. (1973). Interscholastic athletics and educational expectations. *Sociology of Education, 46,* 171-182.

Thomas, J.R. (1980). Acquisition of motor skills: Information processing differences between children and adults. *Research Quarterly for Exercise and Sport, 51,* 158-173.

Thomas, J.R. (1977). Effects of perceptual-motor programs on children. In M. Riley (Ed.), *Echoes of influence for elementary school physical education* (pp. 43-46). Washington, DC: AAHPER.

Thomas, J.R., & Chissom, B.S. (1974). Prediction of first grade academic performance from kindergarten perceptual-motor data. *Research Quarterly, 45,* 148-153.

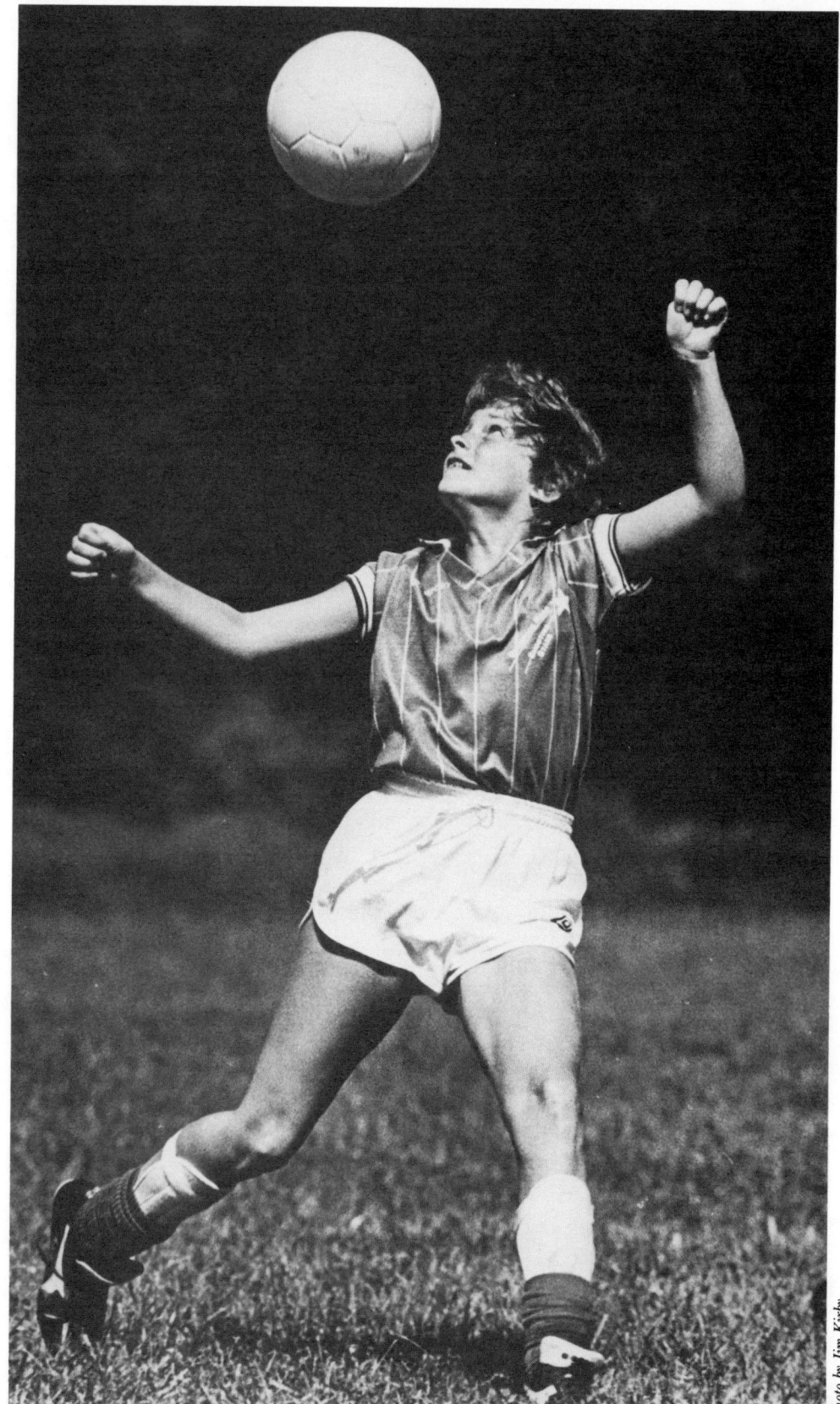

photo by Jim Kirby

CHAPTER EIGHTEEN

Effects of Physical Education Programs on Children

Paul G. Vogel
School of Health Education, Counseling
Psychology, and Human Performance
Michigan State University
East Lansing, Michigan

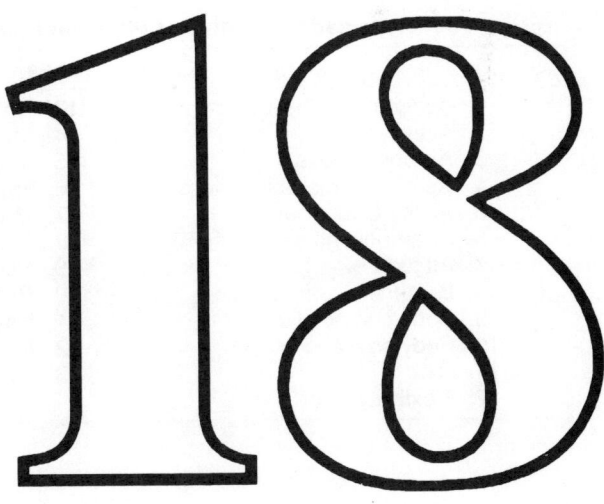

Introduction

Evidence of the effects of activity on human well-being, presented in the other chapters of this book, clearly indicates that participation in various kinds and amounts of physical activity can significantly influence both health and performance. Desirable exercise effects have been demonstrated for children and adults of both genders within what has been assumed to be reasonable levels of risk. Risks associated with activity include physical injury such as sprains, strains, lacerations, and scrapes, and hazards such as dehydration, hypoglycemia, and amenorrhea. Since exercise is typically considered to be healthful, it has essentially been prejudged to result in beneficial, rather than detrimental, effects. Data on the actual risks of participation in exercise programs, however, are essentially non-existant (Koplan, Siscovick, & Goldbaum, 1985).

An important question about the effects of activity on human well-being is, "Can the benefits of participation that have been obtained within the carefully controlled conditions of experimental research be replicated in school settings?" The primary purpose of this chapter is to identify the health or performance-related effects of exercise that have been obtained within the context of school physical education programs. A secondary purpose is to draw implications from the review for improving the current status of physical education programs.

Two major divisions of information and a brief summary are presented. The first division includes evidence on the effects of physical education programs on school children. As indicated in Table 1, many outcomes have been considered to measure the effects of physical education programs on their participants. The review is limited, therefore, to the results obtained in each outcome area by the original authors, with only a brief discussion of the findings.

Table 1
Reported Outcomes of Physical Education Programs

Outcome Areas	
1. Academic achievement	13. Knowledge
2. Activity level	14. Maturation
3. Aerobic fitness	15. Motor performance
4. Aerobic/Anaerobic fitness	16. Muscular endurance
5. Agility/Coordination	17. Muscular power
6. Anaerobic fitness	18. Muscular strength
7. Attitude	19. Perceptual-Motor
8. Balance	20. Personal-Social
9. Body composition	21. Physical fitness
10. Body size and shape	22. Speed
11. Diet	23. Other
12. Flexibility	

The second division of the chapter discusses several implications of the review. This discussion includes a reaction to the quality of the evidence reported, need for evidence of program effectiveness, and criteria that must be met to provide convincing evidence of effectiveness. A brief summary of the effects of activity concludes the chapter.

Effects of Activity in School Settings

All of the outcome areas listed in Table 1 have one or more data based studies that report effects associated with the outcome areas. In each outcome area there are usually one or more effects that use similar outcome measures, but fail to obtain similar results. Equivocal effects of physical education programs, however, should be expected. Student age, gender, socio-economic status, community values, prior experiences, and a host of variables related to the instructional process are commonly known to interact with various treatments. Treatments (programs) are also highly variable in their intended purposes as well as their intensity, duration, frequency, and length. The match (or lack thereof) between the treatment and the outcomes tested can also account for equivocal results. Results indicating effectiveness or ineffectiveness can also be attributed to the design, implementation, and evaluation of the treatment, the environmental context of the study, characteristics of the students and/or instructors, or some combination of the above.

As indicated in the column entitled, "Repeatability," included in Tables 2-24, few of the studies listed can be replicated. This inability to be repeated is a consequence of insufficient description and/or monitoring of the treatment. A study was judged repeatable if there was convincing evidence that it was implemented as intended and that it could be repeated at another site or another time. Because the vast majority of the studies included in the chapter do not meet this criterion, they are not generalizable to other sites or times. Appropriate interpretation of the results of these studies, therefore, must be made by potential users on the basis of judgments regarding the degree to which treatment, contextual, student, teacher, and other variables associated with a given effect are similar to those of the user group.

When such a match is appropriate, or potential users assume that such a program could be implemented, then one can use the reported results as evidence that a similar program effect may occur at another site or point in time. Because the majority of studies do not have evidence supporting their repeatability, they must be viewed as a collection of specific effects, associated with a particular outcome area, rather than as part of the effects of a generic physical education treatment. As such, it is inappropriate to interpret the strength of a program effect in terms of the number of instances that significant or non-significant findings are reported in an outcome area. Clearly, if all of the results in an outcome area are significant (or non-significant) a strong indication about the effectiveness (or ineffectiveness) of physical education is available. It must be remembered, however, that the assessment is based upon a collection of independent occurrences, rather than on an estimate of the chances that implementation of a generic physical education program will result in the given effect. When a small number of significant effects are obtained in an outcome area, there is simply less chance that potential users may find a study that will match their local conditions. There is evidence of transportability of an effect to a local site when a good match is apparent between one or more studies in an outcome area in which significant effects were obtained, and the local conditions of a user. The stronger the compatibility between local conditions and the size of the effect obtained, and the number of studies that obtained significant results that also match local conditions, the stronger the evidence of transportability of the obtained effect.

Appropriate interpretation of Tables 2-24, in terms of the potential of some unknown kind of physical education program to generate a significant effect, is also important. Since the majority of studies must be considered independent events, one significant result may be interpreted as evidence that a significant effect *can* occur. Naturally, this interpretation must be made within the limitations inherent in the design, conduct, and reporting of the independent study. Evidence that a significant program effect has occurred provides a reasonable basis for assuming that it can happen again, and consequently, becomes evidence that some form of physical education program is effective. A reported effect of one high quality study, therefore, provides evidence that physical education programs can produce significant effects on that reported outcome. A larger number of significant effects increases the chances that similar programs can also produce that effect. They do not increase the chances that the effect can be obtained by dissimilar programs.

A lack of unanimity of findings may be explained by reviewing the characteristics of the independent studies. Review of a listed study may reveal that it used a tight experimental design, appropriate measures and data collection techniques, monitored the treatment, analyzed the data in an appropriate manner, and was complete in its reporting of the results. Other studies reported in the same outcome category may be deficient in one or more of these same categories. They may also differ on age, gender, treatment emphasis, instructional time, and/or staffing differences. Comparing the characteristics of studies that achieved significance with those that did not often reveals characteristics of the treatments, students, teachers, context, or research approach that aids in the interpretation of the results.

An overview of the studies cited in Tables 2-24 is included in the Appendix. Each study is listed by first author, publication date, outcome, and the test(s) used to measure each outcome. Age, gender, sample size (N), results (significant or not significant, statistically), and repeatability of the results are also included. More complete information, such as prior experience of the students, geographical setting, student-teacher ratio, intensity, duration, length and frequency of the treatment, specific methodological strengths and weaknesses, and other characteristics of the studies can be obtained from the original sources. When significant (or non-significant) findings are reported in Tables 2-24, use the characteristics associated with the original studies to influence your judgments of worth about specific program effects.

Studies that have reported effects for each outcome area included in Table 1 are presented in the following pages. A brief definition of the outcome area and an overview of how it was measured is included. The author, date, effects, and other pertinent study characteristics are presented in a table format, followed by a brief discussion of the effects reported.

Academic Achievement

Academic achievement includes studies that have measured the effects of physical education programs on student performance in academic, mental ability, or readiness tests. Academic achievement, as used here, refers to student performance in subject matter areas other than physical education, as measured by teacher grades and/or standardized tests. Mental ability refers to intellectual capacity as measured by a standardized intelligence test, and readiness refers to a pupil's state of preparedness for success in subsequent learning tasks. Readiness was reported in two ways: readiness for school and readiness for reading. The results of these studies are included in Table 2.

Results of the studies included in Table 2 are mixed. Shephard, Volle, LaVallee, LaBarre, Jequier, and Rajie (1984) found rather impressive differences between elementary age subjects who participated in a year long, five day a week, one hour a day program of physical education and subjects who participated in a regular physical education program conducted one day per week for 40 minutes. The significant effects occurred even though the extra time allocated to physical education (+400%) was removed from the time formerly devoted to the academic subjects measured. The extra time allocated to physical education was taken from:

Table 2
Effects of Physical Education Programs on Academic Performance

			Characteristics						
			Total Instructional		Subjects		Teacher		Repeat-
Study	Date	Test	Time (hrs.)	Age	Gender	N	Type[a]	Design[b]	Result[c]	ability[d]
Moore	1984	Readiness	31.5	5	M/F	85	CR/Aide	Con.	NS	?
Shephard	1984	Teacher Grades	180	6-12	M/F	546	PE	Comp.	S	?
Thomas	1975	Otis Lennon MAT	50	6	M/F	40	PE	Con.	NS	?
	1975	Teacher Rating	50	6	M/F	40	PE	Con.	NS	?
Lipton	1970	Reading Readiness	12	6	M/F	92	PE	Comp.	S	?

[a] Teacher type: PE = Physical education specialist, CR = Classroom teacher
[b] Design: Comp. = Comparison group, Con. = Control group
[c] Result: S = Statistically significant, NS = Not statistically significant
[d] Repeatability: Yes = Evidence that the program can be replicated, ? = Replication possibilities unknown

Table 3
Effects of Physical Education Programs on Activity Level

			Characteristics						
			Total Instructional		Subjects		Teacher		Repeat-
Study	Date	Test	Time (hrs.)	Age	Gender	N	Type[a]	Design[b]	Result[c]	ability[d]
Gilliam	1982	HR out-of-class	53.5	6-7	M/F	26	PE	Comp.	S	?
	1982	HR in-class	53.5	6-7	M/F	59	PE	Comp.	S	?
Kuntzleman	1984	HR out-of-class	27-39	7-12	M/F	420	?	Comp.	NS	?
	1984	HR in-class	27-39	7-12	M/F	420	?	Comp.	S	?
Shephard	1980a	Dairy	180	10-12	M/F	300	PE	Comp.	S	?

[a] Teacher type: PE = Physical education specialist, ? = Unreported
[b] Design: Comp. = Comparison group
[c] Results: S = Statistically significant, NS = Not statistically significant
[d] Repeatability: Yes = Evidence that the program can be replicated, ? = Replication possibilities unknown

religious instruction (−14 to −17%), French language (−13%), mathematics (−12 to −14%), natural science (0 to −50%) and art and other subjects (−51 to −68%).

Thirty-eight teachers were involved in the study. Of these, 80% were favorable toward the experimental physical education treatment, 20% were neutral and none were negatively disposed. Also, 75% of the teachers thought the program had assisted students with their learning of theoretical material, 78% thought behavior had improved and 76% reported a favorable influence on the character of the students.

Contrary to the results of Shephard's study, Thomas, Chissom, Stewart, & Shelley (1975) found no differences between experimental and control subjects on teacher ratings of academic achievement or mental ability. There are, however, many differences in the characteristics of the Shepard and Thomas studies that could account for the results obtained. Among these differences are the age of the subjects and differences in treatment, type, and duration.

Two of the studies listed in Table 2 measure readiness. Lipton (1970) measured reading readiness, and Moore, Guy, and Reeve (1984) measured academic readiness. Again, the results are conflicting. Teacher type, differences in the treatment, the readiness measures used, and the design characteristics of the studies may account for the different results obtained.

The information included in Table 2 suggests that specific kinds of physical education programs, conducted in specific environmental contexts, with particular kinds of students, may contribute at least indirectly to student performance on academic measures. More importantly, it appears that significantly larger portions of time could be allocated to instruction in physical education with no disadvantage to academic performance.

Activity Level

Physical activity refers to bodily movement produced by skeletal muscles that results in energy expenditure (Casperson, Powell, & Christenson, 1985). Physical activity levels can be measured in terms of duration, frequency, and intensity of participation within and/or outside of physical education classes. Although more than 30 different measures have been used to assess physical activity levels in non-laboratory situations (LaPorte, Montoye, & Casperson, 1985), it is typically measured by monitoring heart rate (HR), completing activity logs, diaries, or questionnaires, or by wearing mechanical devices that detect and record movement.

To the degree that is important for children to engage in vigorous physical activity (i.e. heart rates at or above 60% of the HR range) for the purpose of obtaining health and/or performance benefits, educators should be concerned about the failure of children to voluntarily achieve these activity levels. Only rarely do children naturally engage in activity at or above this level of intensity (Gillium, MacConnie, Greenen Pels, & Freedson, 1982; Bradfield & Chan, 1971; Seliger, Trefny, Bartunkova, & Pauer, 1974). Elsewhere in this book the reader will find abundant evidence that increased levels of physical activity are associated with both health and performance outcomes. Consequenlty, increased activity levels within and outside of physical education classes are important considerations when assessing the outcomes of physical education programs.

Three studies have reported the effects of participation in physical education on student activity levels. Two of the studies used continuous HR monitoring (Gilliam et al., 1982; Kuntzleman, Drake, & Kuntzleman, 1984) and the other study (Shephard, Jequier, LaVallee, LaBarre, & Rajic, 1980a) used a diary to assess participant activity levels. The results of these studies are included in Table

Although Kuntzleman et al. (1984) did not report significant differences in out-of-class heart rates between experimental and comparison groups, there was a significant shift in activity level, favoring the experimental group in the light and moderate category levels in three of four measurements. In the heavy and very heavy activity level category, the shift favored the experimental group in all four measures. The shifts in out-of-class activity levels away from the light and moderate categories and toward the heavy and very heavy activity level categories appear to be important. The non-significant findings reported may be attributed to independently testing the effects within each of the four categories of intensity, rather than testing for an overall effect. Seven of eight shifts that favor the experimental group appears to be more than a chance occurance.

The effects summarized in Table 3 provide convincing evidence that physical education programs can influence desirable shifts in student physical activity levels during periods of time when students are not in structured physical education classes. The gains reported are associated with significantly higher levels of activity within the physical education program. Although the effects of the three studies are similar, the treatments appear dissimilar. Both Gillium's et al. (1982) and Kuntzleman's et al. (1984) treatments included a significant amount of instructional time devoted to cognitive learning associated with why activity is important and how activity relates to health. Encouragement to be active during periods of time outside of the scheduled physical education classes was also provided. Similar emphasis on cognitive learning was not included in Shephard's et al. (1980a) study.

Aerobic Fitness

Aerobic fitness is a label used to describe the body's ability to produce energy in the presence of oxygen. Abundant amounts of energy can be produced aerobically without releasing fatiguing by-products. The system is well suited, therefore, for long duration, low intensity (endurance) activities. The term aerobic fitness, as it is used here, is synonymous with cardiorespiratory endurance.

A large number of tests have been devised to measure aerobic fitness and many of these have been used to investigate the effects of physical education on aerobic fitness. Tests range from elaborate laboratory procedures which use gas analysis to assess metabolic activity, to relatively simple field measures that facilitate the comparison of cohorts similar in age and gender. All are based upon measuring bodily responses to long term activity. Tests are included in this section as measures of aerobic fitness if they required a sustained effort of three or more minutes. Table 4 lists the studies that measured the effects of physical education on aerobic fitness. The effects are grouped into those that measure maximum oxygen uptake (max$\dot{V}O_2$), physical work capacity (PWC), and running performance.

The body's ability to consume large amounts of oxygen (maximum oxygen uptake or max $\dot{V}O_2$) has traditionally been viewed as the premier measure of aerobic fitness. Table 4 includes 11 measures of max $\dot{V}O_2$, obtained from five studies. Six of the 11 tests achieved statistical significance. Within the Goode, Virgin, Romet, Crawford, Duffin, Pallandi, and Woch (1976) study, the conflicting results appear to be related to age and gender. The younger males (12-13) did not achieve significant effects, whereas the older males (14) and females (13-14) did. A similar age difference was reported by Shephard et al. (1980a). Nonsignificant effects were obtained for 6- and 7-year-old males and females and significant effects were obtained for children aged 8 to 12 years. Contrary to the Goode study, significant effects were obtained for younger children. Gaisl and Buchberger (1984) also obtained non-significant differences in max $\dot{V}O_2$. These

Table 4
Effects of Physical Education Programs on Aerobic Fitness

Study	Date	Test	Total Instructional Time (hrs.)	Characteristics Subjects Age	Gender	N	Teacher Type[a]	Design[b]	Result[c]	Repeatability[d]
Gaisl	1984	Max V̇O₂	?	10-14	M	28	?	P/Post	NS	?
Goode	1976	Max V̇O₂	8	12	M	111	CR	Comp.	NS	?
		Max V̇O₂	8	13	M	103	CR	Comp.	NS	?
		Max V̇O₂	8	13	F	103	CR	Comp.	S	?
		Max V̇O₂	8	14	F	103	CR	Comp.	S	?
		Max V̇O₂	8	14	M	103	CR	Comp.	S	?
Mocellin	1972	Max V̇O₂	1.2	9-10	M/F	29	?	P/Post	S	Yes
		Max V̇O₂	.6	8-9	M/F	24	?	P/Post	S	Yes
Sargeant	1985	Max V̇O₂	20	13	M	28	?	Comp.	S	?
Shephard	1980b	Max V̇O₂	180	8-12	M/F	395	PE	Comp.	S	?
		Max V̇O₂	180	6-7	M/F	395	PE	Comp.	NS	?
Bar-Or	1972	HR Reduction	12-24	9-10	M	44	?	Comp.	S	?
	1972	HR Reduction	12-24	9-10	F	48	?	Comp.	NS	?
Gaisl	1984	PWC170	?	10-14	M	28	?	P/Post	S	?
	1984	V̇O₂	?	10-14	M	28	?	P/Post	NS	?
	1984	% V̇O₂ Max	?	10-14	M	28	?	P/Post	NS	?
	1984	V̇O₂	?	10-14	M	28	?	P/Post	S	?
	1984	% V̇O₂ Max	?	10-14	M	28	?	P/Post	S	?
Goode	1976	PWC170	8	12	M	111	CR	Comp.	NS	?
		PWC170	8	14	M	103	CR	Comp.	S	?
		PWC170	8	14	F	103	CR	Comp.	S	?

Author	Year	Test		Age	Sex	N	Teacher	Design	Results	Repeatability
Kuntzleman	1984	PWC HR @ 5 Min	27-39	7-12	M/F	420	?	Comp.	NS	?
	1984	PWC SBP @ 5 Min	27-39	7-12	M/F	420	?	Comp.	NS	?
	1984	PWC Peak Work	27-39	7-12	M/F	420	?	Comp.	S	?
	1984	PWC Total Work	27-39	7-12	M/F	420	?	Comp.	S	?
	1984	PWC HR Recovery	27-39	7-12	M/F	420	?	Comp.	NS	?
Shephard	1980b	PWC170	180	6-7	M/F	395	PE	Comp.	NS	?
	1980	PWC170	180	8-11	M/F	395	PE	Comp.	S	?
Ansorge	1985	1.5 Mile Run	36+	16-17	M/F	385	PE	Comp.	NS	?
Burkett	1984	600 Run	?	14-17	M/F	164	PE/Aid	Comp.	S	Yes
Cooper	1975	12 Min Run	12.5	15	M	1215	PE	Comp.	S	?
Duncan	1983	1 Mile Run	96	10	M/F	34	PE/CR	Comp.	S	?
Goode	1976	12 Min Run	8	12	F	103	CR	Comp.	S	?
		12 Min Run	8	13	M	103	CR	Comp.	S	?
		12 Min Run	8	14	M	103	CR	Comp.	NS	?
Kuntzleman	1984	1 Mile Run	27-39	7-12	M/F	420	?	Comp.	S	?
Mocellin	1972	1000 M. Run	1.2	9-10	M/F	29	?	P/Post	S	?
		800 M. Run	.6	8-9	M/F	24	?	P/Post	S	?
Siegel	1984	1600 Mtr. Run	37	9	M/F	109	CR	Con.	S	?

[a] Teacher type: PE = Physical education specialist, CR = Classroom teacher, ? = Unreported
[b] Design: Comp. = Comparison group, Con. = Control group, P/Post = Pretest/Posttest
[c] Results: S = Statistically significant difference, NS = Not statistically significant
[d] Repeatability: Yes = Evidence that the program can be replicated, ? = Replication possibilities unknown

data are difficult to interpret, however, because the subjects and school were "special"—a pretest-posttest design with a three year treatment interval was used and the treatment was a combination of special physical education and athletic lessions.

There are many reasons that could explain the different results reported when the effects of activity on aerobic fitness are under investigation. It is well known that changes in aerobic fitness are a function of exercise intensity, duration, frequency, and length of treatment. Although the total time devoted to each program is known for all but the Gaisl (1984) study, the times are highly variable (ranging from 0.6 of an hour to something less than 180 hours). It is more important, however, to know what proportion of the total instructional time was devoted to the development of aerobic fitness. Even if the total amount of instructional time allocated to this specific effect was known, the description of the intensity, duration, and frequency of the aerobic activities used is insufficient to repeat the treatment in all but the Mocellin and Wasmund (1974) study. Age, gender, teacher type, design of the study, characteristics of the subjects, the nature of the treatment, and other variables can all significantly alter treatment effects.

In spite of the difficulties inherent in interpreting the effects of the studies, the results provide evidence that aerobic fitness, as measured by maximum oxygen uptake, can be positively influenced within the context of a physical education program. Unfortunately, the characteristics of the programs reported were not sufficiently monitored and described to provide educators with specific information regarding how these effects were obtained.

Tests of physical work capcity (PWC) are also used to measure aerobic fitness. These can be loosely categorized to include the following:

PWC Heart Rate (HR) at Five Minutes: A measure of heart rate five minutes into a standard bout of work.

PWC Systolic Blood Pressure (SBP) at Five Minutes: a measure of systolic blood pressure taken five minutes into a standard bout of work.

PWC Peak Work: A measure of the rate of work achieved at the completion of a test of maximal work ability.

PWC Total Work: A measure of the total amount of work that can be accomplished in a single bout of exercise prior to exhaustion.

PWC Heart Rate Recovery: A measure of the speed with which the heart rate returns to pre-exercise levels subsequent to a standard bout of work.

Oxygen Uptake ($\dot{V}O_2$) & % $\dot{V}O_2$ Max: Measures of the amount of oxygen consumed (work completed) at sub-maximal rates of work.

Measurement of several different kinds of exercise effects resulting from variable treatment types should result in differential results. The PWC measures reported in Table 4 met this expectation. Additional evidence is added, however, to the pool of information which suggests that aerobic changes can be obtained within the context of physical education programs. Further, the effects reported suggest that these changes can be obtained by children between 7 and 14 years of age of both genders. As with the interpretation of the effects of physical education on maximum oxygen uptake, the characteristics of the treatments associated with the PWC studies were insufficiently described to provide specific information on how the effects were obtained.

Measures of aerobic fitness were also obtained from eight studies that used tests of running performance ranging from 600 yards (mainstreamed handicapped children) to 1.5 miles or 12 minutes. Of these measures, seven effects were significant and two were not. Significant changes were associated with males and females 7 to 15 years of age within programs that expended 8 to 96 total instructional hours and were supervised by physical education specialists, classroom teachers, or a combination of these. Again, variable results are associated with the treatment, subjects, context, and design characteristics of the studies reported.

The effects summarized in Table 4 provide convincing evidence that physical education programs can significantly improve the aerobic fitness of their participants. Of the 12 studies that tested aerobic effects, 25 significant effects and 14 non-significant effects are reported. Significant effects were reported when the total instructional time ranged from 0.6 to something less than 180 hours. The actual amount of time devoted to activities considered to be stimulators of aerobic capacity is unknown. Significant effects were not limited to males or females or to a narrow age range. Similarly, significant results were obtained when the physical education programs were conducted by physical education specialists, classroom teachers, or a combination of both.

Determination of program effects was most frequently made by comparing a specified program with a comparison group that received some "other" physical education program. Often the comparison programs reported significant pretest/posttest gains, thereby increasing the difficulty of obtaining significant effects when comparing what may have been two effective programs. The predominant use of this type of experimental design results in conservative estimates of program effects in aerobic fitness, as well as the other outcome areas listed.

Aerobic/Anaerobic Fitness

Anaerobic fitness refers to the capability of the body to produce energy in the absence of sufficient amounts of oxygen. As with other mechanisms of the body, the production of energy associated with a given exercise event, or bout of work, often combines two or more metabolic systems. Events that require high levels of exercise intensity, and are of one to three minutes duration, require both aerobic and anaerobic energy production. Since the duration of the run times associated with the completion of a 600 yard run are one to three minutes, this test was categorized as a measure of aerobic/anaerobic fitness, even though it is often labeled as an aerobic test. The other measures included in Table 5, namely, heart rate reduction and work rate, also require aerobic/anaerobic energy production.

Aerobic/anaerobic improvements in performance are dependent on training methods that stress these energy production systems. The type of overloads necessary (interval training) to improve this capacity are more related to improving athletic performance than to altering health-related fitness. Activities that create this type of overload are rarely included in physical education programs, particularly at the elementary grade levels.

Table 5 summarizes the effects of five studies that measured the effects of various physical education programs on the development of aerobic/anaerobic fitness. Of the nine effects reported, three are significant. The treatment-test match in the Bar-Or and Zwiren study (1972) was very high. For 40 minutes, two, three, or four times per week over a period of nine weeks the subjects participated in interval runs. In Gaisl and Buchberger's (1984) study, the children attended a special sports school that included sport lessons, two weekly training lessons, and preparation lessons for competitions in track, field, and handball. In addition to the special physical program, a pretest, posttest, and a two year treatment interval were used. No control group was used. Because of limitations associated with the pre-post design (particularly when long intervals of time are involved) and the combined athletic-physical education treatment, the Gaisl and Buchberger effects provide little evidence in support of the effects of physical education programs on aerobic/anaerobic fitness. Thaxton, Rothstein, and Thaxton (1977) also reported effects obtained from pretest and posttest scores. The designs of the Gaisl and

Buchberger (1984) and the Thaxton et al. (1977) studies severely limit the interpretation of the findings because arguments for biased selection, maturation, testing, history, and other threats to the validity of the designs provide strong viable alternative explanations for the results obtained (Campbell & Stanley, 1971).

The results reported in Table 5 indicate that there is limited evidence to claim that physical education programs significantly improve aerobic/anaerobic fitness, with the exception of the Bar-Or and Zwiren (1972) study, where significance was limited to 9- and 10-year-old males. The effect obtained is consistent with the interval training treatment administered, and to the degree that similar treatments are successfully implemented, it appears that programs of physical education can significantly effect aerobic/anaerobic fitness. Most physical education programs simply do not assign the same importance to aerobic/anaerobic fitness that is assigned to skill learning or health related fitness. Accordingly, measurement of physical education programs effects that do not include specific activities to develop this type of fitness are unlikely to obtain significant differences in measures which test this capacity.

Agility–Coordination

Agility refers to the ability of the body to rapidly change directions. Coordination may be defined as the ability to skillfully perform complex movement patterns and is often subdivided into eye-hand, eye-foot, and total body coordination. Factors such as agility, balance, and limb speed are involved in coordination and can be improved through practice and experience. Both agility and coordination, like other forms of motor performance, are specific to the task.

As illustrated in Table 6, the most common measure selected by physical educators to measure agility and coordination is the shuttle run. Another type of agility test, often included in obstacle runs, is one in which the subject runs a course that requires several changes of direction. Although the tests are labeled as measures of agility and/or coordination, other capabilities such as speed, power, skill, and past experience also influence the scores obtained.

Table 6 includes the results of seven studies that have tested the effects of physical education on agility and coordination. All but one (Masche, 1970) used the shuttle run. Significant differences were obtained in two of the seven studies. There appears to no systematic effect of age or gender on this outcome area. Burkett (1984) obtained significant effects in a sample of male and female high school students involved in an adaptive physical education program heavily staffed with peer aids. Shephard et al. (1980b) reported significant improvements for males and females ranging in age from 6 through 12 years. Both were long term programs. The activities used to develop these abilities were not reported by Burkett, but evidence suggests that this study can be repeated in other sites. Shephard's study emphasized the development of endurance and muscular strength and included many sports (soccer, touch football, floor hockey, ice skating/hockey, basketball, and others) which were taught five days per week, one hour per day, over several years.

There are many characteristics of the studies included in Table 6 that could account for the differential results obtained. The studies that did not obtain significance varied in their emphasis on skill and fitness activities. Duncan, Boyce, Itami, and Puffenbarger (1983) emphasized fitness. Franks and Moore (1969) emphasized calesthenics and volleyball and Masche (1970) involved the participants in volleyball, basketball, low organization activities, and movement education. Johnson (1969) and Kemper, Verschurr, Koos, Snel, Splinter, and Tavecchio (1978) focused on the effect of five versus two or three days of physical education

Table 5
Effects of Physical Education Programs on Aerobic/Anaerobic Fitness

Study	Date	Test	Total Instructional Time (hrs.)	Characteristics				Design[b]	Result[c]	Repeatability[d]
				Subjects			Teacher Type[a]			
				Age	Gender	N				
Bar-Or	1972	H R Reduction	12-29	9-10	M	44	?	Comp.	S	?
	1972	H R Reduction	12-29	9-10	F	48	?	Comp.	NS	?
Franks	1969	600 Run/Walk	10	7-8	M/F	76	PE	Comp.	NS	?
Gaisl	1984	H R Reduction	?	10-14	M	28	PE	P/Post	S	?
	1984	Work Rate	?	10-14	M	28	PE	P/Post	NS	?
Goode	1976	600 Run	8	13	M	103	CR	Comp.	NS	?
	1976	600 Run	8	13	F	103	CR	Comp.	NS	?
	1976	600 Run	8	14	M	103	CR	Comp.	NS	?
	1976	600 Run	8	14	F	103	CR	Comp.	NS	?
Thaxton	1977	600 Run	6.7	14-17	F	67	PE	P/Post	S	?

[a] Teacher type: PE = Physical education specialist, CR = Classroom teacher, ? = Unreported
[b] Design: Comp. = Comparison group, P/Post = Pretest/Posttest
[c] Results: S = Statistically significant difference, NS = Not statistically significant
[d] Repeatability: Yes = Evidence that the program can be replicated, ? = Replication possibilities unknown

Table 6
Effects of Physical Education Programs on Agility/Coordination

			Characteristics						
			Total Instructional Time (hrs.)	Subjects			Teacher Type[a]	Design[b]	Result[c]	Repeat-ability[d]
Study	Date	Test		Age	Gender	N				
Burkett	1984	Shuttle Run	?	14-17	M/F	164	PE/Aide	Comp.	S	Yes
Duncan	1983	Shuttle Run	96	10	M/F	34	PE/CR	Comp.	NS	?
Franks	1969	Shuttle Run	10	7-8	M/F	76	PE	Comp.	NS	?
Johnson	1969	Shuttle Run	90-180	13	M	372	PE	Comp.	NS	?
Kemper	1978	Shuttle Run	90-180	12-13	M	70	PE	Comp.	NS	?
Shephard	1980b	Shuttle Run	180	6-12	M/F	395	PE	Comp.	S	?
Masche	1970	Obstacle Race	10	7-8	M/F	48	PE	Comp.	NS	?

[a] Teacher type: PE = Physical education specialist, CR = Classroom teacher
[b] Design: Comp. = Comparison group
[c] Results: S = Statistically significant difference, NS = Not statistically significant
[d] Repeatability: Yes = Evidence that the program can be replicated, ? = Replication possibilities unknown

Table 7
Effects of Physical Education Programs on Anerobic Fitness

			Characteristics						
			Total Instructional Time (hrs.)	Subjects			Teacher Type[a]	Design[b]	Result[c]	Repeat-ability[d]
Study	Date	Test		Age	Gender	N				
Grodjinovsky	1984	Peak Power	180	10-14	M/F	65	PE	Comp.	S	?
	1984	Mean Power	180	10-14	M/F	65	PE	Comp.	S	?
Sargeant	1985	Max Peak Power	20	13	M	28	?	Comp.	NS	?

[a] Teacher type: PE = Physical education specialist, ? = Unreported
[b] Design: Comp. = Comparison group
[c] Results: S = Statistically significant difference, NS = Not statistically significant
[d] Repeatability: Yes = Evidence that the program can be replicated, ? = Replication possibilities unknown

per week and did not report a treatment emphasis. Unfortunately, the nature of the physical education activities and the relative emphasis they were given is essentially unknown in all programs except Burkett (1984). It appears, however, that Shephard's et al. (1980a) program contained more activities similar to capabilities tested with a shuttle run than did the activities of the non-significant studies. The importance of a treatment-test match is particularly important for detecting significant effects for agility and coordination and may, in part, account for the non-significant effects obtained in this category of outcomes.

Even though the majority of studies included in Table 6 report non-significant program effects on agility and coordination, evidence does exist that physical education programs can improve these capabilities. The evidence is limited to high school age handicapped students and 6- to 12-year-old students of both genders who are exposed to programs similar to those reported by Burkett (1980) and Shephard (1980b). It is also important to recognize, however, that the effects obtained may have been produced by gains obtained in speed, power, or skill.

Anaerobic Fitness

Anaerobic fitness is a term used to identify the capacity of the body to rapidly produce energy supplies to muscle cells that are working under high intensity loads. The term literally means "in the absence of oxygen." The advantage of rapid energy replacement is offset by reduced efficiency. The anaerobic system can produce 3 units of energy per unit of fuel (carbohydrates), compared with 39 units of energy per unit of fuel (fats, carbohydrates, or proteins) produced by the aerobic system. Another disadvantage associated with rapid production of energy is the relatively short duration of time that energy can be produced (30 seconds to approximately 3 minutes) before the system can no longer function. Anaerobic fitness, therefore, is necessary to support high intensity, short duration bouts of work that are interrupted by short periods of rest.

As with aerobic work, several measures are available to test anaerobic fitness levels. Tests generally measure residual effects of the anaerobic metabolic process or estimate those effects based upon their established linkage to other physiological or performance effects associated with high intensity, short duration, work. Table 7 includes the tests that were used to measure this capacity in the studies investigating the effects of physical education on anaerobic fitness. Of the measures included in Table 7, peak power refers to the highest 5 seconds of work output and mean power refers to the average work output for 30 seconds. Maximal peak power refers to the power generated at the instant of maximal peak force measured at 108 revolutions per minute. All measures were taken using a bycicle ergometer.

As indicated in Table 7, two studies measured the effect of physical education programs on anaerobic fitness. No significant effect was obtained by Sargeant, Dolan, and Thorn (1985) even though the additional 150 minutes per week of physical education instruction was designed to improve short term power and muscular endurance and strength. Although Grodjinovsky and Bar-Or (1984) reported significant differences between the experimental group and the comparison group for peak and mean power, the design of the study limits the interpretability of the reason for the changes. The experimental group was composed of interested children of high sports ability who received six versus two hours of physical education per week. They also received coaching in specialty events three times a week. It is impossible, therefore, to determine whether the changes obtained were due to selection of the participants, the physical education program, the additional coaching, or some combinations of these other influences.

The studies included in Table 7 provide little or no evidence that anaerobic fitness can be significantly improved by participating in programs of physical education. Since anaerobic fitness is more closely aligned with athletic performance than it is with health-related performance, it is rarely emphasized in physical education programs, particularly those conducted in the elementary grades. Accordingly, it would be unusual to find physical education programs that include the intense interval training work that would produce significant differences in this capacity.

Attitude

Attitude refers to how one feels about an event, person, object, program, or state of being. The two studies included in Table 8 use the term to describe attitudes toward physical activity (Burkett, 1984) and attitude toward health and fitness (Osness, undated).

As indicated in Table 8, both studies that measured the effects of physical education on attitude obtained significant effects. Note that other significant effects were also achieved in these studies. In Burkett's (1984) study, other significant effects included agility, speed, muscular power and endurance, motor performance, and flexibility. Osness' study also obtained significant effects on measures of health fitness knowledge and knowledge of exercise and diet. The effects of these two physical education programs on attitude in the absence of significant effects in other outcome areas is unknown.

The information included in the studies reported in Table 8 provide evidence that physical education programs can significantly influence how children feel about physical activity, health, and fitness, at least when other significant effects are also occuring. As with the other effects reported in this chapter, the replication of the results reported in this outcome area are contingent on and limited to the specific characteristics of the independent studies reported.

Balance

Balance, the ability to maintain body position, is usually divided into static and dynamic types. Static balance refers to maintaining body equilibrium while standing in one place and dynamic balance is the ability to maintain equilibrium while moving from one place to another. Some investigators believe that the division of balance into dynamic and static components is an oversimplification, and argue that balance is both complex and highly specific to individual motor tasks. To the degree that this more complex conceptualization of balance is correct, general tests of balance that are not closely matched to the objectives of instruction are unlikely to be suitable measures of program effects. General tests of balance, however, are the only measures that have been reported by investigators who studied the effects of physical education programs on balance.

The studies included in Table 9 measured static balance and both reported significant effects. The effects reported by Masche (1980) and Thomas et al. (1975) were obtained even though the emphasis of the treatment was on activities that required dynamic, as opposed to static, balance abilities.

The effects obtained provide evidence that the static balance ability of 6- to 8-year-old males and females, as measured by the stork stand and the stabilometer, can be significantly influenced by participation in physical education programs similar to those implemented by Masche (1970) and Thomas (1975).

Table 8
Effects of Physical Education Programs on Attitude

			Characteristics							
			Total Instructional Time (hrs.)	Subjects			Teacher Type[a]	Design[b]	Result[c]	Repeatability[d]
Study	Date	Test		Age	Gender	N				
Burkett	1984	Wears Attitude Scale	?	14-17	M/F	164	PE/Aide	Comp. Con./Comp.	S	Yes
Osness	Undated	Health/Fitness	?	10-15	M/F	300	?		S	?

[a] Teacher type: PE = Physical education specialist, ? = Unreported
[b] Design: Comp. = Comparison group, Con. = Control group
[c] Results: S = Statistically significant difference
[d] Repeatability: Yes = Evidence that the program can be replicated, ? = Replication possibilities unknown

Table 9
Effects of Physical Education Programs on Balance

			Characteristics							
			Total Instructional Time (hrs.)	Subjects			Teacher Type[a]	Design[b]	Result[c]	Repeatability[d]
Study	Date	Test		Age	Gender	N				
Masche	1970	Stork Stand	10	7-8	M/F	48	PE	Comp. Con.	S	?
Thomas	1975	Stabilometer	50	6	M/F	40	PE		S	?

[a] Teacher type: PE = Physical education specialist
[b] Design: Comp. = Comparison group, Con. = Control group
[c] Results: S = Statistically significant difference
[d] Repeatability: Yes = Evidence that the program can be replicated, ? = Replication possibilities unknown

Body Composition

Body composition is a health-related component of physical fitness. It refers to the relative proportion of the body that is composed of fat, or lean body tissue (muscle, bone, other). Adult male body weight is comprised of approximately 15% fat and 85% lean body tissue. Approximations of adult female proportions of fat and lean tissue are 25% and 75%, respectively.

Body composition may be influenced by age, gender, diet, and exercise. Age and gender changes are most prominent during puberty, with males depositing more muscle and females depositing more fat. Dietary intake must equal energy consumption in order to maintain weight. Inbalances in exercise and/or diet can cause significant positive or negative shifts in body weight and body composition. Health and performance-related standards for men and women are available for individuals of various body types who wish to obtain or maintain desirable proportions of lean and fat body tissues.

Body fat can be measured in several ways. Since much of the body's fat is stored under the skin, estimates of the body's fat weight can be obtained by measuring skinfold thickness. More accurate estimates, however, are obtained by hydrometry. Electrical impedience methods are also used, but their reliability and validity are still considered unsatisfactory. The effects of physical education programs on body composition reported in Table 10 used skinfolds and hydrometry to estimate body composition.

Table 10 includes measures of body density (the relationship between weight in air and weight underwater), body fat, and lean body mass. Higher measures of body density or lean weight are associated with lower levels of body fat. Within the seven studies that estimate the effects of physical education programs on body composition, 29 results were reported. Of these, 9 were significant and 20 were not.

Significant effects of physical education programs on body composition were found for females within the age range of 7 to 16, with the exception of age 15, where no subjects were tested. Within the group of 16-year-old obese and non-obese females studied by Moody, Wilmore, Girandola, and Royce (1972), all of the significant effects obtained, with one exception, were for the obese rather than the non-obese subjects. Non-significant effects occurred in the 12- and 13-year-old females (Goode et al., 1976; Johnson, 1969) and also for females 16 years old (Moody et al., 1972). For the males, significant effects were obtained for 13-year-old boys (Johnson, 1969; Sargent, Dolan, & Thomas, 1985) and for the age group from 7 to 12 years (Kuntzleman et al., 1984). Non-significant effects were also obtained for males 12 to 14 years old (Goode et al. 1976; Johnson, 1969; Sargent et al., 1985) and 10 to 14 years old (Grodjinovsky & Bar-Or, 1984).

The four studies that obtained significant effects were either designed to influence body composition or involved large quantities of physical activity. Moody's et al. (1972) study was designed specifically as a weight reduction program. Kuntzleman et al. (1984) emphasized both health-related fitness activities and diet. Johnson (1969) measured the effects of a two year program, with classes held five days a week, and Grodjinovsky and Bar-Or (1984) studied a group that was selected for their interest and ability in sport who were also exposed to six hours of physical education per week for one year plus specialized coaching for three additional practices per week.

The studies that did not obtain significant effects were very different in their treatment emphasis. They did not design the programs to influence body composition and the activity levels were much lower.

Table 10
Effects of Physical Education Programs on Body Composition

Study	Date	Test	Total Instructional Time (hrs.)	Characteristics				Design[b]	Result[c]	Repeatability[d]
				Age	Gender	N	Teacher Type			
Goode	1976	Triceps	8	12	M	111	CR	Comp.	NS	?
	1976	Triceps	8	13	M	103	CR	Comp.	NS	?
	1976	Triceps	8	13	F	103	CR	Comp.	NS	?
	1976	Triceps	8	14	M	103	CR	Comp.	NS	?
	1976	Triceps	8	14	F	103	CR	Comp.	NS	?
	1976	Suprailliac	8	12	M	111	CR	Comp.	NS	?
	1976	Suprailliac	8	13	M	103	CR	Comp.	NS	?
	1976	Suprailliac	8	13	F	103	CR	Comp.	NS	?
	1976	Suprailliac	8	14	M	103	CR	Comp.	NS	?
	1976	Suprailliac	8	14	F	103	CR	Comp.	NS	?
	1976	Sub-scapular	8	13	M	103	CR	Comp.	NS	?
	1976	Sub-scapular	8	13	F	103	CR	Comp.	NS	?
	1976	Sub-scapular	8	14	M	103	CR	Comp.	NS	?
	1976	Sub-scapular	8	14	F	103	CR	Comp.	NS	?
Grodjinovsky	1984	Body Composition	180	10-14	M	65	PE	Comp.	NS	?
	1984	Body Composition	180	10-14	F	65	PE	Comp.	S	?
Johnson	1969	Triceps	90-180	13	M	372	PE	Comp.	S	?
	1969	Triceps	90-180	13	F	472	PE	Comp.	NS	?
Kemper	1978	% Fat	90-180	12-13	M	70	PE	Comp.	NS	?
Kuntzleman	1984	Skinfolds	27-39	7-12	M/F	420	?	Comp.	S	?

continued

Table 10 (continued)
Effects of Physical Education Programs on Body Composition

Study	Date	Test	Total Instructional Time (hrs.)	Characteristics						
				Subjects			Teacher Type	Design[b]	Result[c]	Repeatability[d]
				Age	Gender	N				
Moody	1972	Density (H^{2}O) (Nor.)	?	16	F	12	?	P/Post	NS	?
	1972	Density (H^{2}O) (Obese)	?	16	F	28	?	P/Post	S	?
	1972	Lean Wt. (H^{2}O) (Nor.)	?	16	F	12	?	P/Post	NS	?
	1972	Lean Wt. (H^{2}O) (Obese)	?	16	F	28	?	P/Post	S	?
	1972	% Fat (H^{2}O) (Nor.)	?	16	F	12	?	P/Post	NS	?
	1972	% Fat (H^{2}O) (Obese)	?	16	F	28	?	P/Post	S	?
	1972	Skinfolds (Nor.)	?	16	F	12	?	P/Post	S	?
	1972	Skinfolds (Obese)	?	16	F	28	?	P/Post	S	?
Sargeant	1985	Skinfolds	20	13	M	28	?	Comp.	S	?

[a]Teacher type: PE = Physical education specialist, CR = Classroom teacher, ? = Unreported
[b]Design: Comp. = Comparison group, P/Post = Pretest/Posttest
[c]Results: S = Statistically significant difference, NS = Not statistically significant
[d]Repeatability: Yes = Evidence that the program can be replicated, ? = Replication possibilities unknown

The informaton included in Table 10 provides evidence that programs of physical education can significantly alter body composition. These reports also suggest that significant changes in body composition do not occur in all programs. Differences in treatment emphasis between programs that did, or did not, obtain significant effects suggest that relatively large quantities of activity and/or activities specifically designed to achieve or maintain desirable levels of body fat and/or lean body mass are necessary.

Body Size and Shape

Body size and shape is assessed by measuring the height, weight, length, width, girth, and/or surface area of the body or its segments and then determining how the measures vary among individuals, as well as their relationship to one another. Standard measures include standing height, sitting height, shoulder and hip width, leg length, weight, chest, arm, trunk and leg girths, and somatotype. These measures are often used in the study of growth and development and its relationship to motor skill acquisition, fitness, physical health, and other variables of interest to researchers. Measures of body size and shape are commonly used in at least three ways. First, they are used to describe subjects in a way that allows researchers, or individuals considering the use of research or evaluative findings, to determine the similarity of the subjects to other individuals or groups of interest. Second, they are used to determine whether a hypothesized research treatment or other program will alter these variables. Third, they are often used as intervening variables to determine how their variation may interact with other independent and dependent variables of interest.

As indicated in Table 11, most of the studies measuring program effects on these variables obtained non-significant results. Of the 21 comparisons made, only 4 (2 for height and 2 for weight) were significant.

Seven measures of program effect on height were reported. Two were significant while five were not. Significant differences were obtained in the study by Goode et al. (1976) for the 12- and 13-year-old males, but not for the 13-year-old females or the 14-year-old males or females. The analysis conducted on these data (t-test of mean differences on the posttest where pretest differences were not significant) did not adjust the posttest scores for pretest differences; thus, their interpretability is reduced.

Moody et al. (1972) reported the effects of a 15-week program designed specifically for reducing the weight of obese high school females. As indicated in Table 11, there was a significant pre-post effect obtained for the obese, but not for the subjects of normal weight. Girths, however, did not change for either group.

The significant weight effect obtained by Goode et al. (1976) in the posttest scores of the 14-year-old males is likely to be associated with the realtively large mean differences in the pretest between the experimental and comparison groups. In this group the boys in the comparison group were 3 pounds heavier on the pretest, but not statitically different (t = 1.55). Posttest differences show the control boys to be 4.3 pounds heavier than the experimental group (t = 2.32). Although the initial 3 pound difference was not statistically different, it contributed to the significant mean differences when added to the 1.3 pound change observed on the posttest. Data are not provided by Goode to permit calculation of the significance of posttest differences subsequent to a correction based on pretest values. It appears, however, that such a correction would negate the observed differences.

There are no significant program effects on measures of arm, chest, or waist girth nor was there a significant effect when these measures were combined. Even in obese subjects who lost significant amounts of weight, no significant changes in

Table 11
Effects of Physical Education Programs on Body Size and Shape

Study	Date	Test	Total Instructional Time (hrs.)	Characteristics – Subjects Age	Gender	N	Teacher Type[a]	Design[b]	Result[c]	Repeatability[d]
Goode	1976	Height	8	12	M	111	CR	Comp.	S	?
		Height	8	13	M	103	CR	Comp.	S	?
		Height	8	13	F	103	CR	Comp.	NS	?
		Height	8	14	M	103	CR	Comp.	NS	?
		Height	8	14	F	103	CR	Comp.	NS	?
Grodjinovsky	1984	Height	180	10-14	M/F	65	PE	Comp.	NS	?
Wittle	1961	Height	?	12	M	162	?	Comp.	NS	No
Goode	1976	Weight	8	12	M	111	CR	Comp.	NS	?
		Weight	8	13	M	111	CR	Comp.	NS	?
		Weight	8	13	F	111	CR	Comp.	NS	?
		Weight	8	14	M	103	CR	Comp.	S	?
		Weight	8	14	F	103	CR	Comp.	NS	?
Grodjinovsky	1984	Weight	180	10-14	M/F	65	PE	Comp.	NS	?
Moody	1972	Weight (Nor.)	?	16	F	12	?	P/Post	NS	?
		Weight (Obese)	?	16	F	28	?	P/Post	S	?
Wittle	1961	Weight	?	12	M	162	?	Comp.	NS	No
Ansorge	1985	Upper Arm Girth	36+	16-17	M/F	385	PE	Comp.	NS	?
Kemper	1978	Upper Arm Girth	90-180	12-13	M	70	PE	Comp.	NS	?
Kuntzleman	1984	Chest Girth	27-39	7-12	M/F	420	?	Comp.	NS	?
		Waist Girth	27-39	7-12	M/F	420	?	Comp.	NS	?
Moody	1972	Girths (Nor.)	?	16	F	12	?	P/Post	NS	?
		Girths (Obese)	?	16	F	28	?	P/Post	NS	?

[a] Teacher type: PE = Physical education specialist, CR = Classroom teacher, ? = Unreported
[b] Design: Comp. = Comparison group, P/Post = Pretest/Posttest
[c] Results: S = Statistically significant difference, NS = Not statistically significant
[d] Repeatability: Yes = Evidence that the program can be replicated, ? = Replication possibilities unknown

a sum of seven girth measures were detected (Moody et al., 1972). The information reported in the studies included in Table 8 provide little or no evidence that programmatic effects of physical education can significantly alter (either positively or negatively) the height, weight, or girths of normal subjects.

Diet

Nutritionists state that Americans consume more calories, cholesterol, simple carbohydrates, fat, protein, and sodium and less complex carbohydrates, fiber, and potassium than is healthful. The combination of overeating, inactivity, and eating inappropriate foods has led to increasing levels of overweightness, obesity, and ill health. A large body of knowledge substantiates the need for prudence in exercise and dietary habits. Moreover, diet and exercise have been shown to be effective means of weight control. Diet and exercise in combination, however, appear to have combined effects that are greater than merely adding the benefits of diet to the benefits of exercise (American College of Sports Medicine, 1983).

Table 12 includes the effects obtained from dietary surveys conducted to determine whether or not the "Feelin' Good" physical education program (Kuntzleman, 1984) altered dietary patterns. Six effects are reported and two are significant. The results show improvements associated with participation in each of the effects tested, except potassium consumption. Significant effects in favor of the comparison group were obtained on that measure. Only a reduction in simple carbohydrates was significant, in favor of the experimental group.

The information in Table 12 provides little or no evidence that participation in physical education can alter the nutritional practices of students. Although a significant effect was obtained for simple carbohydrates, the effect was counterbalanced by a significant effect in favor of the comparison group for consumption of potassium. Nutrition is a difficult area to alter, even with excellent instruction, because most children are able to effectively control only a small part of their diet. Family nutritional practices, in addition to broad community involvement, is probably necessary to obtain significant gains in this important area.

Flexibility

Flexibility is the range of motion at a joint or sequence of joints. It is specific to the different joints of the body and is primarily limited by the nature of the joint (hinge, ball and socket) and its surrounding soft tissue (muscle, ligaments, and other connective tissues). Flexibility is related to injury prevention, performance, and posture.

There are many ways to measure flexibility. They include the goniometer (a 180° protractor with one stationary and one moveable arm), Leighton flexometer (an instrument with a circular dial that is applied to a joint and subsequently records range of motion), and the electrogoniometer (a devise that provides an electronical output, used to monitor joint angles of subjects while they are stationary or moving).

Table 13 includes the results of four studies that have measured the effects of physical educaton programs on the flexibility of several joints. Two studies reported significant results and two did not. There was a similar division of results within the joints tested. Measures of flexibility taken by Ansorge et al. (1985) were non-significant, while in the Burkett (1984) study they were significant. In Duncan's et al. (1983) study, significant improvements in flexibility, favoring the experimental group, occurred in the sit and reach test. The experimental group also experienced significant decreases in flexibility in the ankle joint. The treatment in this study emphasized aerobic fitness, calesthenics and once-a-week training on items that paralled the AAHPERD performance-related fitness test. Treatment in Whittle's (1961) study is unknown except that the experimental and

Table 12
Effects of Physical Education Programs on Diet

Study	Date	Test	Total Instructional Time (hrs.)	Subjects Age	Subjects Gender	Subjects N	Teacher Type[a]	Design[b]	Result[c]	Repeatability[d]
Kuntzleman	1984	Total Calories	27-39	7-12	M/F	420	?	Comp.	NS	?
	1984	Simple Carbohydrates	27-39	7-12	M/F	420	?	Comp.	S	?
	1984	Sodium	27-39	7-12	M/F	420	?	Comp.	NS	?
	1984	Potassium	27-39	7-12	M/F	420	?	Comp.	S	?
	1984	Fat	27-39	7-12	M/F	420	?	Comp.	NS	?

[a] Teacher type: PE = Physical education specialist, CR = Classroom teacher, ? = Unreported
[b] Design: Comp. = Comparison group
[c] Results: S = Statistically significant difference, NS = Not statistically significant
[d] Repeatability: Yes = Evidence that the program can be replicated, ? = Replication possibilities unknown

Table 13
Effects of Physical Education Programs on Flexibility

Study	Date	Test	Total Instructional Time (hrs.)	Subjects Age	Subjects Gender	Subjects N	Teacher Type[a]	Design[b]	Result[c]	Repeatability[d]
Ansorge	1985	Sit & Reach	36+	16-17	M/F	385	PE	Comp.	NS	?
Burkett	1984	Sit & Reach	?	14-17	M/F	164	PE/Aide	Comp.	S	Yes
Duncan	1983	Ankle	96	10	M/F	34	PE/CR	Comp.	S	?
	1983	Sit & Reach	96	10	M/F	34	PE/CR	Comp.	S	?
Wittle	1961	Trunk	?	12	M	162	?	Comp.	NS	No
	1961	Hip	?	12	M	162	?	Comp.	NS	No
	1961	Ankle	?	12	M	162	?	Comp.	NS	No

[a] Teacher type: PE = Physical education specialist, CR = Classroom teacher, ? = Unreported
[b] Design: Comp. = Comparison group
[c] Results: S = Statistically significant difference, NS = Not statistically significant
[d] Repeatability: Yes = Evidence that the program can be replicated, No = Program replication unlikely, ? = Replication possibilities unknown

control schools were designated as good or poor as a function of their scores on the Laporte Elementary School Score Card (LaPorte, 1955).

Table 13 provides evidence that physical education programs can improve flexibility of the hip and spine. Although the effects are mixed, the one nonsignificant effect (Ansorge et al., 1985) was accompanied by similar findings on all other physical measures incorporated in that study. The results obtained in this study can be attributed to an ineffective intervention, or an effective comparison group, a combination of both, or some other unknown influences. Two other programs obtained significant effects, however, and to the degree that those interventions can be replicated, similar results could be obtained elsewhere. These studies provide no evidence for positive program effects on the flexibility of the ankle, however. In fact, evidence is provided that ankle flexibility may be reduced in programs of physical education.

Knowledge

Knowledge refers to cognitive information, specifically taught as part of the physical education program. It could include information such as how to warm up, cool down, learn a motor skill, or how to develop and/or maintain strength and flexibility. Knowledge was measured using pencil and paper tests or observations of students behaviors.

Table 14 includes three studies that measured the effects of participation in physical education on the acquisition of knowledge. In all cases, the information tested was related to the development of healthy lifestyles. Significant effects were obtained by males and females ranging in age from 7 to 17. In Ansorge's et al. (1985) study, health knowledge was the only significant effect resulting from participation in the experimental program.

The studies included in Table 14 provide strong evidence that knowledge pertinent to healthy lifestyles can be acquired within the context of instruction in physical education. As with other physical education outcomes, relatively greater or lesser knowledge transmission would be expected across different programs, depending upon the complexity of the content and effectiveness of the instruction.

Maturation

Maturation refers to the process of growth and development which leads to achievement of adult characteristics. Although maturation roughly parallels chronological age, there are wide variances among individuals and/or biological systems at any given age level. Early maturing individuals are often at an advantage, in terms of status (Jones and Bayley, 1950) self-confidence (Mussen and Jones, 1957) and performance (Clarke, 1973). According to Malina (chapter 1, this edition), the effects of regular activity on maturation are not well known, but the available evidence suggests little, if any, effect.

Three measures of maturity have been used to investigate the effects of participation in physical education on the biological process (see Table 15). Skeletal age (a measure of bone ossification obtained by comparing an x-ray of the hand and wrist with chronological age standards) is an excellent measure of biological maturity. The McCloy Index I uses age, height, and weight to approximate levels of maturity; and the Wetzel Grid is a measure of maturity based on a plot of height and weight against standards of a peer group, by gender and age.

Results of Wittle's (1961) study include no significant effects on skeletal age, status on the Wetzel Grid, or the McCloy Index I associated with participation in programs rated "good" on the LaPort score card (LaPort, 1955) when compared to programs rated "poor." These results, though limited to boys 12 years of age,

Table 14
Effects of Physical Education Programs on Knowledge Acquisition

| | | | Total Instructional Time (hrs.) | Characteristics | | | | | | |
| | | | | Subjects | | | Teacher Type[a] | Design[b] | Result[c] | Repeatability[d] |
Study	Date	Test		Age	Gender	N				
Ansorge	1985	Health Knowledge	36+	16-17	M/F	385	PE	Comp.	S	?
Kuntzleman	1984	Cardiovascular Health	27-39	7-12	M/F	420	?	Comp.	S	?
Osness	Undated	Health-Fitness Q	?	10-15	M/F	300	?	Comp.	S	?
	Undated	Exercise/Diet Q	?	10-15	M/F	300	?	Comp.	S	?

[a] Teacher type: PE = Physical education specialist, CR = Classroom teacher, ? = Unreported
[b] Design: Comp. = Comparison group
[c] Results: S = Statistically significant difference
[d] Repeatability: Yes = Evidence that the program can be replicated, ? = Replication possibilities unknown

Table 15
Effects of Physical Education Programs on Maturation

| | | | Total Instructional Time (hrs.) | Characteristics | | | | | | |
| | | | | Subjects | | | Teacher Type[a] | Design[b] | Result[c] | Repeatability[d] |
Study	Date	Test		Age	Gender	N				
Wittle	1961	Skeletal Age	?	12	M	162	?	Comp.	NS	No
	1961	Wetzel Grid	?	12	M	162	?	Comp.	NS	No
	1961	McCloy Index I	?	12	M	162	?	Comp.	NS	No

[a] Teacher type: PE = Physical education specialist, CR = Classroom teacher, ? = Unreported
[b] Design: Comp. = Comparison group
[c] Results: NS = Not statistically significant
[d] Repeatability: No = Program replication unlikely

are consistent with other works (Malina, chapter 1, this edition) that have studied the relationship between physical activity and maturation. The information included in Table 15 provides some evidence that participation in physical education neither accelerates nor retards the maturation process.

Motor Performance

Motor performance can be defined as the ability to perform fundamental motor and sport skills. There are many ways that motor performance can be measured ranging from tests of general motor ability through very specific tests of discrete skills. Like the concept of physical fitness, there is general agreement in the profession regarding the uniqueness and importance of instruction in the area of motor performance, but great disagreement about precisely what motor performance is or how it should be measured.

Table 16 summarizes 12 studies that have investigated the effects of physical education programs on motor performance. Within the 12 studies, 28 effects are reported. The effects range from tests that are considered measures of the components of skill to general estimates of motor performance. For example, the first set of tests listed in Table 16 include the shuttle run, and obstacle course. These tests are used as measures to estimate muscular power, speed, agility, and coordination. Because practice can dramatically improve the scores obtained on these measures (up to the point where genetic potential is reached or where limits in necessary strength, power, or other components of skill are reached) it can be concluded that they also contain a motor skill component. The degree to which the scores on these measures represent skilled ability or the underlying components of skill is not clear. Because the test scores are potentially limited by factors other than skill, results obtained on these measures may be an inaccurate estimate of the potential effects of physical education programs on the development of motor performance abilities, particularly those that are more complex.

Of the first seven effects listed in Table 16, two are significant. A discussion of the characteristics of the studies from which these effects were obtained that could account for the differential results obtained is included in the section of this chapter devoted to agility-coordination.

The second set of effects included in Table 16 measures fundamental skills. These tests, in part, are similar to the tests included in the first set of effects, because performance is limited by factors other than skill. For example, high scores on the long jump or vertical jump are limited or enhanced by muscular power as well as motor skill.

There are six studies represented in this second set of tests and 10 effects reported. Of these, seven were significant. There appears to be no influence of gender or age on the significance of the results. Two of the three non-significant effects were reported by Franks and Moore (1969). A review of the treatments involved in their study shows that the program was of short duration (five weeks) and emphasized volleyball, calesthenics, or volleyball and calesthenics. As such, there is little reason to expect significant differences in the performance of the long jump or the softball throw between these three treatments. Johnson's (1969) study focused on testing the effects of five versus two or three days of physical education per week and the treatment emphasis was not specified. The non-significant results obtained in this study can be explained by a weak match between the instructional content and the test, ineffective instruction in the experimental group, effective instruction in the comparison group, or some combination of these or other unknown factors.

The third set of tests in Table 16 are more closely related to the acquisition of skill in specific sports and general (or a collection of specific) skills representing a wide range of motor abilites. Although peformance on these measures is also

Table 16
Effects of Physical Education Programs on Motor Performance

| | | | Total Instructional Time (hrs.) | Characteristics | | | | | | | |
| | | | | Subjects | | | Teacher Type[a] | Design[b] | Result[c] | Repeat-ability[d] |
Study	Date	Test		Age	Gender	N				
Burkett	1984	Shuttle Run	?	14-17	M/F	164	PE/Aid	Comp.	S	Yes
Duncan	1983	Shuttle Run	96	10	M/F	34	PE/CR	Comp.	NS	?
Franks	1969	Shuttle Run	10	7-8	M/F	76	PE	Comp.	NS	?
Johnson	1969	Shuttle Run	90-180	13	M	372	PE	Comp.	NS	?
Kemper	1978	Shuttle Run	90-180	12-13	M	70	PE	Comp.	NS	?
Shephard	1980	Shuttle Run	180	6-12	M/F	395	PE	Comp.	S	?
Masche	1970	Obstacle Race	10	7-8	M/F	48	PE	Comp.	NS	?
Masche	1970	Ball Handling	10	7-8	M/F	48	PE	Comp.	S	?
Franks	1983	Softball Throw	10	7-8	M/F	76	PE	Comp.	NS	?
Masche	1970	Throw	10	7-8	M/F	48	PE	Comp.	NS	?
Franks	1969	Long Jump	10	7-8	M/F	76	PE	Comp.	NS	?
Johnson	1969	Long Jump	90-180	13	M/F	844	PE	Comp.	S	?
Masche	1970	Long Jump	10	7-8	M/F	48	PE	Comp.	S	?
Newfield	1984	Long Jump	?	6-8	M/F	3800	?	Comp.	S	Yes
Shephard	1980b	Long Jump	180	6-12	M/F	395	PE	Comp.	S	?
Johnson	1969	Vert. Jump	90-180	13	M	372	PE	Comp.	NS	?
Wittle	1961	Vert. Jump	?	12	M	162	?	Comp.	S	No

Author	Year	Skill	Length	Age	Sex	N	Teacher[a]	Design[b]	Results[c]	Repeat.[d]
Johnson	1969?	Basketball	90-180	13	F	472	PE	Comp.	NS	?
Thaxton	1977	Foul Shot, Pass, Dribble	6.7	14-18	F	67	PE	P/Post	S	?
Johnson	1977	Mats, Sidehorse	6.7	14-18	F	67	PE	P/Post	S	?
	1977	Trampoline	6.7	14-18	F	67	PE	P/Post	S	?
Johnson	1969	Soccer	90-180	13	M	372	PE	Comp.	S	?
Franks	1969	VB Wall Volley	10	7-8	M/F	76	PE	Comp.	NS	?
	1969	VB Serve	10	7-8	M/F	76	PE	Comp.	NS	?
Johnson	1969	Volleyball	90-180	13	M/F	844	?PE	Comp.	S	?
Kemper	1978	Motor Performance	90-180	12-13	M	70	PE	Comp.	S	?
McAdam	1974	Motor Performance	?	11	M/F	600	PE	Comp.	S	?
Vogel	1981	I CAN Perf. T	?	5-23	M/F	2-15	PE/CR	Comp.	S	?

[a] Teacher type: PE = Physical education specialist, CR = Classroom teacher, ? = Unreported
[b] Design: Comp. = Comparison group, P/Post = Pretest/Posttest
[c] Results: S = Statistically significant difference, NS = Not statistically significant
[d] Repeatability: Yes = Evidence that the program can be replicated, No = Program replication unlikely, ? = Replication possibilities unknown

contingent on strength, power, or other components of skill, they are more complex, require higher levels of skill and, therefore, may be a better representation of the potential that physical education programs have to improve the skilled performance of their participants.

Six studies and 11 effects are included in the third section of Table 16. Of these, eight are significant. The differential results do not appear to be related to gender or age. Again, the effects measured in Franks and Moore (1969) were non-significant. Since the instructional emphasis included volleyball and the tests used to measure program effects were the volleyball serve and volleyball wall volley, an inappropriate treatment-test match does not account for the results. Review of the pre to post differences in mean values, however, shows rather large but untested, positive changes for all three treatment groups across all measures except the serve. The authors note that high pre-test scores precluded large gains on this measure and may be related to obtaining lower posttest means for all three treatment groups. The other non-significant effect occurred on the basketball test administered by Johnson (1969). As indicated elsewhere, the focus on this study was on differences associated with five versus two and three day a week classes and, consequently, characteristics of the instructional treatment are not described.

Of the 28 effects tested in Table 16, 16 are significant and 17 are not. Review of the studies which reported non-significant effects yield no reasons sufficient to discount the significant results obtained in the other studies. There is strong evidence that physical education programs can be effective in improving the motor performance abilities of their participants.

Muscular Endurance

Muscular endurance is the ability of the muscle to repeatedly contract and move a sub-maximal load. It is closely related to capacities such as muscular strength and muscular power. Muscular endurance is a common measure used by investigators when performance- and health-related physical fitness is measured. Typical measurement items include situps, pushups, and the flexed arm hang.

Eight studies have tested the effects of physical education programs on muscular endurance (see Table 17). Fourteen effects were reported and 10 were significant. Each of the four test items used to measure muscular endurance had at least one significant effect. Significant effects were obtained for males and females ranging in age from 6 to 17 years.

The effects included in Table 17 confirm that males and females of elementary and secondary school ages can obtain significant changes in muscular endurance through participation in programs of physical education. Evidence that these effects can be obtained is not provided, however, for females at or near age 13.

Muscular Power

Muscular power is a combination of muscular strength and speed and like muscular endurance, strength and flexibility, it is a common inclusion in tests used to measure performance related physical fitness. Muscular power is defined as the rate at which work can be performed by the involved muscle group(s).

Performers who effectively combine strength and speed of movement are said to be powerful. The vertical and long jumps are activities that require high amounts of power for exceptional performance. Power is measured in the field, therefore, by using activities such as the vertical and horizontal jump. Other activities such as the shuttle run, short dash, and throw for distance have also been used to estimate muscular power. Power can influence the performance of motor skills, as skill can influence the measurement of muscular power. Consequently, the effects obtained from measures such as those included in Table 18 are not as

Table 17
Effects of Physical Education Programs on the Acquisition of Muscular Endurance

			Characteristics							
Study	Date	Test	Total Instructional Time (hrs.)	Age	Gender	N	Teacher Type[a]	Design[b]	Result[c]	Repeatability[d]
Thaxton	1977	Flexed Arm Hang	6.7	14-18	F	67	PE	P/Post	S	?
Burkett	1984	Flexed Arm Hang	?	14-17	M/F	164	PE/Aide	Comp.	S	Yes
Duncan	1983	Flexed Arm Hang	96	10	F	21	PE/CR	Comp.	NS	?
Johnson	1969	Flexed Arm Hang	90-180	13	F	472	PE	Comp.	NS	?
Kemper	1978	Flexed Arm Hang	?	12-13	M	70	PE	Comp.	NS	?
Shephard	1980	Flexed Arm Hang	180	6-12	M/F	395	PE	Comp.	S	?
Burkett	1984	Situps	?	14-17	M/F	164	PE/Aide	Comp.	S	?
Duncan	1983	Situps	96	10	M/F	34	PE/CR	Comp.	S	?
Franks	1969	Situps	10	7-18	M/F	76	PE	Comp.	S	?
Shephard	1980b	Situps	180	6-12	M/F	395	PE	Comp.	S	?
Thaxton	1977	Situps	6.7	14-18	F	67	PE	P/Post	S	?
Johnson	1969	Curl-up	90-180	13	F	472	PE	Comp.	NS	?
Newfield	1984	Curl-up	?	6-8	M/F	3800	?	Comp.	S	Yes
Johnson	1969	Push-up	90-180	13	?M	372	PE	Comp.	S	?

[a] Teacher type: PE = Physical education specialist, CR = Classroom teacher, ? = Unreported
[b] Design: Comp. = Comparison group, P/Post = Pretest/Posttest
[c] Results: S = Statistically significant difference, NS = Not statistically significant
[d] Repeatability: Yes = Evidence that the program can be replicated, ? = Replication possibilities unknown

Table 18
Effects of Physical Education Programs on the Acquisition of Muscular Power

			Characteristics							
			Total Instructional Time (hrs.)	Age	Subjects Gender	N	Teacher Type[a]	Design[b]	Result[c]	Repeatability[d]
Study	Date	Test								
Burkett	1984	Shuttle Run	?	14-17	M/F	164	PE/Aide	Comp.	S	Yes
Duncan	1983	Shuttle Run	96	10	M/F	34	PE/CR	Comp.	NS	?
Franks	1969	Shuttle Run	10	7-8	M/F	76	PE	Comp.	NS	?
Johnson	1969	Shuttle Run	90-180	13	M	372	PE	Comp.	NS	?
Kemper	1978	Shuttle Run	90-180	12-13	M	70	PE	Comp.	NS	?
Shephard	1980b	Shuttle Run	180	6-12	M/F	395	PE	Comp.	S	?
Duncan	1983	Long Jump	96	10	M/F	34	PE/CR	Comp.	NS	?
Franks	1969	Long Jump	10	7-8	M/F	76	PE	Comp.	NS	?
Johnson	1969	Long Jump	90-180	13	M/F	844	PE	Comp.	S	?
Masche	1970	Long Jump	10	7-8	M/F	48	PE	Comp.	S	?
Newfield	1984	Long Jump	?	6-8	M/F	3800	?	Comp.	S	Yes
Shephard	1980b	Long Jump	180	6-12	M/F	395	PE	Comp.	S	?
Johnson	1969	Vertical Jump	90-180	13	M	372	PE	Comp.	NS	?
Wittle	1961	Vertical Jump	?	12	M	162	?	Comp.	S	No
Newfield	1984	Dash	?	6-8	M/F	3000	?	Comp.	S	Yes
Shephard	1980b	50 Yd. Dash	180	6-12	M/F	395	PE	Comp.	S	?

[a] Teacher type: PE = Physical education specialist, CR = Classroom teacher, ? = Unreported
[b] Design: Comp. = Comparison group
[c] Results: S = Statistically significant difference, NS = Not statistically significant
[d] Repeatability: Yes = Evidence that the program can be replicated, No = Program replication unlikely, ? = Replication possibilities unknown

precise as more sophisticated laboratory methods for measuring this performance capacity.

Table 18 lists nine studies that have measured various motor performance items which could be used to estimate muscular power. Sixteen effects are listed and 10 are significant. There is at least one significant effect for each of the measures.

Five of the studies reported significant effects on all of the measures used to assess this capacity, but four of the studies had at least one non-significant effect. Duncan et al. (1983) emphasized aerobic fitness five days per week, including one day per week that incorporated training on the long jump and shuttle run items. Franks and Moore (1969) emphasized volleyball and calesthenics, while Johnson (1969) and Kemper et al. (1978) studied the differential effects of five versus two or three days of physical education. However, Johnson and Kemper et al. did not describe the characteristics of the instructional program. Lack of information about the nature of the treatment involved in these studies prohibits a full understanding of the results. However, little reason is provided to discount the effects obtained in the other five. No gender or age characteristics appear related to incidences of effect significance.

The effects listed in Table 18 provide convincing evidence that physical education programs can significantly improve the muscular power of their participants. This same information highlights the fact that not all physical education programs will produce these outcomes. Rather, certain kinds of activities, in appropriate forms and amounts, in interaction with specific children and contexts, are required to obtain effects such as muscular power.

Muscular Strength

Muscular strength is a primary component in the performance of motor skills. It can be defined as the maximum force that can be exerted by a muscle or muscle group in one repetition. Muscular strength is closely related to muscular power and muscular endurance and it is important for both health-related and performance-related fitness. It is, therefore, a common and important criterion to consider when evaluating the effects of physical education programs on children.

Strength can be measured in many ways. Instruments that have been developed to measure this attribute include hand, back, and leg dynamometers, cable tensiometers, strain guages, cybex type machines and weight machines. Strength can also be measured through various calesthenic activities using little or no equipment. The use of calesthenics or other submaximal loading methods to measure strength (one repetition maximum) is based on the strong relationship that exists between muscular strength and muscular endurance.

Nine different studies are included in Table 19 that have tested the effects of a variety of physical education programs on muscular strength. Within the nine studies, 13 effects are reported, with 8 of those indicating significant changes attributed to the physical education program. Review of these effects indicates that significant gains in strength were obtained by both males and females at elementary and secondary school ages. Activities included in the programs, time allocated to instruction, teaching effectiveness, equipment, facilities, context, and children were all very different among the nine interventions. Even when many differences existed, there were apparently sufficient commonalities in treatment intensity, duration, frequency, and length to obtain a large proportion of success.

The information included in Table 19 provides convincing evidence that muscular strength can be improved within the context of physical education programs. It also provides evidence, however, that physical education programs can be ineffective in producing such changes. No evidence suggests that participating in programs of physical education results in losses of muscular strength.

Table 19
Effects of Physical Education Programs on the Acquisition of Muscular Strength

Study	Date	Test	Total Instructional Time (hrs.)	Characteristics Subjects Age	Gender	N	Teacher Type[a]	Design[b]	Result[c]	Repeatability[d]
Ansorge	1985	Bench Press	36+	16-17	M/F	385	PE	Comp.	NS	?
Newfield	1984	Pushups	?	6-8	M/F	3800	?	Comp.	NS	Yes
Duncan	1983	Pullups	96	10	M	13	PE/CR	Comp.	S	?
Franks	1969	Pullups	10	7-8	M/F	76	PE	Comp.	S	?
Johnson	1969	Pull-up	90-180	13	M	872	PE	Comp.	S	?
Grodjinovsky	1984	Grip	180	10-14	F	65	PE	Comp.	S	?
Grodjinovsky	1984	Grip	180	10-14	M	65	PE	Comp.	NS	?
Kemper	1978	Grip	90-180	12-13	M	70	PE	Comp.	S	?
Wittle	1961	Grip	?	12	M	162	?	Comp.	NS	No
Shephard	1980	Back	180	6-12	M/F	395	PE	Comp.	S	?
Wittle	1961	Back	?	12	M	162	?	Comp.	NS	No
Ansorge	1985	Leg Press	36+	16-17	M/F	385	PE	Comp.	NS	?
Wittle	1961	Leg	?	12	M	162	?	Comp.	S	No

[a] Teacher type: PE = Physical education specialist, CR = Classroom teacher, ? = Unreported
[b] Design: Comp. = Comparison group
[c] Results: S = Statistically significant difference, NS = Not statistically significant
[d] Repeatability: Yes = Evidence that the program can be replicated, No = Program replication unlikely, ? = Replication possibilities unknown

Perceptual-Motor

Due to the correlation that exists between intellectual and psychomotor variables for young, mentally impaired children or those with learning difficulties, psychologists and physical educators have introduced perceptual motor activities to the physical education programs of many elementary schools. According to Seefeldt (1974), the term "perceptual-motor programs" has received wide usage. However, the disparity in its meaning to various groups has rendered the term worthless in representing specific programs, content, or methodology. It can be defined, however, as the practice of using movement in the achievement of academic objectives.

As would be expected, difficulties associated with the definition of the term would also create difficulties for measuring its existence. Consequently, there are many tests of traits associated with the different perceptions of meaning associated with the term. This variability in test items is apparent in Table 20.

According to Seefeldt (1974), the symptoms of perceptual-motor dysfunction include an inabilty to establish balance and postural control, ineffective coordination of body parts, immature judgment of temporal-spatial relationships, and inadequte body image. The most extensive test published to measure attributes such as these is the Purdue Perceptual-Motor Survey (Roach & Kephart, 1966). It requires individual testing by qualified testers and is, therefore, inappropriate for mass testing. Other measures more suitable for mass testing are available in the literature. Although many of those available have suitable reliability, assessments of their validity are unavailable (Baumgartner & Jackson, 1982).

Five studies that have investigated the effects of physical education programs on perceptual-motor skills are included in Table 20. Within the five studies, 12 effects are reported and 8 of these are significant. Significant results were obtained for both males and females. No significant results were obtained, however, by groups over 12 years of age.

The nature of the program, tests selected, characteristics of the participants, and the context within which the study occurred can account for the differential results obtained. There is evidence that programs of physical education can significantly influence measures of perceptual-motor ability. It must be remembered, however, that the purpose for which many perceptual-motor programs are included in school programs revolves around the use of movement to achieve academic objectives. There is no evidence provided in these studies that physical education programs devoted to perceputal-motor activities can significantly alter academic achievement.

Personal-Social

Four studies measured the effects of their treatments on personal-social skills (see Table 21).

A review of Table 21 reveals that none of the effects measured were altered by the experimental treatment beyond the levels attained by the comparison groups. No evidence is provided, therefore, that programs of physical education can influence self-concept or personality.

Physical Fitness

A common goal of the majority of physical education programs is to develop physical fitness. Physical fitness has been defined in many different ways and significant differences of opinion remain regarding what definition is most appropriate. The term, therefore, only has clear meaning when viewed in terms of the specific characteristics that are measured or used in its operational definition.

Table 20
Effects of Physical Education Programs on the Acquisition of Perceptual Motor Skills

Study	Date	Test	Total Instructional Time (hrs.)	Characteristics Subjects Age	Gender	N	Teacher Type[a]	Design[b]	Result[c]	Repeatability[d]
Kemper	1978	Plate Tapping	90-180	12-13	M	70	PE	Comp.	NS	?
Lipton	1970	Purdue PMS	12	6	M/F	92	PE	Comp.	S	?
	1970	Dev. Test of Visual Perception	12	6	M/F	92	PE	Comp.	S	?
Moore	1984	Capon PMT	31.5	5	M/F	85	CR/Aide	Con.	NS	?
Thomas	1975	Shape-O Ball T	50	6	M/F	40	PE	Con.	S	?
Volle	1984	Height Perception	180	6-11	M/F	?	PE	Comp.	S	?
	1984	Arm Span	180	6-11	M/F	?	PE	Comp.	S	?
	1984	Verticality	180	6-11	M/F	?	PE	Comp.	S	?
	1984	Finger Recognition	180	6	M/F	?	PE	Comp.	NS	?
	1984	Finger Recognition	180	7	M/F	?	PE	Comp.	NS	?
	1984	Finger Recognition	180	8	M/F	?	PE	Comp.	S	?
	1984	Finger Recognition	180	9	M/F	?	PE	Comp.	S	?

[a] Teacher type: PE = Physical education specialist, CR = Classroom teacher
[b] Design: Comp. = Comparison group, Con. = Control group
[c] Results: S = Statistically significant difference, NS = Not statistically significant
[d] Repeatability: Yes = Evidence that the program can be replicated, ? = Replication possibilities unknown

Table 21
Effects of Physical Education Programs on the Acquisition of Personal-Social Skills

			Characteristics							
			Total Instructional	Subjects			Teacher			Repeat-
Study	Date	Test	Time (hrs.)	Age	Gender	N	Type[a]	Design[b]	Result[c]	ability[d]
Kuntzleman	1984	Self-Concept	27-39	7-12	F	420	?	Comp.	NS	?
	1984	Self-Concept	27-39	7-12	F	420	?	Comp.	NS	?
	1984	Self-Concept	31.5	5	M/F	85	CR/Aide	Con.	NS	?
Moore	1975	Parker S C Scale	50	6	M/F	40	PE	Con.	?	?
Thomas	1961	Personality	?	12	M	162	?	Comp.	NS	No
Wittle										

[a] Teacher type: PE = Physical education specialist, CR = Classroom teacher, ? = Unreported
[b] Design: Comp. = Comparison group, Con. = Control group
[c] Results: NS = Not statistically significant
[d] Repeatability: Yes = Evidence that the program can be replicated, No = Program replication unlikely, ? = Replication possibilities unknown

Table 22
Effects of Physical Education Programs on Physical Fitness

			Characteristics							
			Total Instructional	Subjects			Teacher			Repeat-
Study	Date	Test	Time (hrs.)	Age	Gender	N	Type[a]	Design[b]	Result[c]	ability[d]
Fabricus	1964	Oregon Motor FT	6.25	10	M/F	162	PE	Comp.	S	?
McAdam	1974	Illinois PFT	?	11	M/F	600	PE	Comp.	S	?
Vogel	1981	I CAN PFT	?	5-23	M/F	2-15	PE/CR	Comp.	S	Yes
Wittle	1961	Rogers PF Index	?	12	M	162	?	Comp.	S	No
	1961	Rogers Strength I	?	12	M	162	?	Comp.	S	No
	1961	Metheny-Johnson	?	12	M	162	?	Comp.	S	No
	1961	Indiana PFT	?	12	M	162	?	Comp.	S	No

[a] Teacher type: PE = Physical education specialist, CR = Classroom teacher, ? = Unreported
[b] Design: Comp. = Comparison group
[c] Results: S = Statistically significant difference
[d] Repeatability: Yes = Evidence that the program can be replicated, No = Program replication unlikely, ? = Replication possibilities unknown

Differentiations are made when assessing health-related fitness versus performance or motor fitness. Many different characteristics are measured when assessing physical fitness. Baumgartner and Jackson (1982) suggested that there are four general categories of information needed to assess fitness. They listed motor fitness, health related fitness, cardiorespiratory function, and body composition. Although the terms health-related and performance-related fitness may reduce miscommunication associated with the general term "physical fitness," they do not discriminate among the components measured in most test items. Independent of the two divisions or four categories suggested above, there is fairly common agreement about the components that are measured. They include: muscular strength, muscular endurance, cardiorespiratory endurance, muscular power, agility, speed, body composition, flexibility, oxygen consumption, and abdominal and low back function.

Tables 4-7, 10, 13, 17-19, 22 and 24 list many studies that have measured the effects of physical education programs on many of the components of physical fitness listed elsewhere in this chapter. The tables prior to and following Table 22 include information specific to the individual components of fitness. Table 22 includes four studies that reported the effects of physical education programs on composite measures of physical fitness. Seven effects were listed and all were significant.

Note that significant results were obtained in all of the measures taken. The programs, tests, characteristics of the participants, experimental contexts, instructors, and other factors within the five studies were different; yet the effects were similar. The program effects on individual components of physical education mentioned elsewhere in this chapter always resulted in a combination of significant and non-significant effects. In several of these studies, mean gains that were not significant were routinely obtained and some of the effects that were significant had very small mean gains. The combination of several components of fitness into a composite score, therefore, may result in an overestimate of independent program effects by masking small changes on individual components of fitness included in the composite score.

The information included in Table 22 provides evidence that programs of physical education can significantly improve physical fitness, as measured by composite physical fitness tests. Although it is not apparent in the table, high scores on some components of the composite could mask small, insignificant gains on other components of the composite measure while maintaining an overall significant effect.

Speed

Speed can be defined as the ability to move rapidly. Rapid movement is important to the performance of most motor skills and speed, therefore, is usually listed among the components of motor fitness. Speed is typically measured using a short dash. Laboratory methods are more sophisticated and many reports have fractionated speed of movement into smaller divisions, such as reaction time and movement time.

Table 23 includes the results of studies that have measured the effect of physical education programs on the shuttle run, short dashes, and a short obstacle course. These measures were selected as indicators of program effects because of their speed requirements. Each of the measures included in Table 23 is also influenced by other components of performance related fitness (muscular power, strength, agility and coordination) and by improvements in skill. True causes of significant differences, therefore, cannot be attributed only to speed.

Eight studies and 11 effects are included in Table 23. Of the 11 effects, 5 were significant and 6 were not. The results do not appear to be related to gender or age

Table 23
Effects of Physical Education Programs on Speed

			Characteristics							
			Total Instructional	Subjects			Teacher			Repeat-
Study	Date	Test	Time (hrs.)	Age	Gender	N	Type[a]	Design[b]	Result[c]	ability[d]
Burkett	1984	Shuttle Run	?	14-17	M/F	164	PE/Aide	Comp.	S	Yes
Duncan	1983	Shuttle Run	96	10	M/F	34	PE/CR	Comp.	NS	?
Franks	1969	Shuttle Run	10	7-8	M/F	76	PE	Comp.	NS	?
Johnson	1969	Shuttle Run	90-180	13	M	372	PE	Comp.	NS	?
Kemper	1978	Shuttle Run	90-180	12-13	M	70	PE	Comp.	NS	?
Shephard	1980b	Shuttle Run	180	6-12	M/F	395	PE	Comp.	S	?
Masche	1970	Obstacle Race	10	7-8	M/F	48	PE	Comp.	NS	?
Duncan	1983	50 Yd Dash	96	10	M/F	34	PE/CR	Comp.	NS	?
Franks	1969	50 Yd Dash	10	7-8	M/F	76	PE	Comp.	S	?
Newfield	1984	Dash	?	6-8	M/F	3800	?	Comp.	S	Yes
Shephard	1980	50 Yd Dash	180	6-12	M/F	395	PE	Comp.	S	?

[a] Teacher type: PE = Physical education specialist, CR = Classroom teacher, ? = Unreported
[b] Design: Comp. = Comparison group
[c] Results: S = Statistically significant difference, NS = Not statistically significant
[d] Repeatability: Yes = Evidence that the program can be replicated, ? = Replication possibilities unknown

because significant results were reported for both elementary and secondary age males and females. Only two of the studies, Burkett (1984) and Newfield and Baumgartner (1984) provided evidence supporting their ability to be replicated in other sites. Lack of descriptive characteristics associated with the other studies mentioned elsewhere in this chapter limits the interpretation of the results.

The studies included in Table 23 provide evidence that appropriately designed and implemented physical education programs can improve the speed of movement of their participants. The information in Table 23 also provides evidence that not all physical education programs are effective in facilitating this capacity. This statement is obviously limited to the treatments, characteristics of the subjects, experimental context and the measures used. No evidence is provided that the participation in physical education programs referred to in Table 23 deters or reduces the development of speed.

Other Effects

Several other variables were measured as part of the studies reporting effects of participation in physical education programs. These effects are reported in Table 24.

Review of Table 24 suggests that the measures of some form of lung volume (Bar-Or, 1972; Kemper, 1978 and Wittle, 1961) were unaltered by participation in the physical education programs studied by those authors. Similarly, Kuntzleman (1984) obtained no significant reduction between experimental and comparison subjects in total triglicerides or systolic blood pressure.

There is evidence that the program implemented by Kuntzleman was significantly more effective than the comparison program for both males and females, aged 7 to 12, when cholesterol levels, HDL-C, risk factors and diastolic blood pressures were tested. Also, Shephard (1980b) found significant differences between experimental and comparison males and females in the quantity of sleep obtained per night, with the experimental subjects sleeping less even though their activity levels were significantly higher than those of the comparison group.

The studies listed in Table 24 provide evidence, within the limitations of their design, implementation and precision of reporting that physical education programs can significantly alter several "other" important outcome variables.

Quality of the Information on the Effects of Programs

Review of the literature describing the effects of physical education on children is both encouraging and discouraging. The encouraging aspect of the review is that many of the effects of activity reported in the research literature have also been obtained as a result of participation in physical education programs. The discouraging aspects of the review are the inferior scientific quality of the studies that have investigated the association between physical education programs and their outcomes. Many of the studies reported have flaws in design, implementation and/or reporting that restrict interpretation of the results.

The most serious flaws in the information reviewed were those resulting from weak experimental designs. Throughout the literature, there is evidence of designs which provide rival interpretations of program effect, that are equally or more convincing than the experimental effect. The consequences of these design problems can range from incorrectly ascribing program effects to the experimental treatment when they were not present, to accepting no experimental effect when a treatment effect was present.

Design invalidities such as maturation, history, and selection (Campbell & Stanley, 1971) are common in the literature. Due to the rapid growth of children and the need for extended treatments to obtain some program effects, studies that

Table 24
Effects of Physical Education Programs on Other Outcomes

Study	Date	Test	Total Instructional Time (hrs.)	Characteristics				Teacher Type[a]	Design[b]	Result[c]	Repeatability[d]
				Subjects							
				Age	Gender	N					
Bar-Or	1972	Vital Capacity	12-24	9-10	M/F	91		?	Comp.	NS	?
Wittle	1961	Vital Capacity	?	12	M	162		?	Comp.	NS	No
Bar-Or	1972	Forced Expiratory Vol	12-24	9-10	M/F	91		?	Comp.	NS	?
	1972	Max VE	12-24	9-10	M/F	91		?	Comp.	NS	?
	1972	FEV%	12-24	9-10	M/F	91		?	Comp.	NS	?
Kemper	1978	FEV%	90-180	12-13	M	70		PE	Comp.	NS	?
Kuntzleman	1984	Cholesterol	27-39	7-12	M/F	420		?	Comp.	S	?
	1984	+ Shift in Risk Factor	27-39	7-12	M/F	420		?	Comp.	S	?
	1984	Systolic BP	27-39	7-12	M/F	420		?	Comp.	NS	?
	1984	Diastolic BP	27-39	7-12	M/F	420		?	Comp.	S	?
Shephard	1980	Sleep	180	10-12	M/F	300		PE	Comp.	S	?

[a] Teacher type: PE = Physical education specialist, CR = Classroom teacher, ? = Unreported
[b] Design: Comp. = Comparison group
[c] Results: S = Statistically significant difference, NS = Not statistically significant
[d] Repeatability: Yes = Evidence that the program can be replicated, No = Program replication unlikely, ? = Replication possibilities unknown

do not control for maturation provide little or no usable evidence. The control of history is also critical to appropriate interpretation of effects. Whittle, in 1961, published evidence of the important influence that participation in youth sport programs has on achievement in physical education. In recent years, the potential for subjects to be affected by such programs has dramatically increased; yet studies are continually designed which do not control for this effect. Improper selection of study samples also limits interpretation. Several instances of effects were reported for individuals who were skilled performers, interested in a given sport and selected on the basis of skill. These subjects were then assigned to a special school, where additional time for sports and physical education was provided. The individuals were then compared to students in regular programs. Data obtained from such a study is severely restricted for determining program effects of a physical education program.

Selection of control and/or comparison groups also influences the interpretation of results. The vast majority of studies investigating the effects of physical education programs compare the results of an experimental treatment with an alternative treatment. Such comparisons are useful when making a choice between two or more programs (or program components) when the effectiveness of the comparison group is known or can be assumed. Without such evidence, investigators have frequently concluded that non-significant differences indicates that no effects were present, when in fact, the experimental and comparison programs may both be effective, but not significantly different in their effects.

Research studies and program evaluations require considerable effort, whether or not the design of the study is well conceived. Appropriate design and planning facilitates all aspects of the work and provides opportunities for clear, potential use of the results. Such evidence, which clarifies the strengths and weaknesses that may exist within physical education programs, is critically needed to advance the status of our programs.

Need for Effectiveness Information

Persons who are responsible for appropriating resources to programs of physical education are interested in understanding the extent to which their appropriations influence important outcomes. In many schools it is assumed that when children are active participants in a program of physical activities, significant outcomes in fitness, skills, attitudes, and knowledge will occur. The differential effects reported in the studies included in this chapter and observation of the performance qualities of graduates from our programs provide strong evidence that this assumption is false. We can argue that our individual programs are effective, but can we support our assertions with evidence? Individuals who have observed our performance are skeptical. Iverson, Fielding, Crow, and Christenson (1985), reporting in a special section of Public Health Reports on public health aspects of physical activity and exercise, think not. They state, "It appears that a major opportunity to influence favorable physical activity in the United States is being missed in the schools. A large majority of students are enrolled in physical education classes, but the classes appear to have little effect on the current physical fitness levels of children and, furthermore, have little impact on developing life-long physical activity skills."

There is evidence that programs of physical education can be effective. Some of that evidence is cited in previous sections of this chapter and is briefly summarized below. Rarely, however, is evidence of effectiveness available to the taxpayers, administrators, board members, or others in local communities who are responsible for allocation of funds. These individuals are much more interested in details associated with educational "outcomes" than educational "inputs." Programs must be able to provide evidence that they are effective facilitators of outcomes that the community views as important or the resources necessary to support them will continue to erode.

Criteria for Obtaining Evidence of Program Effectiveness

There are many criteria that can be used to judge the evidence of effectiveness in support of an educational program. As suggested by Tallmadge (1977), convincing evidence of effectiveness is accumulated when studies are conducted in a such a way that each of the following questions can be answered affirmatively:
1. Did a change occur?
2. Was the effect consistent enough and observed often enough to be statistically significant?
3. Was the effect educationally significant?
4. Can the intervention be implemented in another location with a reasonable expectation of comparable impact?
5. How likely is it that observed effects resulted from the intervention?
6. Is the evidence presented believable and interpretable?

Other criteria that have traditionally been used to assess program quality have focused on program "inputs" (facilities, equipment, staffing, time) and/or program "processes" (content selection and placement, methods of instruction, frequency and duration of classes, and others). For example, of 36 evaluative items included in the Assessment Guide for Secondary School Physical Education (American Alliance for Health, Physical Education and Recreation, 1977), none address questions related to providing evidence of program effectiveness. Although it is important to document selected input and process variables, they must be studied in relation to "program outcomes" before one can interpret their meaning for improving physical education programs.

By following the suggestions outlined by Tallmadge (1977), it is possible to answer questions of effectiveness with data that is convincing to those responsible for allocating resources. Without such evidence, programs will continue to lose support, and prospects for demonstrating significant effects will diminish. This chapter provides evidence, with abundant examples that such evidence can be acquired. The responsibility to make it happen belongs to the members of our profession, not educators or administrators. If we do not accept the responsibility, others less knowledgeable about the profession will do so.

Summary of Effects

All of the effects included in Tables 2-24 may not be obtainable by individuals participating in a specific school district. The time allocated to instruction for all the effects reported here would, no doubt, far exceed what is commonly available in a single program. The effects obtained are also associated with unique program treatments, student characteristics, school and community contexts, design limitations, instructional effectiveness, limitations of the treatment-measurement match, degree to which the instruments represent the capacities they were selected to measure, quality of data collection procedures, data analysis, and reporting accuracy. The mixed results typical within each outcome area underscore that the effects observed do not occur in all physical education programs. Programs must be appropriately designed, implemented, and evaluated in accordance with what is known about the uniqueness of circumstances within which significant or non-significant effects were obtained.

The statements listed below serve as a summary of the evidence reported in the outcome areas listed elsewhere in this chapter. These statements must be interpreted in terms of the strengths and weaknesses of the studies they represent. As such they provide an indication of what can occur when programs are conducted in a manner similar to those from which the significant effects were obtained.

1. There is evidence that participation in physical education programs can contribute (probably indirectly) to student performance on academic measures. More importantly, it appears that more time could be allocated to instruction in physical education with no disadvantage to academic performance.
2. There is convincing evidence that participation in physical education programs can influence desirable shifts in student physical activity levels.
3. There is convincing evidence that participation in physical education programs can improve aerobic fitness.
4. There is little evidence that participation in physical education programs can improve aerobic/anaerobic fitness.
5. There is limited or no evidence that participation in physical education programs can improve agility-coordination.
6. There is little or no evidence that participation in physical education programs can improve anaerobic fitness.
7. There is evidence that participation in physical education programs can significantly influence how children feel about physical activity and health-fitness.
8. There is evidence that participation in physical education programs can improve static balance.
9. There is evidence that participation in physical education programs can positively alter body composition.
10. There is little or no evidence that participation in physical education programs can significantly alter height, weight, or girth.
11. There is little or no evidence that participation in physical education programs can alter nutritional practices.
12. There is evidence that participation in physical education programs can improve flexibility of the hip and spine. There is also evidence that flexibility of the ankle may be reduced with physical education participation.
13. There is convincing evidence that participation in physical education programs can improve knowledge relative to healthy lifestyles.
14. There is no evidence that participation in physical education programs can accelerate or retard the maturation process.
15. There is convincing evidence that participation in physical education programs can improve motor performance.
16. There is convincing evidence that participation in physical education programs can improve muscular endurance.
17. There is convincing evidence that participation in physical education programs can improve muscular power.
18. There is convincing evidence that participation in physical education programs can improve muscular strength.
19. There is evidence that participation in physical education programs can improve performance on selected measures of perceptual ability. There is no evidence, however, that these effects directly improve academic achievement.
20. There is no evidence that participation in physical education programs can improve self-concept or personality.
21. There is convincing evidence that participation in physical education programs can improve physical fitness.
22. There is evidence that participation in physical education programs can improve movement speed.
23. There is evidence that participation in physical education programs can improve several other important outcome areas, including blood cholesterol, HDL-C, risk factor reduction, and diastolic blood pressure.

References

American Alliance for Health, Physical Education and Recreation. (1977). *Assessment guide for secondary school physical education programs*. Reston, VA: Author.

American College of Sports Medicine. (1983). Position stand on proper and improper weight loss programs. *Medicine and Science In Sports and Exercise, 15*(1), ix-x.

Ansorge, C.J., Schier, J.K., Wandzilak, T., Potter, G., Schmidt, R., & Petrakis, E. (1985). *Effects of a model 11-week physical education program on fitness, body fat, strength, flexibility, and health knowledge*. Unpublished manuscript.

Bar-Or, O., & Zwiren, L.D. (1972). Physiological effects of increased frequency of physical education classes and of endurance conditioning on 9 to 10 year old girls and boys. In O. Bar-Or (Ed.), *Pediatric Work Physiology: Proceedings of the Fourth International Symposium* (pp. 183-198). Natanya, Israel: Wingate Institute.

Baumgartner, T.A., & Jackson, A.S. (1982). *Measurement for evaluation in physical education*. Dubuque, IA: Brown.

Bradfield, R.B., Chan, H., Bradfield, N.E., & Payne, P.R. (1971). Energy expenditures and heart rates of Cambridge boys at school. *American Journal of Clinical Nutrition, 24*, 1461-1466.

Burkett, L.N. (1984). *PEOPEL impact data results, 1983-1984*. Unpublished report. Arizona State University, Department of Physical Education, Tempe, Arizona.

Campbell, D.T., & Stanley, J.C. (1971). *Experimental and quasi-experimental designs for research*. Chicago: Rand McNally.

Caspersen, C.J., Powell, K.E., & Christenson, G.M. (1985). Physical activity, exercise, and physical fitness: Definitions and distinctions for health-related research. *Public Health Reports, 100*, 126-130.

Clarke, H.H. (1973). Individual differences, their nature, extent and significance. *Physical Fitness Research Digest, 3*(4), 1-23.

Cooper, K.H., Purdy, J.G., Friedman, A., Bohannon, R.L., Harris, R.A., & Arends, J.A. (1975). An aerobics conditioning program for the Fort Worth, Texas school district. *Research Quarterly, 46*, 345-350.

Duncan, B., Boyce, W.T., Itami, R., & Puffenbarger, N. (1983). A controlled trial of a physical fitness program for fifth grade students. *Journal of School Health, 53*(8), 467-471.

Fabricus, H. (1964). Effect of added calisthenics on the physical fitness of fourth grade boys and girls. *Research Quarterly, 35*, 135-140.

Franks, B.D., & Moore, G.C. (1969). Effects of calisthenics and volleyball on the AAHPER fitness test and volleyball skill. *Research Quarterly, 40*(2), 288-292.

Gaisl, G., & Buchberger, J. (1984). Changes in the aerobic-anaerobic transition in boys after 3 years of special physical education. In J. Ilmarinen & I. Vaelimaeki (Eds.), *Children and sport: Paediatric work physiology* (pp. 156-161). Berlin: Springer-Verlag.

Gilliam, T.B., MacConnie, S.E., Greenen, D.L., Pels, A.E., & Freedson, P.S. (1982). Exercise program for children: A way to prevent heart disease? *The Physician and Sportsmedicine, 10*(9), 96-101, 105-106, 108.

Goode, R.C., Virgin, A., Romet, T.T., Crawford, P., Duffin, J., Pallandi, T., & Woch, Z. (1976). Effects of a short period of physical activity in adolescent boys and girls. *Canadian Journal of Applied Sport Sciences, 1*, 241-250.

Grodjinovsky, A., & Bar-Or, O. (1984). Influence of added physical education hours upon anaerobic capacity, adiposity, and grip strength in 12-13 year old children enrolled in a sports class. In J. Ilmarinen, and I. Vaelimaeki (Eds.), *Children and sport: Paediatric work physiology* (pp. 162-169). Berlin: Springer-Verlag.

Iverson, D.C., Fielding, J.E., Crow, R.S., & Christenson, G.M. (1985). The promotion of physical activity in the United States population: The status of programs in medical, worksite, community and school settings. *Public Health Reports, 100,* 212-224.

Johnson, L.C. (1969). Effects of 5-day-a-week vs. 2-and-3-day-a-week physical education class on fitness, skill, adipose tissue and growth. *Research Quarterly, 40,* 93-98.

Jones, M.C. & Bayley, N. (1950). Physical maturity among boys as related to behavior. *Journal of Educational Psychology, 41,* 129-148.

Kemper, H.C.G., Verschurr, R., Koos, G.A.R., Snel, J., Splinter, P.G., & Tavecchio, L.W.R. (1978). Investigation into the effects of two extra physical education lessons per week during one school year upon the physical development of 12-13-year old boys. *Medicine Sport, 11,* 159-166.

Koplan, J.P., Siscovick, D.S., & Goldbaum, G.M. (1985). The risks of exercise: A public health view of injuries and hazards. *Public Health Reports, 100,* 189-195.

Kuntzleman, C.T., Drake, D.A., & Kuntzleman, B.A. (1984). *Feelin' good: Youth fitness report—summary.* Spring Arbor, MI: Fitness Finders.

LaPort, R.E., Montoye, H.J. & Caspersen, C.J. (1985). Assessment of physical activity in epidemiologic research: Problems and prospects. *Public Health Reports, 100,* 131-146.

LaPort, W.D. (1955). *Health and physical education score card number one for elementary schools.* Los Angeles: University of Southern California Press.

Lipton, E.D. (1970). A perceptual-motor development program's effect on visual perception and reading readiness of first grade children. *Research Quarterly, 41,* 402-405.

Malina, R.M. (1986). Physical growth and maturation. In V.D. Seefeldt (Ed.), *Physical Activity and Well-being.* Reston, VA: American Alliance for Health, Physical Education, Recreation and Dance.

Masche, K.A. (1970). Effects of two different programs of instruction on motor performance of second grade students. *Research Quarterly, 41,* 406-411.

McAdam, R. (1974, Winter). One small step. *Illinois Journal,* p. 17.

Mocellin, R. & Wasmund, V. (1972). Investigations on the influence of a running-training program on the cardiovascular and motor performance capacity in 53 boys and girls of a second and third primary school class. In O. Bar-Or (Ed.), *Pediatric work physiology: Proceedings of the Fourth International Symposium* (pp. 279-285). Natanya, Israel: Wingate Institute.

Moody, D.L., Wilmore, J.H., Girandola, R.N., & Royce, J.P. (1972). The effects of a jogging program on the body composition of normal and obese high school girls. *Medicine and Science in Sports, 4,* 210-213.

Moore, J.B., Guy, L.M., & Reeve, T.G. (1984). Effects of the capon perceptual-motor program on motor ability, self-concept, and academic readiness. *Perceptual and Motor Skills, 58,* 71-74.

Mussen, P.H., & Jones. M.C. (1957). Self-conceptions, motivations and interpersonal attitudes of late and early maturing boys. *Child Development, 28,* 242-256.

Newfield, J., & Baumgartner, T. (Undated). *Every child a winner impact study: 1982-83 final evaluation report.* Ocilla, GA: Irwin County Schools.

Osness, W. (Undated). *Sunflower project follow up study.* Unpublished manuscript. University of Kansas, Department of Physical Education, Lawrence.

Roach, E.G., & Kephart, N.C. (1966). *The Purdue Perceptual-Motor Survey.* Columbus: Merrill.

Sargeant, A.J., Dolan, P., & Thorne, A. (1985). Effects of supplemental physical activity on body composition, aerobic and anaerobic power in 13-year-old boys. In R.A. Binkhorst, H.C.G. Kemper, & W.H.M. Saris (Eds.), *Children and exercise XI* (pp. 135-139). Champaign, IL: Human Kinetics.

Seefeldt, V. (1974). Perceptual-motor programs. *Exercise and Sport Sciences Re-*

views, 2, 265-288.

Seliger, V., Trefany, S., Bartunkova, S., & Paver, M. (1974). The habitual activity and physical fitness of twelve year old boys. *Acta Paediatrica Belg., 28,* 54-59.

Shephard, R. J., Jequier, J.C., Lavallee, H., LaBarre, R., & Rajic, M. (1980). Habitual physical activity: Effects of sex, milieu, season and required activity. *Journal of Sports Medicine, 20,* 55-66.

Shephard, R.J., Lavallee, H., Jequier, J.C., Rajic, M., & LaBarre, R. (1980). Additional physical education in the primary school: A preliminary analysis of the Trois-Rivieres regional experiment. In M. Ostyn, G. Beunen, and J. Simmons (Eds.), *Kinanthropometry II: International Series on sport science, volume 9* (pp. 306-316). Baltimore, MD: University Park Press.

Shephard, R.J., Volle, M., Lavallee, H. LaBarre, R., Jequier, J.C., & Rajic, M. (1984). Required physical activity and academic grades: A controlled study. In J. Ilmarinen & I. Vaelimaeki (Eds.), *Children and sport: Paediatric work physiology* (pp. 58-63). Berlin: Springer-Verlag.

Siegel, J.A., & Manfredi, T.G. (1984). Effects of a ten month fitness program on children. *The Physician and Sportsmedicine, 12*(5), 91-97.

Thaxton, A.B., Rothstern, A.L., & Thaxton, N.A. (1977). Comparative effectiveness of two methods of teaching physical education to elementary school girls. *Research Quarterly, 48,* 420-427.

Tallmadge, G.K. (1977). *The joint dissemination review panel ideabook* (DHEW Publication). Washington, D.C.: U.S. Government Printing Office.

Thomas, J.R., Chissom, B.S., Stewart, C., & Shelley, F. (1975). Effects of perceptual motor training on preschool children: A multivariate approach. *Research Quarterly, 46,* 505-513.

Vogel, P., & Wessel, J. (1981, November). *Evidence of Effectiveness of the I CAN instructional physical education system.* Occasional Report. Michigan State University, Health and Physical Education Department, East Lansing.

Volle, M., Tisal, H., LaBarre, R., Lavallee, H., Shephard, R.J., Jequier, J.C., & Rajic, M. (1984). Required physical activity and psychomotor development of primary school children. In J. Ilmarinen & I. Vaelimaeki (Eds.), *Children and sport: Paediatric Work Physiology* (pp. 53-57). Berlin: Springer-Verlag.

Wittle, H.D. (1961). Effects of elementary school physical education upon aspects of physical, motor and personality development. *Research Quarterly, 32,* 249-260.

Appendix
Overview of the Studies in Tables 2 through 24
Listed Alphabetically by Author

Author	Date	Outcome	Test	Age	Gender	N	Result
Ansorge	1985	Body Size/Shape	U Arm Girth	16-17	M/F	385	NS
	1985	Knowledge	Health Knowledge	16-17	M/F	385	S
	1985	Aerobic Fitness	1.5 Mile Run	16-17	M/F	385	NS
	1985	Flexibility	Sit & Reach	16-17	M/F	385	NS
	1985	M. Strength	Leg Press	16-17	M/F	385	NS
	1985	M. Strength	Bench Press	16-17	M/F	385	NS
Bar-Or	1972	Other Biological	Vital Capacity	9-10	M/F	91	NS
	1972	Other Biological	Forced Expiratory Vol.	9-10	M/F	91	NS
	1972	Other Biological	Max VE	9-10	M/F	91	NS
	1972	Aerobic Fitness	HR Reduction	9-10	M	44	S
	1972	Aerobic/Anaerobic Fit.	HR Reduction	9-10	M	44	S
	1972	Aerobic Fitness	HR Reduction	9-10	F	48	NS
	1972	Aerobic/Anaerobic Fit.	HR Reduction	9-10	F	48	NS
	1972	Other	Vital Capacity (FEV)	9-10	M/F	92	NS
Burkett	1984	Agility/Coordination	Shuttle Run	14-17	M/F	164	S
	1984	Speed	Shuttle Run	14-17	M/F	164	S
	1984	M. Power	Shuttle Run	14-17	M/F	164	S
	1984	Motor Performance	Shuttle Run	14-17	M/F	164	S
	1984	M. Endurance	Flexed Arm Hang	14-17	M/F	164	S
	1984	M. Endurance	Situps	14-17	M/F	164	S
	1984	Flexibility	Sit & Reach	14-17	M/F	164	S
	1984	Attitude	Wears Attitude Scale	14-17	M/F	164	S
	1984	Aerobic Fitness	600 Run	14-17	M/F	164	S
Cooper	1975	Aerobic Fitness	12 Min Run	15	M	1215	S
Duncan	1983	Flexibility	Ankle	10	M/F	34	S
	1983	Flexibility	Sit and Reach	10	M/F	34	S
	1983	M. Strength	Pullups	10	M	13	S
	1983	M. Endurance	Flexed Arm Hang	10	F	21	NS
	1983	M. Endurance	Situps	10	M/F	34	S
	1983	M. Power	Long Jump	10	M/F	34	NS
	1983	Agility/Coordination	Shuttle Run	10	M/F	34	NS
	1983	Speed	Shuttle Run	10	M/F	34	NS
	1983	M. Power	Shuttle Run	10	M/F	34	NS
	1983	Motor Performance	Shuttle Run	10	M/F	34	NS
	1983	Speed	50 Yd Dash	10	M/F	34	NS
	1983	Aerobic Fitness	1 Mile Run	10	M/F	34	S
Fabricus	1964	Physical Fitness	Oregon Motor Ft	10	M/F	162	S
Franks	1969	Motor Performance	VB Wall Volley	7-8	M/F	76	NS
	1969	Motor Performance	Long Jump	7-8	M/F	76	NS

Appendix (continued)
Overview of the Studies in Tables 2 through 24
Listed Alphabetically by Author

Author	Date	Outcome	Test	Age	Gender	N	Result
Franks	1969	Motor Performance	Shuttle Run	7-8	M/F	76	NS
	1969	Motor Performance	VB Serve	7-8	M/F	76	NS
	1969	Motor Performance	Softball Throw	7-8	M/F	76	NS
	1969	M. Endurance	Situps	7-8	M/F	76	S
	1969	M. Endurance	600 Run/Walk	7-8	M/F	76	S
	1969	M. Strength	Pullups	7-8	M/F	76	S
	1969	Speed	50 Yd Dash	7-8	M/F	76	S
	1969	Agility/Coordinating	Shuttle Run	7-8	M/F	76	NS
	1969	Speed	Shuttle Run	7-8	M/F	76	NS
Franks	1969	M. Power	Shuttle Run	7-8	M/F	76	NS
	1969	M. Power	50 Yd Dash	7-8	M/F	76	S
	1969	M. Power	Long Jump	7-8	M/F	76	NS
	1969	Aerobic/Anaerobic Fit.	600 Run/Walk	7-8	M/F	76	NS
Gaisl	1984	Aerobic Fitness	Max $\dot{V}O_2$	10-14	M	28	NS
	1984	Aerobic Fitness	PWC170	10-14	M	28	S
	1984	Aerobic Fitness	$\dot{V}O_2$	10-14	M	28	NS
	1984	Aerobic Fitness	% $\dot{V}O_2$ Max	10-14	M	28	NS
	1984	Aerobic/Anaerobic Fit.	H R Reduction	10-14	M	28	S
	1984	Aerobic/Anaerobic Fit.	Work Rate	10-14	M	28	NS
	1984	Anaerobic Fitness	$\dot{V}O_2$	10-14	M	28	S
	1984	Anaerobic Fitness	% $\dot{V}O_2$ Max	10-14	M	28	S
Gilliam	1982	Activity Level	H R out-of-class	6-7	M/F	26	S
	1982	Activity Level	H R in-class	6-7	M/F	59	S
Goode	1976	Aerobic Fitness	Max $\dot{V}O_2$	12	M	111	NS
	1976	Aerobic Fitness	PWC170	12	M	111	NS
	1976	Aerobic Fitness	PWC170	14	M	103	S
	1976	Aerobic Fitness	PWC170	14	F	103	S
	1976	Body Size & Shape	Height	12	M	111	S
	1976	Body Size & Shape	Height	13	M	103	S
	1976	Body Size & Shape	Height	13	F	103	NS
	1976	Body Size & Shape	Height	14	M	103	NS
	1976	Body Size & Shape	Height	14	F	103	NS
	1976	Body Size & Shape	Weight	12	M	111	NS
	1976	Body Size & Shape	Weight	13	M	111	NS
	1976	Body Size & Shape	Weight	13	F	111	NS

Appendix (continued)
Overview of the Studies in Tables 2 through 24
Listed Alphabetically by Author

Author	Date	Outcome	Test	Age	Gender	N	Result
Goode	1976	Body Size & Shape	Weight	14	M	103	S
	1976	Body Size & Shape	Weight	14	F	103	NS
	1976	Body Composition	Triceps	12	M	111	NS
	1976	Body Composition	Triceps	13	M	103	NS
	1976	Body Composition	Triceps	13	F	103	NS
	1976	Body Composition	Triceps	14	M	103	NS
	1976	Body Composition	Triceps	14	F	103	NS
	1976	Body Composition	Suprailliac	12	M	111	NS
	1976	Body Composition	Suprailliac	13	M	103	NS
	1976	Body Composition	Suprailliac	13	F	103	NS
	1976	Body Composition	Suprailliac	14	M	103	NS
	1976	Body Composition	Suprailliac	14	F	103	NS
	1976	Body Composition	Sub-scapular	13	F	103	NS
	1976	Body Composition	Sub-scapular	13	M	103	NS
	1976	Body Composition	Sub-scapular	14	F	103	NS
	1976	Body Composition	Sub-scapular	14	M	103	NS
	1976	Aerobic Fitness	12 Min Run	12	F	111	S
	1976	Aerobic Fitness	Max $\dot{V}O_2$	13	M	111	NS
	1976	Aerobic/Anaerobic Fit.	600 Run	13	M	103	NS
	1976	Aerobic/Anaerobic Fit.	600 Run	13	F	103	NS
	1976	Aerobic/Anaerobic Fit.	600 Run	14	F	103	NS
	1976	Aerobic/Anaerobic Fit.	600 Run	14	M	103	NS
	1976	Aerobic Fitness	12 Min Run	13	M	103	S
	1976	Aerobic Fitness	12 Min. Run	14	M	103	NS
	1976	Aerobic Fitness	Max $\dot{V}O_2$	13	F	103	S
	1976	Aerobic Fitness	Max $\dot{V}O_2$	14	F	103	S
	1976	Aerobic Fitness	Max $\dot{V}O_2$	14	M	103	S
Grodjinovsky	1984	Anaerobic Fitness	Peak Power	10-14	M/F	65	S
	1984	Anaerobic Fitness	Mean Power	10-14	M/F	65	S
	1984	M. Strength	Grip	10-14	F	65	S
	1984	M. Strength	Grip	10-14	M	65	NS
	1984	Body Composition		10-14	M	65	NS

Appendix (continued)
Overview of the Studies in Tables 2 through 24
Listed Alphabetically by Author

Author	Date	Outcome	Test	Age	Gender	N	Result
Grodjinovsky	1984	Body Composition		10-14	F	65	S
	1984	Body Size/ Shape	Height	10-14	M/F	65	NS
	1984	Body Size/ Shape	Weight	10-14	M/F	65	NS
Johnson	1969	Body Composition	Triceps	13	M	372	S
	1969	Body Composition	Triceps	13	F	472	NS
	1969	Aerobic/ Anaerobic Fit.	600 Run Walk	13	M/F	844	NS
	1969	M. Power	S Long Jump	13	M/F	844	S
	1969	M. Power	Vertical Jump	13	M	372	NS
	1969	M. Power	Shuttle Run	13	M	372	NS
	1969	M. Endurance	Curl-up	13	F	472	NS
	1969	M. Endurance	Flexed Arm Hang	13	F	472	NS
	1969	M. Endurance	Push-up	13	M	372	S
	1969	M. Strength	Pull-up	13	M	372	S
	1969	Motor Performance	Long Jump	13	M/F	844	S
	1969	Motor Performance	Vertical Jump	13	M	372	NS
	1969	Motor Performance	Shuttle Run	13	M	372	NS
	1969	Motor Performance	Volleyball	13	M/F	844	S
	1969	Motor Performance	Basketball	13	F	472	NS
	1969	Motor Performance	Soccer	13	M	372	S
	1969	Speed	Shuttle Run	13	M	372	NS
	1969	Agility/ Coordination	Shuttle Run	13	M	372	NS
Kemper	1978	M. Strength	Grip	12-13	M	70	S
	1978	Motor Performance		12-13	M	70	S
	1978	Other Biological	FEV %	12-13	M	70	NS
	1978	Body Size/ Shape	Upper Arm Girth	12-13	M	70	NS
	1978	Body Composition	% Fat	12-13	M	70	NS
	1978	Perceptual Motor	Plate Tapping	12-13	M	70	NS
	1978	Agility/ Coordination	Shuttle Run	12-13	M	70	NS
	1978	Speed	Shuttle Run	12-13	M	70	NS
	1978	M. Power	Shuttle Run	12-13	M	70	NS
	1978	Motor Performance	Shuttle Run	12-13	M	70	NS
	1978	M. Endurance	Flexed Arm Hang	12-13	M	70	NS
	1978	Aerobic Fitness	PWC170	12-13	M	70	NS
Kuntzleman	1984	Body Composition	Skinfolds	7-12	M/F	420	S

Appendix (continued)
Overview of the Studies in Tables 2 through 24
Listed Alphabetically by Author

Author	Date	Outcome	Test	Age	Gender	N	Result
Kuntzleman	1984	Body Size/Shape	Chest Girth	7-12	M/F	420	NS
	1984	Body Size/Shape	Waist Girth	7-12	M/F	420	NS
	1984	Aerobic Fitness	1 Mile Run	7-12	M/F	420	NS
	1984	Aerobic Fitness	PWC HR 5 Min.	7-12	M/F	420	NS
	1984	Aerobic Fitness	PWC SBP 5 Min.	7-12	M/F	420	NS
	1984	Aerobic Fitness	PWC Peak Work	7-12	M/F	420	S
	1984	Aerobic Fitness	PWC Total Work	7-12	M/F	420	S
	1984	Aerobic Fitness	PWC HR Recovery	7-12	M/F	420	NS
	1984	Other	Cholesterol	7-12	M/F	420	S
	1984	Other	HDL-C	7-12	M/F	420	S
	1984	Other	+ Shift in Risk Factor	7-12	M/F	420	S
	1984	Other	Total Triglycerides	7-12	M/F	420	NS
	1984	Other	Systolic BP	7-12	M/F	420	NS
	1984	Diet	Total Calories	7-12	M/F	420	NS
	1984	Diet	Simple Carbohydrates	7-12	M/F	420	S
	1984	Diet	Sodium	7-12	M/F	420	NS
	1984	Diet	Potassium	7-12	M/F	420	S
	1984	Diet	Fat	7-12	M/F	420	NS
	1984	Other	Diastolic BP	7-12	M/F	420	S
	1984	Activity Level	HR out-of-class	7-12	M/F	420	NS
	1984	Activity Level	HR in-class	7-12	M/F	420	S
	1984	Self Concept		7-12	F	420	NS
	1984	Self Concept		7-12	F	420	NS
	1984	Knowledge	Cardiovascular Health	7-12	M/F	420	S
Lipton	1970	Perceptual Motor	Purdue PMS	6	M/F	92	S
	1970	Visual Perception	Dev. Test of VP	6	M/F	92	S
	1970	Academic	Reading Readiness	6	M/F	92	S
Masche	1970	Motor Performance	Ball Handling	7-8	M/F	48	S
	1970	Motor Performance	Long Jump	7-8	M/F	48	S
	1970	Motor Performance	Obstacle Race	7-8	M/F	48	NS
	1970	M. Power	Obstacle Race	7-8	M/F	48	NS
	1970	Speed	Obstacle Race	7-8	M/F	48	NS
	1970	Motor Performance	Throw	7-8	M/F	48	S
	1970	M. Power	Long Jump	7-8	M/F	48	S
	1970	Agility/Coordination	Obstacle Race	7-8	M/F	48	NS
	1970	Motor Performance	Stork Stand	7-8	M/F	48	S
	1970	Balance	Stork Stand	7-8	M/F	48	S
McAdam	1974	Physical Fitness	Illinois PFT	11	M/F	600	S
	1974	Motor Performance		11	M/F	600	S

Appendix (continued)
Overview of the Studies in Tables 2 through 24
Listed Alphabetically by Author

Author	Date	Outcome	Test	Age	Gender	N	Result
Mocellin	1972	Motor Performance	1000 Mtr. Run	9	M/F	29	S
	1972	Motor Performance	800 Mtr. Run	8-9	M/F	24	S
	1972	Aerobic Fitness	Max $\dot{V}O_2$	9-10	M/F	29	S
	1972	Aerobic Fitness	Max $\dot{V}O_2$	8-9	M/F	24	S
Moody	1972	Body Composition	Density (H2O) (Nor.)	16	F	12	NS
	1972	Body Composition	Density (H2O) (Obese)	16	F	28	S
	1972	Body Composition	Lean Wt. (H2O) (Nor.)	16	F	12	NS
	1972	Body Composition	Lean Wt. (H2O) (Obese)	16	F	28	S
	1972	Body Composition	% Fat (H2O) (Nor.)	16	F	12	NS
	1972	Body Composition	% Fat (H2O) (Obese)	16	F	28	S
	1972	Body Composition	Skinfolds (Nor.)	16	F	12	NS
	1972	Body Composition	Skinfolds (Obese)	16	F	28	S
	1972	Body Size/Shape	Weight (Nor.)	16	F	12	NS
	1972	Body Size/Shape	Weight (Obese)	16	F	28	S
	1972	Body Size/Shape	Girths (Nor.)	16	F	12	NS
	1972	Body Size/Shape	Girths (Obese)	16	F	28	NS
Moore	1984	Perceptual Motor	Capon PM	5	M/F	85	NS
	1984	Self Concept	Capon PM	5	M/F	85	NS
	1984	Academic	Readiness	5	M/F	85	NS
Newfield	1984	Physical Fitness	Wash State PFT	6-8	M/F	3800	S
	1984	M. Power	Long Jump	6-8	M/F	3800	S
	1984	M. Power	Dash	6-8	M/F	3800	S
	1984	Speed	Dash	6-8	M/F	3800	S
	1984	M. Strength	Pushups	6-8	M/F	3800	S
	1984	M. Endurance	Curlup	6-8	M/F	3800	S
	1984	Motor Performance	Long Jump	6-8	M/F	3800	S
	1984	Motor Performance	Dash	6-8	M/F	3800	S
Osness	?	Attitude	Questionnaire	10-15	M/F	300	S
	?	Knowledge	Health-Fitness Q	10-15	M/F	300	S
	?	Knowledge	Exercise/Diet Q	10-15	M/F	300	S
Sargeant	1985	Aerobic Fitness	Max $\dot{V}O_2$	13	M	28	S
	1985	Anaerobic Fitness	Max Peak Power	13	M	28	NS
	1985	Body Composition	Skinfolds	13	M	28	S

Appendix (continued)
Overview of the Studies in Tables 2 through 24
Listed Alphabetically by Author

Author	Date	Outcome	Test	Age	Gender	N	Result
Shephard	1980a	Activity Level	Diary	10-12	M/F	300	S
	1980a	Other	Sleep	10-12	M/F	300	S
	1980b	Aerobic Fitness	Max $\dot{V}O_2$	8-12	M/F	395	S
	1980b	Aerobic Fitness	Max $\dot{V}O_2$	6-7	M/F	395	NS
	1980b	Aerobic Fitness	PWC170	6-7	M/F	395	NS
	1980b	Aerobic Fitness	PWC170	8-11	M/F	395	S
	1980b	M. Strength	Back	6-12	M/F	395	S
	1980b	Motor Performance	Situps	6-12	M/F	395	S
	1980b	Motor Performance	Long Jump	6-12	M/F	395	S
	1980b	Motor Performance	Shuttle Run	6-12	M/F	395	S
	1980b	M. Endurance	Situps	6-12	M/F	395	S
	1980b	M. Endurance	Flexed Arm Hang	6-12	M/F	395	S
	1980b	M. Endurance	300 Yard Run	6-12	M/F	395	S
	1980b	M. Power	50 Yd. Dash	6-12	M/F	395	S
	1980b	M. Power	Long Jump	6-12	M/F	395	S
	1980b	M. Power	Shuttle Run	6-12	M/F	395	S
	1980b	Speed	50 Yd. Dash	6-12	M/F	395	S
	1980b	Speed	Shuttle Run	6-12	M/F	395	S
	1980b	Agility/ Coordination	Shuttle Run	6-12	M/F	395	S
	1984	Academic	Teacher Grades	6-12	M/F	546	S
Siegel	1984	Aerobic Fitness	1600 Mtr. Run	9	M/F	109	S
Thaxton	1977	Motor Performance	Trampoline	14-17	F	67	S
	1977	Motor Performance	Foul Shot, Pass, Dribble	14-17	F	67	S
	1977	Motor Performance	Mats, Sidehorse	14-17	F	67	S
	1977	M. Endurance	Situps	14-17	F	67	S
	1977	M. Endurance	Flexed Arm Hang	14-17	F	67	S
	1977	Aerobic/ Anaerobic Fit.	600 Run	14-17	F	67	S
Thomas	1975	Perceptual Motor	Shape-O Ball T	6	M/F	40	S
	1975	Balance	Stabilometer	6	M/F	40	S
	1975	Self Concept	Parker S C Scale	6	M/F	40	NS
	1975	Academic	Otis Lennon MAT	6	M/F	40	NS
	1975	Academic	Teacher Rating	6	M/F	40	NS
Vogel	1981	Physical Fitness	I CAN Fitness T	5-2	M/F	2-15	S
	1981	Motor Performance	I CAN Performance T	5-2	M/F	2-15	S
Volle	1984	Perceptual Motor	Height Perception	6-11	M/F	?	S
	1984	Perceptual Motor	Arm Span	6-11	M/F	?	S
	1984	Perceptual Motor	Verticality	6-11	M/F	?	S
	1984	Perceptual Motor	Finger Recognition	6	M/F	?	NS
	1984	Perceptual Motor	Finger Recognition	7	M/F	?	NS
	1984	Perceptual Motor	Finger Recognition	8	M/F	?	S

Appendix (continued)
Overview of the Studies in Tables 2 through 24
Listed Alphabetically by Author

Author	Date	Outcome	Test	Age	Gender	N	Result
Volle	1984	Perceptual Motor	Finger Recognition	9	M/F	?	S
Wittle	1961	Maturation	Skeletal Age	12	M	162	NS
	1961	Maturation	Wetzel Grid	12	M	162	NS
	1961	Maturation	McCloy Index I	12	M	162	NS
	1961	Body Size/Shape	Height	12	M	162	NS
	1961	Body Size/Shape	Weight	12	M	162	NS
	1961	Fitness	Rogers PF Index	12	M	162	S
	1961	Fitness	Rogers Strength I	12	M	162	S
	1961	Fitness	Metheny-Johnson	12	M	162	S
	1961	Fitness	Indiana PFT	12	M	162	S
	1961	Personal-Social	Cal. Test of	12	M	162	NS
	1961	M. Power	Vertical Jump	12	M	162	NS
	1961	Motor Performance	Vertical Jump	12	M	162	S
	1961	M. Strength	Grip	12	M	162	NS
	1961	M. Strength	Leg	12	M	162	S
	1961	M. Strength	Back	12	M	162	S
	1961	Flexibility	Trunk	12	M	162	NS
	1961	Flexibility	Hip	12	M	162	NS
	1961	Flexibility	Ankle	12	M	162	NS
	1961	Other	Lung Capacity	12	M	162	NS